PHARMACEUTICAL DOSAGE FORMS: TABLETS

PHARMACEUTICAL DOSAGE FORMS: TABLETS
Third Edition

Volume 1:
Unit Operations and Mechanical Properties

Edited by

Larry L. Augsburger
University of Maryland
Baltimore, Maryland, USA

Stephen W. Hoag
University of Maryland
Baltimore, Maryland, USA

informa
healthcare

New York   London

Informa Healthcare USA, Inc.
52 Vanderbilt Avenue
New York, NY 10017

© 2008 by Informa Healthcare USA, Inc.
Informa Healthcare is an Informa business

No claim to original U.S. Government works
Printed in the United States of America on acid-free paper
10 9 8 7 6 5 4 3 2 1

ISBN-13: 978-0-8493-9014-2 (v. 1 : hardcover : alk. paper)
ISBN-10: 0-8493-9014-1 (v. 1 : hardcover : alk. paper)
ISBN-13: 978-0-8493-9015-9 (v. 2 : hardcover : alk. paper)
ISBN-10: 0-8493-9015-X (v. 2 : hardcover : alk. paper)
ISBN-13: 978-0-8493-9016-6 (v. 3 : hardcover : alk. paper)
ISBN-10: 0-8493-9016-8 (v. 3 : hardcover : alk. paper)

International Standard Book Number-10: 1-4200-6345-6 (Hardcover)
International Standard Book Number-13: 978-1-4200-6345-5 (Hardcover)

This book contains information obtained from authentic and highly regarded sources. Reprinted material is quoted with permission, and sources are indicated. A wide variety of references are listed. Reasonable efforts have been made to publish reliable data and information, but the author and the publisher cannot assume responsibility for the validity of all materials or for the consequence of their use.

No part of this book may be reprinted, reproduced, transmitted, or utilized in any form by any electronic, mechanical, or other means, now known or hereafter invented, including photocopying, microfilming, and recording, or in any information storage or retrieval system, without written permission from the publishers.

For permission to photocopy or use material electronically from this work, please access www.copyright.com (http://www.copyright.com/) or contact the Copyright Clearance Center, Inc. (CCC) 222 Rosewood Drive, Danvers, MA 01923, 978-750-8400. CCC is a not-for-profit organization that provides licenses and registration for a variety of users. For organizations that have been granted a photocopy license by the CCC, a separate system of payment has been arranged.

Trademark Notice: Product or corporate names may be trademarks or registered trademarks, and are used only for identification and explanation without intent to infringe.

Library of Congress Cataloging-in-Publication Data

Pharmaceutical dosage forms. Tablets. – 3rd ed. / edited by Larry L. Augsburger, Stephen W. Hoag.
  p. ; cm.
  Includes bibliographical references and index.
  ISBN-13: 978-0-8493-9014-2 (v. 1 : hardcover : alk. paper)
  ISBN-10: 0-8493-9014-1 (v. 1 : hardcover : alk. paper)
  ISBN-13: 978-0-8493-9015-9 (v. 2 : hardcover : alk. paper)
  ISBN-10: 0-8493-9015-X (v. 2 : hardcover : alk. paper)
  ISBN-13: 978-0-8493-9016-6 (v. 3 : hardcover : alk. paper)
  ISBN-10: 0-8493-9016-8 (v. 3 : hardcover : alk. paper)
  1. Tablets (Medicine) 2. Drugs–Dosage forms. I. Augsburger, Larry L. II. Hoag, Stephen W. III. Title: Tablets.
  [DNLM: 1. Tablets–pharmacology. 2. Drug Compounding. 3. Drug Design. 4. Drug Industry–legislation & jurisprudence. 5. Quality Control. QV 787 P536 2008]
  RS201.T2P46 2008
  615'.1901–dc22   2007048891

For Corporate Sales and Reprint Permissions call 212-520-2700 or write to:
Sales Department, 52 Vanderbilt Ave., 16th floor, New York, NY 10017.

Visit the Informa web site at
www.informa.com

and the Informa Healthcare Web site at
www.informahealthcare.com

To my loving wife Jeannie,
the light and laughter in my life.
—Larry L. Augsburger

To my dear wife Cathy and my children Elena
and Nina and those who helped me
so much with my education:
My parents Jo Hoag and my late father
Jim Hoag, Don Hoag, and Edward G. Rippie.
—Stephen W. Hoag

Foreword

We are delighted to have the privilege of continuing the tradition begun by Herb Lieberman and Leon Lachman, and later joined by Joseph Schwartz, of providing the only comprehensive treatment of the design, formulation, manufacture and evaluation of the tablet dosage form in *Pharmaceutical Dosage Forms: Tablets*. Today the tablet continues to be the dosage form of choice. Solid dosage forms constitute about two-thirds of all dosage forms, and about half of these are tablets.

Philosophically, we regard the tablet as a drug delivery system. Like any delivery system, the tablet is more than just a practical way to administer drugs to patients. Rather, we view the tablet as a system that is designed to meet specific criteria. The most important design criterion of the tablet is how effectively it gets the drug "delivered" to the site of action in an active form in sufficient quantity and at the correct rate to meet the therapeutic objectives (i.e., immediate release or some form of extended or otherwise modified release). However, the tablet must also meet a number of other design criteria essential to getting the drug to society and the patient. These include physical and chemical stability (to assure potency, safety, and consistent drug delivery performance over the use-life of the product), the ability to be *economically* mass produced in a manner that assures the proper amount of drug in each dosage unit and batch produced (to reduce costs and provide reliable dosing), and, to the extent possible, patient acceptability (i.e., reasonable size and shape, taste, color, etc. to encourage patient compliance with the prescribed dosing regimen). Thus, the ultimate goal of drug product development is to design a system that maximizes the therapeutic potential of the drug substance and facilitates its access to patients. The fact that the tablet can be uniquely designed to meet these criteria accounts for its prevalence as the most popular oral solid dosage form.

Although the majority of tablets are made by compression, intended to be swallowed whole and designed for immediate release, there are many other tablet forms. These include, for example, chewable, orally disintegrating, sublingual, effervescent, and buccal tablets, as well as lozenges or troches. Effervescent tablets are intended to be taken after first dropping them in water. Some modified release tablets may be designed to delay release until the tablet has passed the pyloric sphincter (i.e., enteric). Others may be designed to provide consistent extended or sustained release over an extended period of time, or for pulsed release, colonic delivery, or to provide a unique release profile for a specific drug and its therapeutic objective.

Since the last edition of *Pharmaceutical Dosage Forms: Tablets* in 1990, there have been numerous developments and enhancements in tablet formulation science and technology, as well as product regulation. Science and technology developments include new or updated equipment for manufacture, new excipients, greater understanding of excipient functionality, nanotechnology, innovations in the design of modified release tablets, the use of artificial intelligence in formulation and process development, new initiatives in real time and on-line process control, and increased use of modeling to understand and optimize formulation and process parameters. New regulatory initiatives include the Food and Drug Administration's SUPAC (scale up and post approval changes) guidances, its risk-based Pharmaceutical cGMPs for the 21st Century plan, and its PAT (process analytical technology) guidance. Also significant is the development, through the International Conference on Harmonization of proposals, for an international plan for a harmonized quality control system.

Significantly, the development of new regulatory policy and new science and technology are not mutually exclusive. Rather, they are inextricably linked. The new regulatory initiatives serve as a stimulus to academia and industry to put formulation design, development, and manufacture on a more scientific basis which, in turn, makes possible science-based policies that can provide substantial regulatory relief and greater flexibility for manufacturers to update and streamline processes for higher efficiency and productivity. The first SUPAC guidance was issued in 1995 for immediate release oral solid dosage forms (SUPAC-IR). That guidance was followed in 1997 with SUPAC-MR which covered scale-up and post approval changes for solid oral modified release dosage forms. These guidances brought much needed consistency to how the Food and Drug Administration deals with post approval changes and provided substantial regulatory relief from unnecessary testing and filing requirements. Major underpinnings of these two regulatory policies were research programs conducted at the University of Maryland under a collaborative agreement with the Food and Drug Administration which identified and linked critical formulation and process variables to bioavailability outcomes in human subjects. The Food and Drug Administration's Pharmaceutical cGMPs for the 21st Century plan seeks to merge science-based management with an integrated quality systems approach and to "create a robust link between process parameters, specifications and clinical performance"[1] The new PAT guidance proposes the use of modern process analyzers or process analytical chemistry tools to achieve real-time control and quality assurance during manufacturing.[2] The Food and Drug Administration's draft guidance on Q8 Pharmaceutical Development[3] addresses the suggested contents of the pharmaceutical development section of a regulatory submission in the ICH M4 Common Technical Document format.

A common thread running through these newer regulatory initiatives is the building in of product quality and the development of meaningful product specifications based on a high level of understanding of how formulation and process factors impact product performance.

Still other developments since 1990 are the advent of the internet as a research and resource tool and a decline in academic study and teaching in solid dosage forms. Together, these developments have led to a situation where there is a vast amount of formulation information widely scattered throughout the literature which is unknown and difficult for researchers new to the tableting field to organize and use. Therefore, another objective to this book to integrate a critical, comprehensive summary of this formulation information with the latest developments in this field.

Thus, the overarching goal of the third edition of *Pharmaceutical Dosage Forms: Tablets* is to provide an in-depth treatment of the science and technology of tableting that

---

[1] J. Woodcock, "Quality by Design: A Way Forward," September 17, 2003.

[2] http://www.fda.gov/cder/guidance/6419fnl.doc

[3] http://www.fda.gov/cder/guidance/6672dft.doc

Foreword

acknowledges its traditional, historical database but focuses on modern scientific, technological, and regulatory developments. The common theme of this new edition is DESIGN. That is, tablets are delivery systems that are engineered to meet specific design criteria and that product quality must be built in and is also by design.

No effort of this magnitude and scope could have been accomplished without the commitment of a large number of distinguished experts. We are extremely grateful for their hard work, dedication and patience in helping us complete this new edition.

Larry L. Augsburger
Stephen W. Hoag

Preface

The development of a successful tablet formulation can be a substantial challenge, because formulation scientists are often confronted with a bewildering array of formulation and process variables that can interact in complex ways. These interactions will primarily be discussed in Volume 2, but to understand these interactions the reader must first have a good understanding of the different unit operations involved in making a tablet, the physicochemical and mechanical properties of the active drug substance, and the causes of drug product instability.

Unit operations such as drying, milling, granulating, mixing, and compaction use physical and chemical processes that take the raw materials in a formulation and convert them into a useful product or the intermediate needed to make the product. Successfully setting up and controlling a unit operation requires an understanding of the basic physical and chemical phenomena that a particular unit operation uses to process a formulation. The first three chapters cover key concepts in powder science which are necessary in order to understand the different unit operations. The first chapter discusses sampling. The second chapter covers micrometrics or powder science and addresses particles, particle populations and population statistics, methods of particle size characterization, powder beds, and the interactions of powders in a powder bed. The third chapter covers powder flow and basic solids handling principles. The unit operations chapters that follow cover all the basic unit operations needed to make tablets, granules, and pellets. These include milling, blending and blend uniformity, drying, wet and dry granulation, extrusion and spheronization, compaction, and coating. These chapters all have a similar structure: introduction, significance, specific theory, methods, equipment and equipment operation, and process control.

In addition, this volume contains chapters on preformulation testing, drug product stability, and tablet testing using a compaction simulator. Preformulation testing is the first step in the rational development of dosage forms. It should result in a "portfolio of information" that provides guidance in formulation design. With its comprehensive review of unit operations, physicochemical and mechanical properties, the causes of drug product instability, and testing, Volume 1 provides the essential background upon which formulation design and manufacture are based.

Larry L. Augsburger
Stephen W. Hoag

Contents

Dedication iii
Foreword v
Preface ix
Contributors xiii

1. Principles of Sampling for Particulate Solids *1*
   Patricia L. Smith

2. Particle and Powder Bed Properties *17*
   Stephen W. Hoag and Han-Pin Lim

3. Flow: General Principles of Bulk Solids Handling *75*
   Thomas Baxter, Roger Barnum, and James K. Prescott

4. Blending and Blend Uniformity *111*
   Thomas P. Garcia and James K. Prescott

5. Milling *175*
   Benjamin Murugesu

6. Drying *195*
   Cecil Propst and Thomas S. Chirkot

7. Spray Drying: Theory and Pharmaceutical Applications *227*
   Herm E. Snyder and David Lechuga-Ballesteros

8. Pharmaceutical Granulation Processes, Mechanism, and the Use of Binders *261*
   Stuart L. Cantor, Larry L. Augsburger, Stephen W. Hoag, and Armin Gerhardt

9. Dry Granulation *303*
   Garnet E. Peck, Josephine L. P. Soh, and Kenneth R. Morris

10. The Preparation of Pellets by Extrusion/Spheronization *337*
    J. M. Newton

11. Coating Processes and Equipment *373*
    David M. Jones

12. Aqueous Polymeric Film Coating *399*
    Dave A. Miller and James W. McGinity

13. The Application of Thermal Analysis to Pharmaceutical Dosage Forms *439*
    Duncan Q. M. Craig

14. Preformulation Studies for Tablet Formulation Development *465*
   Raghu K. Cavatur, N. Murti Vemuri, and Raj Suryanarayanan

15. Stability Kinetics *485*
   Robin Roman

16. Compaction Simulation *519*
   Michael E. Bourland and Matthew P. Mullarney

17. Compression and Compaction *555*
   Stephen W. Hoag, Vivek S. Dave, and Vikas Moolchandani

Index 631

Contributors

Larry L. Augsburger School of Pharmacy, University of Maryland, Baltimore, Maryland, U.S.A.

Roger Barnum Jenike & Johanson, Inc., Tyngsboro, Massachusetts, U.S.A.

Thomas Baxter Jenike & Johanson, Inc., Tyngsboro, Massachusetts, U.S.A.

Michael E. Bourland Pfizer, Inc., Groton, Connecticut, U.S.A.

Stuart L. Cantor School of Pharmacy, University of Maryland, Baltimore, Maryland, U.S.A.

Raghu K. Cavatur Sanofi-Aventis, Bridgewater, New Jersey, U.S.A.

Thomas S. Chirkot Patterson-Kelley, Division of Harsco Corp., East Stroudsburg, Pennsylvania, U.S.A.

Duncan Q. M. Craig School of Chemical Sciences and Pharmacy, University of East Anglia, Norwich, U.K.

Vivek S. Dave School of Pharmacy, University of Maryland, Baltimore, Maryland, U.S.A.

Thomas P. Garcia Pfizer, Inc., Groton, Connecticut, U.S.A.

Armin Gerhardt Libertyville, Illinois, U.S.A.

Stephen W. Hoag School of Pharmacy, University of Maryland, Baltimore, Maryland, U.S.A.

David Lechuga-Ballesteros Aridis Pharmaceuticals, San Jose, California, U.S.A.

Han-Pin Lim School of Pharmacy, University of Maryland, Baltimore, Maryland, U.S.A.

David M. Jones Ramsey, New Jersey, U.S.A.

James W. McGinity College of Pharmacy, University of Texas at Austin, Austin, Texas, U.S.A.

Dave A. Miller College of Pharmacy, University of Texas at Austin, Austin, Texas, U.S.A.

Vikas Moolchandani School of Pharmacy, University of Maryland, Baltimore, Maryland, U.S.A.

Kenneth R. Morris   Department of Industrial and Physical Pharmacy, College of Pharmacy, Nursing and Health Sciences, Purdue University, West Lafayette, Indiana, U.S.A.

Matthew P. Mullarney   Pfizer, Inc., Groton, Connecticut, U.S.A.

Benjamin Murugesu   Quadro Engineering Corp., Waterloo, Ontario, Canada

J. M. Newton   The School of Pharmacy, University of London, and Department of Mechanical Engineering, University College London, London, U.K.

Garnet E. Peck   Department of Industrial and Physical Pharmacy, College of Pharmacy, Nursing and Health Sciences, Purdue University, West Lafayette, Indiana, U.S.A.

James K. Prescott   Jenike & Johanson, Inc., Tyngsboro, Massachusetts, U.S.A.

Cecil Propst   SPI Pharma, Grand Haven, Michigan, U.S.A.

Robin Roman   GlaxoSmithKline, R&D, King of Prussia, Pennsylvania, U.S.A.

Patricia L. Smith   Alpha Stat Consulting, Lubbock, Texas, U.S.A.

Herm E. Snyder   Nektar Therapeutics, San Carlos, California, U.S.A.

Josephine L. P. Soh   Department of Industrial and Physical Pharmacy, College of Pharmacy, Nursing and Health Sciences, Purdue University, West Lafayette, Indiana, U.S.A.

Raj Suryanarayanan   University of Minnesota, Minneapolis, Minnesota, U.S.A.

N. Murti Vemuri   Sanofi-Aventis, Bridgewater, New Jersey, U.S.A.

1
Principles of Sampling for Particulate Solids

Patricia L. Smith
Alpha Stat Consulting, Lubbock, Texas, U.S.A.

INTRODUCTION

When addressing the sampling of particulate solids, discussion of the physical act of sampling is often missing. Specific guidance for consistent sampling techniques is needed to increase the likelihood of obtaining unbiased and more consistent results. In contrast, the statistical principle of random sampling is well known and is applied without difficulty. It works well when individual units of the population or lot can be identified, and it gives us confidence that the sampling process is fair and unbiased. The method of identifying individual units breaks down, however, when sampling particulates. Imagine trying to distinguish separate powder particles to apply this classical statistical technique!

In this chapter, we extend the idea of random sampling to particulate solids. The theory we present is that of Gy (1,2), who first started developing his ideas when confronted with sampling problems in the mining industry. Fortunately, his expanded theory applies to all solids sampling as well as to liquids and gases. He identified seven sampling errors, which separate total sampling variation into component parts. The basic principles can be applied to any sampling situation. Further, the ideas complement those in classical statistical sampling theory and have many parallels.

We begin with the principle of correct sampling, which provides an analogy to the idea of randomness. It is perhaps the most important idea in the chapter. Next we discuss the concept of sampling dimension, which is important for the actual physical definition and selection of the sample. Then, we provide some background information on sampling frequency and sampling mode, which are used when sampling over time or space. With these ideas as a foundation, we present Gy's seven sampling errors and ways to minimize them.

PRINCIPLE OF CORRECT SAMPLING

Classical statistical sampling theory uses the ideas of randomness and unbiasedness. The base case, simple random sampling (SRS), states that every individual unit in the population, or lot, has the same chance of being in the sample. Since we cannot identify individual particles in a bulk material, we need another approach. The analogy in bulk sampling is correctness: (*i*) Every equal-sized portion of the lot has the same chance of being in the sample. In addition, because the characteristic of interest may change from the time the sample is taken to the time it is analyzed, sample handling is important. So in the case of bulk material, we have an additional requirement for correctness: (*ii*) The integrity of the sample is preserved during and after sampling. While sample preservation does not appear to apply to SRS, there is actually an analogy in reverse. Any mistake in recording or transferring data could be considered a violation of the integrity of the sample.

Therefore, sampling correctness has a special meaning in Gy's theory. When we talk about a correct sample, we mean that the principle of correct sampling has been followed. Note that correctness is a process, which we have some control over. We do not have control, however, over the accuracy of a sample value, which is a result. This is no different than SRS, where we can control the method by which we obtain a subset of the population of individual units using a random technique. But we are "stuck with" the resulting sample and its value of the characteristic of interest.

Equipped now with knowledge of this very important principle, we can now evaluate sampling instruments, systems, and procedures for correctness. Here are a few examples, and we will provide more later on in the chapter. A "grab" sample of particles from one side of conveyor belt is not correct, since material on the opposite side has no chance of being in the sample. A grab sample is really just a sample of convenience. A round bottom scoop, which might be used to get a cross-stream sample of stationary material, will not give a correct sample because it under-selects particles at the bottom and over-selects particles at the top. A probe collecting material from one location inside a pipe cannot obtain a correct sample. The use of hand samplers is typically not correct because we cannot consistently control their speed passing through a falling "stream" of material, which allows one side of the stream to be favored.

A violation of the second part of the principle of correct sampling occurs if, for example, we are interested in the weight percent of fines, and some fines escape from the sample. Sieves and grinders, if not cleaned, may retain material from one sample and thus allow contamination of the next. Some samples not refrigerated or not analyzed within a specified amount of time might degrade. The sample container itself may alter the characteristic of interest, such as when analyzing for trace amounts of sodium from a sample stored in a soft glass container. A chemist is the best resource for evaluating whether the sample integrity has been compromised and to help us avoid the cause or minimize the effect.

SAMPLING DIMENSION

SRS means selecting individual units or particles one at a time, at random, and with equal probability. Repeated samples will be different, but in general, the variation of unbaised estimates of population values will be minimized. The classical approach is to assign a number to each unit, generate a set of random numbers, and select the units with those numbers. Gy calls this zero-dimensional sampling. All units are identifiable and accessible, and the order or arrangement of the units in time or space is not important. If the order of the units makes sense and is known, then further analysis should be performed and SRS should not be applied. Zero-dimensional sampling is rare in practice for bulk solids unless the entire container is of interest. Examples include the selection of vials of a standard for instrument calibration or the selection of individual tablets for further analysis. Even when zero-dimensional sampling takes place, it is often only one step in the sampling protocol, which usually requires several sampling and subsampling steps. The problem, of course, is that the particles are not individually identifiable, and time order or spatial arrangement may be important. In the former case, SRS is impossible; in the latter case, it is inappropriate.

Generally, we are confronted with three-dimensional lots, such as material in a production batch or in a lab container. How do we apply SRS to these lots? We might think about identifying a "random" point in the lot and taking material surrounding it. We would want the probability of selection from the point to be the same in all directions, so "enlarging" this point generates a sphere. This works only in theory, however. We neither can really identify a "random" point and the resulting sphere inside a pile of bulk material, nor can we extract exactly what we think we have identified. So our idea of randomness does not actually work in practice. With three-dimensional sampling, we cannot achieve our objective of a random sample (Fig. 1). Alternatives are to perform one- or two-dimensional sampling, discussed next.

One way to avoid the problem of sampling a three-dimensional lot is to perform two-dimensional sampling. Our sample is taken by extracting material completely through one dimension of the lot, which is still three-dimensional. The most common situation is sampling through the vertical dimension, taking a core sample from a drum from top to bottom, for instance. In this case, we look at the lot from the top and see only two dimensions. We select a point at random and generate a circle by going in all directions with equal probability. By "moving" the circle down through the third dimension, we generate a cylinder, which is the correct geometry for two-dimensional sampling. While this sample is theoretically correct since every core of material has the same chance of being the core sample, the method is difficult to achieve in practice. Core sampling with a thief (Fig. 2), for example, disturbs material as it passes through, and "particles of different sizes often flow unevenly into the thief cavities" (3). For a drum, a thief will not get material at the very bottom because of its pointed end.

Reducing the sampling dimension from three to two improves our chances of getting a correct sample and thus reduces our overall sampling error. A further improvement can often be made with one-dimensional sampling. In this case, we sample across two dimensions of the material. For example, rather than addressing the material as a pile, we can flatten and lengthen the pile into a narrow "stream," which we consider a one-dimensional line. We pick a point at random along the length of the line and generate an interval by measuring equal amounts on both sides. By "moving" the interval completely across the stream, we are sampling completely across the remaining two dimensions: the height and depth of the material. We have thus generated a "slice," with parallel sides, which is the correct geometry for one-dimensional sampling (Fig. 3). This technique applies to nonstationary material as well. Material moving along a conveyor belt, for example, can be considered a one-dimensional stream. If we sample completely across it and include the full height, then we have one-dimensional sampling. Sampling material during transfer, before it becomes a stationary three-dimensional pile, is an alternative to three-dimensional sampling.

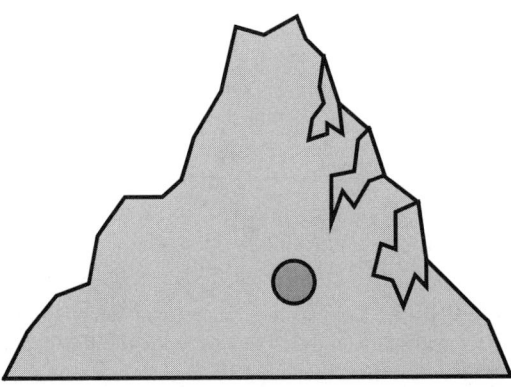

FIGURE 1 A correct three-dimensional sample is impossible to obtain.

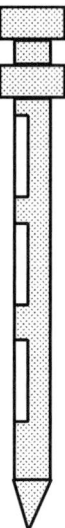

FIGURE 2 A thief probe can take a vertical core sample but cannot get material from the very bottom of the container.

A correct alternative to the one-dimensional cross-stream slice with parallel sides is a cutter (sampling tool) that rotates around an axis in a circular fashion. In such a case, the cutter must have a radial shape, that is, it must be wedge-shaped, with the cutter edges converging towards the axis of rotation (Fig. 4). This design ensures that material on the outside of the arc, where the cutter moves faster, has the same chance of being in the sample as material near the center, where the cutter moves more slowly.

With zero-dimensional lots, we can apply SRS. All other lots of bulk material are three-dimensional and thus impossible to sample correctly. By reducing the sampling dimension, we can reduce our overall sampling error.

SAMPLING FREQUENCY AND MODE

When collecting several samples over time or space, we must decide on sampling frequency and mode. Inappropriate sampling frequency or mode can produce deceptive results and lead to inappropriate actions and bad outcomes.

Sampling frequency can be too often or too infrequent. If we sample too often, then sampling is inefficient, time consuming, and costly. Random variation, the natural variation of the process, might be interpreted as a process upset, and a temptation arises to

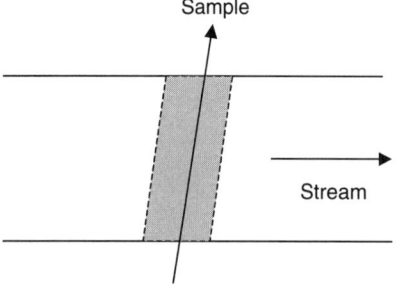

FIGURE 3 Correct one-dimensional sampling is a slice with parallel sides and includes the full height and width of the stream.

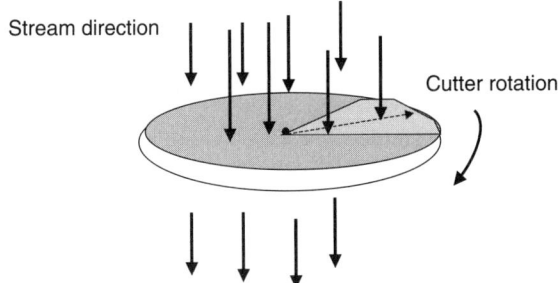

FIGURE 4 The correct geometry for a rotational sampler (*cutter*) is wedge-shaped with the cutter edges converging toward the axis of rotation.

make unnecessary changes. Overcontrol and increased process variation will result. On the other hand, if we sample too infrequently, then trends cannot be detected in time to take corrective action. Consequently, too much off-spec product may be manufactured, contaminant amounts may exceed regulations, and process cycles, if they exist, remain hidden. With "just right" sampling frequency, drifts are detected in time to take corrective action, process cycles can be discovered, and sampling is efficient and worthwhile.

The most common sampling modes are SRS, discussed previously, stratified random sampling, and systematic random sampling. SRS over time or space consists of identifying times or places totally at random to take the samples. The great disadvantage of this approach is that certain portions of the lot or production times may be under or over represented, and process stability cannot be monitored effectively. Consequently, we do not recommend SRS for long-term examination of lot characteristics.

Both stratified random sampling and systematic random sampling require dividing the lot into strata, over time or space, whichever is appropriate. The definition of each stratum should make sense. For example, taking samples every hour or every few hours is logical in production environments where frequent results are required to control the process within a narrow range. For spatial lots, strata should be located along logical geographic divisions, taking into account the characteristics of the spatial area.

For stratified random sampling, a random time or spatial point is identified for every stratum, and a sample is taken from each one. For systematic random sampling, a random time or spatial point is identified for the sample for the first stratum only. Samples from all other strata are taken at the same relative time or from the same relative spatial point. For example, if samples are to be taken every hour, and the first time is randomly selected as 21 min past the hour, then every sample after that is also taken at 21 min past the hour.

Systematic random sampling is very convenient both in a manufacturing environment and in the field because it is simple to implement and can easily be incorporated into a work schedule. A drawback, however, is that a long-term cycle will remain hidden if the selected times or points in space are synchronous (coincide) with that cycle. If cycles are suspected or need to be ruled out, then stratified random sampling should be used.

OVERVIEW OF THE SEVEN SAMPLING ERRORS OF GY

Intuitively, we can think of the total sampling error as the discrepancy between the sample value and the "true" but unknown lot value. Gy parses it into component parts, allowing us to reduce this total error by eliminating one or more of the components or moderating their effects. In some cases the word "error" means mistake; in other cases it means variation. Mistakes can be avoided and variation can be reduced. We will point out these differences as we discuss Gy's "errors."

Gy's first error is the fundamental error (FE). It is unavoidable because it arises from variation in the material itself: the constitution heterogeneity. Since no material is completely homogeneous, each sample will be different. The FE corresponds to the error resulting from classical statistical random sampling (SRS). It can be reduced but not eliminated.

The second error, the grouping and segregation error (GE), is also related to the material variation, in this case the distribution heterogeneity. At the level of the small scale where we actually take a sample, particles may segregate by particle size or shape. If we cannot select material totally at random, then our sample will be biased. In addition, we sample groups of particles, not one at a time as in SRS. So in addition to the unavoidable FE, we have an additional component in bulk sampling that contributes to our total sampling error. The GE is not present in classical SRS.

Gy's next three errors, the delimitation error (DE), extraction error (EE), and preparation error (PE), result from not following the principle of correct sampling. The first part of this principle requires that every equal-sized portion of the lot have the same chance of being in the sample. This means we must first determine the sampling dimension and identify specifically the material we intend to collect. The DE arises from not defining the sample correctly. In two dimensions, for example, a DE would occur if we defined a section of material other than a core. The analogy of sample definition in SRS is using random numbers to identify those units in the population that will make up the sample. Exempting certain units from the random number assignment would be an example of a DE for SRS. After defining the intended sample, we incur an EE if we do not actually extract the designated material. This can happen, for example, if we use an incorrect collection tool or use a correct tool incorrectly. In SRS, obtaining those individual items identified for the sample is not usually a problem, though there are exceptions; selecting particular bags or drums stacked in a warehouse can be a big logistical problem. The second part of the principle of correct sampling requires that we preserve the integrity of the sample. Failure to do so results in what is commonly referred to as a handling error. Gy calls this the PE. It includes but is not limited to sample preparation in the lab. Each of these errors contributes to the total variation in our sample results, but they are also errors (mistakes).

Gy's last two errors address large scale non-random variation in sampling over time or space: the long-range nonperiodic heterogeneity fluctuation error and the long-range periodic heterogeneity fluctuation error. While developing his sampling theory over the years, Gy has used other terms, such as continuous selection errors or integration errors. We will refer to these two long-range errors as (*i*) shifts and trends and (*ii*) cycles. Industrial processes, for example, may experience non-random increases or decreases over time in the measured characteristic of interest. Changes in ambient temperature can result in non-random periodic fluctuations.

FUNDAMENTAL ERROR

Material in every lot is heterogeneous because of its diverse composition; its particles differ by size, shape, or density, or by the chemical or physical characteristics of interest. This constitution heterogeneity gives rise to different physical samples that we may obtain and thus makes it unusual for any of these samples to be exactly representative of the entire lot. In other words, the sample is unlikely to be a microcosm of the lot. We thus

Principles of Sampling for Particulate Solids

generate an error: the discrepancy between the content of the sample and the content of the lot. This is the total sampling error. It is also the FE, if all of Gy's other sampling errors and the analytical error are zero. The FE is thus the minimum error we could possibly have in particulate sampling. It also corresponds to SRS in classical statistical sampling because no other errors are present in that case.

For a given sample, the result of the chemical or physical analysis is a fixed number, which is our estimate of the characteristic of interest in the lot. Also of importance is how the number might change with different samples, because the magnitude of these changes gives us an idea of how consistent our sampling process is. We are thus concerned with the sampling variation, that is, the variance of the FE, Var(FE).

In the classical statistical framework, the variance of an estimate $\bar{x}$ of the true population average μ changes with the number n of units sampled: $\text{Var}(\bar{x}) = \sigma^2/n$, where the population variance σ^2 can be estimated from the current sample or from a previously obtained sample. This formula can be used in two different ways. If there is a certain variance ($\pm$ error) we can tolerate on our estimate $\bar{x}$, then we can calculate how many units (n) must be in the sample. On the other hand, for any number n of units, we can find the variance that will result. Because of their inverse relationship, the variation in $\bar{x}$ from different samples can be reduced by increasing the number n of units in the sample.

The variation corresponding to $\text{Var}(\bar{x})$ for particulate sampling is the Var(FE). Because his initial ideas for bulk sampling theory were for mining, Gy focuses on measurements of weight percent and uses the term *critical content*: c_s for the sample (rather than $\bar{x}$) and c_L (rather than μ) for the lot. Also, since weight percents are a relative measure, he defines the total sampling error as a relative value: $(c_s - c_L)/c_L$. When all the other sampling errors and the analytical error are zero, this quantity consists entirely of the FE.

Formulas for Var(FE)

Pitard (4) presents two formulas relating an estimate of the Var(FE) to the weight of the sample and the particle size. One case is fairly general; the other is for particle size distribution. In each case, physical characteristics of the particles are used: a size factor and a density factor. By characterizing the type of material being sampled, we can determine if our sample weight is sufficient to get a desired low variance of the estimate, and if not, what we can to do reduce that variance. Because the characterizations are made on a preliminary examination of the material, these formulas are an order of approximation only.

General Formula for Var(FE)

In the general case, where we wish to estimate the critical content, we have the following formula, estimating the variance of the FE:

$$\text{Var}(\text{FE}) \approx (1/M_S - 1/M_L)\, d^3 f\, g\, c_F \ell \tag{1}$$

The mass of the sample in grams is denoted by M_S, and the mass of the lot in grams is M_L. Values for d, f, g, c_F, and ℓ are based on both experimental evidence and mathematical theory. We give here a brief explanation of each, with common values given in Tables 1–4, derived from Gy (1) and Pitard (4).

The quantities d, f, and g combine to make up the size factor. The value d is the diameter in cm of the size of the opening of a screen retaining 5% by weight of the lot to be sampled. So d represents the largest particles. Because all particles do not have this

TABLE 1 Shape or Form Factor f

Shape	Value	Comment
Flakes	0.1	
Nuggets	0.2	
Sphere	0.5	Most common
Cube	1	Basis for calculations
Needles	(1,10)	Length divided by width
		In the formula below, d = diameter of needle

Notes: Calculated: f = (Volume of particle with diameter d) / (Volume of cube of side d).

TABLE 2 Granulometric or Size Distribution Factor g

Type	Value	Comment
Non-calibrated	0.25	From a jaw crusher
Calibrated	0.55	Between two consecutive screen openings
Naturally calibrated	0.75	Cereals, beans, rice,...
Perfectly calibrated	1	All particles exactly the same size

Notes: Calculated: g = (Diameter of smallest 5% of material) / (Diameter of largest 5% of material).

TABLE 3 Liberation Factor l

Type	Value	Comment
Almost homogeneous	0.05	Not liberated
Homogeneous	0.1	
Average	0.2	
Heterogeneous	0.4	
Very heterogeneous	0.8	Nearly liberated
Liberated	1	Completely liberated

Calculated (based on critical content of particles):
ℓ = (Maximum critical content − average critical content)/(1 − average critical content) or
ℓ = SQRT{(Diameter at which particle is completely liberated)/(Current particle diameter)}

size but are smaller, we "down weight" the contribution of d in the formula by a particle size distribution or granulometric factor g, a number between 0 and 1. The more varied the particle sizes are, the more d needs to be dampened, so the smaller g is. The shape or form factor f is the volume of the particles with diameter d relative to a cube with all sides d in length, which would fit perfectly through a mesh screen with openings d in size.

TABLE 4 Mineralogical or Composition Factor c_F in g/cm³

For $c < 0.1$	For $0.1 < c < 0.9$	For $c > 0.9$
$c_F \cong \lambda_m/c$	$c_F = [(\lambda_m(1-c)^2)/c] + [\lambda_g(1-c)]$	$c_F \cong \lambda_g(1-c)$

Abbreviations: λ_m, density of the material of interest (in g/cm³); λ_g, density of everything but the material of interest (in g/cm³); c, content as a weight proportion of the material of interest.

Principles of Sampling for Particulate Solids

So for example, for spherical particles having diameter d and volume $(4/3)\pi(d/2)^3$, the value of f would be $(4/3)\pi(d/2)^3/d^3 \approx 0.5$.

The values c_F and ℓ make up the density factor. The mineralogical or composition factor c_F is a sort of weighted average of the density and critical content of the material of interest and everything else (the gangue). Its value is calculated based on the case when the material consists only of two types of particles: those containing only the ingredient of interest and those containing only the gangue. In other words, the particles have the maximum amount of heterogeneity between them, resulting in a maximum value for c_F. In this case, the material of interest can be identified as separate particles, which are said to be completely "liberated." When the material of interest does not appear as separate particles, we need to reduce the effect of using the maximum value for c_F. So we multiply it by a number between 0 and 1, the liberation factor ℓ, which accounts for less particle to particle variation. Just as the granulometric factor g was used to adjust for the fact that not all particles had the large diameter d, the liberation factor ℓ is the dampening effect for c_F. When the material of interest is completely liberated, then the calculated value of c_F is appropriate and $\ell = 1$. In the opposite extreme, if there are essentially no particle to particle differences, we may assign ℓ a value of 0.05 or 0.1.

From Equation (1) we see that the Var(FE) is inversely related to the sample mass M_S and directly proportional to the particle size d. This provides two approaches to reduce the Var(FE). First, we could take a larger sample, that is, increase the total sample weight. Second, we could grind the particles in the lot to reduce the maximum particle size d. Unfortunately, there may be drawbacks to each of these approaches. Taking a larger weight sample will probably necessitate one or more additional subsampling stages, which may increase the overall sampling error. Pitard (4) illustrates how to control the overall error by using a nomograph. Reducing the particle size by grinding will result in a PE if the material tends to adhere to the sampling equipment.

Example Calculation of Var(FE)

A filler and active ingredient are mixed in a ratio targeted at 24:1 by weight and then granulated. The granules are approximately spherical and 2.0 mm maximum in diameter, having been passed through a mesh screen. The density of the active ingredient is 0.4 g/cm^3. As a quality control measure before proceeding to the next formulation step, a 500-g sample of granules is taken and delivered to the lab for evaluation. The lab takes a 10-g subsample for analysis. What is the Var(FE) in this subsampling step for estimating the percent weight of the active ingredient?

$M_L = 500$ g (lot size)
$M_S = 10$ g (sample size)
$d = 0.2$ cm (particle size)

From Tables 1–4 we have:
$f = 0.5$ (spherical shape)
$g = 0.55$ (calibrated granules)
$\lambda_m = 0.4$ g/cm^3 (density of material of interest, the active ingredient)
$c = 1/25 = 0.04$ (average relative weight of active ingredient)
$c_F = \lambda_m / c = (0.4 \text{ g/cm}^3) / 0.04 = 10$ g/cm^3 (composition factor)
$\ell = 0.1$ (granules very similar; small granule to granule variation)

From Equation (1), we have the following result.
   Var(FE) $\approx (1/10 - 1/500) * 0.2^3 (0.5)(0.55)(10)(0.1) \approx 0.0002156 = 0.022\%$
   SD(FE) $\approx$ SQRT(0.0002156) $= 0.01468 = 1.5\%$.

Var(FE) for Particle Size Distribution

In the case where we are sampling to determine particle size distribution, the formula for estimating the Var(FE) is the following:

$$\text{Var(FE)} \approx [(1/M_S) - (1/M_L)] \, f \, \lambda \{[(1/c_1) - 2] \, d_1^3 + g \, d_2^3\} \qquad (2)$$

where M_S, M_L, and f are the same as in Equation (1), λ is the density (in g/cm3) of the material, c_1 is the proportion of the particle size class of interest in the lot, d_1 is the average particle size (in cm) for the particle size class of interest, and d_2 is the near maximum particle size (in cm) for all other particle size classes combined.

We need to calculate Var(FE) for each particle size class. Then we must take the maximum sample weight to guarantee achieving the level of variation desired for each particle size class.

Summary

We can reduce the variance of the FE by increasing the weight of the sample, regardless of how many increments make up the sample. If appropriate, we can reduce the particle size of the lot material before sampling.

GROUPING AND SEGREGATION ERROR

The GE is a source of sampling variation at the "local level," that is, at the small scale where the sample is actually taken. It is not present in classical SRS. The GE is due to (*i*) the distribution heterogeneity of the material, which is random at the small scale area where we take our sample, (*ii*) the selection of groups of particles, rather than individual particles, and (*iii*) the segregation of material at the short range where we take the sample.

Recall that the FE is the minimum sampling error we would incur if we had no other errors. It corresponds to SRS: sampling particles one at a time with equal probability and at random. If we could sample particles one at a time, then we would not have an error due to grouping. And if we could sample randomly, then we would not have an error due to material segregation. This observation leads to two ways to minimize the GE. First, the smaller the groups (or increments) of particles we collect to form the sample, the closer we come to the ideal of "one at a time." So it is preferable for us to take many small increments to form the sample rather than taking the entire amount for the sample in one portion. Second, mixing the material will reduce the material segregation.

A few examples will illustrate these ideas. A spinning riffler takes many small increments to form the sample and works well for a wide variety of material. The lot is divided into anywhere from 6 to 12 containers, which are filled by several rotations under a steady falling stream of the material. Each rotation corresponds to one increment for each container, and the more rotations, the greater the number of increments. One or more containers are selected at random to form the sample, and repeated subsampling can be carried out to achieve the desired sample size for analytical purposes. Fractional shoveling is a similar manual technique, where the entire lot is moved to smaller piles using one small shovelful at a time to each pile in sequence, one after the other, until the entire lot has been divided. One or more piles are selected at random to form the sample. To mix material, stirring, rotating, and shaking are common techniques. It is best to verify that the chosen method is effective because some materials actually segregate when shaken. Fill levels and rotation speed can also affect mixing performance (5). Coning and quartering (6) is a poor sampling technique because it violates both of the minimization criteria. Each sample consists of only one or two increments of the material: one quarter or two opposite quarters, depending on the protocol. The performance is worse if the material is not well mixed, which is very hard to accomplish with some materials.

With this understanding of the underlying idea behind the GE, the futility of "grab" (convenience) sampling is now clear. Because mixing is imperfect and transitory, there is always some degree of segregation. Thus, taking our sample in one big portion from the top of the local area of interest will result in a biased sample. The notion that "the material is homogeneous (or well-mixed) so it does not matter how or where we sample" is erroneous. For instance, since different particle types segregate at transfer points, it is a mistake to sample after transfer of previously mixed material (3).

The variance of the GE can be larger, and in some cases, much larger, than the variance of the FE. This means that incorrect sampling from lots with large distribution heterogeneity will produce very different results for separate samples. An excellent example of this phenomenon is a laboratory experiment performed by Pitard (7). Three approximately equal-sized lots of material were divided into 16 parts (samples) each using a different sampling technique for each lot. Each of the $16 \times 3 = 48$ samples was then analyzed for lead concentrate. Averages of 8.250%, 8.326%, and 8.300% for the three lots indicate very close agreement. In contrast, the lead concentrate values for the 16 samples within each lot varied substantially. The total relative standard deviations were 0.358, 0.114, and 0.110, respectively. This difference in sampling variation is due to the variance of the GE, because the analytical variation and variance of the FE are constant and do not depend on the sampling technique used. Grab sampling was used to subdivide the first lot and produced fairly poor results compared to the other two cases where a riffle splitter was used, one without prior mixing and one with prior mixing. This example illustrates that even on a small scale in the laboratory, variation between sub-samples in the measured characteristic can be very big. We can imagine that the variation is substantially larger when the initial or secondary sampling takes place, which is outside the laboratory and more difficult to perform correctly.

In summary, we can decrease the GE by collecting several increments at random in the local area of interest and combining them to form the sample. We can also reduce this error by mixing the material and ensuring it does not resegregate prior to collecting the sampl.

DELIMITATION ERROR

The DE is one of the three errors arising from violating the principle of correct sampling. It addresses activity on a small scale, at the level where we *define* the sample we wish to take. We first must determine the sampling dimension. The smaller this is, the better chance we have of defining and obtaining a correct sample. Three-dimensional sampling should be avoided. We have seen that the correct geometry in this case is a sphere, which is impossible to obtain. For one- and two-dimensional sampling, we know that the correct geometries are a line and a circle, respectively. Extending these through the remaining dimensions produces a cross-stream sample for one-dimensional sampling and a cylinder (core) for two-dimensional sampling. As we saw earlier, a different and still correct type of one-dimensional cross-stream sample can be obtained using a V-shaped cutter when movement across the stream is circular.

Two-dimensional sampling is a substantial improvement over three-dimensional sampling. Even so, correct sample definition and extraction are difficult. When a correct core sample cannot be obtained, as with a thief (6), for example, then reducing the sampling dimension to one is advisable. Rather than using a thief to puncture a bag and collect material (incorrectly) as is sometimes done in acceptance sampling, a riffle splitter might be used to obtain a correct subsample to be analyzed.

In one-dimensional sampling, grab samples from the side of a conveyor belt produce a DE. The sample has not been correctly defined because material on the other side will have no chance of being collected. Any segregation across the stream will result in a biased sample (Fig. 5). Collecting a sample by diverting a stream may get more material from one side than the other. A true cross-stream sample may be impossible to define if the material is enclosed. Grab samples in this environment are common: probes that collect material only from the side of the stream or tubes that collect material only from the center, for instance (Fig. 5). In such cases, though we still have a DE, mixing the material before taking a "spot" sample will reduce the GE and thus the total sampling error. Use of a static mixer upstream of the sample collection is one way to do this (Fig. 6). Another option is "swirling" the material before siphoning off the sample (8).

In summary, to minimize the DE, reduce the sampling dimension, if possible. Define a correct sample for that sampling dimension. Consider the type of tool that will be used for extraction. Condition (mix) a one-dimensional enclosed stream upstream of the sampling point.

EXTRACTION ERROR

While defining a correct sample is straightforward in theory, sample extraction is difficult to carry out in practice because of the sampling dimension, the tools used, and how they are used. The sampling tool must be compatible with the boundaries defined, and the tool must be used correctly. When the sample defined is not the same as the sample extracted, we incur an EE, another of the three errors arising from violating the principle of correct sampling.

Two-dimensional sampling is very common, and even though correct, core samples are difficult to obtain. A thief probe, for example, does not extract a core but rather material only at the probe windows. Of course, taking material from various levels is better than taking a grab sample from the top, as is often the case with a three-dimensional lot. But we

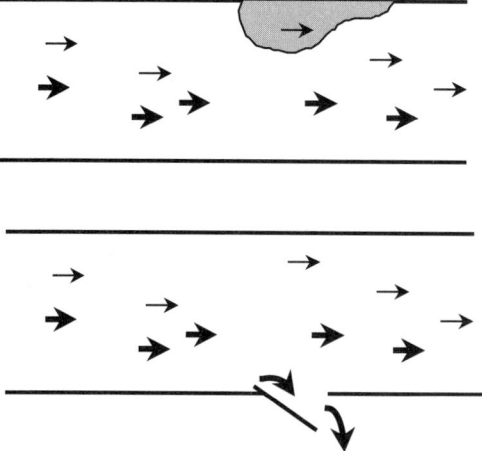

FIGURE 5 Material taken from only one side of a stream (such as a conveyor belt or enclosed pipe) will result in a sample with bias, which will increase with more heterogeneity across the stream.

Principles of Sampling for Particulate Solids

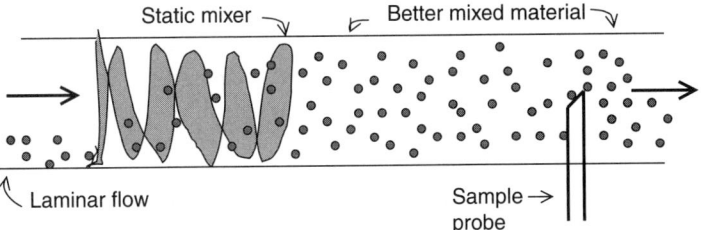

FIGURE 6 Mixing upstream of the sample collection reduces the segregation error when a correct, cross-stream sample cannot be obtained.

must be aware of the drawbacks. Another problem with a thief probe is that the pointed end does not allow material at the bottom to be part of the sample. Any vertical segregation will produce biased results. Fraud may also be perpetrated. Gy (1) gives an example of a supplier who covered the bottom of its delivery containers with rocks. The supplier knew its customer sampled vertically with a thief. The result was huge monetary losses for the customer.

One-dimensional sampling is preferred, and many tools are available for correct delimitation and extraction. As we have seen, correct delimitation for one-dimensional sampling is defined by either a cross-stream sample or a circular rotation with a wedge-shaped cutter. Even with a correct tool, however, an EE can occur. A few examples illustrate this point. The sampling tool must not slow down or speed up as it advances across a moving stream, since material on the opposite side will not have the same chance of being in the sample as material on the near side. A bias will occur if the cutter does not pass all the way through the stream before starting back. In the laboratory, round bottom scoops will under represent material at the bottom as it passes through the material. Spatulas will under represent material at the top, since it forms a rounded cone at the top.

A controlled laboratory experiment by Allen and Kahn (9) compared the total sampling variation of five tools and techniques: coning and quartering, scooping, a table sampler, a Jones riffler, and a spinning riffler. To compare these methods in the presence of particle size differences, they used a 60/40 mixture of coarse and fine sand. To compare the methods in the presence of density differences, they used a 60/40 mixture of sand and sugar. Each method performed about the same for both particle size and density. Scoop sampling and coning and quartering were the worst with a standard deviation of the major component between 5% and 7%. The table sampler was just over 2%, and the Jones riffle splitter produced about 1%. The best was a spinning riffler with 0.2%.

In summary, to avoid EEs, use a correct tool, and use it correctly.

PREPARATION ERROR

When the sample integrity has not been preserved during or after sampling, we incur a PE. While a PE is not a sampling error per se, Gy includes it because it is part of the whole sampling protocol, whether in the field or lab. We should not confuse this terminology with sample preparation in the lab. Gy's PE is much broader. A common and perhaps more descriptive term is sample handling. Handling errors may occur during transfer, storage, drying, and grinding. They include sample contamination, loss, chemical or physical alteration, unintentional mistakes, and, unfortunately, intentional tampering. A chemist is the best resource to help with protocols, tools, and containers that will ensure preserving the sample integrity.

Contamination occurs when extraneous material is added to the sample during the sampling process or after the sample is taken but before the chemical or physical analysis. For example, if a sampling tool, container, or system is not cleaned between the collection of samples, material from a previous batch will contaminate the current sample. If a sampling system is not purged before a sample is taken, then the sample line contains old material that is collected with the current sample. Contamination occurs when grinding tools, screens, or meshes are not cleaned. An uncovered container may allow moisture absorption. A sampling tool or container having trace amounts of the critical component will affect the analysis: metal scoops, rifflers, or holding trays containing the metal of interest, for instance.

One cause of loss is through abrasion, which may occur during transport. Improper temperature controls may lead to loss of volatiles or changes in chemical or physical properties. Grinding tools, screens, or meshes may retain material, and material may get caught in the elbows of sampling lines. Fines may be lost from the effects of static electricity on scoops, bags, or containers, or from uncovered containers during sampling or transfer.

Chemical alteration includes oxidation, addition or loss of water, fixation or loss of carbon dioxide, and chemical reactions. Physical alterations include a change in state, changes in particle size, and the addition or loss of water.

Unintentional mistakes may also occur. These include mislabeling, missing labels, samples taken from the wrong place, samples mixed up with other samples, spills, and, if required, no chain of custody. Intentional tampering (fraud) is also a PE. Examples include selective selection of material to be in the sample, not taring containers, using containers made of the component of interest, and falsified chemical or physical analysis. While we do not think of PEs as applying to SRS, both unintentional mistakes and fraud occur.

To avoid or minimize a PE, preserve the integrity of the sample.

LONG-RANGE NONPERIODIC HETEROGENEITY FLUCTUATION ERROR

The previous errors addressed heterogeneity on a small scale. Now we examine heterogeneity on a large scale: the scale of the lot over time or space. The long-range nonperiodic heterogeneity fluctuation error is nonrandom and results in trends or shifts in the measured characteristic of interest as we track it over time or over the extent of the lot in space. For example, measured characteristics of a chemical product may decrease due to catalyst deterioration. Particle size distribution may be altered due to machine wear. Samples from different parts of the lot may show trends due to lack of mixing.

The best way to identify process shifts and trends is by plotting the sample measurements over time or by location. Adding control limits can help spot outliers. Interestingly, changes in sampling technique can make a process appear to have undergone a shift or trend, when in fact it has not. For instance, if material is more thoroughly mixed now than in the past before a sample is taken, then results will be different, either higher or lower, than the biased results previously observed.

A tool used to identify variation in the measurements over time is a variogram. Since this is a quite complicated calculation and analysis, we refer the reader to books by Gy (1) and Pitard (4).

Principles of Sampling for Particulate Solids

LONG-RANGE PERIODIC HETEROGENEITY FLUCTUATION ERROR

The long-range periodic heterogeneity fluctuation error is the result of nonrandom periodic changes in the critical component as we track it over time or over the entirety of the lot in space. For instance, certain measurements may show periodic fluctuations due to different control of the manufacturing process by various shifts of operators. Batch processes that alternate raw materials from two different suppliers may show periodicity in measurements.

A time series plot can help identify cycles. As in the case of shifts and trends, the sampling mode or frequency can affect our interpretation of sample measurements. As a case in point, if we use systematic random sampling that is in sync with a cycle, then we do not see the entire variation in our process. So if our measurements are taken at the low end of the process cycle, we do not see high values that may be outside the specification limits of our customers or outside regulatory limits. If our sampling is too infrequent, we may observe a long-term cycle that is not process related at all (Fig. 7). Incorrect sampling due to DEs or EEs can also make a process look like it has a cycle over time. For example, suppose the critical content varies across a conveyor belt and alternate samples are taken on opposite sides. Then every second result will be lower than the others, which will be higher. This observed heterogeneity is local, however, not temporal.

Cyclic fluctuations may or may not be avoidable, but they should be identified and their variation assessed.

ADDITIONAL REMARKS

An estimate of the combined variation from the first five sampling errors and the analytical error can be obtained by taking several samples very close together in time, just seconds or minutes apart. Controlling process variation below this amount will be impossible unless the variation due to these errors is reduced. The long-term periodic and nonperiodic variation will presumably not be present in these samples because the process will not have changed much during this short span. Since analytical variation for specific methods is typically known, it can be subtracted out to get an estimate of the contribution from the first five errors.

Sampling safely should be a primary concern. So it is important to know the hazards of the material, the capabilities and limitations of the equipment, and the environment where the sample will be taken. In many cases, government regulations will apply, and protective clothing may be necessary.

Finally, a plan for reducing the total sampling error can be started in a straightforward way. Using the information in this chapter, you can audit sampling procedures,

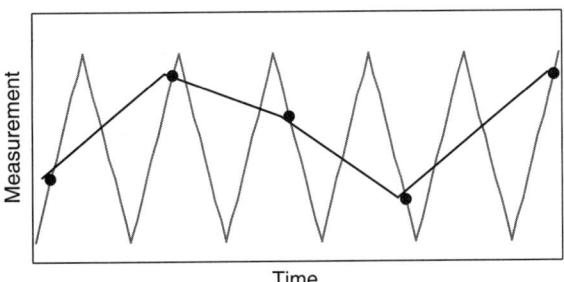

FIGURE 7 In the presence of an underlying cycle, sampling too infrequently can lead to the appearance of a longer cycle, which is purely artificial.

practices, and equipment for correctness and safety. An assessment of the findings can then proceed, with actions taken to address the shortcomings. In some cases, actions will be easy and inexpensive. In other cases, more extensive investigations will be required. More details can be found in Smith (10).

REFERENCES

1. Gy PM. Sampling of Heterogeneous and Dynamic Material Systems: Theories of Heterogeneity, Sampling and Homogenizing. Amsterdam: Elsevier, 1992, pp. 1–653.
2. Gy PM. Sampling for Analytical Purposes. Chichester: Wiley, 1998, pp. 1–153.
3. Muzzio FJ, Robinson P, Wightman C, Brone D. Sampling practices in powder blending. Int J Pharm 1997; 155:153–78.
4. Pitard FF. Pierre Gy's Sampling Theory and Sampling Practice: Heterogeneity, Sampling correctness, and Statistical Process Control. 2nd ed. Boca Raton, FL: CRC Press, 1993, pp. 1–488.
5. Llusa L, Muzzio F. The Effect of shear Milling on the Blending of Cohesive Lubricant and Drugs, http://www.pharmtech.com/pharmtech/article/articleDetail.jsp?id=283906&searchString=llusa (accessed February 2008).
6. Venables HJ, Wells JI. Powder sampling. Drug Dev Ind Pharm 2002; 28(2):107–17.
7. Pitard FF. Unpublished course notes. 1989.
8. Sprenger GR. Continuous Solids Sampler, GR Sprenger Engineering, Inc., http://www.grsei.com (accessed February 2008).
9. Allen T, Khan AA. Critical Evaluation of Powder Sampling Procedures. Chem Eng 1970; 238:108ff.
10. Smith PL. A Primer for Sampling Solids, Liquids, and Gases: Based on the Theory of Pierre Gy. Philadelphia: The Society for Industrial and Applied Mathematics, 2001, pp. 55–60.

2
Particle and Powder Bed Properties

Stephen W. Hoag and Han-Pin Lim
*School of Pharmacy, University of Maryland, Baltimore,
Maryland, U.S.A.*

INTRODUCTION

Micromeritics is the study of the science and technology of small particles (1); this includes the characterization of important properties such as particle size, size distribution, shape, and many other properties. All dosage forms from parenterals to tablets at some point in their manufacture involve particle technology and the performance of these dosage forms is much dependent upon the particle size of the drug and excipients. Given the central role played by the particle properties in tablet production, this chapter is devoted to the subject of characterizing particle properties; other chapters will examine the physical and rheological properties of particles in powder beds and tablet production.

One reason for the importance of particle size is that the surface area to volume ratio (often called the surface to volume ratio) is dependent upon particle size. The surface to volume ratio is the ratio of the surface area divided by the volume (V) of a spherical particle and is given by

$$V = \frac{\pi d^3}{6} \tag{1}$$

and the surface area (S) of a spherical particle is given by

$$S = \pi d^2 \tag{2}$$

where d is the diameter of the particle. Hence, the surface to volume ratio can be defined as:

$$\frac{S}{V} = \frac{6}{d} \tag{3}$$

Figure 1 plots the surface to volume ratio in Equation (3) versus the particle diameter; this graph shows that as the particle size decreases, the surface to volume ratio tends towards infinity. In other words, the total surface area of a set of particles is greatly affected by the particle size. Thus, phenomena that occur at a particle's surface, such as dissolution, will occur at a faster rate for particles with a higher surface to volume ratio, because there is more surface area available for interaction with the surroundings; conversely slower reactions will occur for particles with a lower surface to volume ratio. As shown in Figure 1, the effect of particle size can be very significant as particle size decreases. For example, particles with diameter of 1 μm will yield a surface to volume

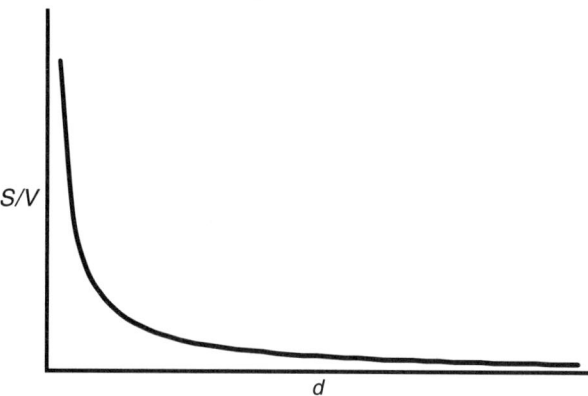

FIGURE 1 Surface to volume ratio versus the particle diameter. The particle size decreases as the surface to volume ratio tends towards infinity.

ratio of $6\,\mu m^{-1}$ while particles with diameter of $100\,\mu m$ will only yield a surface to volume ratio of $0.06\,\mu m^{-1}$.

One important particle property affected by total surface area is solute dissolution, i.e., drug release rate. The drug release rate from a solid as described by the Noyes–Whitney equation is:

$$\frac{dM}{dt} = \frac{SD_k(C_s - C_b)}{h} \tag{4}$$

where M is the mass, t is time, dM/dt is the drug release rate, D_k is the diffusion coefficient, C_s is the drug solubility at the same conditions as the particle surface, C_b is the concentration in the bulk dissolution medium, and h is the thickness of the boundary or diffusion layer (Fig. 2). According to Equation (4), drug release is directly proportional to the total surface area; thus, increasing the particle surface area will increase the drug release rate. Changes in particle size that affect the release rate can influence the bioavailability of a dosage form (2). Thus, for some drugs, e.g., low-solubility drugs, controlling particle size is essential for reliable therapeutic outcomes.

In addition to drug dissolution and bioavailability, the properties of a powder bed can be strongly influenced by particle size. As the particle size decreases, the number of contact points between particles in a given volume of material drastically increases. For example, if 1 g of material with a density $1\,g/cm^3$ were densely packed with six contact points per particle, then 10 and $100\,\mu m$ diameter spherical particles would have about 11.5×10^9 and 11.5×10^6 contact points/g, respectively. In other words, the smaller

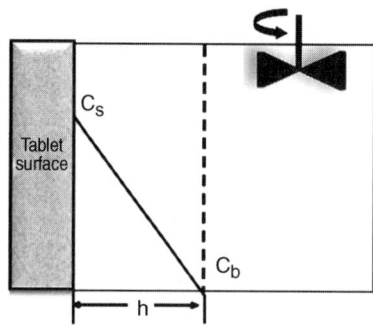

FIGURE 2 Noyes–Whitney dissolution model where C_s is the drug solubility at the same conditions as the particle surface, C_b is the concentration in the bulk dissolution medium and h is the thickness of the boundary or diffusion layer.

Particle and Powder Bed Properties

particles would have a thousand times more contact points per gram compared to the larger particles. If each contact point is associated with cohesive forces then the powder bed with smaller particles would be much more cohesive. As a result, the degree of powder bed cohesion is heavily influenced by particle size, and the degree of cohesion affects powder flow, segregation propensity, and the consolidation properties of the powder bed. Many literature reports have shown that decreasing particle size generally decreases the powder flowability while increasing the tablet mechanical strength as smaller particles have more surface area exposed for particle bonding (3–6).

For unit operations like milling and granulation the key output is a material with a certain particle size. Given the significance of particle size, it is critical for formulation development and quality control to be able to quantitatively and qualitatively characterize and accurately measure particle size, which will be discussed in detail in this chapter.

The first step of the particle size characterization process is acquiring a representative sample from a batch or lot of material. The issue of bulk sampling is complex; the first chapter of this book is devoted to sampling theory. Any analysis of particle size is only as good as the sample used for the measurement and any errors in sampling will lead to erroneous results.

Overview of Particle Size Characterization

For the sake of presentation, the measurement and the determination of particle size will be broken into three sections: first, characterizing the size of individual particles, second, statistically summarizing groups of particles, and third, a discussion of the methods for particle size measurement.

The problem of determining a reliable particle size is illustrated by Figure 3, which shows a set of particles. The goal of any particle size analysis is to summarize this set of particles in a manner which provides the maximum useful information that relates to the particle's properties during dosage form manufacturing and in the final dosage form.

According to United States Pharmacopeia (USP) <776>, a particle is defined as the smallest discrete unit, and collections of particles can be described by their degree of association such as aggregates, agglomerates, lamellar, conglomerates and spherulites. An aggregate is a mass of adhered particles, agglomerates are fused or cemented

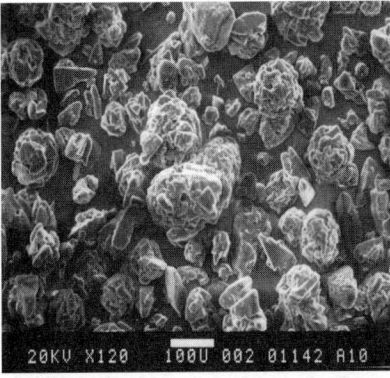 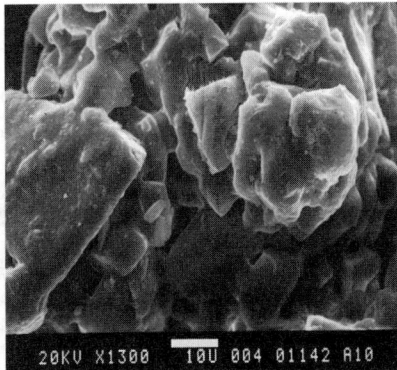

FIGURE 3 A set of irregularly shaped particles.

particles, lamellar is a stack of plates, conglomerates are a mixture of two or more types of particles, and spherulites are radial clusters (7). In many references, the term primary particle is used, for this text the term is synonymous with the USP definition of particle.

One of the key elements for meaningful particle size determinations is defining the type of particle (primary particle or group of particles) that can best represent the application and properties of interest. For example, when studying a granulation process the particle size of the agglomerate is the critical size needed for characterizing the granulation. On the other hand, if the dissolution profile of the drug is being characterized then the particle size of the primary particle is the critical size. Knowing the type of particle to be measured is critical because certain sample preparation techniques and analysis conditions can influence the degree of particle aggregation.

DEFINITION OF PARTICLE SIZE

The first step in the statistical analysis of particle size is to define the radius or diameter of the particle in question. For spherical particles the diameter or radius is easy to measure and can be defined by a unique number that is characteristic of a sphere. If the diameter of a sphere is known then the surface area, volume, mass (using true density), and sieve diameter of that particle can be determined, which is useful for assessing properties such as dissolution rate. However, most particles used in tablet manufacturing are not perfect spheres with an easily defined diameter. For example, the irregular shaped particle in Figure 4A has an infinite number of different diameters which could be drawn; in addition, none of these diameters gives any information about the surface area or volume of the particle, which decreases the usefulness of the determined particle size. Ideally the diameter should uniquely define the particle and give information about its surface area and or volume. Currently, the two most popular methods for defining particle size are the equivalent diameters and the statistical diameters; these two methods are discussed in the following two sections.

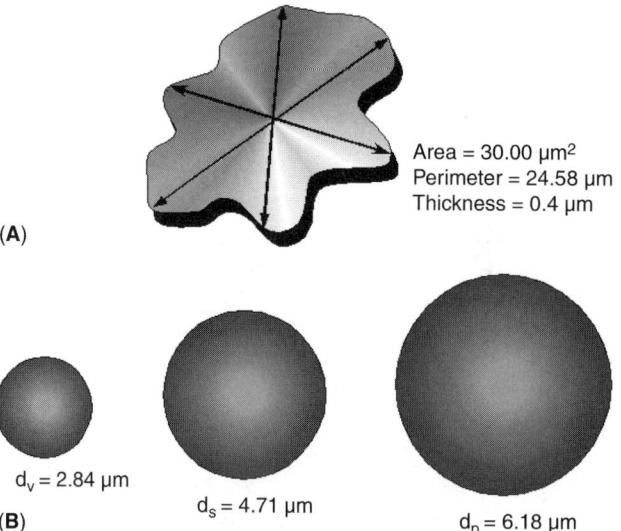

FIGURE 4 (**A**) An irregularly shaped particle with an infinite number of diameters. (**B**) The equivalent volume, surface, and projected area diameter of (A).

Particle and Powder Bed Properties

Equivalent Diameters

The concept of equivalent diameters can be used to uniquely define particle size of an irregularly shaped particle. Equivalent diameters are based either on geometry or physical properties. While the equivalent geometry could be based upon a cube, sphere or other regular shapes for reasons of convenience the equivalent spherical diameter is typically based on a spherical geometry. Thus, the equivalent spherical diameter of a particle is the diameter of a sphere with equivalent geometric or physical properties as the particle in question. For example, if a microscope was used to measure the projected area diameter (i.e., the two-dimensional projection of a particle onto a microscope slide) of the irregular particle shown in Figure 4A, the equivalent projected area diameter would be determined by first measuring the projected area of the particle and then using this area to calculate the diameter of a sphere with an equivalent projected area as the particle shown in Figure 4A. The equation for the projected area of a sphere is:

$$A_p = \frac{\pi}{4} d_p^2 \tag{5}$$

and the equivalent projected area diameter can be calculated using:

$$d_p = \sqrt{\frac{4A_p}{\pi}} \tag{6}$$

In addition, to the projected area, an equivalent diameter could also be calculated based upon the particle's surface area. The equation for the surface area of a sphere is:

$$S = \pi d_s^2 \tag{7}$$

hence, the equivalent surface area diameter is:

$$d_s = \sqrt{\frac{S}{\pi}} \tag{8}$$

Likewise, an equivalent diameter could be calculated based upon the particle's volume; the volume of a sphere equals:

$$V = \frac{\pi}{6} d_v^3 \tag{9}$$

and this yields an equivalent volume diameter of:

$$d_v = \sqrt[3]{\frac{6V}{\pi}} \tag{10}$$

Another useful equivalent diameter is the equivalent sieve diameter, it is the diameter of the largest sphere which can pass through a given sieve aperture. It should be noted that the equivalent diameter of a particle always has dimension of length.

An advantage of equivalent diameters is that they provide a unique characterization of particle size for the given method of measurement. In addition, the diameter gives information about the particle properties. For example, the equivalent surface diameter would give information about the surface area of the particle and the equivalent volume diameter would give information about the volume. Thus, if the density of the particles is known, the mass and properties important to pharmaceutical applications can be calculated. The numerical value for equivalent diameters derived from different geometric properties will only be identical in the case of perfectly spherical particles, and if the particle irregularity increases so will the differences between the different equivalent diameters.

Example 1. Calculate the equivalent projected area diameter, surface area diameter and volume diameter of a particle with a projected area of 30.00 μm², perimeter of 24.58 μm, and thickness of 0.40 μm as shown in Figure 4A.

Using Equation (6), the equivalent projection diameter is:

$$d_p = \sqrt{\frac{4A_p}{\pi}} = \sqrt{\frac{4(30)}{\pi}} = 6.18 \, \mu m$$

The surface area of the particle can be calculated using the projection area, A_p, perimeter, P, and thickness, t as follows:

$$S = (P \times t) + 2A_p = (24.58 \times 0.40) \, \mu m^2 + 2 \, (30.00 \, \mu m^2) = 69.83 \, \mu m^2.$$

Thus, according to Equation (8), the equivalent surface diameter is:

$$d_S = \sqrt{\frac{S}{\pi}} = \sqrt{\frac{69.84 \, \mu m}{\pi}} = 4.71 \, \mu m$$

The volume of the particle is simply the projection area multiplied by the thickness:

$$V = 30.00 \, \mu m^2 \times 0.40 \, \mu m = 12.00 \, \mu m^3.$$

Hence, Equation (10) yields the equivalent volume diameter of:

$$d_v = \sqrt[3]{\frac{6V}{\pi}} = \sqrt[3]{\frac{6(12)}{\pi}} = 2.84 \, \mu m$$

This example shows that an irregularly shaped particle can have different values for the different equivalent diameters when they are calculated from different geometric properties, i.e., each type of equivalent diameter weights the particle based upon the property that was measured (Fig. 4B).

In addition to equivalent diameters based on geometric properties there are also equivalent diameters that are based on the physical properties of the particle. For example, the Stokes' diameter uses Stoke's law to calculate the diameter of a sphere with the same settling velocity as the particle in question. The terminal velocity (V_s) of a sphere settling in a fluid can be described by Stokes' law:

$$V_s = \frac{h}{t} = \frac{d^2(\rho_p - \rho_m)g}{18\eta} \tag{11}$$

upon rearrangement, the Stokes' diameter can be defined as:

$$d_{st} = \sqrt{\frac{18\eta v_s}{(\rho_p - \rho_m)g}} \tag{12}$$

where ρ_p is the density of the particles, ρ_m is the density of the fluid medium, g is the acceleration of gravity and η is the viscosity of the medium.

Example 2. The settling velocity of a newly discovered drug, XYZ2007, with a density of 3.80 g/cm³, is 0.021 cm/sec as measured by an Andreasen apparatus at 25°C. Water is used as the medium and the viscosity and density of water at 25°C is 0.01 poise (0.01 g/cm sec) and 1.0 g/cm³, respectively. Calculate the Stokes' diameter of this drug.

Using Equation (12), yields,

$$d_{st}(16 \, min) = \sqrt{\frac{18(0.01 \, g/cm \, sec)(0.021 \, cm/sec)}{(3.80 - 1.0 \, g/cm^3)(981 \, cm/sec^2)}} = 11.73 \times 10^{-4} \, cm \, or \, 11.73 \, \mu m$$

Particle and Powder Bed Properties

Another example is the aerodynamic diameter; this diameter is used to characterize aerosolized particles for which the density is difficult to determine. Thus, one assumes that the particle density equals 1 and does the Stokes' Law calculations for the sphere of unit density and having the same settling velocity as the particle in question (8).

Statistical Diameters

Statistical diameters are often used in microscopy as they can be easily and rapidly measured, but the disadvantage is that they do not give information about the particle properties such as volume, mass, or surface area. However, for quality control applications this information may not be important. Figure 5 illustrates the most commonly used diameters. The USP <776> defines Martin's and Feret's diameter and other less commonly used diameters as (7):

Feret's diameter: The distance between imaginary parallel lines tangent to a randomly oriented particle and perpendicular to the ocular scale also called a graticule.
Martin's diameter: The diameter of the particle at the point that divides a randomly oriented particle into two equal projected areas.
Length: The longest dimension from edge to edge of a particle oriented parallel to the ocular scale.
Width: The longest dimension of the particle measured at right angles to the length.

Note, many of these diameters assume a random particle orientation relative to the ocular scale or graticule. This is important for sample preparation because anything that biases the orientation of the particles on the microscope slide will bias the results. For example, to uniformly cover a microscope slide with particles one could usually swipe a spatula over the slide which could potentially induce a preferred orientation to the particles, especially for needle shaped particles.

Diameters Summary

In summary, not all equivalent diameters are equivalent to each other, unless the particles are perfect spheres; this highlights the importance of reporting the type of particle size and method of measurement. Different equivalent diameters emphasize different properties of the particle as shown in Example 1, and these differences become more significant as the particles become more irregular. The choice of diameter is in part determined by the method of measurement, because different methods measure different

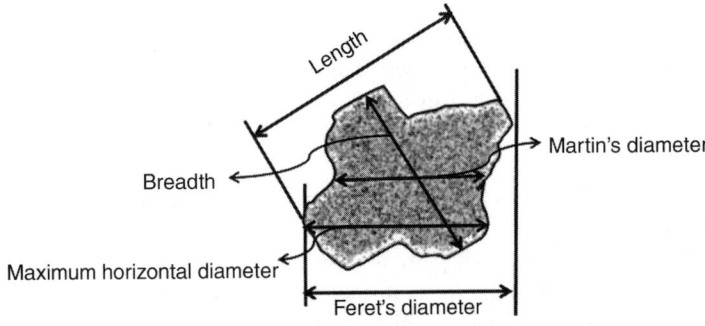

FIGURE 5 The most commonly used diameters.

particle properties. For example, in microscopy the projected area of a particle is measured; thus, the projected area diameter of a particle is the logical diameter to use. For the measurement of particle volume, a Coulter counter or laser diffraction instrument is commonly used to measure the volume diameters. Because there are as many different types of diameters as there are methods of measurement, one should select a measurement method that gives the most information about the properties of interest. Ideally, the properties of interest should guide the selection of the measurement method and hence the type of diameter to be used. As always, practical considerations such as the instrument availability, cost, convenience and many other factors often intercede and affect the choice of analysis method. Given these differences in diameters, there have been methods developed for converting from one type of diameter to another; these methods will be discussed in the Hatch–Choate equations and in the section Particle Shape.

STATISTICS OF PARTICLE SIZE

Following the progression of the particle size analysis we first obtained a representative sample, then a unique characterization of the particle size and now we must summarize assemblies or sets of particles often called the population by statisticians. The statistical methods used to summarize the particles that make up our samples will be covered in this section. For a set or particles in a sample like those shown in Figure 3, the goal of a statistical analysis is to summarize a large amount of data into a usable form while losing as little information as possible about the original population. However, before continuing, it is worth reviewing some statistical concepts that are critical to the discussion of particle populations.

Types of Probability Distributions

For this section, histograms will be used to illustrate the concept of a probability distribution. For example, if we were to summarize the particles shown in Figure 3 using a histogram we would divide the particle size range into equally spaced intervals and then calculate the frequency or fraction of particles that fall into each interval; this frequency is then plotted versus particle size (Fig. 6A). Generally, histograms are very good summaries of a population of particles. However when constructing a histogram one has to be careful not to distort the nature of the population by selecting an inappropriate interval size. For example, a skewed distribution could appear symmetric as a result of choosing the wrong interval size. See the textbook by Allen for guidance on the construction of histograms (9).

Typically, the intervals used to construct a histogram are based on practical considerations such as the sieve sizes used when collecting data. However, if the experiment was repeated using a larger sample size and a finer interval size one would see a refined histogram, which better reveals the underlying distribution that gives rise to the population characteristics, and if we kept increasing the measurement resolution the distribution would converge to an underlying distribution characteristic of that population (Fig. 6B).

This underlying distribution is the state of nature dictated by the intrinsic properties of the particles, and particles with different intrinsic properties will be best described by different types of distributions. For example, particles formed by granulation will often have a different type of distribution from particles formed by milling, because the nature of the formation processes produces populations with different characteristics, which are reflected in the distribution of particle size.

Particle and Powder Bed Properties

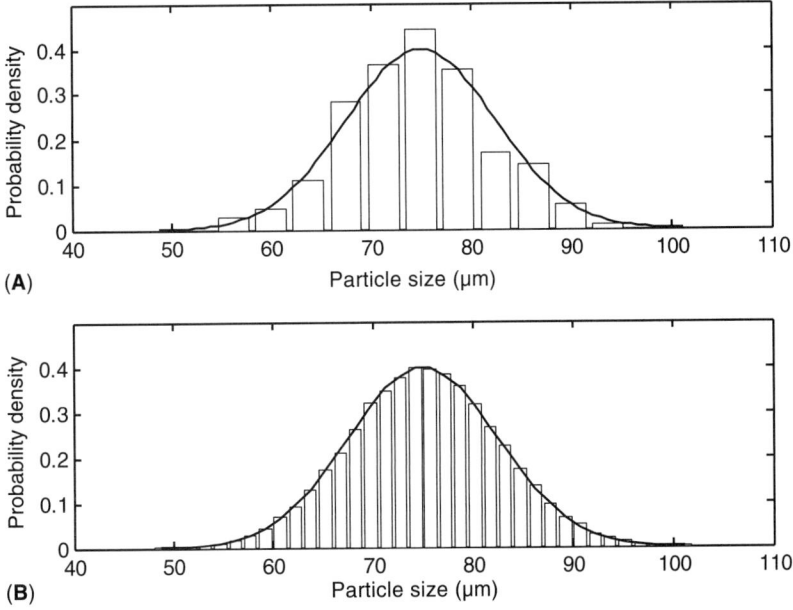

FIGURE 6 (A) Frequency versus particle size for a set of irregularly shaped particles similar to those in Figure 3. (B) A normal distribution is obtained when using a larger sample size and a finer interval size.

The most common probability distribution in nature is the normal or Gaussian distribution (Fig. 6B). The normal distribution has been used to describe the distribution of everything from particle size to shoe size. The equation for the normal distribution is:

$$f(x) = \frac{1}{\sigma\sqrt{2\pi}} e^{-\frac{1}{2\sigma^2}(x-\mu)^2} \tag{13}$$

where x is the particle size, σ^2 is the variance of the distribution, σ is the standard deviation, and μ is the mean. The function $f(x)$ is called the probability density function or just the density function, which gives the frequency of occurrence or fraction of a population of a particle size, x. The shorthand notation for the distribution of x is $x \sim N(\mu, \sigma)$, which can be read as x is distributed normally with mean, μ and standard deviation, σ. As implied by this notation, the normal distribution can be completely described by the mean, μ, and the standard deviation, σ. These parameters will be discussed in more detail below.

The Gaussian distribution is symmetric and has a domain from minus infinity to plus infinity and ranges over the probabilities from 0 to 100%. In general, larger particles formed by granulation can be described by the normal distribution. However, smaller particles formed by fracture, e.g., milling, often have asymmetric distributions that cannot be described by a normal distribution. The log normal distribution is one asymmetric distribution which generally works well for particles formed by fracture. The equation of the log normal distribution is:

$$f(x) = \frac{1}{x \ln \sigma_g \sqrt{2\pi}} e^{-\frac{(\ln x - \ln x_g)^2}{2 \ln^2 \sigma_g}} \tag{14}$$

where ln is the natural logarithm, σ_g and x_g are the geometric standard deviation and geometric mean, respectively; a graph of the log normal distribution is shown in Figure 7.

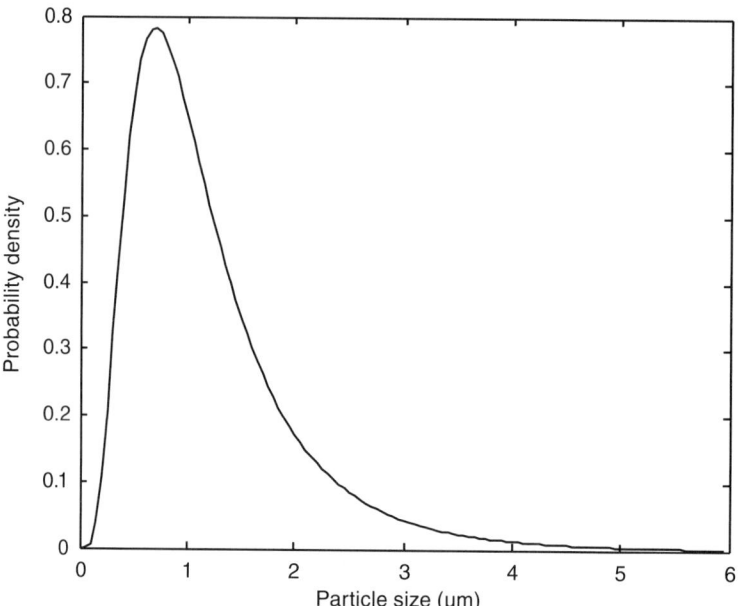

FIGURE 7 A graph of the log normal distribution.

For asymmetric particle populations the log normal distribution is one of the most commonly used distributions.

Because particle populations have such varied properties depending upon how the particles were formed, there are many other types of distributions that can be used to describe particle populations. A partial summary of these distributions is given in Table 1 (9).

All probability distributions can be characterized by two parameters, the mean and the standard deviation. The mean or average gives the location of distribution, and the standard deviation gives the spread or degree of variability in the distribution. The variance is also a measure of the degree of variability in a distribution, it is the square of the standard deviation hence its symbol σ^2 indicating this relationship. The units of the variance are length squared but the standard deviation, which has units of length is more commonly used. Figure 8 illustrates populations with different means and standard deviations.

Two other statistical terms used are the median and the mode. The median is the point where half the population is above the median and half the population is below the median. The median is less influenced by a small number of extreme values. The mode is the most frequently occurring value and is shown in Figure 8. For the normal distribution where the distribution is symmetrical, the mean, median, and the mode are all the same value. However, for other distributions such as a log normal distribution this is not true.

Probability Density Function and Cumulative Probability Distribution

Figure 9 shows the normal frequency or density distribution and the cumulative distribution function. Both of these plots can be used to illustrate a distribution; transformations of the cumulative distribution function will be used later in this chapter.

Particle and Powder Bed Properties

TABLE 1 Summary of Some Commonly Used Density Distribution Functions

Distribution functions	Equation	Range of x
Normal	$\frac{1}{\sigma\sqrt{2\pi}} e^{-\frac{(x-\mu)^2}{2\sigma^2}}$	$[-\infty, +\infty]$
Log normal	$\frac{1}{x \ln \sigma_g \sqrt{2\pi}} e^{-\frac{(\ln x - \ln x_g)^2}{2 \ln^2 \sigma_g}}$	$[0, +\infty]$
Poisson's	$\frac{e^{-m} m^x}{x!}$	$[0, +\infty]$
Binomial	$\frac{n!}{(n-x)! x!} P^x (1-P)^{n-x}$	$[0, +\infty]$
Rosin–Rammler	$Cx^{n-1} e^{-bx^n}$	$[0, +\infty]$
Gaudin–Schuman	Cx^{n-1}	$[0, x_{max}]$
Gaudin–Meloy	$C[1 - n(1 - Cx)^{n-1}]$	$[0, x_{max}]$
Roller	$C\left[\frac{0.5}{\sqrt{x}} + \frac{b}{\sqrt[3]{x^2}}\right]$	$[0, x_{max}]$
Harris	$Cx^{s-1}[1 - bx^s]$	$[0, x_{max}]$
Martin	$Cx^3 e^{-bx}$	$[0, +\infty]$
Gamma function	$Cx^{P-1} e^{-x}$	$[0, +\infty]$
Weinig	$Cx^a e^{-bx^2}$	$[0, +\infty]$
Heywood	$Cx^3 e^{-bx^n}$	$[0, +\infty]$
Griffith	$Cx^{-a} e^{-bx^{-1}}$	$[0, +\infty]$
Klimpel–Austin	$Cx^2[1 - n(1 - Cx)^3]$	$[0, x_{max}]$
Beta function	$Cx^{p-1}[1 - n(1 - Cx)^{q-1}]$	$[0, x_{max}]$

Source: Adapted from Ref. 9.

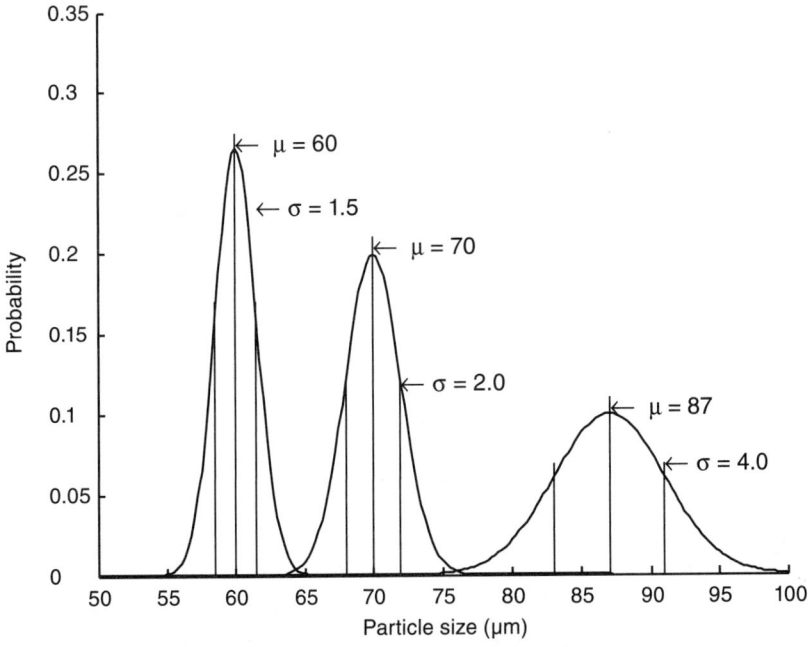

FIGURE 8 Populations with different means and standard deviations.

The density function $f(x)$ in Figure 9 was generated using Equation (13). The cumulative distribution function $F(x)$ is obtained by integrating the density function:

$$\phi = F(x) = \int_{-\infty}^{x} f(x)dx \tag{15}$$

There are some general properties of all distribution functions irrespective of the type of distribution. For example, $F(x) \geq 0$ is a practical constraint because negative probabilities have no meaning. Typically, the probability distribution functions are normalized, i.e., the density function integrated over the entire domain of the density function has a total area under the curve of one:

$$\int_{-\infty}^{\infty} f(x)dx = 1 \tag{16}$$

where $f(x) > 0$. In addition, the probability of a random variable x occurring between x_i and x_{i+1} can be calculated by integrating the density function:

$$P[x_i < x < x_{i+1}] = \int_{x_i}^{x_{i+1}} f(x)dx \tag{17}$$

This is a very useful property for determining the probabilities of certain events occurring. For the discrete case:

$$\frac{n_i}{N}(x_i, x_{i+1}) = P[x_i < x < x_{i+1}] = \int_{x_i}^{x_{i+1}} f(x)dx \tag{18}$$

where n_i is the number of particles in the ith interval and N is the total number of particles in all intervals. Note, the notation n_i divided by N is equivalent to the integral

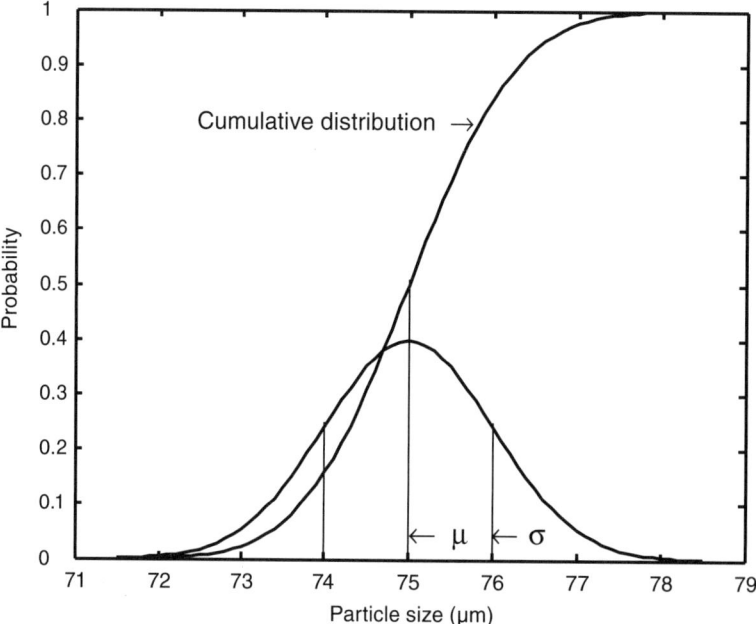

FIGURE 9 Normal frequency or density distribution and the cumulative distribution function used to illustrate a distribution and transformations of the cumulative distribution function.

Particle and Powder Bed Properties

between x_i and x_{i+1}, in other words, the probability of a particular particle being within that interval.

Characterization of a Distribution

Given that a probability distribution can be characterized by a mean and variance, this section will discuss the nature of these parameters. The following section will discuss how to estimate these parameters from a sample. For virtually any probability density function, the average or mean and variance can be determined by the calculation of expected values. The expected value of x for the distribution $f(x)$ is given by:

$$E(x) = \int_{-\infty}^{\infty} x f(x) dx \qquad (19)$$

where $E(x)$ is the expected value of x, which equals the mean μ of the distribution. The expected value formula for x is analogous to the center of mass and moments of the inertia calculations in physics. For example, a teeter totter or seesaw will balance when the weight downwards times the distance from the fulcrum (or average in this example) is equal for each side. The balance point can be found by calculating the average position of all the weights on the teeter totter. By analogy, if you think of a distribution as a thin uniform plate shaped like a normal distribution, then the average is the point where this plate balances, which can be determined by calculating the average position of all the weights of the distribution. The average can be calculated by summing up (integrating) the weights multiply by the position of the weight, i.e., $x f(x)$. A more detailed explanation can be found in engineering and statistics books. The average is called the first moment of the distribution. In summary, the balance point or center of mass of a distribution is equivalent to the mean of that distribution and gives the location of the distribution.

In general any moment of the distribution can be calculated by:

$$E\left((x-b)^k\right) = \int_{-\infty}^{\infty} (x-b)^k f(x) dx \qquad (20)$$

where k is an integer called the order or the kth moment of the random variable x about the point where $x = b$. If b in Equation (20) is the mean (μ) then the moment is called the central moment. The first ($k = 1$) central moment is always zero:

$$E(x - \mu) = \int_{-\infty}^{\infty} x f(x) - \mu f(x) dx = E(X) - E(\mu) = 0 \qquad (21)$$

The second central moment gives the spread or dispersion of the distribution which is the variance; in this moment notation the variance can be calculated using:

$$\text{Var}(x) = \sigma^2 = E\left((x-\mu)^2\right) = \int_{-\infty}^{\infty} (x-\mu)^2 f(x) dx \qquad (22)$$

It can be shown (10) that Equation (22) can also be expressed as:

$$\text{Var}(x) = E\left((x-\mu)^2\right) = E(x^2) - (E(x))^2 \qquad (23)$$

The third moment gives the skewness of the distribution, in other words whether the distribution is symmetric or asymmetric. The fourth moment or kurtosis of the distribution is a measure of the "peakeness" of the distribution and this describes to what extent the distribution is, whether it is tall and skinny or short and squat.

Example 3. For the throw of two fair dice (i.e., each number has 1/6 probability of occurring), let x be a random variable that is equal to the sum of the numbers: then

$P(x=2) = P((1,1)) = 1/36$
$P(x=3) = P((1,2), (2,1)) = 2/36$
$P(x=4) = P((1,3), (2,2), (3,1)) = 3/36$
$P(x=5) = P((1,4), (2,3), (3,2), (4,1)) = 4/36$
$P(x=6) = P((1,5), (2,4), (3,3), (4,2), (5,1)) = 5/36$
$P(x=7) = P((1,6), (2,5), (3,4), (4,3), (5,2), (6,1)) = 6/36$
$P(x=8) = P((2,6), (3,5), (4,4), (5,3), (6,2)) = 5/36$
$P(x=9) = P((3,6), (4,5), (5,4), (6,3)) = 4/36$
$P(x=10) = P((4,6), (5,5), (6,4)) = 3/36$
$P(x=11) = P((5,6), (6,5)) = 2/36$
$P(x=12) = P((6,6)) = 1/16$

where P stands for probability of x equaling some number which is the sum of the two dice. Using expectations calculate the mean and variance of the above distribution. Equation (19) can be used to calculate the mean and notice that n_i/N takes the place of $f(x)$ when going from a continuous variable as in Equation (18) to a discrete variable; thus the mean is equal to:

$$E(x) = 2 \cdot \frac{1}{36} + 3 \cdot \frac{2}{36} + 4 \cdot \frac{3}{36} + 5 \cdot \frac{4}{36} + 6 \cdot \frac{5}{36} + 7 \cdot \frac{6}{36}$$
$$+ 8 \cdot \frac{5}{36} + 9 \cdot \frac{4}{36} + 10 \cdot \frac{3}{36} + 11 \cdot \frac{2}{36} + 12 \cdot \frac{1}{36} = 7$$

Next, Equation (23) can be used to calculate the variance. First, the $E(x^2)$ must be calculated:

$$E(x^2) = 4 \cdot \frac{1}{36} + 9 \cdot \frac{2}{36} + 16 \cdot \frac{3}{36} + 25 \cdot \frac{4}{36} + 36 \cdot \frac{5}{36} + 49 \cdot \frac{6}{36}$$
$$+ 64 \cdot \frac{5}{36} + 81 \cdot \frac{4}{36} + 100 \cdot \frac{3}{36} + 121 \cdot \frac{2}{36} + 144 \cdot \frac{1}{36} = 54.8$$

Plugging in to Equation (23) yields:

$$\text{Var}(x) = E(x^2) - (E(x))^2 = 54.8 - 49 = 5.83$$

Particle size averages: This section describes how to calculate the arithmetic ($\bar{d}$), geometric (d_g) and harmonic (d_h) means. The derivation of optimal estimates is beyond the scope of this chapter but the interested reader can consult any good statistic book (1,9). The most commonly used averages are the arithmetic averages. The standard formulas for estimating the arithmetic or average diameter and the standard deviation are:

$$\bar{d} = \frac{\sum n_i d_i}{\sum n_i} \tag{24}$$

where n_i is the number of particles in the ith interval and d_i is the diameter of the ith interval, typically the mid point of the interval is used for d_i. The variance is estimated by:

$$\sigma^2 = \frac{\sum n_i (d_i - \bar{d})^2}{(N-1)} \tag{25}$$

Particle and Powder Bed Properties

and the standard deviation is the square root of Equation (25):

$$\sigma = \sqrt{\frac{\sum n_i (d_i - \bar{d}_{av})^2}{(N-1)}} \tag{26}$$

where the total number of particles is given by:

$$N = \sum_{0}^{\infty} n_i \tag{27}$$

The geometric mean can be calculated using:

$$d_g = \sqrt[N]{d_1 d_2 d_3 \ldots d_N} \tag{28}$$

The log transformation of Equation (28) yields:

$$\log d_g = \frac{\sum n_i \log d_i}{\sum n_i} \tag{29}$$

as before n_i is the number of particles in the ith interval of size d_i. Note that the log of the geometric mean is like the arithmetic average for the log normal distribution. The geometric mean is less than or equal to the arithmetic mean ($d_g \leq \bar{d}$) and the geometric standard deviation, σ_g is estimated by:

$$\ln \sigma_g = \sqrt{\frac{\sum n_i (\ln d_i - \ln d_g)^2}{\sum n_i - 1}} \tag{30}$$

The harmonic mean can be calculated by:

$$\frac{N}{d_h} = \frac{1}{d_1} + \frac{1}{d_2} + \frac{1}{d_3} + \ldots + \frac{1}{d_N} \tag{31}$$

$$\frac{1}{d_h} = \frac{1}{\sum n_i} \sum \frac{n_i}{d_i} \tag{32}$$

$$d_h = \left[\frac{1}{\sum n_i} \sum \frac{n_i}{d_i} \right]^{-1} \tag{33}$$

as before n_i is the number of particles in the ith interval of size d_i. The harmonic mean is less than both the geometric and arithmetic mean:

$$d_h \leq d_g \leq \bar{d} \tag{34}$$

Sometimes when working with powders the harmonic and geometric means are more representative of the properties of a powder than the arithmetic mean. For example, when working with the log normal distribution the geometric mean is the appropriate mean for characterizing the distribution. Another example is the specific surface area (also called weight specific surface area), S_w, which is the surface area divided by the particle weight. Here the weight of the specific surface area is best described by the harmonic mean:

$$S_w = \frac{S}{W} = \frac{S}{V\rho} \tag{35}$$

where W is the weight, V is the volume and ρ is the true density. Combining Equations (35), (7), and (9) yields:

$$S_w = \frac{6}{\rho d_h} \tag{36}$$

For calculations dealing with the specific surface area the harmonic mean would best summarize the data. The harmonic mean is weighted towards the smaller particles because the reciprocal $1/d_i$ is larger for smaller diameters, which have a higher surface to mass ratio. Thus, if the properties of interest are affected by the surface area, e.g., drug dissolution, then a more representative mean diameter would weight the smaller particles more heavily than the larger particles which have a much smaller specific surface area.

Example 4. The number of particles that fall between different size ranges are counted using a microscope and shown in Table 2. The arithmetic, geometric, and harmonic mean diameters along with their arithmetic and geometric standard deviations can be calculated using Equations (24)–(33) and is shown in Table 2.

Weighted diameter averages: Most people are very comfortable calculating the arithmetic mean diameter as discussed earlier [Equation (24)]. In micromeritics, the arithmetic mean is often called the number–length mean diameter, d_{NL}; however, it is not always the best representation of a powder's properties. For example, when we talked about specific surface area, the appropriate mean diameter is proportional to one over the diameter as in the calculation of a harmonic mean. Another example is if tablet content uniformity is important then the larger particles relative to their number hold a disproportionate share of the mass in the distribution and averages based upon particle volumes (d^3) would be more representative of these larger particles. Therefore, to better reflect a powder's properties often weighted averages are used.

There are many formulas for the calculation of weighted averages. For example, the number–surface mean diameter calculates the mean diameter based upon the surface area and number of particles:

$$d_{NS} = \sqrt{\frac{\sum S_i}{\sum n_i}} \tag{37}$$

Since the surface area is proportional to d^2:

$$S \propto \sum n_i d_i^2 \tag{38}$$

Thus, the number–surface mean diameter can be calculated using:

$$d_{NS} = \sqrt{\frac{\sum n_i d_i^2}{\sum n_i}} \tag{39}$$

This mean diameter weighs the effect of total surface area more than just the length. Another diameter is the length–surface mean diameter which measures the total surface area divided by the length:

$$d_{LS} = \frac{\sum S_i}{\sum n_i d_i} \tag{40}$$

thus, combining Equation (38), yields:

$$d_{LS} = \frac{\sum n_i d_i^2}{\sum n_i d_i} \tag{41}$$

TABLE 2 Method of Determining the Arithmetic, Geometric and Harmonic Mean Diameter with Standard Deviation

Particle size range (μm)	Mean of particle size range, d_i (μm)	Number of particles, n_i	$n_i d_i$	$(d_i - \bar{d})^2$	$n_i(d_i - \bar{d})^2$	$\ln d_i$	$n_i \ln d_i$	$\frac{n_i}{d_i}$	$n_i(\ln d_i - \ln d_g)^2$
0–10	5	2	10	2857.8	5715.5	1.6094	3.22	0.4000	11.43
10–20	15	4	60	1888.6	7554.4	2.7081	10.83	0.2667	6.67
20–30	25	15	375	1119.4	16791.5	3.2189	48.28	0.6000	9.14
30–40	35	33	1155	550.3	18159.1	3.5553	117.33	0.9429	6.51
40–50	45	53	2385	181.1	9599.2	3.8067	201.75	1.1778	1.97
50–60	55	67	3685	12.0	801.1	4.0073	268.49	1.2182	0.00
60–70	65	62	4030	42.8	2653.5	4.1744	258.81	0.9538	1.89
70–80	75	43	3225	273.6	11766.5	4.3175	185.65	0.5733	4.34
80–90	85	22	1870	704.5	15498.6	4.4427	97.74	0.2588	4.32
90–100	95	13	1235	1335.3	17359.2	4.5539	59.20	0.1368	3.99
100–110	105	7	735	2166.2	15163.1	4.6540	32.58	0.0667	3.00
		321	18765		121061.7		1283.89	6.5950	53.28

$$\bar{d} = \frac{\sum n_i d_i}{\sum n_i} = 58.5\ \mu m,\ \sigma^2 = \frac{\sum n_i(d_i - \bar{d})^2}{(N-1)} = 378.3\ \mu m,\ \sigma = \sqrt{\sigma^2} = 19.4\ \mu m$$

$$\ln d_g = \frac{\sum n_i \ln d_i}{\sum n_i} = 3.9997,\ d_g = e^{3.9997} = 54.6\ \mu m,\ \ln \sigma_g = \sqrt{\frac{\sum n_i (\ln d_i - \ln d_g)^2}{\sum n_i - 1}} = 0.4080,\ \sigma_g = 1.5\ \mu m$$

$$d_h = \left[\frac{1}{\sum n_i} \sum \frac{n_i}{d_i} \right]^{-1} = 48.7\ \mu m$$

Similarly, if the volume and length are important, one may consider the length–volume mean diameter shown in Equations (42)–(44):

$$d_{\text{LV}} = \frac{\sum V_i}{\sum n_i d_i} \tag{42}$$

and since

$$V \propto \sum n_i d_i^3 \tag{43}$$

$$d_{\text{LV}} = \frac{\sum n_i d_i^3}{\sum n_i d_i} \tag{44}$$

There is also a mixture of number and volume mean diameter given by Equation (45) where it gives information about the mean diameter in terms of the total number of particles in the total volume:

$$d_{\text{NV}} = \sqrt[3]{\frac{\sum V_i}{\sum n_i}} \tag{45}$$

combining Equation (43) yields,

$$d_{\text{NV}} = \sqrt[3]{\frac{\sum n_i d_i^3}{\sum n_i}} \tag{46}$$

Another important mean diameter in the pharmaceutical industry that weighs the effects of both the total surface area and volume is the surface–volume mean diameter. This mean diameter can be very useful when the specific surface area is desired as it is inversely related to the specific surface area.

$$d_{\text{SV}} = \frac{\sum n_i d_i^3}{\sum n_i d_i^2} \tag{47}$$

Other mean diameters include the volume-moment (d_{VM}) or weight-moment (d_{WM}) mean diameter:

$$d_{\text{VM}} = d_{\text{WM}} = \frac{\sum n_i d_i^4}{\sum n_i d_i^3} \tag{48}$$

A general notation for the different types of averages is given by:

$$\bar{x} = \sum x_i P(x) \tag{49}$$

where

$$P(x) = \frac{n_i}{N} \tag{50}$$

while

$$x^p = \sum x^p P(x) \tag{51}$$

and

$$x^{-q} = \sum x^q P(x) \tag{52}$$

Particle and Powder Bed Properties

Thus,

$$\frac{\overline{x^{-q}}}{\overline{x^p}} = \frac{\sum x^q P(x)}{\sum x^p P(x)} \tag{53}$$

A summary of these different types of averages can be found in Table 3.

Example 5. Using the particle count data given in Example 4 and Table 2, compute the statistical mean diameters for the number–length, number–surface, number–volume, length–surface, length–volume, surface–volume, volume-moment and weight-moment mean diameters.

Using the equations from Table 3, the mean diameters for number–length, number–surface, number–volume, length–surface, length–volume, surface–volume, volume-moment and weight-moment mean diameters are calculated as shown in Table 4.

Log Normal Distribution

The log normal distribution has many special properties that merit additional discussion, and the log normal distribution is particularly important, because many particle formation

TABLE 3 Summary of Statistical Mean Diameters

Mean diameters	Formula	Where used	Comments
Number–length	$\bar{d} = d_{NL} = \dfrac{\sum n_i d_i}{\sum n_i}$	Comparison, evaporation	Good for narrow and normal particle size distributions but rarely found in pharmaceutical powders
Number–surface	$d_{NS} = \sqrt{\dfrac{\sum n_i d_i^2}{\sum n_i}}$	Absorption	Refers to particles having an average surface area
Number–volume	$d_{NV} = \sqrt[3]{\dfrac{\sum n_i d_i^3}{\sum n_i}}$	Comparison, hydrology atomizing	Refers to particles having an average weight and it is inversely related to the number of particles per gram of material
Length–surface	$d_{LS} = \dfrac{\sum n_i d_i^2}{\sum n_i d_i}$	Absorption	Not significant to pharmaceutical use
Length–volume	$d_{LV} = \dfrac{\sum n_i d_i^3}{\sum n_i d_i}$	Evaporation, molecular diffusion	Not significant to pharmaceutical use
Surface–volume	$d_{SV} = \dfrac{\sum n_i d_i^3}{\sum n_i d_i^2}$	Efficiency studies	Ideal to use when specific surface per unit volume is important since it is inversely related to the specific surface
Volume–moment, Weight–moment	$d_{VM} = d_{WM} = \dfrac{\sum n_i d_i^4}{\sum n_i d_i^3}$	Combustion, equilibrium	Refers to the particle having an average size based on the weight of the particle

Source: Modified from Refs. 9, 36.

TABLE 4 Calculation of the Number–Length, Number–Surface, Number–Volume, Length–Surface, Length–Volume, Surface–Volume, Volume–Moment and Weight–Moment Mean Diameter

Particle size range (μm)	Mean of particle size range, d_i (μm)	Number of particles, n_i	$n_i d_i$	$n_i d_i^2$	$n_i d_i^3$	$n_i d_i^4$
0–10	5	2	10	50	250	1250
10–20	15	4	60	900	13500	202500
20–30	25	15	375	9375	234375	5859375
30–40	35	33	1155	40425	1414875	49520625
40–50	45	53	2385	107325	4829625	217333125
50–60	55	67	3685	202675	11147125	613091875
60–70	65	62	4030	261950	17026750	1106738750
70–80	75	43	3225	241875	18140625	1360546875
80–90	85	22	1870	158950	13510750	1148413750
90–100	95	13	1235	117325	11145875	1058858125
100–110	105	7	735	77175	8103375	850854375
Total		321	18765	1218025	85567125	6411420625

$$d_{NL} = \frac{\sum n_i d_i}{\sum n_i} = 58.5 \, \mu m, \, d_{NS} = \sqrt{\frac{\sum n_i d_i^2}{\sum n_i}} = 61.6 \, \mu m, \, d_{NV} = \sqrt[3]{\frac{\sum n_i d_i^3}{\sum n_i}} = 64.4 \, \mu m$$

$$d_{LS} = \frac{\sum n_i d_i^2}{\sum n_i d_i} = 64.9 \, \mu m, \, d_{LV} = \frac{\sum n_i d_i^3}{\sum n_i d_i} = 67.5 \, \mu m, \, d_{SV} = \frac{\sum n_i d_i^3}{\sum n_i d_i^2} = 70.3 \, \mu m$$

$$d_{VM} = d_{WM} = \frac{\sum n_i d_i^4}{\sum n_i d_i^3} = 74.9 \, \mu m$$

methods, such as milling, produce particle distributions best described by the log normal distribution. The log normal distribution shown in Figure 7 is a skewed distribution. For these types of distributions the mean, mode, and median are not equal; i.e., mean ≠ mode ≠ median.

For the log normal distribution, it turns out that if d is distributed log normally then the log transformation of d is normally distributed. In fact the log normal distribution can be defined by stating that a variable d is log normally distributed if $z = \ln(d)$ is normally distributed; hence the name log normal distribution. This transformation is plotted in Figure 10. The transformation is based upon the properties of the natural logarithm of d (Fig. 11). As d approaches zero the logarithm $z(d)$ asymptotically approaches minus infinity, which expands the lower end of the distribution. As d increases, the logarithm $z(d)$ tends towards infinity at a slow rate, which compresses the upper end of the distribution. The combination of the expansion of the low end and compression of the high end of the distribution makes the asymmetric log normal distribution symmetrical. An advantage of the log normal distribution is that the log transformation of d is normally distributed; thus, much of what can be statistically done with the normal distribution can also be done with the log normal distribution.

Particle and Powder Bed Properties

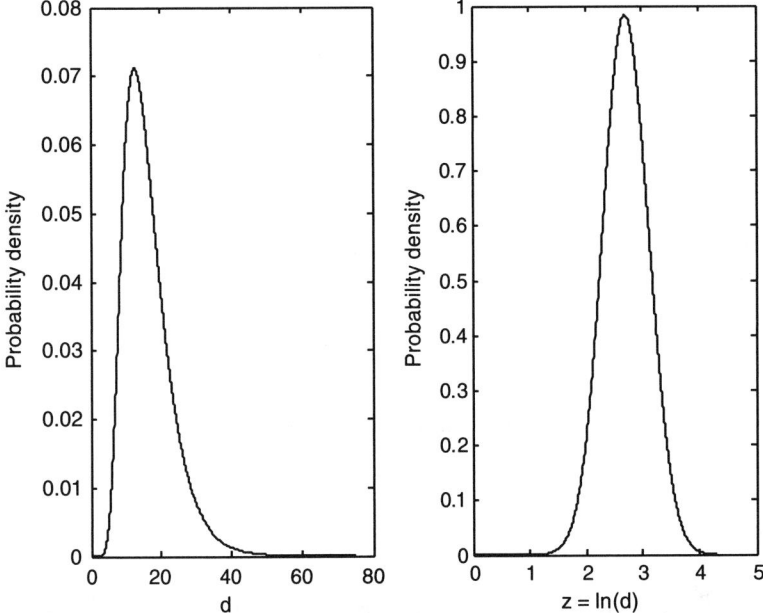

FIGURE 10 Log normal distribution.

The fact that d or z can be used as the independent variable for the log normal distribution creates confusion among students because the log normal density function can take on different forms depending on which variable is used. Thus, if we let x be the actual particle size and z be the ln transformation then we have the following relationships:

$$z = \ln(x), \quad \bar{z} = \ln x_g \text{ and } \quad \sigma_z = \ln \sigma_g \tag{54}$$

where x_g is the geometric mean and σ_g is the geometric standard deviation, as discussed in Equations (28)–(30). The probability distribution function of the log normal distribution expressed in terms of the transformed variable z is given by:

$$\frac{d\varphi(z)}{dZ} = f(z) = \frac{1}{\sigma_z \sqrt{2\pi}} e^{-\frac{1}{2\sigma_z^2}(z-\bar{z})^2} \tag{55}$$

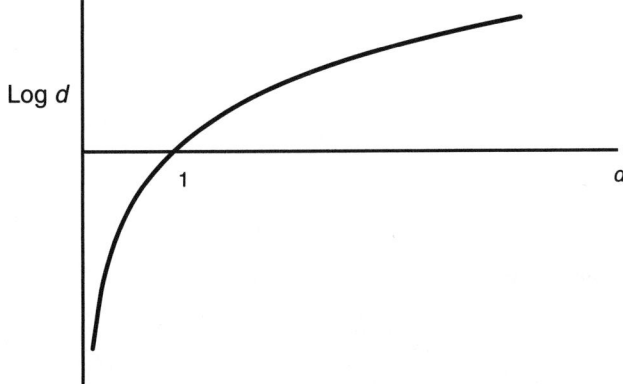

FIGURE 11 Log d versus d. As d approaches zero the log d asymptotically approaches minus infinity. This expands the lower end of the distribution while log d tends towards infinity at a slower rate as d increases.

This probability distribution can also be expressed in terms of x:

$$\frac{d\varphi(\ln x)}{d\ln x} = \frac{1}{\ln \sigma_g \sqrt{2\pi}} e^{-\frac{1}{2\ln^2 \sigma_g}(\ln x - \ln x_g)^2} \tag{56}$$

Recall the chain rule for composite functions $f(Z(x))$:

$$\frac{df(Z(x))}{dx} = \frac{df(Z(x))}{dZ}\frac{dZ}{dx} \tag{57}$$

Applying the chain rule to Equation (56) we obtain:

$$\frac{d\varphi(x)}{dx} = \frac{d(\varphi(z))}{dZ}\frac{dZ}{dx} = \frac{d\varphi(z)}{d(\ln x)}\left(\frac{1}{x}\right) \tag{58}$$

By substitution of Equation (54) into Equation (56) yields:

$$\frac{d\varphi}{dx} = f(x) = \frac{1}{x \ln \sigma_g \sqrt{2\pi}} e^{-\frac{1}{2}\left(\frac{\ln x - \ln x_g}{\ln \sigma_g}\right)^2} \tag{59}$$

Thus, Equations (59) and (56) are equivalent key equations expressing the log normal density function and are plotted in Figure 10. Care should be taken not to confuse these two subtly different forms of the log normal distribution.

Probability paper and linearization of the cumulative distribution curve: In general, when calculating an average one uses the diameter d_i at the midpoint of an interval times the number or weight of particles in that interval for the equations summarized in Table 3. However, there are situations where this is not possible; e.g., when one considers sieve data the midpoint of the interval for the largest sieve size is not defined, all that is known is how much material passes through the top sieve. Thus, to analyze this type of data one cannot use the standard methods illustrated in the previous examples.

One way of determining the average particle size is to plot the cumulative size distribution in manner such that the distribution is linearized, and from this plot the mean and standard deviation can be graphically determined. For example, if we had a random variable x which was distributed:

$$x \sim N(\mu, \sigma) \tag{60}$$

which is described by the density function Equation (13), we can standardize this distribution by making the substitution:

$$t = \frac{x - \bar{x}}{\sigma} \tag{61}$$

$$\frac{dt}{dx} = \frac{1}{\sigma} \tag{62}$$

$$dx = \sigma dt \tag{63}$$

Plugging this into Equation (13) yields:

$$f(t) = \frac{d\varphi}{dt} = \frac{1}{\sqrt{2\pi}} e^{-\frac{t^2}{2}} \tag{64}$$

Particle and Powder Bed Properties

which is distributed $t \sim N(0,1)$. The cumulative distribution for t is given by:

$$F(t) = \int_{-\infty}^{t} d\varphi = \frac{1}{\sqrt{2\pi}} \int_{-\infty}^{t} e^{-\frac{t^2}{2}} dt \tag{65}$$

Based upon the properties of the normal distribution the following values for Equation (65) can be calculated:

$$\varphi = \int_{-\infty}^{\mu} d\varphi = \frac{1}{\sqrt{2\pi}} \int_{-\infty}^{\mu} e^{-\frac{t^2}{2}} dt = \int_{\mu}^{\infty} d\varphi = 0.5 \tag{66}$$

$$\varphi = \int_{-\infty}^{\sigma} d\varphi = 15.87\% \tag{67}$$

$$\varphi = \int_{-\infty}^{\mu+\sigma} d\varphi = 84.13\% \tag{68}$$

$$\varphi = \int_{\mu-\sigma}^{\mu+\sigma} d\varphi = 68.26\% \tag{69}$$

These values are plotted on the cumulative distribution (Fig. 12), from this graph we could read off the mean ($\mu = 75 \, \mu m$) and standard deviation ($\sigma = 75 - 74 = 1 \, \mu m$); however, with real data that contains error this is not an optimal statistical method. A better statistical method would be to linearize the plot of the cumulative distribution $F(x)$ shown in Figure 13. The plot could be linearized by scaling the cumulative probability axis so that the cumulative distribution would be linear when plotted versus the

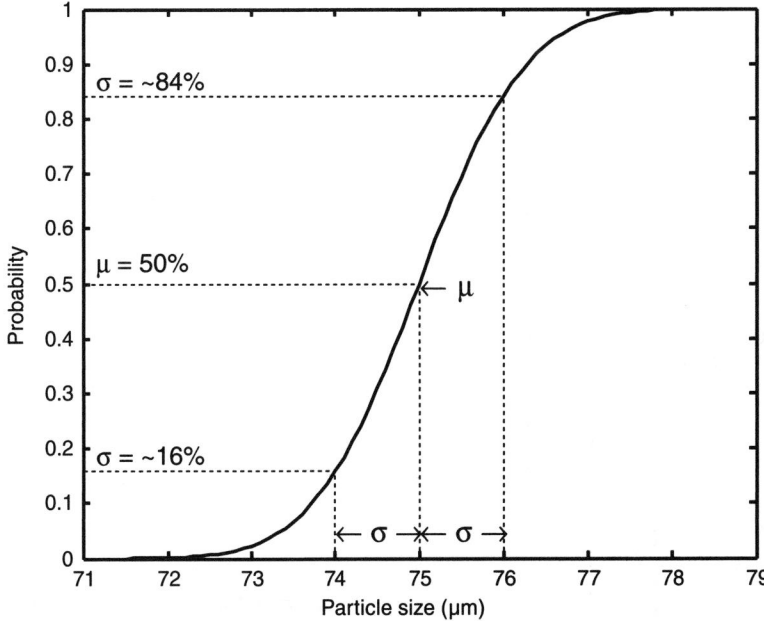

FIGURE 12 A cumulative distribution plot where the mean and standard deviation can be read off directly from the graph.

particle size using arithmetic probability paper (Fig. 13), and notice the probability axis scaling. The details of how this axis is constructed can be found in Allen (9). The use of probability paper can be extended to the log normal distribution by changing the linear arithmetic axis to a log scale axis (Fig. 14). Linearizing the cumulative data plot has two main advantages, (*i*) any error in the data can be averaged out by drawing a best fit line and (*ii*) the linearity or lack of linearity would indicate how well the data fit the normal distribution. Recall that to characterize a population of particles one needs to know the average, standard deviation and type of distribution. With arithmetic and log probability paper a plot's linearity is an excellent indication of goodness of fit to the normal or log normal distribution, respectively. The lack of fit can be due to lack of fit to the distribution (e.g., non-normality for arithmetic probability paper) or a bimodal distribution.

Table 5 shows the sieve data of two batches of materials prepared by milling. These materials with a wide distribution exhibit a linear plot when plotted on log probability paper. When the percent cumulative undersize is plotted on the log probability paper, Batch# S0903 shows a linearized log normal distribution. Hence, the value for the geometric mean ($\mu = 115\,\mu m$) can be obtained directly from the graph in Figure 14. The geometric standard deviation can also be easily obtained from the graph by the following equation:

$$\ln \sigma_g = \ln x_{84} - \ln x_{50} = \ln x_{50} - \ln x_{16} \tag{70}$$

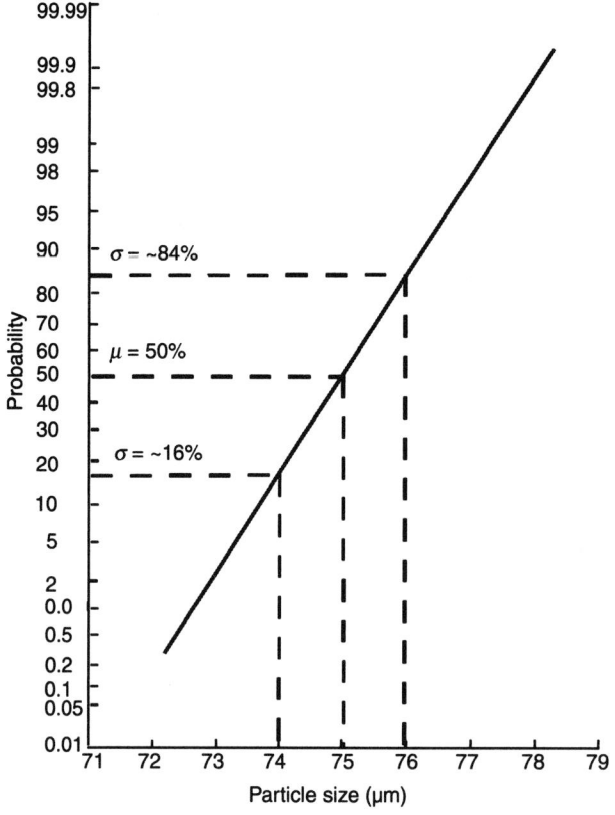

FIGURE 13 A linearized cumulative distribution from Figure 12 when plotting on arithmetic probability paper.

Particle and Powder Bed Properties

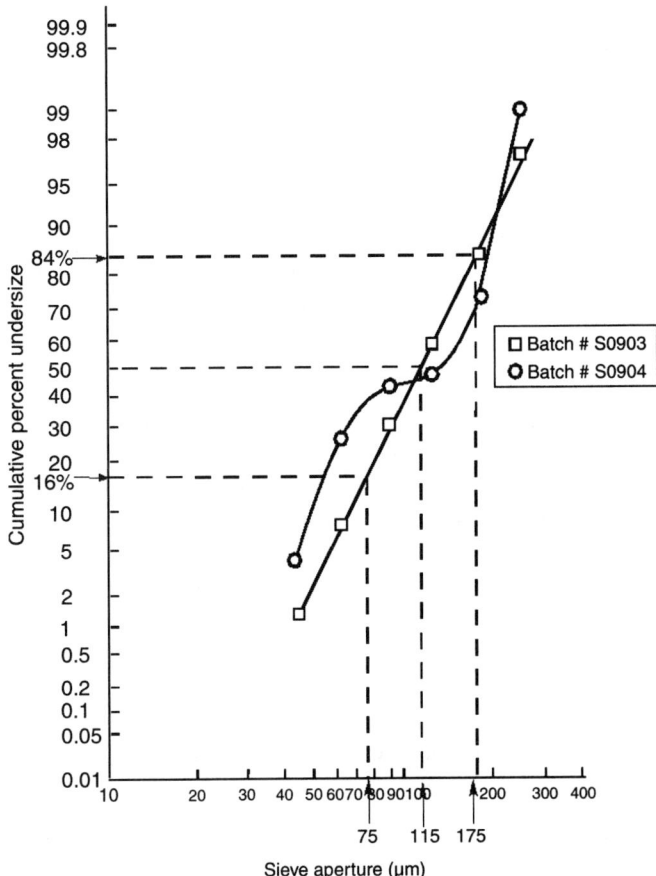

FIGURE 14 Percent cumulative undersize of Batch #S0903 and Batch #S0904 plotted on log probability paper.

TABLE 5 Particle Size Distribution of Batch #S0903 and Batch #S0904 Obtained from Sieving Analysis

Sieve aperture size (μm)	Batch #S0903			Batch #S0904		
	Weight retained (g)	% Retained	% Cumulative undersize	Weight retained (g)	% Retained	% Cumulative undersize
Fine collector	0.12	1.2	–	0.4	4	–
45	0.83	8.3	1.2	2.4	24	4
63	2.1	21	9.5	1.5	15	28
90	2.75	27.5	30.5	0.4	4	43
125	2.9	29	58	2.6	26	47
180	1	10	87	2.6	26	73
250	0.3	3	97	0.1	1	99
Total	10	100	100	10	100	100

Recall, multiplication and division become addition and subtraction in logarithms, thus, from Figure 14 the standard deviation can be directly read of the graph:

$$\sigma_g = \frac{x_{84}}{x_g} = \frac{x_g}{x_{16}} = \frac{115}{75} = 1.53 \, \mu m \tag{71}$$

Bimodal distributions are very evident when plotted on log probability paper, which is the case of Batch# S0904. As seen in Figure 14, the bimodal distribution will have two slopes on the log probability paper. The mean and standard deviation of the bimodal distribution can be estimated by drawing the slopes. Details of computing the mean and standard deviation of a bimodal distribution can be found in Allen (11).

Hatch–Choate Equations

An advantage of the log normal distribution is that multiplication becomes addition and exponential terms become multiplicative. As a result of the properties of logarithms, the geometric standard deviation is the same for the number–length, number–surface, number–volume, etc. distributions. This fact allows one to calculate the relationships between different averages for the log normal distribution, and these equations are called the Hatch–Choate equations. For example, the number length diameter can be expressed as:

$$\bar{d}_{NL} = \frac{\sum n_i d_i}{\sum n_i} = \frac{1}{\ln \sigma_g \sqrt{2\pi}} \int_{-\infty}^{\infty} d \cdot e^{-\frac{(\ln d - \ln d_g)^2}{2 \ln^2 \sigma_g}} \, d \ln d \tag{72}$$

Upon much manipulation, see Allen for details (9), the following relationship can be deduced from Equation (72):

$$d_{NL} = d_g e^{0.5 \ln^2 \sigma_g} \Rightarrow \ln d_{NL} = \ln d_g + 0.5 \ln^2 \sigma_g \tag{73}$$

Thus, for log normal distributions if one mean diameter is known, equations like Equation (73) can be used to find the other mean diameters. Such equations enable one to convert between number and mass means. A summary of these mean diameter conversions can be found in Table 6. These equations are very useful for comparing different types of data, e.g., microscopy and light scattering data, but these conversions assume a perfect log normal distribution and deviations from this assumption can cause erroneous results.

TABLE 6 Hatch–Choate Equations for Different Diameters

Mean diameters	Formula
Surface	$\ln d_S = \ln d_g + 2.0 \ln^2 \sigma_g$
Volume	$\ln d_V = \ln d_g + 3.0 \ln^2 \sigma_g$
Number–length	$\ln d_{NL} = \ln d_g + 0.5 \ln^2 \sigma_g$
Number–surface	$\ln d_{NS} = \ln d_g + 1.0 \ln^2 \sigma_g$
Number–volume	$\ln d_{NV} = \ln d_g + 1.5 \ln^2 \sigma_g$
Length–surface	$\ln d_{LS} = \ln d_g + 1.5 \ln^2 \sigma_g$
Length–volume	$\ln d_{LV} = \ln d_g + 2.0 \ln^2 \sigma_g$
Surface–volume	$\ln d_{SV} = \ln d_g + 2.5 \ln^2 \sigma_g$
Volume-moment, weight-moment	$\ln d_{VM} = \ln_{WM} = \ln d_g + 3.5 \ln^2 \sigma_g$

Particle and Powder Bed Properties

PARTICLE SHAPE

The shape of a particle is defined by its external morphology, i.e., the form or overall shape, the roundness or smoothness and the surface texture (12–14). Particle shape is important because it can influence many critical powder properties such as the powder flowability, compactibility, content uniformity, dissolution, drug release, bioavailability, and stability; these factors ultimately affect the safety and efficacy of a dosage form (4,15–24). Particles with different shapes can have the same size (i.e., volume or surface area) but very different properties. For instance, spherical particles tend to have greater flowability than irregularly shaped particles as the irregularly shaped particles can interlock with each other resulting in poor flow and bridging in hoppers, etc. The interlocking properties of the irregular particles can also affect the blend uniformity of the formulation, which can lead to inconsistency of content uniformity. See Table 7 for a summary of the flow properties for several general particle shapes for powder particles greater than 74 µm. The flowability of powder particles less than this size is usually more affected by surface properties such as static charge and adsorbed moisture (25).

On the other hand, it has been reported that materials with larger irregularly shaped particles which fragment to a limited degree during compression have higher compactibility (3,19,25). Irregularly shaped particles have a higher number of interparticulate contact points thereby allowing more interparticulate bonding. The edges and corners of the irregularly shaped particles can undergo higher degree of deformation due to the existence of lattice defects and primarily dislocations thus allowing higher bonding strength between compact particles. As the surface roughness of the particle increases, the possibility for a particle to find a position at an adjacent surface which promotes bond formation will increase thus more force is needed to break these bondings which yields a higher crushing strength (3).

Particle shape can also influence particle size analysis. The particle size distribution measured by sieve analysis can be influenced by particle shape, because irregularly shaped particles take longer to reach their final sieve. Biased results will be reported if the test is stopped before the particles reach their final sieve.

Particle size can be characterized in terms of length, width, breadth, radius, diameter, etc., but particle shape is dimensionless. It is easy to define a commonly seen regular shape such as a sphere, cube, or cylinder but it is more complicated to define irregular shapes. For instance, a sphere is a three-dimensional circle that is round and the distance from any point on the surface to the center of the sphere is the same. Thus, any three-dimensional solid that has this characteristic can be defined as a sphere. To characterize the shape of a complicated irregularly shape particle can be challenging as there are no definite characteristics for the irregular particle. Thus, there have been many methods developed and reported in the literature to quantitatively characterize the shape factor of a particle. These methods will be reviewed in this section. The most commonly used shape factors are those derived from regular shapes such as spheres, cubes, triangles, etc. However, due to the complexity of an irregularly shaped particle, no one method can quantitatively characterize the shape factor of all particles, and it is very difficult to characterize the form, roundness, and surface texture of an irregular particle using just one equation or mathematical model.

Besides the numerical calculation of shape factors, there are also qualitative descriptions of shape. For example, certain pharmacopoeias define shapes such as an agglomerate, needle, etc. Since no one method is best in all applications, the best method for determining particle shape depends on the application and nature of the particle being examined.

TABLE 7 Effect of Some General Particle Shapes on Powder Flow

General shapes	Effects on powder flow
(a) Spherical shape 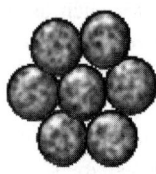	Often produces good flowability
(b) Oblong shape with smooth edges 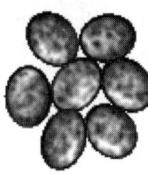	Often produces good flowability
(c) Equidimensional shape with sharp edges 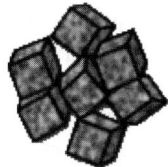	Less flowable than (a) or (b)
(d) Irregularly shaped interlocking particles 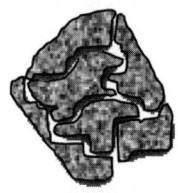	Often shows poor flowability and causes bridging
(e) Irregularly shaped two-dimensional particles such as flakes 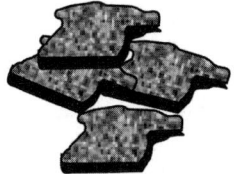	Often produces greater flowability than (d) but less flowability than (a), (b), and (c) and may cause bridging
(f) Fibrous particles 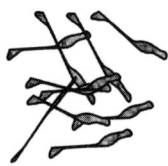	Shows very poor flowability and bridges easily

Source: Adapted from Ref. 25.

Particle and Powder Bed Properties

Quantitative Shape Factors

Characterizing the shape of an irregular particle can be complicated; to address this problem a lot of research by many different groups has been done to find a numerical value that can quantitatively characterize the shape of an irregular particle. Collectively, these numerical values are often referred to as the shape factor; the goal of a shape factor is to define the shape of an irregular particle. For instance, how spherical or square a particle is or how different is the irregular particle from a commonly seen shape using a mathematical model.

This section will discuss some of the commonly used and cited shape factors in the pharmaceutical industry; the shape factors discussed in this section are: Wadell's true sphericity and circularity, rugosity coefficient, correction factor, Dallavalle's shape factor, Heywood's shape factor, Schneiderhöhn's aspect ratio, one plane critical stability (OPCS), and Podczeck's two- and three-dimensional factor. There are also many other shape factors but they are beyond the scope of this chapter (11,14,26–31).

Wadell's True Sphericity and Circularity

One of the earliest particle shape factors used in the pharmaceutical industry was Wadell's true spheritcity, ψ_w. The true sphericity defines the proximity of the irregular particle measured to a perfect sphere and the relationship between the irregular particles to the perfect sphere is given by:

$$\psi_w = \frac{S'}{S} = \left(\frac{d_v}{d_s}\right)^2 \tag{74}$$

where S' is the surface area of a sphere having the same volume as the particle and S is the actual surface area of the particle. ψ_w is 1.0 when the particle is a perfect sphere and is less than 1.0 for all other shapes; the smaller the value the less spherical the particles is. This true sphericity is not the roundness of a particle as roundness is only a sense of smoothness or the sharpness of the corners. While roundness is an intrinsic property of a sphere, many other circular forms (e.g., an ellipse) can show some degree of roundness but yet they are not considered as a sphere (14,32). Hence, roundness and the true sphericity are two independent variables.

The inverse of Wadell's true sphericity is known as the rugosity coefficient by some researchers to express any lack of smoothness in a particle's perimeter (27,33,34). Hence, the rugosity coefficient, γ, can be use to describe the roughness of a particle and is defined as:

$$\gamma = \frac{S}{S'} = \frac{A_{BET}}{A_g} \tag{75}$$

where A_{BET} is the measured specific surface area usually obtained by nitrogen adsorption while A_g is the surface area of a sphere having the same volume as the particle and it is usually obtained by microscopy or sieve analysis.

Wadell also defined the degree of circularity, ϕ, to determine the proximity of a particle outline to a circle. This relationship can be described by:

$$\phi = \frac{C'}{C} = \frac{P^2}{4\pi A} \tag{76}$$

where C' is the circumference of a circle having the same cross-sectional area as the particle, C is the actual perimeter of the cross section, P is the perimeter of the particle outline, and A is the cross-sectional or projection area of the particle outline. This circularity is very similar to the circularity developed by Cox (35) in an earlier work where Wadell's circularity is the inverse of Cox's circularity. Thus, the type of circularity should be reported to avoid confusion.

Correction Factor

Martin et al. have shown that a volume factor, α_v, and a surface factor, α_s, can be assigned as a correction factor to the chosen statistical diameter, d, of the irregular particle of interest when estimating its volume and surface (36). One can then write the surface area and volume as:

$$V = \frac{\pi d_v^3}{6} = \alpha_v d^3 \tag{77}$$

and

$$S = \pi d_s^2 = \alpha_s d^2 \tag{78}$$

The volume and surface factor can also be used in the specific surface (S_w) equation, when S_w is of interest. Therefore, for 1 g compound, the volume and surface equation can be written as:

$$V = \frac{1}{\rho N_m} = \alpha_v d_v^3 = N_m \rho \alpha_v d_v^3 \tag{79}$$

and

$$S = N_m \alpha_s d_s^2 \tag{80}$$

where ρ is the true density of the compound for N_m number of particles per unit-weight of compound. Thus,

$$S_w = \frac{S}{W} = \frac{N_m \alpha_s d_s^2}{N_m \rho \alpha_v d_v^3} \tag{81}$$

substituting the statistical surface–volume mean diameters from Equation (47) into Equation (81) leads to:

$$S_w = \frac{S}{W} = \frac{\alpha_s}{\rho \alpha_v d_{sv}} \tag{82}$$

Example 6. Calculate the volume, surface factor and specific surface for a perfect sphere with density of $1.0 \, \text{g/cm}^3$ and surface–volume mean diameter of $100 \, \mu\text{m}$.

Since the statistical diameter, d, chosen for a perfect sphere is equal to d_v and d_s, the volume and surface factor are:

$$\alpha_v = \frac{\pi d_v^3}{6d} = \frac{\pi}{6}$$

$$\alpha_s = \frac{\pi d_s^2}{d^2} = \pi$$

and the specific surface is:

$$S_w = \frac{S}{W} = \frac{\alpha_s}{\rho \alpha_v d_{sv}} = \frac{(\pi)}{(1 \, \text{g/cm}^3)(\pi/6)(100 \, \mu\text{m})} = 6 \times 10^{-6} \, \text{cm}^2/\text{g}$$

Particle and Powder Bed Properties

Understanding this correction factor is important as it is widely used in the pharmaceutical industry, and many other researchers have further modified these correction factors for different applications. Some of these modifications will be discussed in the following sections.

Dallavalle's Shape Factor

Dallavale defined a new shape factor that is modified from the correction factor. The Dallavalle shape factor can be useful for a log normal distribution because the shape of the size–frequency (density distribution) curve can be taken into account when combining Martin's correction factor with the Hatch–Choate equation (1,34,37). Applying the Hatch–Choate equation of d_v and d_s from Table 6 to N_m in Equation (79) and S_w in Equation (81) yields,

$$\ln[N_m] = \ln\left[\frac{1}{\rho\alpha_v}\right] - 3\ln[d_g] - 4.5\ln^2[\sigma_g] \tag{83}$$

$$\ln[S_w] = \ln\left[\frac{\alpha_s}{\rho\alpha_v}\right] - \ln[d_g] - 2.5\ln^2[\sigma_g] \tag{84}$$

and if the specific surface is defined in terms of the surface area per unit volume instead of per unit weight, Equation (84) becomes,

$$\ln[S_v] = \ln\left[\frac{\alpha_s}{\alpha_v}\right] - \ln[d_g] - 2.5\ln^2[\sigma_g] \tag{85}$$

A specific shape factor, α_{sv} is also discussed by Dallavele which can be used to describe N number of particles with a specific weight, W. Combining the density equation with Equation (77) where projection diameter, d_P, is used yields,

$$d_P = \sqrt[3]{\frac{V}{\alpha_v}} = \sqrt[3]{\frac{W}{N\rho\alpha_v}} \tag{86}$$

Then, substituting Equation (86) into the surface area equation (78) gives,

$$S = \alpha_s d_P^2 = \alpha_s \left(\frac{W}{N\rho\alpha_v}\right)^{\frac{2}{3}} = \alpha_{sv}\left(\frac{W}{N\rho}\right)^{\frac{2}{3}} \tag{87}$$

where the specific shape factor, α_{sv}, is now:

$$\alpha_{sv} = \frac{\alpha_s}{(\alpha_v)^{\frac{2}{3}}} \tag{88}$$

Heywood's Surface Coefficient, Flatness Ratio and Elongation Ratio

The shape factors developed by Heywood for rock studies are still widely employed by many researchers in various industries including the pharmaceutical industry. These shape factors are based on the proximity of a particle to a geometrical or approximate form. The geometrical forms used by Heywood to derive this shape factor are the ellipsoids, prisms, and tetrahedrons while their approximate forms are angular (tetrahedral or prismodal), sub-angular, and rounded (38). This method's utility comes from the ability to combine the information from a three-dimensional irregularly shaped particle based on the measurement of length, l, breadth, b, (which is the maximum distance between two points that is perpendicular to the length), and thickness, t, on three mutually perpendicular axes into a surface coefficient, f (38–40):

$$f = 1.57 + c\left(\frac{k_e}{m}\right)^{\frac{4}{3}}\frac{(n+1)}{n} \qquad (89)$$

where c and k_e are the coefficients of geometric form selected from Table 8, m is defined as Heywood's flatness ratio and n is the Heywood's elongation ratio.

$$m = \frac{b}{t} \qquad (90)$$

$$n = \frac{l}{b} \qquad (91)$$

Note that the values for c and k_e need to be selected by an operator manually depending on the particle form appearing in the microscope. Hence, an untrained operator may report biased results when selecting these coefficients as there is no clear cut definition of an irregular particle and of which form it should be classified in.

The inverse of Heywood's elongation ratio is also known as the aspect ratio, AR, suggested by Schneiderhöhn (41):

$$\text{AR} = \frac{b}{l} \qquad (92)$$

Despite their popularity, many criticize the elongation ratio and aspect ratio for their inability to truly reflect the shape of a particle as both the elongation and aspect ratios are equal to 1 for any symmetrical shape such as a circle, square, etc., since the length and breath is the same for these symmetrical shapes (42,43).

Fractal Dimension

The concept of fractal geometry was first introduced by Mandelbrot and it refers to a rough or fragmented geometric shape that is composed of many smaller copies that have the same shape but different sizes of the whole figure and fractal dimension is a statistical tool to measure how the fractal object fills the space (44).

The principle of fractal analysis is based on the fact that the perimeter measured is dependent upon the scaling length or the step size chosen. For instance, if the perimeter of an irregularly shaped particle shown in Figure 15 is measured

TABLE 8 Heywood's Coefficient of Geometric Form

Form group	k_e	c
Geometric forms		
Tetrahedral	0.328	4.36
Cubical	0.696	2.55
Spherical	0.524	1.86
Approximate forms		
Angular-tetrahedral	0.38	3.3
Angular-prismoidal	0.47	3.0
Sub-angular	0.51	2.6
Rounded	0.54	2.1

Source: Adapted from Ref. 38.

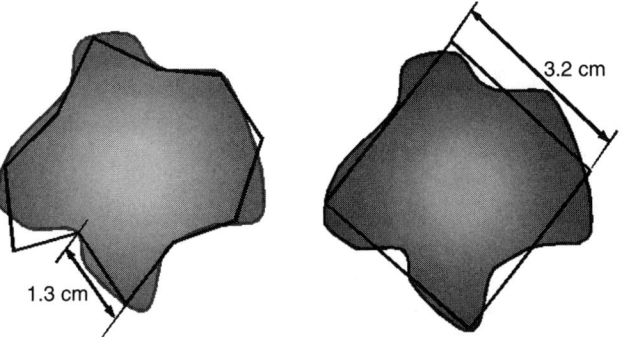

FIGURE 15 Different step size (1.3 and 3.2 cm) used to measure the perimeter of an irregular particle.

using step sizes of 1.3 and 3.2 cm, then the perimeter will be equal to 14.3 and 12.8 cm, respectively. Thus, the smaller the step size, the larger the perimeter measured. An ideal fractal particle that is made up from many smaller copies of that same shape but different sizes of the whole particle should yield a linear plot at any resolution when the log [perimeter] is plotted against the log [step size] and the slope of the straight line is defined as (45):

$$\text{Slope} = 1 - D \tag{93}$$

where D defines the fractal dimension. Thus, the fractal dimension shows the degree of irregularity or ruggedness of the particle. For a line the fractal dimension is between 1 and 2; while for a surface, the fractal dimension is between 2 and 3. The more irregular the surface, the higher its fractal dimension (9). Therefore, a particle with a fractal dimension of 2 will have a less rugged or smoother boundary than a particle with a fractal dimension of 3. Despite the uniqueness of fractal geometry, it did not gain popularity in the pharmaceutical industry because it cannot distinguish between spherical, polygonal, or unorganized particles (46).

One Plane Critical Stability

OPCS is a two-dimensional shape factor developed by Chapman et al. to characterize the roundness of a particle. OPCS is the minimum angle between a horizontal plane and the plane where the particle is lying on and that is necessary to be raised to shift the center of gravity of the particle outside of the boundary so that it would start rolling (Fig. 16) (47). OPCS is defined as:

$$\theta = \sin^{-1} \max\left(\left|\frac{||u(j+1)| - |u(j)||}{u(j) - u(j+1)}\right|\right) \tag{94}$$

where $u(j)$ and $u(j+1)$ are the segment base of a triangle drawn from the center of gravity of the particle (Fig. 17). Chapman et al. had shown that this method is particularly applicable to spherical particles (47). However, it only detects minor differences in roundness and it requires individual measurements of particles with a specialized computer system (46).

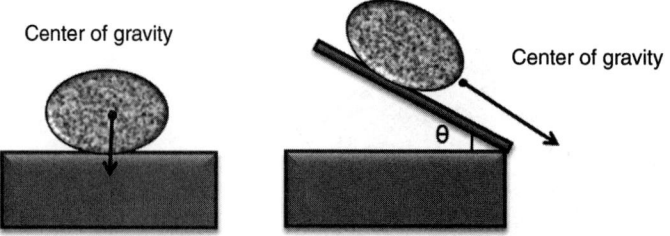

FIGURE 16 OPCS is the minimum angle between a horizontal plane and the plane where the particle is lying on and that is necessary to be raised to shift the center of gravity of the particle outside of the boundary so that it would start rolling. *Abbreviation*: OPCS, one plane critical stability. *Source*: Adapted from Ref. 47.

Podczeck Two- and Three-Dimensional Shape Factor

There are two- (46) and three-dimensional (43) shape factors suggested by Podczeck et al. to describe how the form of spherical particles approaches a true spheroid (46). The two-dimensional shape factor e_R derived from an ellipse is:

$$e_R = \frac{2\pi r_e}{P_m f} - \sqrt{1 - \left(\frac{b}{l}\right)^2} \tag{95}$$

where

$$f = 1.008 - 0.231\left(1 - \frac{b}{l}\right) \tag{96}$$

and

$$r_e = \frac{\sum d_\alpha}{n} \tag{97}$$

where b and l are the breadth and length of the particle, respectively, f is the correction factor for surface roughness of an ellipse, P_m is the perimeter of the particle measured and r_e is the mean radius between the center of gravity to the perimeter from n measurements of α angle between every distance measurement.

Though Podczeck et al. claim that this method is able to detect small deviations from circularity and differentiates the degree of elliptical figures, they later developed an improved three-dimensional shape factor based on this two-dimensional model:

$$e_{c3} = \frac{(2\pi r_e/P_m f)_1 + (2\pi r_e/P_m f)_2}{2} - \sqrt{2 - \left(\frac{b}{l}\right)^2 - \left(\frac{t}{l}\right)^2} \tag{98}$$

where t is the thickness of the particle and the subscript of 1 and 2 represent the two measurements taken from two different points at 90° from each measurement (Fig. 18).

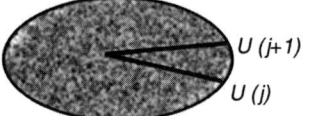

FIGURE 17 $u(j)$ and $u(j+1)$ are the segment base of a triangle draw from the center of gravity of the particle. *Source*: Adapted from Ref. 47.

Particle and Powder Bed Properties

Using this equation, a perfect sphere will give an e_{c3} value of 1 while the value is less than 1 for non-spherical particles and it goes onto negative infinity as the irregularity of the particle increases.

Qualitative Shape Description

Besides the quantitative mathematical definition of shape factor there are also qualitative descriptions for some commonly seen irregularly shaped particles such as acicular, columnar, flake, plate, lath, and equant. A summary of the description specified in USP <776> is shown in Table 9 (9).

Summary of Shape Factors and Description

Besides the various shape factors and descriptions discussed above, there are many other methods reported in the literature with the goal of finding a universal shape factor that is widely applicable. Despite these efforts, there still does not exist a general shape factor that is applicable to all particles. Thus, the best shape factor and description really depends on the application. The more sophisticated models for shape factors may more accurately define the shape of an irregular particle but are more complex and time consuming to compute. Thus, one must choose the method that is most suitable for their particular application.

MEASUREMENT

Following the progression of particle size analysis, so far we have gotten a perfect sample, uniquely characterized the particle size and done the statistical parameter estimates; now we have the tools to look at actual data and methods of measurement. There are many methods for the characterization of particle size and shape; however, in this section we will only include methods commonly used by researchers in tableting. The methods covered are microscopy, sieving, and laser diffraction.

Microscopy

Microscopy is the only method that is capable of directly observing a particle. This allows for the simultaneous measurement of individual particle properties such as size, shape, degree of aggregation, etc., which is very useful because indirect methods of measurements can sometimes have artifacts that lead to erroneous results. Thus, when

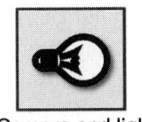
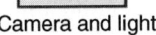
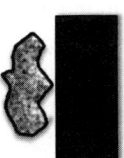

FIGURE 18 Two measurements taken from two different points at 90° from each measurement. *Source*: Modified from Ref. 46.

TABLE 9 Qualitative Shape Characterization Specified by USP

Particle shape	Definitions
Acicular	Slender, needle-like particle of similar width and thickness
Columnar	Long, thin particle with a width and thickness that are greater than those of an acicular particle
Flake	Thin, flat particles of similar length and width
Plate	Flat particles of similar length and width but with greater thickness than flakes
Lath	Long, thin, and blade-like particle
Equant	Particles of similar length, width, and thickness; both cubical and spherical particles are included

Source: Adapted from Ref. 7.

developing a new indirect method for particle size measurement it is always a good idea to use microscopy to confirm the method and sample preparation techniques. For example, particles or granules that are very friable may undergo attrition during sieving due to the aggressive vibration, tapping, and gyratory motion of the sieves. Thus, the particle size reported will be less than the true particle or granule size. This artifact may pose serious consequences for formulation development and product reproducibility. Thus, detection of particle attrition in method development is critical. However, detecting this underestimation of particle size using only sieve analysis would be very difficult or impossible, but cross-checking the sieve data using microscopy will help to discover particle attrition and the extent of particle deaggregation.

Some light scattering measurements require knowledge of a particle's optical properties. The light scattering analysis uses these optical properties in a model for the calculation of particle size, and for accurate results you need to choose a model that best represents these optical properties. Picking an improper model will yield inaccurate results. Microscopy only requires a small amount of material and can be used to quickly measure these optical properties.

Another advantage of microscopy is that it can also identify the nature of the particle. For example, if there is a contaminant in a tablet or powder there are well developed forensic techniques that can be used to identify the particle source, e.g., a packaging machine, and being able to identify the source will help eliminate the problem. In addition, recent advances in combining microscopy with chemical imaging using near-infrared spectroscopy really extends the range of analysis that can be done using a microscope. Using these methods one can acquire a spectrum containing quite detailed chemical and physical information about the particle and particle heterogeneity in a tablet or powder, and this has proven to be a very powerful technique. Please see the chemical imaging section for a more detailed discussion.

Even though there are many positive aspects of microscopy, there are also some disadvantages. In particular, microscopy is a very slow and tedious analysis method if manual counting is done. It can take a long time to count the 200–500 particles that are necessary for a statistically valid analysis. In addition, manual counting requires an experienced operator. If the operator is not well trained, inaccurate results can occur due to systematic biases that are common to the human eye (9,40). There is also a reproducibility issue between different operators.

Some of these drawbacks have been reduced by new developments with automated sample counting using an automated microscope and image analysis software. For these systems an image of the sample is transmitted to a computer system, and the number of pixels which make up a particle is counted by the image analysis software. The size of each pixel is converted to micrometers for the calculation of average particle size, size distribution, and particle shape by the image analysis software (48). Depending upon the level of automation and sophistication of the software these systems can become expensive. In addition, the data obtained are very dependent on the mathematical model and operator entered parameters used by the image analysis software; often this software is proprietary in nature and may vary from vendor to vendor and operator to operator; thus, the reproducibility of the data may be a problem when using different systems and operators.

Microscopes

The principle of a light microscope is based upon the ability to magnify an object using combinations of lenses and is shown in Figure 19. An image is formed on the lens' focal plane as the light from the object passes through the lens. The focal plane is the plane on which the image is formed for a given lens type. The magnification of a lens is the magnified image size divided by the actual object size. In other words, it defines how many times bigger the image one sees is than the actual size of the object itself. The magnification, M, for a single lens is given by (Fig. 19):

$$M = \frac{\text{Image size}}{\text{Object size}} = \frac{\text{Image distance}}{\text{Object distance}} \tag{99}$$

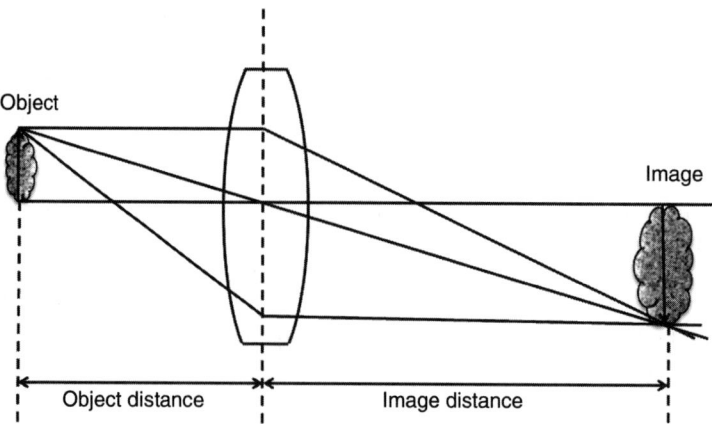

FIGURE 19 Principle of a light microscope. An image is formed on the lens' focal plane as the light from the object passes through the lens.

Due to the limitations of any specific lens, a modern microscope is based on a combination of multiple lenses where subsequent lenses will further magnify the image from the first lens to enhance the magnification and image quality. The total magnification of multiple lenses is:

Total magnification = Magnification of 1st × Magnification of 2nd (100)

Figure 20 is a simplified example of this combination of lenses.

It is worth introducing some key terminology (Fig. 20 and 21); the objective lens is the first lens closest to the object being magnified. The objective lens produces the primary image, which is an intermediate image within the microscope. The eyepiece or ocular lens then magnifies the primary image to create the secondary image or virtual image as seen by the eye (Fig. 20). For modern microscopes, this schematic is greatly oversimplified. Modern microscopes have many more lenses and are much more complicated than the scope of this chapter. However, this section covers the key terminology and use of microscopes. As illustrated in Figure 21, the key features of an optical microscope are the light source, the condenser, and the lenses.

There are three common types of lens aberrations. An aberration is the failure of a lens to produce an exact point-to-point correspondence between an object point and an image point, or in other words, an image distortion. The types of aberrations are spherical, chromatic, and curvature of field as illustrated in Figure 22A–22C. Spherical aberration is the failure of the lens to focus light onto the same focal plane (Fig. 22A). Chromatic aberration is when the different colors focus on different focal planes (Fig. 22B), which makes the image appears blurry. Curvature of field is when the plane of sharpest focus is curved; due to this image curvature the whole image cannot be in focus (Fig. 22C).

These aberrations can be corrected by coatings and proper lens design, but the corrections increase the cost of the lens, thus lens designers offer lenses with different degrees of correction and consequently cost. The most common corrections are achromats, semi-apochromats and aprochromats. Table 10 gives examples of the different types of corrections done for commercially available lenses.

The objective lens is the most important lens having the greatest impact on the image quality. Magnification depends on the focal length as discussed previously, hence,

Particle and Powder Bed Properties

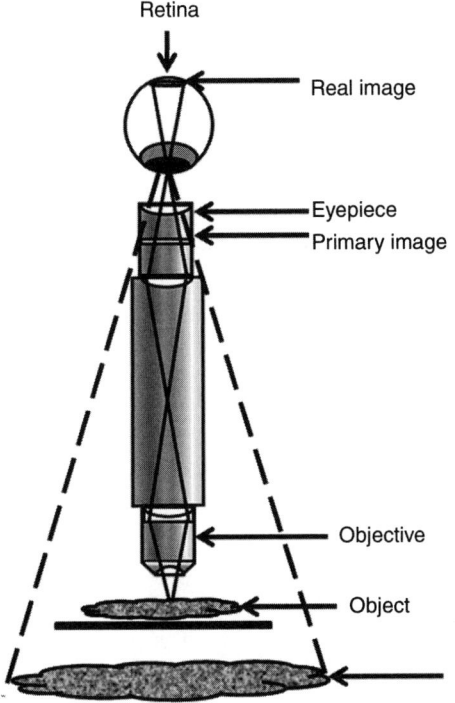

FIGURE 20 Schematic of a modern microscope that shows a combination of multiple lenses. *Source*: Modified from Ref. 40.

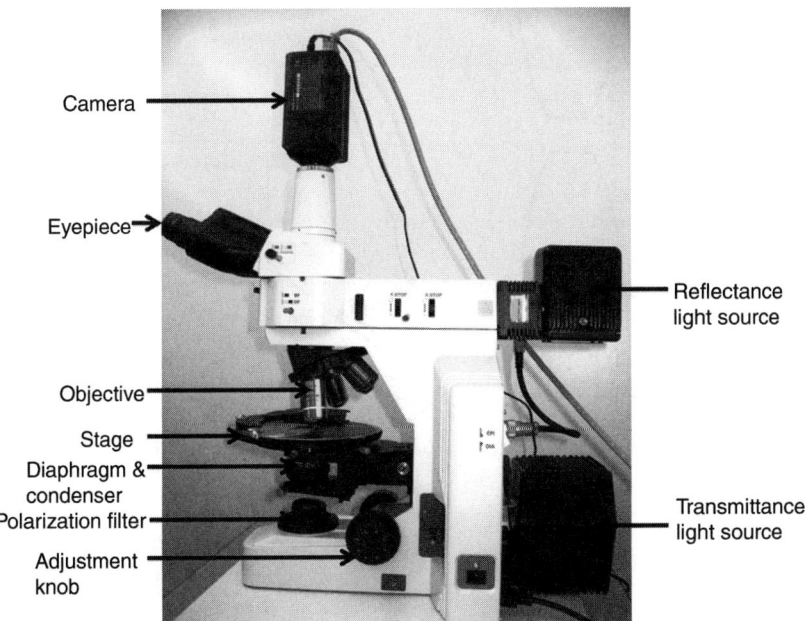

FIGURE 21 A metallurgical microscope with combination of reflectance and transmittance light source. Other key features of the microscope include the eyepiece, objective and condenser.

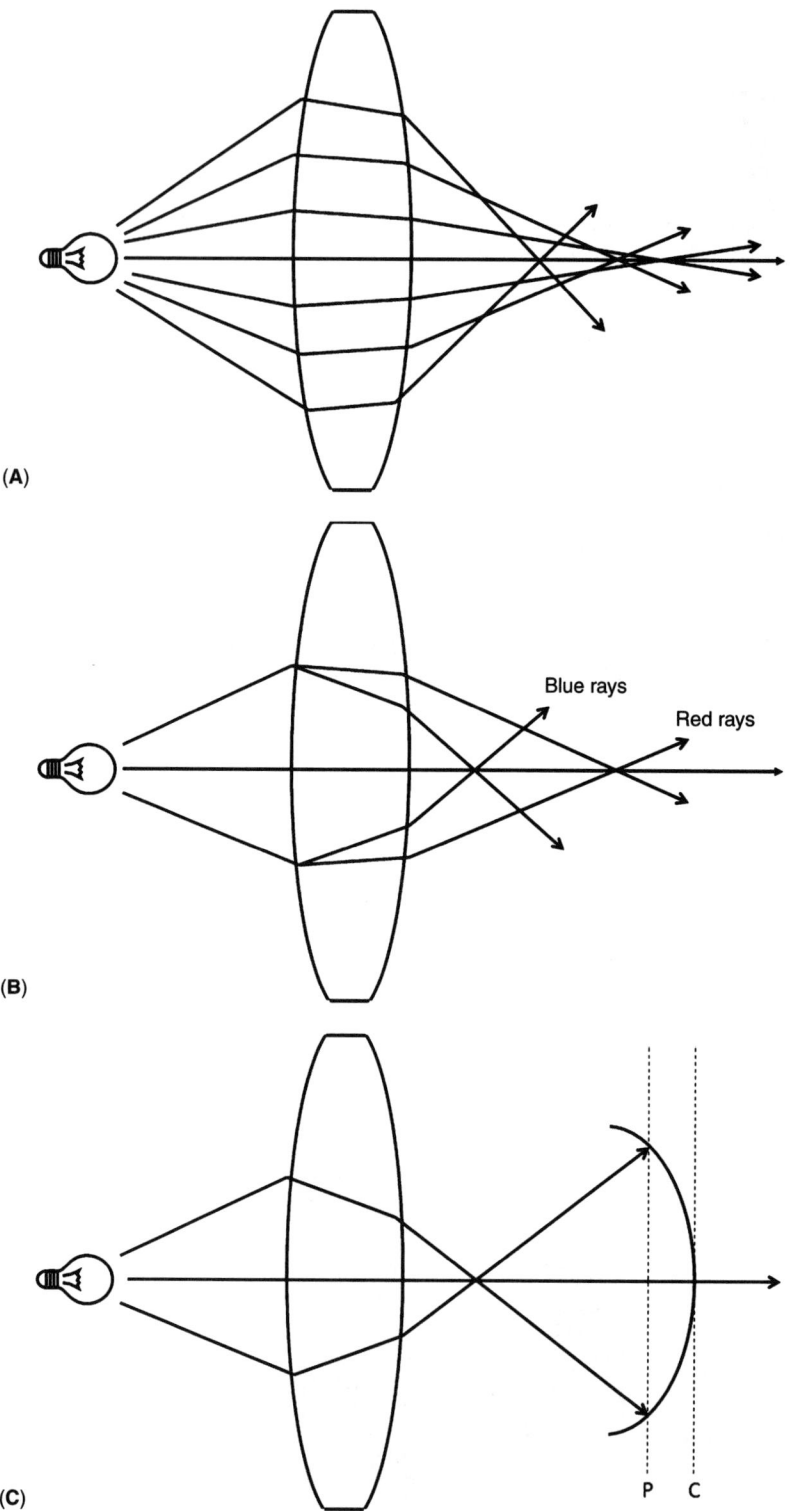

FIGURE 22 The three common types of lens aberration: (**A**) spherical aberration; (**B**) chromatic aberration; (**C**) curvature of field.

Particle and Powder Bed Properties

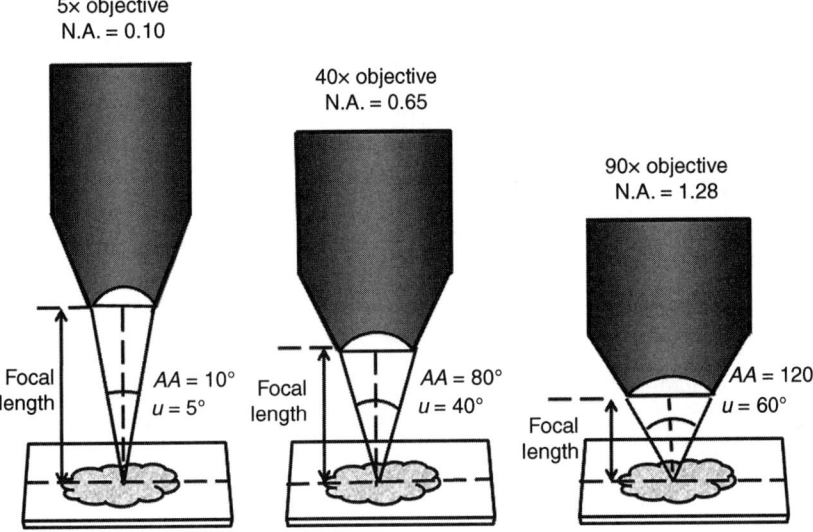

FIGURE 23 The relationship between the focal length, angular, and numerical apertures of objectives.

the greater the magnification power of the objectives, the shorter the focal length needed for magnification (Fig. 23).

This figure also shows that the greater the angular aperture, AA, and numerical aperture, NA, the greater the ability to gather light. This relationship can be summarized as:

$$\text{NA} = n \sin\left(\frac{\text{AA}}{2}\right) \text{ or } \text{NA} = n \sin u \tag{101}$$

where, u is half of the angular angle, AA, and the refractive index n is the c divided by v which is the speed of light in the medium of interest divided by the speed of light in a vacuum.

While this information may seem like arcane trivia it is actually very important in the proper utilization of a microscope because it determines how the lens is used. For example, the maximum value of the numerical aperture of air is equal to 1 since the refractive index for air is 1 and the maximum value for the sine function is 1. Thus, a different media with the refractive index that is greater than 1 must be employed to overcome this limitation. Oil which has a refractive index of 1.4 is commonly used to increase the maximum numerical aperture to 1.4; this shows how the magnification can be increased by changing the media used. The numerical aperture is often printed on the objective, thus, numerical apertures less than 1 suggest that it is designed to be used

TABLE 10 Examples of the Different Types of Corrections Done for Commercially Available Lenses

	Chromatic	Spherical
Achromats	2 colors	1 color
Semi-apochromats	2 colors	2 colors
Aprochromats	3 colors	2 colors

without the oil. If the numerical aperture is greater than 1, then this lens is designed to be used with oil. Using a lens not designed for oil immersion can damage the lens, and using a lens designed for oil immersion without oil will result in a degraded image quality.

Resolutions: Resolution is another key aspect of optical microscopy which affects the sharpness and clarity of an image. Similar to a digital camera, a higher resolution microscope will yield a better image quality. The resolution of the microscope can be increased by decreasing the wavelength of the light or by increasing the numerical aperture since the limit of resolution, R_L, that is the smallest distance between two elements that can be determined from an optical microscope is,

$$R_L = \frac{\lambda f}{2NA} \quad (102)$$

where λ is the wavelength of the light, NA is the numerical aperture and f is the factor to correct the inefficiency of the system which is usually about 0.6. Hence, if λ is 1000 nm, NA is 1.2 and f is 0.61. Then,

$$R_L = \frac{\lambda f}{2NA} = \frac{1000\,\text{nm} \times 0.61}{2 \times 1.2} = 254\,\text{nm} = 0.25\,\mu\text{m}$$

It is important that one be aware of the microscope resolution because if the particles are smaller than the optical resolution limit, the particles will appear to be blurry and it may affect the particle size analysis as a number of smaller particles may look like a single larger particle. This artifact will result in overestimation of the size distribution.

Oculars (eyepiece): The ocular or eyepiece is the second optical lens that magnifies the primary image from the objective lens. The magnification size of an ocular is usually between $5\times$ and $30\times$ and the optimum magnification size of the oculars is dependent on the numerical aperture of the objective since the total magnification on a microscope is usually about $1000\times$ the numerical aperture of the objective (40). For instance, if the numerical aperture of the objective would be 10, then, the maximum magnification size of the ocular should be $10\times$ since the magnification beyond this value will not further improve the quality of the image but will unnecessarily waste money.

Illumination: Two types of microscope illumination are the reflectance and transmittance illumination. Reflectance illumination is where the light source illuminates the sample from above, bounces off the walls and is reflected off the sample. This type of illumination is useful for opaque samples where light cannot penetrate through. It is also useful to examine larger particles or to get the surface details of particles. On the other hand, the light from the transmittance illumination method goes through the sample but outside of the silhouette of particles. The reflectance and transmittance illumination light source are often combined in a single microscope known as a metallurgical microscope (Fig. 21). Optical microscopes are well suited for measuring particles from about 0.8–150 μm. Larger particles are better off counted by a stereoscope or a lower magnification device with a greater viewing area.

When using a microscope it is important to understand the depth of field especially when taking an image of a three-dimensional object that has front to back depth. One has to remember that not all depth will be able to be focused on the focal plane into a sharper image. This whole range of clear focus on to the focal plane is called the depth of field. Anything closer than the depth of field or further than the depth of field will be blurry. This is important because blurry particles may seem larger than their actual size. For example, if one has a microscope slide with a lot of particles present and these particles vary in size, it is possible that some of the smaller particles will be outside of the depth of field. In fact the microscope will be focusing on the larger particles and thus the smaller

Particle and Powder Bed Properties

particles will appear to be larger than their actual size because they are outside of the depth of field.

The above discussion illustrates the importance of operator training. If the operator is not well trained there would be various human perception tendencies that can bias the counting and the particle size distribution calculated will be inaccurate due to these issues. Unfortunately, we do not have time to cover all of these concerns in this section but see the reference from Allen for a more complete discussion of operator training for microscopy (9).

Sample Preparation

Sample preparation must be done carefully because biases in sample preparation will lead to inaccurate results. The statistical diameters that are popular for characterizing particles in microscopy are based on a random orientation; thus, biases in orientation due to improper sample preparation will affect the values. Any factors that cause the particles to preferentially orient on the microscope slide will affect the results. For example, spreading the particles out with a spatula may causes a preferential orientation. Another example is particles dispersed in a liquid; when the liquid is sprayed or poured onto the microscope slide the particles could orient themselves with the flow lines of the liquid and this could lead to their non-random orientation.

Samples used in microscopes can be placed on the slide dry or wet. Typical liquids used for wet-immersion are non-aqueous based like Nujol® (International Crystal Laboratories, Garfield, New Jersey, U.S.A.), which is liquid paraffin, or Sirax, which is cedar wood oil. Again, there are many practical aspects of preparing samples for microscopy and the requirement of proper microscope settings can be found in Refs. 7, 9, 40.

Sieving

Sieving is one of the oldest and most reliable methods for particle size characterization even though there are many sophisticated particle size characterization instruments currently available. A key advantage of this method is its ability to measure large quantities of particles at the same time, low instrument and maintenance cost, and ease of use. Though sieving is a reliable method, the aggressive motion of the sieving instrument can be very harsh for friable particles. Friable particles may undergo attrition if the sieving process is not optimized.

Sieving serves two purposes; the first is to separate or deagglomerate the powder into fractions of desired size, and the second purpose, often referred to as analytical sieving, is to determine the particle size. It is important to note that the sieves used for these two different applications are very different in construction. Analytical sieves should not be used to separate or deagglomerate powders because this process often requires forcing the powders through the sieve and this can damage the analytical sieves. Damage or wear will introduce error for the measured particle size and consequently it may contribute to poor results.

The basic set up for a sieving instrument usually involves a top cover, a stack of 2–6 different sieves with ascending order of opening size and a fines collector. The sieves are often made of wire woven with different aperture sizes and the particle size of the powder is characterized by the size of the sieve aperture.

The basic idea of sieve analysis is very simple, a sample with a predetermined weight is placed on the top sieve and will be divided into multiple sieve fractions by the shaking, tapping, vibration, or air movements of the sieve instrument. The shaking, vibration and air movements of the sieve instrument causes the particles to move around and potentially pass through the sieve aperture (this process continues until the particles can no longer pass through the apertures of the sieve at which it is resting on). Particles that are smaller than the aperture size of the sieve will pass through the aperture while particles that are bigger than the aperture size of the sieve will be retained on the sieve. Thus if the particle passes through a 120-μm sieve aperture but is retained on a 75-μm sieve aperture then the particle size is between 75 and 120 μm. Often, the particle size can also be characterized by an equivalent diameter called the sieve diameter, d_A, that is the minimum screen aperture size which the particle can pass through. Note that the size obtained from sieve analysis is a function of the maximum breadth and maximum thickness only as length does not affect the particle size obtained (Fig. 24). Thus, if the length of a particle is extremely long, as in acicular needles, then the size reported from the sieve analysis may not represent the actual size of the particles.

Thus, using a stack of sieves with an ascending order of aperture sizes one can separate the powder sample into the various sizes. By weighing the amount of powders

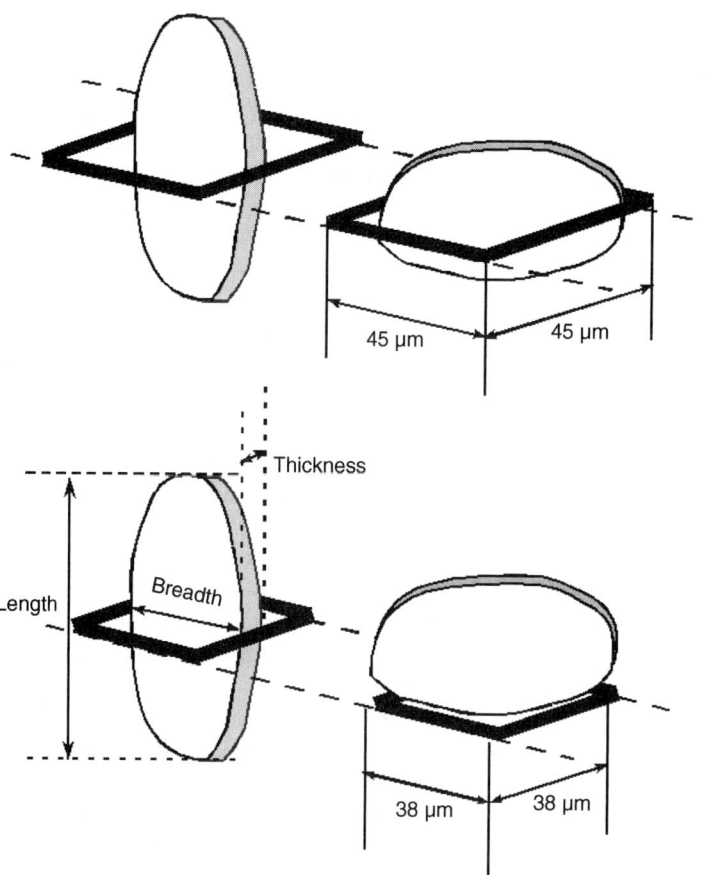

FIGURE 24 An irregularly shaped particle passing through an U.S. ASTM #324 mesh sieve (45 μm) and U.S. ASTM #400 mesh sieve (38 μm). Size obtained from sieve analysis is a function of the maximum breadth and maximum thickness, however, particle shape can affect the sieving end point.

Particle and Powder Bed Properties

that are retained on each sieve one can plot the particle size versus the amount retained or cumulative retained on the sieves to obtain a particle size distribution. A detailed description of how to conduct this analytical sieving is given in the USP<786> (7). In this section, we will discuss the types of sieves, method of sieving, how to obtain reliable data and some specifications from the regulatory chapters in the pharmacopoeias.

Sieves

The sieves are often made of woven wire, with different aperture sizes ranging from 20 μm to 125 mm (7,9). There are many different standards for sieves such as the original Tyler standard, the U.S. standard of American Society for Testing Material (ASTM), the International Organization for Standardization (ISO), German standard of Deutsches Institut für Normung e.V. (DIN), British standard (IMM), Japanese standard, and several others. These standard sieves are slightly different in the sieve size name and the sieve aperture size. In most cases, the sieve size can either be referred to by the aperture size, the sieve number, or mesh number. The sieve and mesh number of the U.S. ASTM standards, Tyler standards, and Japan standards refers to the number of wires per linear inch while the European sieve number refers to the actual sieve aperture size. For instance, a U.S. ASTM sieve number of 45 (written #45), refers to the sieve with 45 wires per linear inch and an aperture size of 355 μm while the European sieve #45 refers to a sieve with an aperture size of 45 μm. Besides the differences in naming nomenclature, there is also a slight difference in the aperture size between different standards, i.e., the aperture sizes of U.S. ASTM sieves #12 and #14 is 1.7 and 1.4 mm, respectively, while the aperture sizes of Japan sieves #12 and #14 is 1.4 and 1.18 mm, respectively. Hence, the standard used for particle size analysis should always be specified to avoid confusion especially for an international drug company. A summary of the different sieve sizes commonly used in the pharmaceutical industry from a few different standards can be found in Table 11.

Figure 25 shows a U.S. ASTM #400 mesh sieve with an aperture size of 38 μm. For this mesh size, the nominal wire thickness is 25.5 μm; thus, only 35.81% of the total area is open for the particles to pass through because the rest of the area is taken up by the wire. This example illustrates that as the sieve size decreases, the open area for particles to pass through also proportionally decreases because more and more of the area is taken up by the wire mesh. Thus, sieving smaller particles takes longer because the efficiency of sieving decreases as the aperture size decreases.

Besides the different types of standard sieves, structures and composition of sieves can also subtly affect the particle size measured. In general, the three types of sieves are woven wire, punched plate, and micromesh. Woven wire sieves are usually made from phosphor bronze, brass, and mild steel wires and the wires are mounted to the bottom of a cylindrical container (9). The basic types of woven sieves are plain, twilled and braided. Each of these woven sieves will have a slightly different aperture due to the difference in the geometry of the wires surrounding the aperture. Figure 26 illustrates some differences in woven sieves. Plate sieves are made by punching holes in a flat plate to create circular apertures. Due to their construction, plate sieves tend to be stronger. Micron mesh sieves are made from a photo-etching process where the desired sieve aperture size and pattern are first photographically applied on a metal sheet and then etched away (9). A detailed description of the construction and specifications of these types of sieves can be found in Allen (9), ASTM E11-04, ASTM E323-80, and ASTM E161-00.

Care must be taken when handling the analytical sieves to ensure accurate and reproducible particle size analysis. It should be noted that anything that may move the

TABLE 11 Sieve Standards Specified by USP and Tyler

ISO nominal aperture							
Principal sizes	Supplementary sizes		U.S. sieve no.	Recommended USP sieves (mesh)	European sieve no.	Japan sieve no.	Tyler mesh no.
R 20/3	R 20	R 40/3					
11.20 mm	11.20 mm	11.20 mm					
	10.00 mm						
		9.50 mm					
	9.00 mm						
8.00 mm	8.00 mm	8.00 mm					
	7.10 mm						
		6.70 mm					
	7.10 mm						
		6.70 mm					
	6.30 mm						
5.60 mm	5.60 mm	5.60 mm			5600	3.5	
	5.00 mm						
		4.75 mm	4			4	4
	4.50 mm						
4.00 mm	4.00 mm	4.00 mm	5	4000	4000	4.7	5
	3.55 mm						
		3.35 mm	6			5.5	6
	3.15 mm						
2.80 mm	2.80 mm	2.80 mm	7	2800	2800	6.5	7
	2.50 mm						
		2.36 mm	8			7.5	8
	2.24 mm						
2.00 mm	2.00 mm	2.00 mm	10	2000	2000	8.6	9
	1.80 mm						
		1.70 mm	12			10	10
	1.60 mm						
1.40 mm	1.40 mm	1.40 mm	14	1400	1400	12	12
	1.25 mm						
		1.18 mm	16			14	14
	1.12 mm						
1.00 mm	1.00 mm	1.00 mm	18	1000	1000	16	16
	900 μm						
		850 μm	20			18	20
	800 μm						
710 μm	710 μm	710 μm	25	710	710	22	24
	630 μm						
		600 μm	30			26	28
	560 μm						
500 μm	500 μm	500 μm	35	500	500	30	32
	450 μm						
		425 μm	40			36	35

(*Continued*)

TABLE 11 Sieve Standards Specified by USP and Tyler (*Continued*)

ISO nominal aperture			U.S. sieve no.	Recommended USP sieves (mesh)	European sieve no.	Japan sieve no.	Tyler mesh no.
Principal sizes R 20/3	Supplementary sizes R 20	R 40/3					
355 μm	400 μm 355 μm 315 μm	355 μm	45	355	355	42	42
		300 μm	50			50	48
250 μm	280 μm 250 μm 224 μm	250 μm	60	250	250	60	60
		212 μm	70			70	65
180 μm	200 μm 180 μm 160 μm	180 μm	80	180	180	83	80
		150 μm	100			100	100
125 μm	140 μm 125 μm 112 μm	125 μm	120	125	125	119	115
		106 μm	140			140	150
90 μm	100 μm 90 μm 80 μm	90 μm	170	90	90	166	170
		75 μm	200			200	200
63 μm	71 μm 63 μm 56 μm	63 μm	230	63	63	235	250
		53 μm	270			282	270
45 μm	50 μm 45 μm 40 μm	45 μm	325	45	45	330	325
		38 μm	400		38	391	400

Source: Adapted from Ref. 7 and Tyler.

wires of the sieve around will cause the aperture size to change. This is particularly important in an environment where analytical sieves are used to sieve powders for deagglomeration or deaggregation purposes as this process usually involve forcing particle through the sieve aperture. Forcing particles through the sieve apertures of an analytical sieve can slightly change the sieve aperture size and daily handling and cleaning can also damage the sieves. Hence, it is important to inspect sieves to ensure the apertures are uniform in size and there is no damage on the wire mesh prior to any test. Calibration of the sieve should be done routinely to ensure the functionality of the sieve. It can be done visually to estimate the average opening size, opening variability, distortion and fractures, or standard glass spheres ranging in size from 212 to 850 μm can be used. The details of the calibration and recalibration of test sieves can be found in the USP <786> (7) and ISO 3310-1.

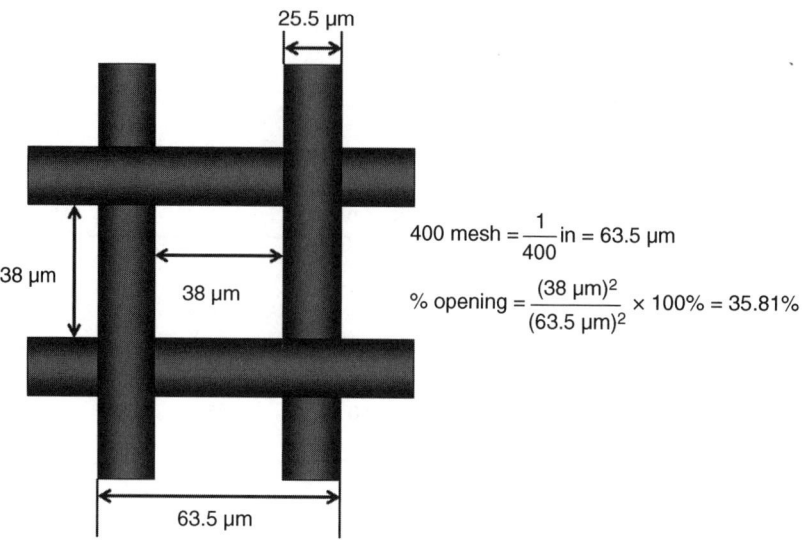

FIGURE 25 U.S. ASTM #400 mesh sieve with an aperture size of 38 μm.

Sieving Methods

A key aspect of sieving is how the particles are set in motion. Particles can be set in motion manually or by an instrument. Sieving by hand is not popular because it varies from operator to operator, which makes reliable data collection difficult. Both manual and automatic sieving analysis use at least two sieves with different aperture sizes. The sieve with the larger aperture is placed at the top while the sieve with the smaller apertures is placed at the bottom. The motion created either by hand or by the instrument will allow the particles to pass through the sieves and be retained on the sieve that has an aperture that is smaller than the particle size. The weight of the sample powder and the sieves are predetermined prior to the test and the sieve weights are again measured after the test. Hence, the percentage of particles retained on a sieve can be calculated and plotted versus the sieve aperture size. The percentage retained is often transformed to the cumulative percentage retained using the statistical method as discussed previously.

Due to the differences between sieve analysis methods, the method of sieve analysis used must be indicated according to USP <786> as the different of types and magnitude of agitation produced by different sieving instruments will yield different results (7).

Manual sieving: Hand sieving is time consuming and it may yield inconsistent results between different operators. However, there are instances when hand sieving is required, such as when samples are limited or when very refined sieving is needed. In a hand sieving operation, the fines are usually pre-removed using the sieve with smallest aperture size intended for that particular analysis. Pre-sieving can reduce the time for sieving since the fines would not have to pass through every sieve. Then, fines collected from the pre-sieving can be kept separately while the particles retained from the finest sieve can be transferred to the sieve with largest aperture size intended to use in that particular analysis with a top cover on top and collection pan at the bottom. Particles that are bigger than the coarsest sieve will be fractionated out by tapping the sieve at about 150 taps per minute and rotated 1/8 of a turn after every 25 taps until less than 0.2% of the original charge passes through the sieve (9). Then, the weight of the particles retained from the

Particle and Powder Bed Properties

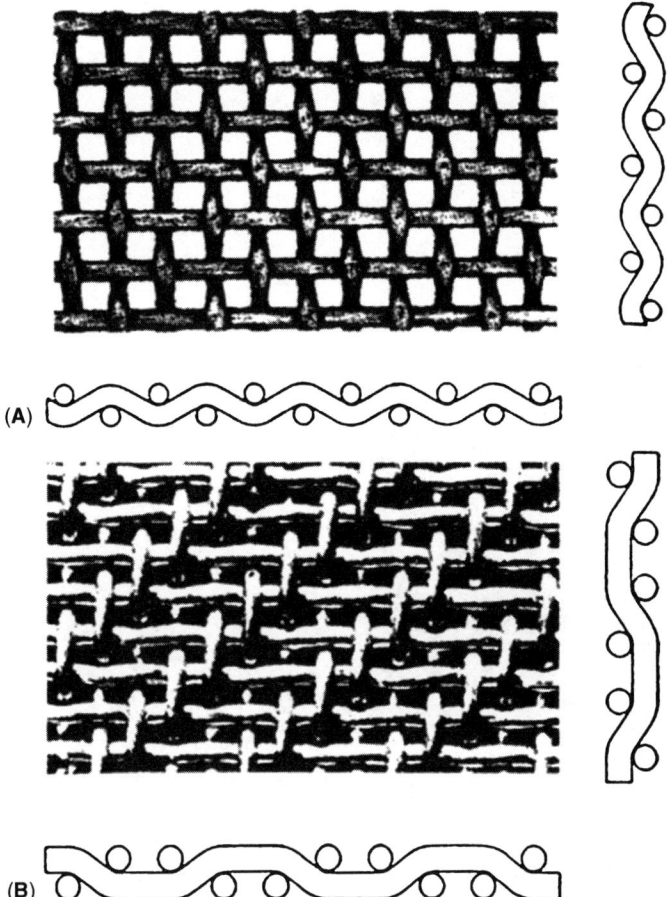

FIGURE 26 (A) Plain weave and (B) twilled weave woven sieves. *Source*: Adapted from Ref. 50.

sieves is measured and the particles from the collection pan are transferred to another sieve with a smaller aperture size and the process is repeated with sieves of decreasing aperture size. Finally, the percentage retained or the percentage of cumulative retained can be calculated from taking the sample and sieve weights before and after the test.

Automatic sieving: Most sieve instruments use either mechanical agitation or air entrainment methods to set the particles in motion. The mechanical agitation method is more aggressive since it uses movements such as gyratory, shaking, tapping, and jolting while the air entrainment method uses air or sonic movement to set the particles in motion and to avoid sieve blinding.

Ro-Tap®. A Ro-Tap® machine (Hauer and Boecker, Germany) (Fig. 27) is one of the most commonly used mechanical sieve shakers in industry and uses aggressive mechanical agitation to set the particles in motion. The sieves are shaken or gyrated in a circular motion and then tapped from the top along the axial direction. Both of these motions set the particles in motion and help them flow down through the progression of sieves to reach their final resting spot. The typical test times for a Ro-Tap are in the order of 20 min. However, this should be checked by taking intermediate sieve weight to ensure that the sieve weight is not changing too much and the losses should not exceed 0.5%.

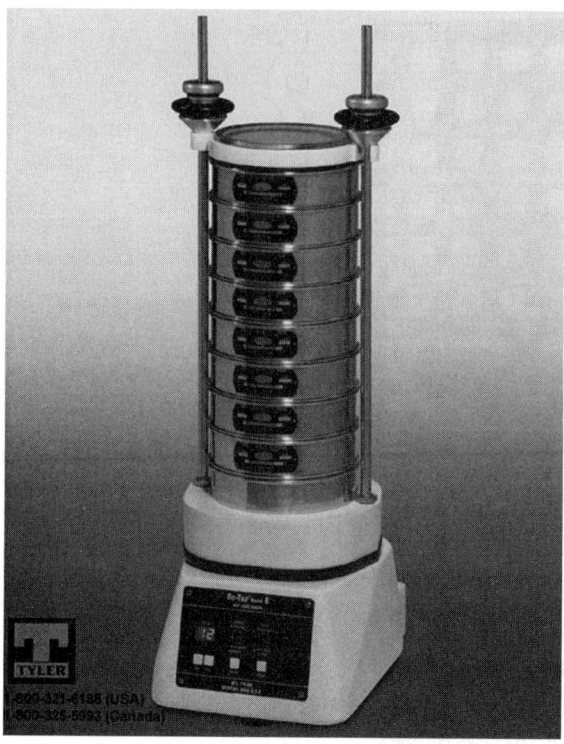

FIGURE 27 Ro-Tap® automatic sieving apparatus.

The test should be repeated if losses are greater than 0.5%. Typically, the sample size required for this method is about 25–50 g depending on the bulk density of the material and the diameter of the sieves; however, this is only a general statement. The Ro-Tap is not suitable for friable materials as the aggressive gyratory and jolting movement will reduce its particle size. Hence, a gentler sieving instrument such as the sonic sifter can be employed.

Sonic Sifter. The sonic sifter is one of the most popular and powerful sieving methods that uses oscillating air to set the particles in motion and a vertical mechanical pulse to shear the aggregates and reorient the particles in the air column allowing particles to pass through the sieves efficiently. The oscillating air can also reduce sieve blinding. The sonic sifter is often preferred over the Ro-Tap as the former method is much quieter and faster. Besides, it produces very little abrasion and particle breakage. It typically uses sample sizes on the order of 1–5 g while sieve times are on the order of 5–10 min.

As seen in Figure 28, the basic set up of the sonic sifter usually involves a column lock, a top diaphragm, a top cone, a stack of 2–6 sieves with an ascending order of aperture size or spacer to fill the gap if less than six sieves are needed, a fines collector, and a fines collector holder. The sonic sifter has the function that allows the user to select either sift action only or sift and pulse action and this allowing the user to optimize the analysis process for particles of different densities (Fig. 28). When the sift and pulse function is selected, a vertical pulse or shock wave will impact the sieve stack to reorient the particles and break down softly clinging or aggregated particles every 4 seconds. Besides, the sonic sifter also has an amplitude control to adjust the amplitude of vibration during the operation and a timer to preset the test time. The light and see-through window

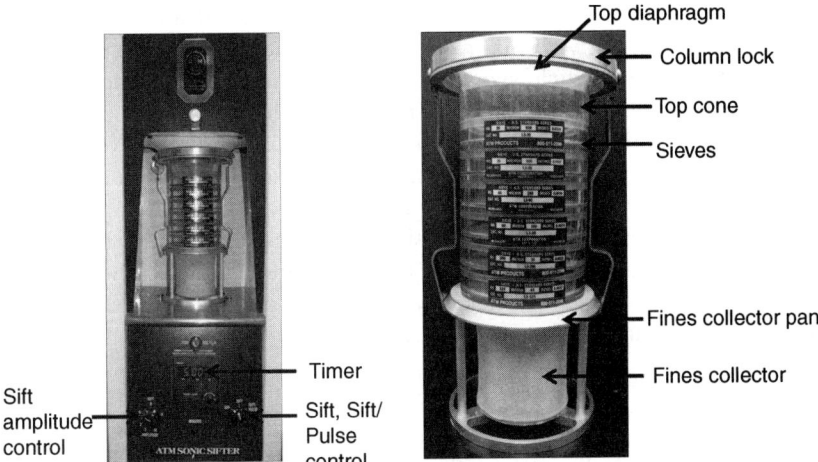

FIGURE 28 Sonic sifter with the typical setup.

allows one to see the particle motion and adjust the settings when necessary. When performing the sieve analysis using a sonic sifter, the amplitude of the vibration should not be too high as the particles that bounce too high tend to fly around and thus not pass through the sieve. On the other hand, if the amplitude is too low, the particles will actively vibrate on the sieve and this may result in attrition from the sieve wires. Thus, it is important to optimize and develop standard method for particles of different properties in order to yield consistent results from batch to batch.

Data Collection Issues

Though sieving analysis is a simple and reliable particle size analysis method, there are some data collection issues that one must be aware of and control in order to obtain reproducible results. Factors that may affect data accuracy include sieve properties, sieve motion and powder properties, sieve time and load, and errors of experimental method and environment. This section will discuss the effects and methods to reduce data collection errors.

Sieve properties: As discussed previously, there are a number of sieve types and sieve standards. These sieves all slightly vary in size, shape, and construction, and they may affect the results obtained. For instance, using a sieve with aperture sizes of 180 and 90 μm to measure the sieve diameter for particles that have a mean diameter of 100 μm will yield a sieve diameter of 180 μm, which clearly shows an over estimate of the particle size. Hence, selecting the proper sieves that can best represent the sample particle size is critical. Selecting sieves that cover the entire range of particle sizes at a $\sqrt{2}$ progression is recommended (7). Thus, for particles with a mean diameter of 100 μm, selecting a stack of six sieves with aperture sizes of 45, 63, 90, 125, 180, and 250 μm can give a good idea about the particle size distribution at the beginning of method development. Upon obtaining the size distribution, one can further modify and optimize the method depending on whether the size distribution is narrow or wide. Using microscopy to measure the particle size prior to the sieving analysis can help in selecting the sieve size required as one would not know the mean diameter of a sample prior to any test.

The material of the sieves can be important as well. One should make sure the sample analyzed is not reacting with the material of the sieve to avoid any unforeseen reaction that may change the particle size or shape during the analysis. Other than the sieve size and sieve materials, wear on the sieve can also result in data inaccuracy. Thus, it is important that one examines the sieve for wear and tear prior to the sieve analysis. Calibration of the sieves should also be done routinely to ensure data accuracy.

Sieve motion and powder properties: One of the reasons for obtaining inaccurate data from any sieving method is when sieve blinding occurs. Sieve blinding is when one particle become permanently lodged in an aperture and blocks the aperture. Blinding will decrease the sieving efficiency because particles can no longer pass through that blinded aperture. Sieving efficiency can be calculated by,

$$\text{efficiency} = \frac{\%\,\text{material actually passing}}{\%\,\text{total capable of passing}} \tag{103}$$

Hence, the efficiency of the sieve will substantially decrease as the number of apertures blocked is increased. This problem is more severe for smaller sieve sizes since the efficiency of a smaller sieve is lower due to the high percentage of mesh in the sieve. In addition, for irregularly shaped particles which are elongated or needle-like, blinding can be more of an issue because these particles can become permanently trapped in the aperture. A method of preventing or mitigating blinding is to employ sieve motion such as jolting or tapping to remove the particle from the sieve aperture. The sieve motion in both the Ro-Tap and sonic sifter, that is the jolting, gyratory, oscillating, tapping and vibration can help to dislodge the blinded particles from the apertures.

However, if one uses aggressive sieve motion on friable particles, it may result in particle attrition during the sieving process and result in the underestimation of particle size. Thus, a balance between sieve efficiency and the particle properties should be considered when selecting a method of analysis.

There are times when the sample is static which results in particles adhering to the sieve wall and not passing through the sieve aperture or particles tending to form granules during the sieving process. In cases like that, adding a small amount of excipient such as a fatty acid, talc, or silicon dioxide may help to reduce the cohesiveness of the particles.

Sieve time and load: Another common error when conducting particle size analysis is when data is obtained prior to the particles falling into their smallest sieve. The sieving endpoint is greatly dependent on the test time and sample load. If sieve loading is too high there are too many particles for the number of the apertures or the area to pass through. This effect decreases the number of particles that can pass through the sieve because the particles are competing to pass through the apertures. Thus if loading is increased, one should run the sieving analysis for a longer time in order to compensate for the higher loading. However, an increase in sieving times may lead to particle attrition and thus it may change the distribution of particles being measured.

In a study discussed by Allen (11), the number of particles that passed through the sieve as a function of time was measured. One can see from Figure 29 that the sieving process occurs in two phases. In the first phase, particles quickly fall through the apertures, but in the second phase the rate of passage through the apertures decreases. This biphasic behavior can be understood by considering the statistics of particles passing through an aperture. When a smaller particle is on a larger sieve, no matter how the particle lands on the sieve as it is being vibrated, it will pass through the aperture. However, as the particle gets closer to its smallest aperture size, it will not pass through with every vibration as shown in Figure 24 and it may only be able to pass through on 1

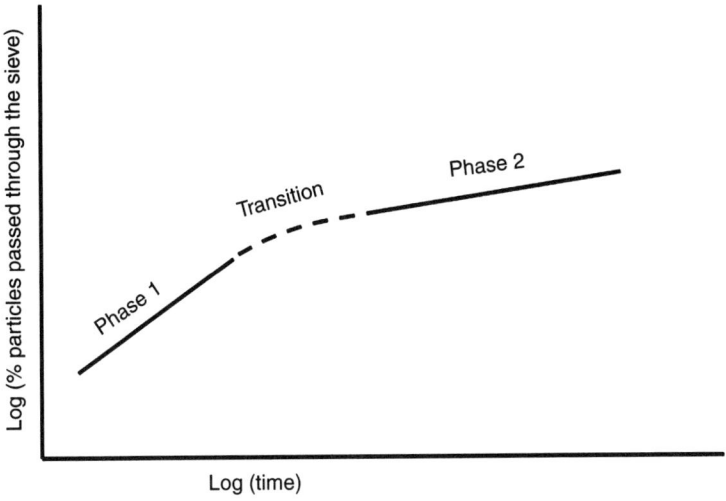

FIGURE 29 The rate of particles passing through the sieve. *Source*: Adapted from Ref. 11.

in 100 vibrations when the narrow dimensions of the particle finally aligns with the sieve opening. Thus, when the particles pass through a larger sieve, they have 100% chance of falling through the aperture if they land in the aperture opening. However, when particles are on a smaller sieve with a smaller aperture, then they may have only 50% chance of passing through the aperture. As a result of this and the fact that the particles are vibrated up and down at a fixed frequency due to the motion of the sieve; one can see that the rate of passage will slow down for these particles.

This behavior is critical to understand and to obtain accurate results. As one can see in Figure 29, that if the sieving time was set in the region where any slight variations in either sieve time or sample loading would affect the passage of the particles and yield drastically different results as the particle size distribution is very much dependent upon the sieving time.

However in phase two region we can see that we are in a much more stable region and the sieve size distribution is not nearly as dependent on sieving time. Thus, when setting specifications it is important to use the data from phase two region, sometimes called the near mesh size region. This is why the USP requires sieve analysis to be done at two different time points to ensure that the actual sieve weights do not change from time to time and that the data will be rugged (7).

The recommended particle size analysis endpoint determination method is to run the particle size analysis for 5 min, and carefully to remove the sieves and collection pan to obtain their weights without losing any material. Then, the sieves and collection pan are reassembled to repeat the test for another 5 min. According to USP<786>, the analysis is considered as complete only when the weight change on any of the sieves is not more than 5% or 0.1 g on the previous weight of that sieve. The test should be repeated with a longer test time if it is more than 5%. On the other hand, the endpoint of the sieve analysis should be increased to a weight change of not more than 20% from the previous weight on that sieve if it is less than 5% (7). Additionally, Allen et al. found that for smaller sieve sizes the effect of loading was much more pronounced so this is a factor which also must be controlled (11). A summary of the factors influencing the sieve analysis can be found in Table 12.

TABLE 12 Summary of Factors Influencing the Sieving Analysis

Factors affecting the probability of a particle to present itself at an sieve aperture	Factors affecting the probability of a particle passing through the sieve aperture when presenting at the sieve aperture
Powder particle size distribution	Sieving duration
Sieve load	Variation of sieve aperture
Physical properties of the particles	Sieve condition (e.g., wear)
Method of sieving motion	Sampling errors
Particle dimension and shape	Observation and experiment errors.
Types, size, and geometry of the sieves	Types of sieve instrument and operation method

Source: Adapted from Ref. 11.

Laser Diffraction

Laser diffraction has become one of the most widely used and reliable techniques for measuring the particle size for a wide range of samples due to its efficient and rapid measurement, ease of use, and this technique can be used to measure samples presented from different physical forms such as dry powders, suspensions, spray dispersions, emulsions, etc. (7,49).

Light scattering is based on the principle that all particles will scatter light at different angles with different intensities depending on the size of the particles. Large particles scatter light at smaller angles with higher intensities while small particles scatter light at wider angles with lower intensities. Therefore, the particle size can be calculated based on the particle's scattering pattern.

The newer laser diffraction instrument allows measurement for particle sizes ranging from 0.1 µm to 8 mm (7). Most of the laser diffraction instruments in the pharmaceutical industry use the optical model based on several theories, either Fraunhofer, (near-) forward light scattering, low-angle laser light scattering, Mie, Fraunhofer approximation, or anomalous diffraction. These laser diffraction instruments assume that the particles measured are spherical. Hence, the instrument will convert the scattering pattern into an equivalent volume diameter. A typical laser diffraction instrument consists of a laser, a sample presentation system, and a series of detectors.

Figure 30 shows a simple model of a typical laser diffraction instrument where the diffraction pattern of light scattered at various angles from the sample particles that pass through the He–Ne laser beam is measured by different detectors and recorded as numerical values relating to the scattering pattern. These numerical values are then converted to the particle size distribution in terms of the equivalent volume diameter using a mathematical model from the instrument's software.

Since the reported diameter is an equivalent volume diameter, proper consideration must be taken when comparing the results with other particle size analysis methods. For instance, the equivalent volume diameter reported for any non-spherical shaped particle will generally be higher than the particle size reported by sieve analysis, as the equivalent volume diameter is based on the volume of a perfect sphere. This theory becomes apparent if one compares the equivalent volume diameter with the sieve diameter of a square that has dimensions of 200 µm by 200 µm by 200 µm and that passes through a U.S. ASTM sieve # 70 (212 µm) and is retained on a U.S. ASTM sieve # 80 (180 µm). In this case, the sieve diameter reported will be 212 µm but the

Particle and Powder Bed Properties

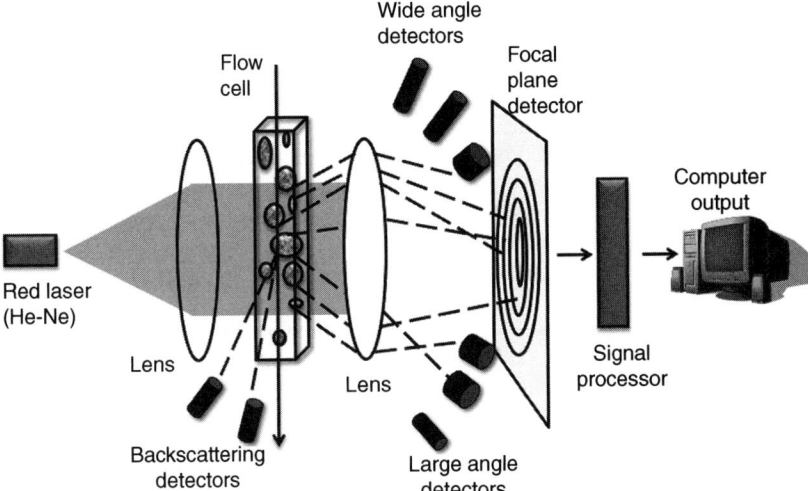

FIGURE 30 A simple model for a typical laser diffraction instrument.

equivalent volume diameter will be 248 μm. The detailed calculation for the equivalent volume diameter is shown:

$$V = (200 \times 200 \times 200)\mu m^3 = 8 \times 10^6 = \frac{\pi d_v^3}{6}$$

$$d_v = 248.14\,\mu m$$

Laser diffraction cannot distinguish primary particles from agglomerates. Hence, it is a good idea to cross-check the results with a microscope. Besides, the high pressure used in laser diffraction may break down the granules if the proper settings are not used. Another common mistake made during particle size measurement when using laser diffraction is the amount of sample used. Large amounts of sample can lead to high obscuration of the laser beam which causes multiple light scattering and results in overestimation of fine particles (49). Even though laser diffraction has some disadvantages, it is particularly useful when the relationship between the mass or volume distribution of particles of different sizes is of interest.

REFERENCES

1. Dallavalle JM. Micromeritics. Chicago: Pitman Publishing Company, 1943.
2. Hoener B, Benet LZ. Factors influencing drug absorption and drug availability. In: Banker GS, Rhodes CT, eds. Modern pharmaceutics, 3rd ed., Vol. 72. New York: Marcel Dekker, Inc., 1996: 121–53.
3. Alderborn G. Particle dimensions. In: Alderborn G, Nyström C, eds. Pharmaceutical Powder Compaction Technology, 1st ed. Vol. 71. New York: Marcel Dekker, Inc., 1996: 245–82.
4. Kaerger JS, Edge S, Price R. Influence of particle size and shape on flowability and compactibility of binary mixtures of paracetamol and microcrystalline cellulose. Eur J Pharm Sci 2004; 22(2–3):173–9.
5. Nagel KM, Peck GE. Investigating the effects of excipients on the powder flow characteristics of theophylline anhydrous powder formulations. Drug Dev Ind Pharm 2003; 29(3):277.

6. Patel S, Kaushal A, Bansal A. Effect of particle size and compression force on compaction behavior and derived mathematical parameters of compressibility. Pharm. Res. 2007, 24(1), 111–24.
7. The United States Pharmacopeia. 2007: Rockville, MD.
8. Reist PC. Aerosol Science and Technology. 2nd ed. New York: McGraw-Hill, 1993.
9. Allen T. Particle Size Measurement. 5th ed. Vol. 1. London: Chapman & Hall, 1997.
10. Ross SM. Introduction to Probability Models. 6th ed. San Diego: Academic Press, 1997.
11. Allen T. Particle Size Measurement. 4th ed. London: Chapman & Hall, 1990.
12. Griffiths JC. Scientific method in analysis of sediments. Technometrics 1967; 11(2):406.
13. Sneed ED, Folk RL. Pebbles in the lower Colorado River, Texas, a study in particle morphology genesis. J Geol 1958; 66:114–50.
14. Barrett PJ. The shape of rock particles, a critical review. Sedimentology 1980; 27:291–303.
15. Flament M-P, Leterme P, Gayot A. The influence of carrier roughness on adhesion, content uniformity and the in vitro deposition of terbutaline sulphate from dry powder inhalers. Int J Pharm 2004; 275(1–2):201–9.
16. Ohta KM, Fuji M, Chikazawa M. Effect of geometric structure of flow promoting agents on the flow properties of pharmaceutical powder mixture. Pharm Res 2003; 20(5):804–9.
17. Swaminathan V, Kildsig D. The effect of particle morphology on the physical stability of pharmaceutical powder mixtures: The effect of surface roughness of the carrier on the stability of ordered mixtures. Drug Dev Ind Pharm 2000; 26(4):365.
18. Swaminathan V, Kildsig D. Polydisperse powder mixtures: Effect of particle size and shape on mixture stability. Drug Dev Ind Pharm 2002; 28(1):41–8.
19. Shotton E, Obiorah BA. Effect of particle shape and crystal habit on properties of sodium chloride. J Pharm Pharmacol 1973; 25(Suppl.):37P–43P.
20. Podczeck F, Miah Y. The influence of particle size and shape on the angle of internal friction and the flow factor of unlubricated and lubricated powders. Int J Pharm 1996; 144(2):187–94.
21. Podczeck F, Sharma M. The influence of particle size and shape of components of binary powder mixtures on the maximum volume reduction due to packing. Int J Pharm 1996; 137(1):41–7.
22. Ridgway K, Rupp R. Effect of particle shape on powder properties. J Pharm Pharmacol 1969; 21(Suppl):30S–39S.
23. Kawashima Y, Cui F, Takeuchi H, et al. Improvements in flowability and compressibility of pharmaceutical crystals for direct tabletting by spherical crystallization with a 2-solvent system. Powder Technol 1994; 78(2):151–7.
24. Martino PD, Censi R, Malaj L, et al. Influence of metronidazole particle properties on granules prepared in a high-shear mixer-granulator. Drug Dev Ind Pharm 2007; 33(2):121–31.
25. Lantz RJ. Size reduction. In: Lieberman HA, Schwartz JB, eds. Pharmaceutical Dosage Forms, 2nd ed. Vol. 2. New York: Marcel Dekker, Inc., 1990: 107–200.
26. Almeida-Prieto S, Blanco-Mendez J, Otero-Espinar FJ. Image analysis of the shape of granulated powder grains. J Pharm Sci 2004; 93(3):621–34.
27. Hawkins AE. The Shape of Powder-Particle Outlines. Vol. 1. New York: John Wiley & Sons Inc., 1993.
28. Bouwman AM, Bosma JC, Vonk P, et al. Which shape factor(s) best describe granules? Powder Technol 2004; 146(1–2):66–72.
29. Lin CL, Miller JD. 3D characterization and analysis of particle shape using x-ray microtomography (xmt). Powder Technol 2005; 154(1):61–9.
30. Realpe A, Velazquez C. Pattern recognition for characterization of pharmaceutical powders. Powder Technol 2006; 169(2):108–13.
31. Taylor MA. Quantitative measures for shape and size of particles. Powder Technol 2002; 124(1–2):94–100.
32. Wadell H. Sphericity and roundness of rock particles. J Geol 1933; 41:310–31.
33. Robertson RHS, Emödi BS. Rugosity of granular solids. Nature 1943; 152:539–40.
34. Carstensen JT. Pharmaceutical Preformulation. 1st ed. Vol. 1. Lancaster, Pennsylvania: Technomic Publishing Company, Inc., 1998: 197–333.

35. Cox EP. A method of assigning numerical and percentage values to the degree of roundness of sand grains. J Paleontol 1927; 1:179–83.
36. Sinko PJ. Martin's Physical Pharmacy and Pharmaceutical Sciences. 5th ed. Philadelphia: Lippincott Williams & Wilkins, 2006: 533–60.
37. Carstensen JT. Advanced Pharmaceutical Solids. 1st ed. Vol. 110. New York: Marcel Dekker, Inc., 2001: 63–88.
38. Heywood H. The evaluation of powders. J Pharm Pharmacol 1963; 15(Suppl):56T–74T.
39. Heywood H. Particle shape coefficients. J Imp Coll Eng Soc 1954; 8:25–33.
40. Barber TA. Pharmaceutical Particulate Matter. Buffalo Grove, IL: Interpharm Press, 1993.
41. Schneiderhöhn P. Eine verleichendestudie über methoden zur quantitativen bestimmung von abrundung und form and sandkörnern. Heidelberger Beiträge Mineralogie Petrographie 1954; 4:172–91.
42. Beddow JK, Meloy TP. Testing and Characterization of Powders and Fine Particles. Particulate Science and Technology. 1980; 1:101–123.
43. Podczeck F, Newton JM. The evaluation of a 3-dimensional shape factor for the quantitative assessment of the sphericity and surface-roughness of pellets. Int J Pharm 1995; 124(2): 253–9.
44. Mandelbrot BB. Fractals, Forms, Chance, and Dimension. San Francisco: W. H. Freeman, 1977.
45. Thibert R, Akbarieh M, Tawashi R. Application of fractal dimension to the study of the surface ruggedness of granular solids and excipients. J Pharm Sci 1988; 77(8):724–6.
46. Podczeck F, Newton JM. A shape factor to characterize the quality of spheroids. J Pharm Pharmacol 1994; 46(2):82–5.
47. Chapman SR, Rowe RC, Newton JM. Characterization of the sphericity of particles by the one plane critical stability. J Pharm Pharmacol 1988; 40(7):503–5.
48. Brittain HG, Bogdanowich SJ, Bugay DE, et al. Physical characterization of pharmaceutical solids. Pharm Res 1991; 8(8):963–73.
49. Shekunov BY, Chattopadhyay P, Tong HHY, et al. Particle size analysis in pharmaceutics: Principles, methods and applications. Pharm Res 2007; 24(2):203–27.
50. Rippie EG. Powders. In: Gennaro AR, Chase GD, Gibson MR et al., eds. Remington's Pharmaceutical Sciences, 17th ed. Easton, Pennsylvania: MACK Publishing Company, 1985: 1585–602.

3
Flow: General Principles of Bulk Solids Handling

Thomas Baxter, Roger Barnum, and James K. Prescott
Jenike & Johanson, Inc., Tyngsboro, Massachusetts, U.S.A.

INTRODUCTION

The primary focus of this chapter is to provide guidance in designing bulk solids handling equipment to provide consistent, reliable "flow." The principles discussed in this chapter can be applied to analyzing new or existing equipment designs, as well as comparing different bulk solids using the various test methods discussed. The chapter will focus on the equipment used from the final blend step to the press/encapsulation machine/etc. (i.e., machine used to create the unit dose), though the technologies apply to almost any bulk solids handling process. The chapter is divided into six primary sections, including:

1. *Introduction*: A review of introductory concepts, such a defining "flowability."
2. *Common Bulk Solids Handling Equipment*: A description of the common handling equipment and the equipment parameters that affect flowability.
3. *Typical Flow Problems and Flow Patterns*: An assessment of common flow problems (e.g., no flow due to arching and ratholing, etc.) and the two primary flow patterns (mass flow vs. funnel flow).
4. *Measurement of Flow Properties*: A summary of the flow properties that need to be measured to obtain the equipment design parameters required for consistent, reliable flow.
5. *Factors that Affect Flow Properties*: An overview of the primary factors that affect the bulk solid flow properties.
6. *Basic Equipment Design Techniques for Reliable Flow*: A review of the basic design techniques for the blender-to-press equipment.

This chapter will provide a working knowledge of what flow properties need to be measured, how to measure them, and how to apply them to analyze or design handling equipment for reliable flow. Substantial portions of pharmaceutical processes include bulk solids handling, such as blending, transfer, storage, feeding, compaction, and fluidization. Therefore, a full understanding of bulk solids flow behavior is essential when designing new equipment or developing corrective actions for existing equipment. There are several instances where the robustness of a process is adversely affected by flow problems that develop. Common flow problems can have an adverse effect upon:

1. *Production costs* due to reduced production rates (e.g., tableting rate limitations, required operator intervention), restrictions on raw ingredient selection (e.g.,

percentage of lubrication used), method of manufacturing (wet granulation vs. dry granulation vs. direct compression), equipment selection (type of blender, bin, press) and overall yield.
2. *Product quality* due to variation of tablet properties (weight, hardness, etc.) or segregation/content uniformity concerns (discussed in another chapter but affected by flow).
3. *Time to market* due to delays in product/process development, validation, or failed commercial batches since flow problems may not occur until the process has been scaled-up.

Defining Flowability

A bulk solid is defined as a collection of discrete solid particles. A "powder" is an example of a fine bulk solid, and this term will be used predominantly throughout this chapter. The concepts discussed in this chapter apply to many types of bulk solids, whether fine or coarse, such as dust, granulations, and granules, either as a single substance or a multi-component blend.

A simple definition of "flowability" is the ability of a powder to flow through equipment reliably. By this definition, there is often a tendency to define flowability as a one-dimensional characteristic of a bulk solid ranked on a scale from "free-flowing" to "non-flowing." Unfortunately, a single parameter such as this is not sufficient in fully defining a bulk solid's handling characteristics or providing the design parameters required to fully address common handling concerns encountered by the formulator and equipment designer. Since bulk solids flow behavior is multi-dimensional, a full range of *flow properties* will need to be measured to fully characterize the bulk solid, as discussed in another section of this chapter. Flow properties are the specific bulk characteristics and properties of a powder that affect flow that can be measured.

In addition, the "flowability" of a bulk solid is a function of the bulk solids flow properties and the design parameters of the handling equipment. For example, "poor flowing" bulk solids can be handled reliably in properly designed equipment, and "good flowing" bulk solids may develop flow problems in improperly designed equipment. As such, a more accurate definition of flowability is the ability of powder to flow in a desired manner in a specific piece of equipment.

It is important that the flow properties of the bulk solid be measured in a way that has meaning with respect to the application so that *quantitative* and *scalable* design parameters can be obtained for developing new existing designs or for evaluating potential corrective actions for existing equipment. Flow property data, which refer to the powder alone, do not refer to specific equipment that may handle the powder, and therefore, should not be confused with flowability. The terms "powder flow" and "powder flow properties" should not be used synonymously since they define different characteristics. "Powder flow" is an observation and should refer to a description as to how material will (or did) flow in a given piece of equipment (e.g., the powder flow through the press hopper was consistent). The term "powder flow properties" should refer to test results of the powder (e.g., the loose density of the final blend is 0.6 g per cc). In discussing or reporting flowability, both the powder flow properties and the handling equipment must be included. This means that one must connect a measurement of the properties of the material to predicted behavior in specific equipment.

Therefore, this chapter focuses on flow properties that are measured on a bench-scale basis in a lab and the factors that may affect these flow properties such as particle

Flow: General Principles of Bulk Solids Handling

size, temperature, etc. In addition, the key process and equipment parameters that affect flowability, typical flow problems and patterns, and basic equipment design techniques are also reviewed.

COMMON BULK SOLIDS HANDLING EQUIPMENT

The primary objective of this section is to describe the common handling equipment used in pharmaceutical processes. In particular, we will review the following common handling equipment and process steps that may affect "flowability":

1. processing steps prior to final blending, such as milling, screening, drying and granulation;
2. final blending;
3. discharge from the final blender;
4. intermediate bulk containers (IBC, totes, bins);
5. transfer from the IBC to the press;
6. feed from the press hopper to the die cavity.

For each of these different process steps, we will review the key equipment parameters that affect the flowability of a bulk solid. These typical handling steps serve as good examples to illustrate the concerns with powder handling; but virtually any solids handling application analyzed the same way.

Processing Steps Prior to Final Blending

Understanding the physical properties of the raw ingredients (API, excipients) and how they affect the flowability of the final blend is crucial in selecting and designing equipment that reliably handles the final blend. Therefore, the preblending process steps and equipment parameters are often critical to the flowability of the final blend. There are several common preblending process steps that may affect the final blend's flowability, including:

- *Storage conditions of the raw ingredients* such as the temperature, relative humidity, and days stored at rest (inventory control) can all influence the flowability of the final blend, especially if any of the raw ingredients are hygroscopic.
- *Milling and screening steps* that alter the raw ingredients', and thus the final blend's, particle size, shape, and distribution. Therefore, milling and screening process parameters such as the mill type, mill speed, screen size, mill/screen feed method (controlled vs. non-controlled feed) may all have an influence on the flowability of the final blend, especially in a dry blending process.
- *Granulation* (dry roller compaction, wet granulation, fluid bed granulation) of the API together with select excipients can often have a positive effect on the flowability of the final blend, especially for blends with high active loadings. The granulation parameters, especially those that influence particle size/shape/distribution, will have a significant effect on flowability. For dry granulation (roller compaction), the process parameters that dictate the particle size distribution (PSD) and shape distribution of the final blend may include the roller compactor speed, roll compactor pressure, and the screen size. The wet granulation process parameters that affect PSD and shape, as well as the moisture content, are often critical to flowability. Therefore, wet granulation parameters such as the blade and impeller design/speed,

binder addition rate and method and end point determination (impeller load vs. set time) are critical to flowability. Similarly, the fluid bed granulation parameters that affect the moisture content and particle size, such as the binder addition rate/method, inlet air flow rate and temperature, drying time, end point determination (target moisture, powder temperature, exhaust air temperature), and fluidization behavior for the powder bed are all critical to flowability.

- *Preblending of selected raw materials,* such as preblending a cohesive bulk solids with a less cohesive bulk solid to reduce the likelihood of flow problems during subsequent handling steps.

The primary factors that affect the flowability of the final blend (or almost any powder), such as moisture content, particle shape/size/distribution, temperature/humidity and others, are discussed in more detail later in this chapter. Note that the measurement of flow properties and the design parameters they provide can also be applied to troubleshooting and developing corrective actions for flow problems in the preblending steps.

Final Blending

The effect of the final blend step upon the flowability of the blend is discussed below. For dry blending (tumble blending), the process parameters that affect the uniformity of the final blend (e.g., order of addition, fill level, number of rotations, etc.) can also effect the flowability of the blend, especially if it is an ordered blending process in which bonding between key ingredients is critical to the flowability. For example, if a glidant such as fumed silica is added, but is not effectively distributed among the other ingredients, the final blend may have poor flowability (e.g., higher cohesive strength). Also, an agitator may be used in a tumble blending process to reduce the likelihood of agglomeration, but could also result in a finer PSD if there are friable ingredients; a reduction in a blend's PSD may result in poorer flowability.

Discharge from a Blender or Processing Vessel

Powder that has been blended must be discharged from the blender for further processing. In many dry blending processes (tumble blending), the discharge is driven by gravity alone. As an example, the final blend step may be conducted in a V-blender or a double-cone blender. In these cases, the blender geometry often consists of a converging cross section to the outlet, through which the powder must be discharged reliably. In these cases, the blender is essentially acting as a "bin," so the equipment parameters that are crucial to a bin design, which are discussed in the following section, must be considered.

For fluid bed granulation processes, it is not uncommon for a conical hopper to be attached to the "bowl" of a fluid bed granulator, inverted, and discharged to a downstream process step via gravity. For wet granulators, the final blend may be discharged using mechanical agitation by continuing to operate the plow blade (typically at a lower speed) to discharge the final blend through a central or side outlet. Although the plow blade typically ensures that the blend discharged from the granulator "bowl" reliably, the transition equipment from the blender to the downstream process will be critical, especially if it is "flood-loaded" (non-metered gravity feed resulting in a full cross section) and has a converging cross section, such that it is essentially acting as a "bin."

When a blender/vessel is discharged manually (hand-scoping), flowability may not be a primary concern, but other factors (e.g., production rate concerns, operator exposure and safety) may limit the extent to which a blender/vessel can be manually unloaded.

Flow: General Principles of Bulk Solids Handling

Intermediate Bulk Containers

The flowability of the final blend is especially critical during storage and discharge from an IBC. The IBC may be a bin (tote) or even a drum that is used to store and transfer the final blend from the blender to the press. When a drum is used, an attachment such as a conical "hopper" may be attached to the cone to mate the drum to downstream equipment with a smaller inlet (e.g., press hopper). In both cases, the IBC consists of two primary sections (Fig. 1):

1. a *cylinder* or straight-sided section with a constant cross-sectional area that is often rectangular (with or without radiussed corners) or circular;
2. a *hopper* section with a changing cross-sectional area that is often a converging conical or pyramidal hopper.

IBCs are often used to store the blend, during which time the flowability may get worse as the blend is subjected to consolidation pressures due to its own weight during storage at rest. In addition, IBCs may be used to move the blend from one process step to another, during which time the blend may be subjected to vibration that may adversely affect flowability. Therefore, it is important to determine what consolidation pressures will act on the powder as it is stored and transferred in an IBC.

The key IBC equipment parameters with respect to flowability include:

- the cylinder cross-sectional area and height, which along with other parameters such as the fill height, will affect the consolidation pressure acting on the blend;

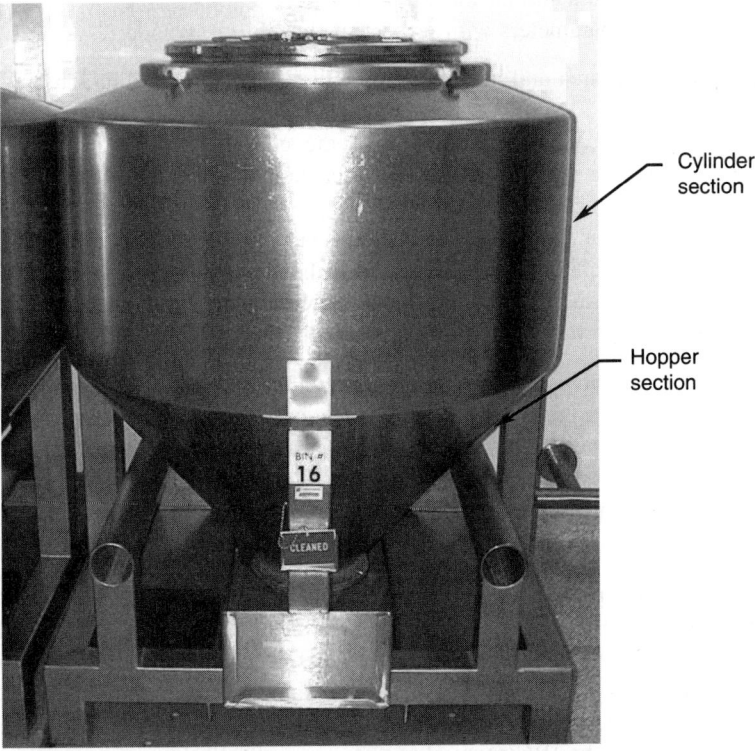

FIGURE 1 Intermediate bulk container (IBC, bin, tote).

- the hopper geometry (planar vs. circular) and angles, which will affect the flow pattern that develops during discharge;
- the interior surface finish of the hopper section, which will affect the flow pattern that develops during discharge;
- the IBC outlet size and shape (slotted vs. circular), which will affect whether the blend will discharge reliably without arching or ratholing;
- general flow impediments such as upward facing ledges or partially opened valves that may act as flow obstructions.

The measurement of the flow properties that are used to obtain the key IBC design parameters are discussed later in this chapter. The application of these design parameters to provide reliable flow from an IBC is discussed later in this chapter.

Transfer from IBCs to the Press

The flowability of the final blend is also critical during transfer from the IBC to the press/encapsulation machine/etc. This transfer step may be a manual transfer (hand-scooping), in which case flowability may not be a primary concern. The transfer step may also be conducted via pneumatic conveying, in which case the flowability of the blend may not be a primary concern, but equipment and material parameters affecting conveying (conveying gas pressure and flow rate, conveying line diameter and layout, etc.) need to be considered.

The transfer step may also be conducted via gravity transfer via a single or bifurcated chute (Fig. 2), depending on the press configuration. Since these chutes are often operated in a flood-loaded manner (full cross section) and may consist of converging sections where the cross-sectional area of the chute is reduced, they often need to be designed for reliable flow in a similar manner as the IBCs.

The key transfer chute parameters with respect to flowability include:

1. The chute cross-sectional area and height, which will effect the consolidation pressure acting on the blend.
2. For converging and non-converging sections of the chute, the chute geometry, angles, and interior surface finish, which will affect the flow pattern that develops during discharge through the chute.
3. For converging sections of the chute, the outlet shape and size that will affect whether the blend will discharge reliably without arching or ratholing.
4. General flow impediments such as upward facing ledges (mismatched flanges), sight glasses, level probes, or partially opened valves that may act as flow obstructions.

The measurement of the flow properties that are used to obtain the key chute design parameters are discussed later in this chapter. The application of these design parameters to provide reliable flow from the IBC to the press is discussed later in this chapter.

Feed from the Press Hopper to the Die Cavity

Once the final blend has been transferred to the press hopper reliably, it is important to ensure that press hopper also provides reliable flow. Most modern presses consist of a small press hopper that is, in essence, a miniature IBC designed to provide a small amount of surge capacity. The press hopper often consists of a cylinder section and a hopper section similar to a larger IBC, but the hopper section may be asymmetric (Fig. 3) as opposed to the symmetric hopper designs commonly used for IBCs. The press hopper is typically flood-loaded from the IBC/chute above via gravity feed. However, in some instances, the material level in the press hopper may be controlled via a feeder at the IBC

Flow: General Principles of Bulk Solids Handling

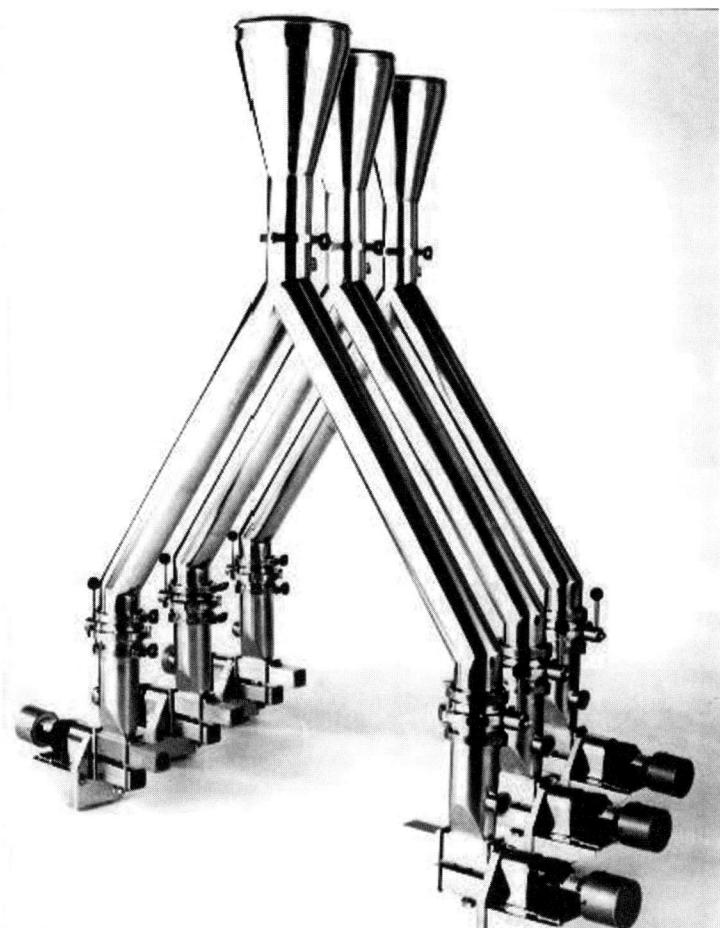

FIGURE 2 Bifurcated press feed chute.

outlet (e.g., rotary valve or screw feeder). Some modern presses do not have press hoppers with a converging hopper, but instead consist of vertical, non-converging chutes from the press inlet to the feed frame inlet.

The key equipment parameters with respect to flowability, which are outlined in the preceding section for IBCs/bins, are also applicable to the press hopper. It is worth noting that since the press hopper outlets are often much smaller than an IBC outlet, flow problems such as arching or ratholing may be more pronounced. As a result, press hoppers may also included mechanical agitators used to assist gravity discharge, such as a rotating agitator mounted to a vertical shaft.

The same design parameters used for a reliable IBC design can also be used to design a press hopper.

TYPICAL FLOW PROBLEMS AND FLOW PATTERNS

Flow Problems

A number of problems can develop as powder flows through equipment such as bins, chutes, and press hoppers. If the powder is cohesive, an arch or rathole may form. Erratic

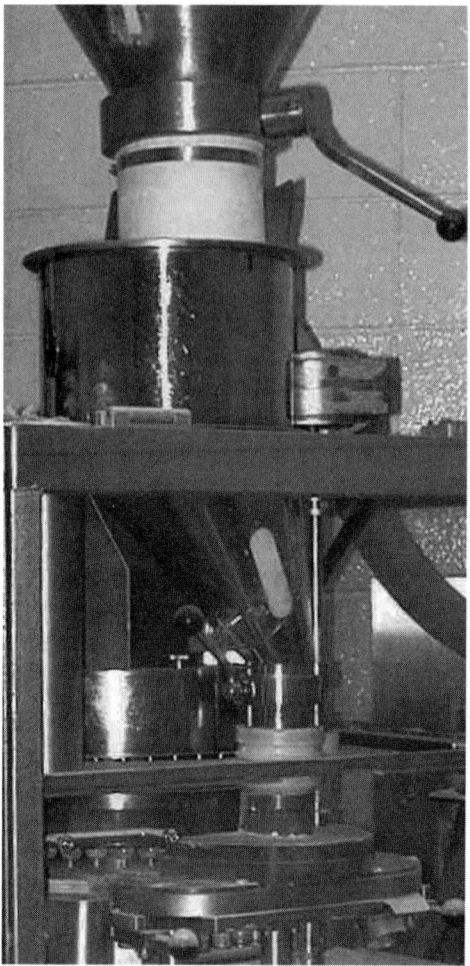

FIGURE 3 Asymmetric press feed hopper.

flow can result, while "flooding" (the aerated powder "flushes" through an opening in a liquid-like manner) or uncontrolled discharge may occur if a rathole spontaneously collapses. On the other hand, a deaerated bed of fine powder may experience flow rate limitations or no-flow conditions. Each of these flow problems is discussed in more detail below.

No-flow from a bin/hopper is a common and significant solids handling problem. In production, it can result in problems such as starving downstream equipment, production delays, and the requirement for frequent operator intervention to reinitiate flow. No-flow can be due to either arching (sometime referred to as "bridging" or "plugging") or ratholing.

Arching occurs when an obstruction in the shape of an arch or a bridge forms above the bin outlet and prevents any further material discharge. It can be an interlocking arch, where the particles mechanically lock to form the obstruction, or a cohesive arch. An interlocking arch occurs when the particles are large compared to the outlet size of the hopper. A cohesive arch occurs when particles pack together to form an obstruction (Fig. 4). Both of these problems are strongly influenced by the outlet size of the hopper the material is being fed through. Material properties will govern the occurrence of these

Flow: General Principles of Bulk Solids Handling

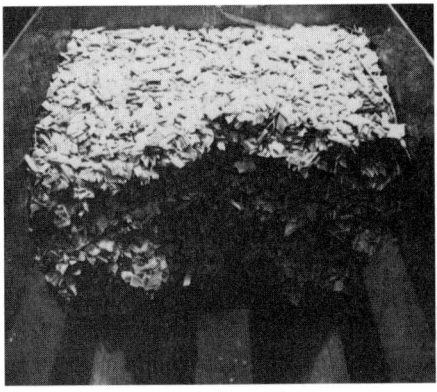 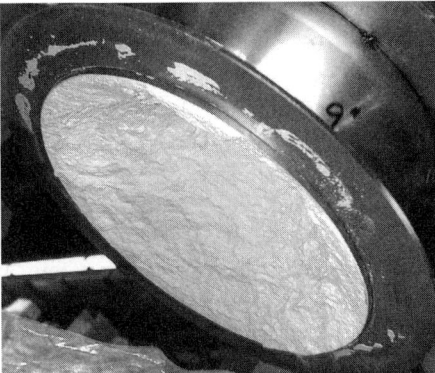

Interlocking arch   Cohesive arch

FIGURE 4 Examples of arching.

problems as well. In particular, the amount of cohesive strength a powder has will dictate what size outlet it can arch over.

Ratholing can occur in a bin when a flow channel though stationary material empties, leaving a hole through the material. Ratholing is influenced by the hopper geometry and outlet size the material is being fed through. Similar to the problem of arching, this problem will arise if the material has sufficient cohesive strength. In this case, no more of the material will discharge once the flow channel empties (Fig. 5).

Erratic flow is the result of obstructions alternating between an arch and a rathole. A rathole may collapse due to an external force, such as vibrations created by surrounding equipment, or a flow-aid device such as an external vibrator. While some material is likely to discharge, falling material often impacts over the outlet and forms an arch. An arch may break due to a similar external force, and material flow may resume until the flow channel is emptied and a rathole is formed again.

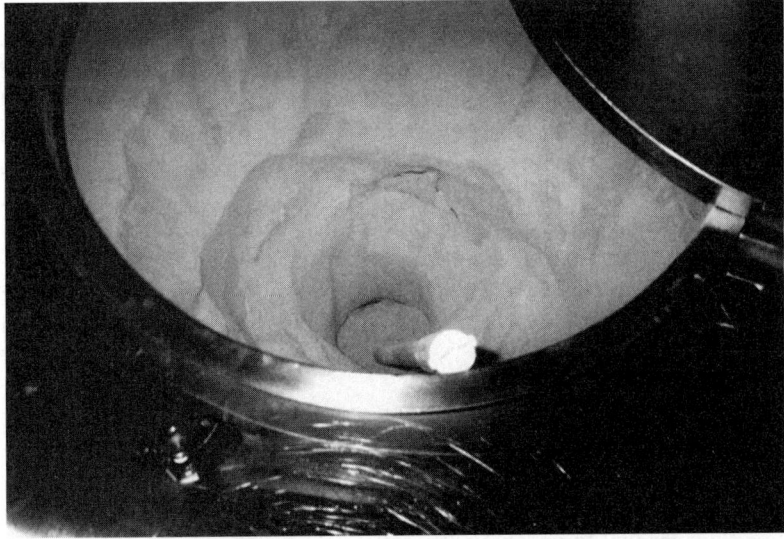

FIGURE 5 Example of ratholing.

Additional flow concerns can arise when handling *fine powders*, generally in the range below 100 μm in average particle size. These concerns are due to the interaction of the material with entrained air or gas, which becomes significant in describing the behavior of the material, bringing about two-phase (bulk solid: interstitial gas) flow effects. There are three modes that can occur when handling fine powders that are susceptible to two-phase flow effects: steady flow, flooding, and a flow rate limitation (2). These three flow modes are discussed in more detail below.

Steady flow will occur with fine powders if the target flow rate (feed rate through the system) is below the "critical flow rate" that occurs when the solids stress is balanced by the air pressure at the outlet. The target flow rate is often controlled by a feeder, such as at the inlet to a compression machine (press feed frame). The critical flow rate, and the flow properties tests used to determine it, is described in more later in this chapter. At target flow rates exceeding the critical flow rate, unsteady flow can occur by two different modes described below.

Flooding is an unsteady two-phase flow mode that can occur as falling particles entrain air and become fluidized. Since powder handling equipment often cannot contain fluids, material can flood through the equipment (feeders, seals) uncontrollably. Flooding can also occur when handling fine powders in small hoppers with high fill and discharge rates. In such situations, the powder does not have sufficient residence time to deaerate, resulting in flooding through the feeder.

A *flow rate limitation* is another unsteady two-phase flow mode that can occur with fine powders. Fine powders have very low permeability, and are affected by any movement of the interstitial air (air between the particles). This air movement will occur due to the natural compression and dilation of the powder bed that takes place as it flows through the cylindrical and hopper geometries; as the material is compressed in the cylinder air is squeezed out, while when it dilates as it flows through the outlet, additional air must be drawn in. The air pressure gradients caused as a result of this air movement can retard discharge from a hopper, significantly limiting the maximum achievable rates.

During unsteady two-phase flow modes, the material's bulk density can undergo dramatic variations, negatively impacting downstream packaging or processing operations. Problems can result such as excessive tablet weight variations, a required reduction in filling speeds, and even segregation (discussed in Chapter 4 of this book). Equipment and process parameters will govern whether such problems occur and are further discussed later in this chapter. These parameters include hopper geometry and outlet size, applied vacuum and other sources of air pressure differences (such as dust collection systems), material level, time since filling, and of course the target feed rate. Material properties such as permeability and compressibility will also play important roles, as will variations in the material's state of aeration that can occur based on its residence time or degree of compaction from external forces and handling.

One of the most important factors in determining whether a powder will discharge reliably from a hopper is establishing what flow pattern will develop, which is discussed below.

Flow Patterns

Two flow patterns can develop in a bin or hopper: *funnel* and *mass flow*. In funnel flow (Fig. 6), an active flow channel forms above the outlet, which is surrounded by stagnant material. This is a first-in, last-out flow sequence. It generally occurs in equipment with

Flow: General Principles of Bulk Solids Handling

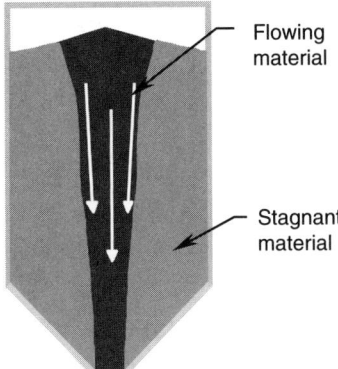

FIGURE 6 Funnel flow schematic.

relatively shallow hoppers. Common examples of funnel flow bins are shown in the accompanying photographs (Fig. 7), and include hopper geometries such as asymmetric cones and rectangular-to-round transitions (which are pyramidal in shape). As the level of powder decreases in funnel flow, stagnant powder may fall into the flow channel if the material is sufficiently free flowing. If the powder is cohesive, a stable rathole may develop. Funnel flow occurs if the powder is unable to flow along the hopper walls, due to the combination of friction against the walls and hopper angle.

In *mass flow* (Fig. 8), all of the powder is in motion whenever any is withdrawn. Powder flow occurs throughout the bin, including at the hopper walls. Mass flow provides a first-in first-out flow sequence, eliminates stagnant powder, provides a steady discharge with a consistent bulk density, and provides a flow that is uniform and well-controlled. Ratholing will not occur in mass flow, as all of the material is in motion.

Requirements for achieving mass flow include sizing the outlet large enough to prevent arch formation, and ensuring the hopper walls are steep and smooth enough to allow the powder to flow along them. An important distinction must be made regarding the occurrence mass flow, as it describes a relationship between a given powder and a given hopper geometry, including the interior surface finish of that hopper. Several flow properties are relevant to making such predictions, which are described in the following section of this chapter.

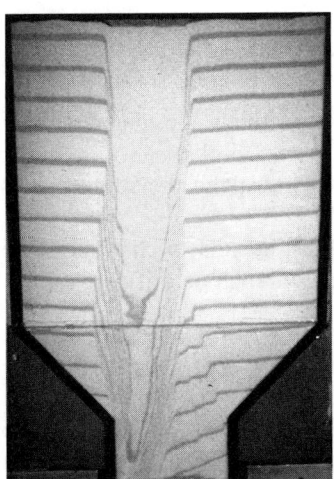 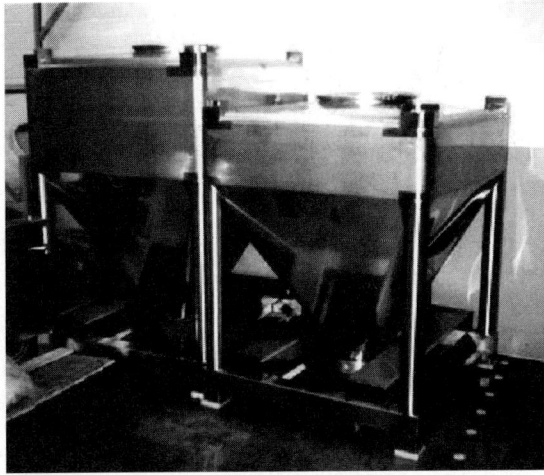

FIGURE 7 Examples of funnel flow bins.

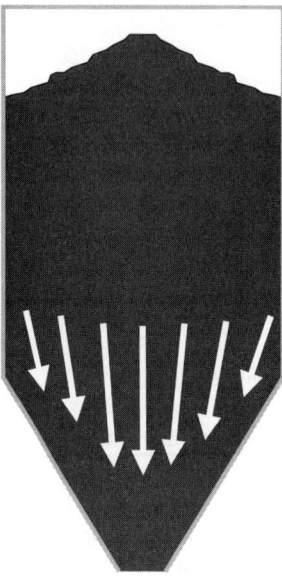

FIGURE 8 Mass flow schematic.

MEASUREMENT OF FLOW PROPERTIES

The primary objective of this section is to provide a description of the *quantitative* flow properties that should be measured and the calculation of equipment parameters required for consistent, reliable flow in handling equipment for gravity discharge. This section will address the question "which test method(s) should I use to predict the flow behavior that will occur in my application?"

This section will review the following primary topics:

1. *Introductory concepts*: A review of the differences between fluids and bulk solids.
2. *Cohesive strength tests*: A review of different shear test methods, the Jenike Direct Shear Test method, and the calculation of the design parameters to prevent arching and ratholing.
3. *Wall friction tests*: A review of the Jenike Direct Shear Test method for measuring wall friction and the calculation of the design parameters to provide mass flow (mass flow hopper angles).
4. *Bulk density test*: A review of different bulk density test methods, the compressibility test method, and the application of the compressibility test results.
5. *Permeability*: A review of the permeability test method and application of the results (critical flow rate).
6. *Additional test methods*: A brief review of additional test methods such as the angle of repose, Hausner ratio and Carr Index, and flow rate through an orifice.

Introductory Concepts: Bulk Solids vs. Liquids

Prior to beginning the discussion of the measurement of flow properties, it is beneficial to review how bulk solids are different than liquids. Since one of our primary concerns with bulk solids handling is "flow," a term that is commonly associated with liquids, it is often assumed that the principles of fluid mechanics may be used to describe the behavior of

Flow: General Principles of Bulk Solids Handling

bulk solids. In fact, this is not the case. Bulk solids cannot be described using fluid mechanics principles, since bulk solids differ from fluid in several key ways (1):

- Bulk solids can transfer shear stresses while at rest and have a static angle of friction greater than zero, but liquids do not.
- Bulk solids possess cohesive strength when consolidated and can retain a shape under loading, unlike liquids.
- The shear stress that occurs in a deforming (i.e., flowing) bulk solid is dependent upon the major consolidating stresses (pressures) acting on the bulk solid but independent of the rate of shear. Conversely, for a liquid, generally the shear stress is dependent upon the rate of shear and independent of the major consolidating pressure.

Therefore, when Jenike developed his methods to mathematically model the flow of bulk solids, he concluded that a bulk solid must be modeled as a plastic, and not a visco-elastic, continuum of solid particles (1). This approach included the postulation of a "flow–no-flow" criterion that states the bulk solid would flow from a bin when the *stresses* applied to the bulk solid exceed the *strength* of the bulk solid. The terms stress and strength are further discussed in this section on cohesive strength tests below. The flow properties test methods discussed are used to obtain the equipment parameters required to provide consistent, reliable flow.

Cohesive Strength Tests: Preventing Arching and Ratholing

Test Methods

One of the primary flow problems that can develop is a "no-flow" obstruction due to the formation of a cohesive arch or rathole. The required outlet size to prevent a stable cohesive arch or rathole from forming is determined from the results of a cohesive strength test by applying the "flow–no-flow" criterion. In order to apply the "flow–no-flow" criterion we need to determine:

1. The cohesive *strength* of the material as a function of the major consolidation pressure acting on the material, since the consolidation pressure acting on the bulk solid changes throughout the bin height. The cohesive strength can be measured as a function of major consolidating pressure using the test methods described in this section.
2. The *stresses* acting on the material acting to induce flow, e.g., gravity pulling downwards on a potential arch that may form. The stresses acting on the bulk solid can be determined using mathematical models (1).

To further illustrate the concepts of *strength* and *consolidation pressure*, consider an "idealized" strength test, as shown in Figure 9. In this idealized test, the cohesive strength of the bulk solid is measured in two distinct steps:

1. *Consolidation of the bulk solid*: The bulk solid is consolidated using a prescribed consolidation pressure (P). In the idealized test shown, the sample is contained in a frictionless cylinder and the consolidation pressure is applied from the top.
2. *Fracture of the bulk solid*: Once the consolidation pressure is applied, the cylinder containing the bulk solid would be removed in some manner without disturbing the sample (middle step shown Fig. 9), so that the strength of the bulk solid can be measured. A pressure would then be applied until the bulk solid fails or fractures. The applied pressure at which the bulk solid failed is referred to as the *unconfined yield strength* (F) (cohesive strength). This idealized test could be repeated several

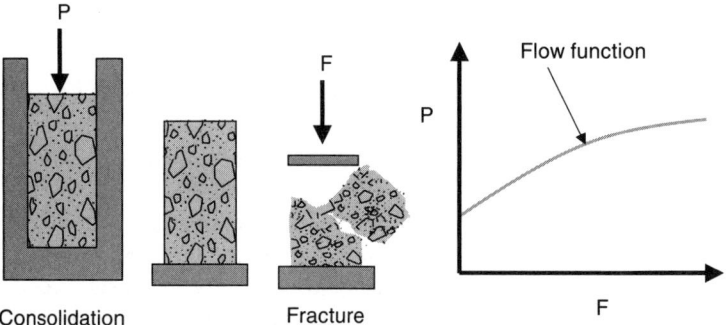

FIGURE 9 Schematic of "idealized" strength test.

times to develop a "flow function," which is a curve illustrating the relationship between the unconfined yield strength (F) and the major consolidation pressure (P).

Since this idealized strength test is not possible for the broad range of bulk solids that might be tested, several different cohesive strength test methods have been developed, and their respective strengths and weaknesses have been assessed (3,4). Although many different test methods can be used to measure cohesive strength, this section focuses specifically upon the Jenike direct shear test method since it is the most universally accepted method. The Jenike direct shear test method is described in ASTM standard D 6128 (5). It is important that these tests be conducted at representative handling conditions such as temperature, relative humidity, and storage at rest, since all these factors can affect the cohesive strength. An arrangement of a cell used for the Jenike direct shear test is shown in Figure 10. The details of this method are provided in Ref. 1, including the generation of a Mohr's circle to plot the shear stress (τ) versus the consolidation pressure (σ), the generation of the effective yield locus, and the generation of a flow function.

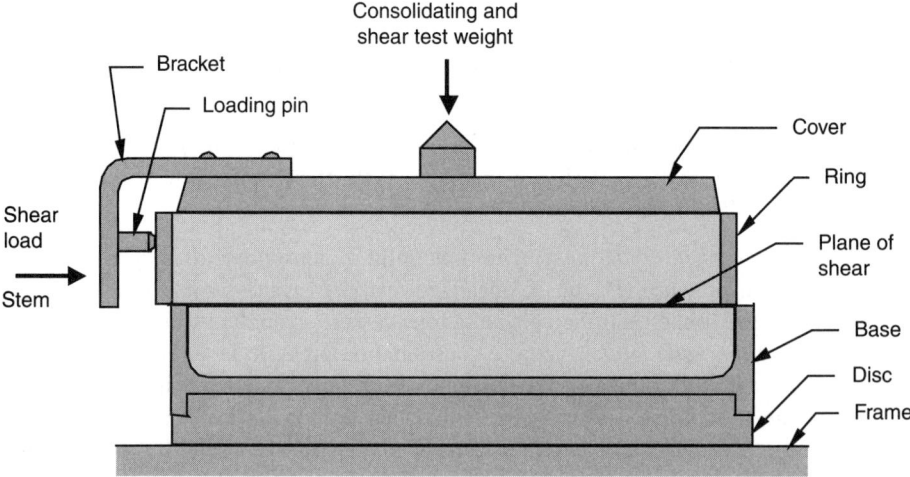

FIGURE 10 Jenike direst shear test, cohesive strength test set-up.

Flow: General Principles of Bulk Solids Handling

The data generated experimentally from the Jenike direct shear test can be used to determine the following derived parameters:

1. The flow function that describes the cohesive strength (unconfined yield strength, F_c) of the powder as a function of the major consolidating pressure (σ_1). The flow function is one of the parameters used to calculate the minimum outlet diameter/width for bins, press hoppers, blender outlets, etc. to prevent arching and ratholing. The calculation of the minimum outlet diameter/width is discussed in more detail below.
2. The effective angle of internal friction (δ) that is also used to calculate the minimum outlet to prevent arching and the required hopper angles for mass flow (described in the following section).
3. The static angle of internal friction (ϕ_1), which is used to calculate the minimum outlet to prevent ratholing (described in the following section).

Other testing methods exist that utilize the same principles of consolidation and shearing to determine the cohesive strength of a bulk powder. Annular (ring) shear testers produce rotational displacement between cell halves containing material, rather than a lateral displacement. Because of the unlimited travel that can be achieved with this type of test cell, the loading and shearing operations are more readily adapted to automation. The successful use of this test method to measure cohesive strength (generate a flow function), as relating to handling characteristics, has been discussed in the industry (6–9).

Calculation of Minimum Required Outlet Dimensions to Prevent Arching (Mass Flow Bin)

The flow behavior of bulk solids through bins and hoppers can be predicted by a complete mathematical relationship. If gravity discharge is used, the minimum outlet size that is required to prevent arching is dependent upon the flow pattern that occurs. Regardless of the flow pattern, the outlet size required to prevent a cohesive arch or rathole from forming can be calculated. This section focuses on calculating the minimum outlet dimension for a bin with a circular outlet or a slotted outlet. For a circular outlet, the minimum outlet diameter (B_c) is used to size the outlet to prevent a cohesive arch from forming in mass flow. For a slotted outlet, in which the length:width ratio exceeds 3:1, the minimum outlet width (B_p) is used to size the outlet to prevent arching in mass flow. Since the majority of bins used in pharmaceutical process utilize hoppers with circular outlets, we will focus our discussion on the calculation of the B_c parameter. It is worth noting that the required outlet width (B_p) will typically be approximately 1/2 of the B_c, and the calculation of B_p is provided in Ref. 1.

For mass flow, the required minimum outlet diameter to prevent arching (B_c) is calculated as:

$$B_c = H(\theta')f_{crit}/\gamma \qquad (1)$$

where $H(\theta')$ is a dimensionless function derived from first principles and is given by Figure 11, and the complete derivation of $H(\theta')$ is beyond the scope of this chapter but is provided in Ref. 1. The parameter f_{crit} (units of force/area) is the unconfined yield strength at the intersection of the hopper "flow factor" and the experimentally derived flow function, as shown in Figure 12. The flow factor is a mathematically determined value that represents the minimum available stress available to break an arch. The calculation of the flow factor is also beyond the scope of this chapter, but is provided in Ref. 1 and is a function of the flow properties and the hopper angle (θ'). "Gamma" (γ) is

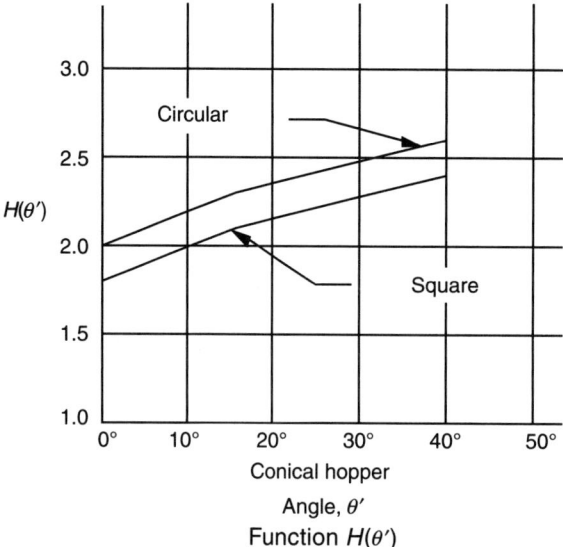

FIGURE 11 Plot of derived function $H(\theta')$ used to calculate arching dimensions for mass flow bins.

the bulk density (units of mass/volume). Therefore, Figure 12 is the visual representation of the "flow–no-flow" criterion with the *strength* of the powder represented by the flow function and the *stress* available to fail an arch represented by the flow factor. The bulk density (γ), with units of weight/volume, is the bulk density determined by compressibility tests described in a following section. This calculation yields a dimensional value of B_c in units of length, which is *scale-independent*. Therefore, for a mass flow bin, the opening size required to prevent arching is not a function of the diameter of the bin, height of the bin, or the height-to-diameter ratio.

As a formulation is developed, a cohesive strength test can be conducted early in the development process to determine the cohesive strength (flow function). This material-dependent flow function, in conjunction with Equation (1), will yield a minimum opening (outlet) size in order to avoid arching in a mass flow bin. For example, this opening size may be calculated to be 8 inches. This 8-inch diameter will be required whether the bin holds 10 kg or 1000 kg of powder and is scale-independent. In this example, since an 8-inch diameter opening is required, feeding this material through a

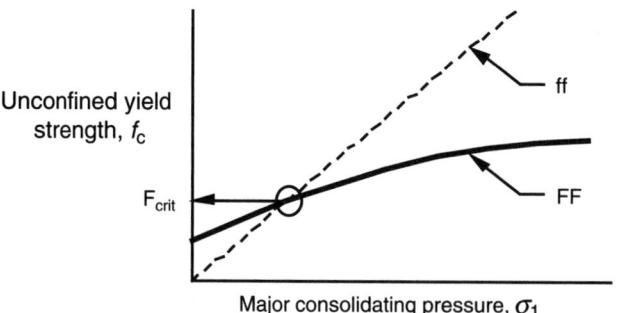

FIGURE 12 Example of flow function and flow factor intersection, showing F_{crit} at their intersection. *Abbreviations*: FF, flow function; ff, flow factor.

press hopper or similarly small openings would pose problems with an arch developing over the outlet. This information could then be used early in the development process to consider reformulating the product to reduce the cohesive strength and improve flowability.

Calculation of Minimum Required Outlet Dimensions to Prevent Ratholing (Funnel Flow Bin)

If the bin discharges in funnel flow, the bin outlet diameter should be sized to be larger than the *critical rathole diameter* (D_f) to prevent a stable rathole from forming over the outlet. For a funnel flow bin with a circular outlet, sizing the outlet diameter to exceed the D_f will also ensure that a stable arch will not form (since a rathole is inherently stronger than an arch). The D_f value is calculated in Equation (2), and additional details of the calculation are provided in Ref. 1.

$$D_f = G(\phi_t) f_c(\sigma_1)/\gamma \qquad (2)$$

where $G(\phi_t)$ is also a mathematically derived function from first principles and is given by Figure 13. The $f_c \sigma_1$ parameter, the unconfined yield strength of the material, is determined by the flow function at the actual consolidating pressure σ_1. The consolidation pressure σ_1 is a function of the head or height of powder above the outlet of the bin, as derived by Janssen (16), and calculated as:

$$\sigma_1 = (\gamma R/\mu k)(1 - e^{(-\mu k h/R)}) \qquad (3)$$

where R is the hydraulic radius (area/perimeter), μ is the coefficient of friction (μ = tangent ϕ'; ϕ' is determined from the wall friction test discussed in the next section), k is the ratio of horizontal to vertical pressures (often, 0.4 is used for a straight sided section), and h is the depth of the bed of powder within the bin. This relationship in Equation (2) cannot be reduced further (e.g., to a dimensionless ratio), as the function $f_c(\sigma_1)$ is highly material dependent.

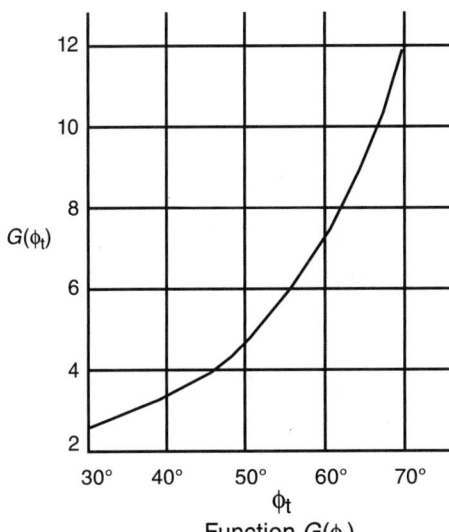

FIGURE 13 Plot of derived function $G(\phi_t)$ used to calculate critical rathole diameter for funnel flow bins.

The application of these parameters (B_c, D_f) to design new equipment or develop corrective equipment modifications is further discussed later in this chapter.

Wall Friction

Test Method

The wall friction test is crucial in determining whether a given bin will discharge in mass flow or funnel flow. Used in a continuum model developed by Jenike (1), wall friction (caused by particles sliding along a surface) is expressed as the wall friction angle (ϕ') or coefficient of sliding friction (μ = tangent ϕ'). The lower the coefficient of sliding friction, the shallower the hopper or chute walls need to be for powder to flow along them. This coefficient of friction can be measured by shearing a sample of powder in a test cell across a stationary wall surface using a Jenike direct shear tester (1,5). One arrangement of a cell used for the wall friction test is shown in Figure 14. In this case, a coupon of the wall material being evaluated is held in place on the frame of the tester, with a cell of powder placed above. The coefficient of sliding friction is the ratio of the shear force required for sliding to the normal force applied perpendicular to the wall material coupon. A plot of the measured shear force as a function of the applied normal pressure (σ_n) generates a relationship known as the *wall yield locus* (Fig. 15).

This flow property is a function of the powder handled and the wall surface in contact with it, as further discussed later in this chapter. Variations in the bulk solid, handling conditions (e.g., temperature/RH), and/or the wall surface finish (including orientation of directional finishes) can have a dramatic effect on the resulting friction coefficient (10). The results of the wall friction test are used to determine the hopper angles required to achieve mass flow, as discussed in the following section.

Calculation of Recommended Mass Flow Hopper Angles

Design charts (1) have been developed to determine which flow pattern is be expected to occur using inputs such as the hopper angle (θ_c or θ_p, as measured from vertical), wall friction angle (ϕ') and internal friction (δ) of the material being handled. Our focus will be on the calculation of the recommended mass hopper angles for a conical hopper (θ_c)

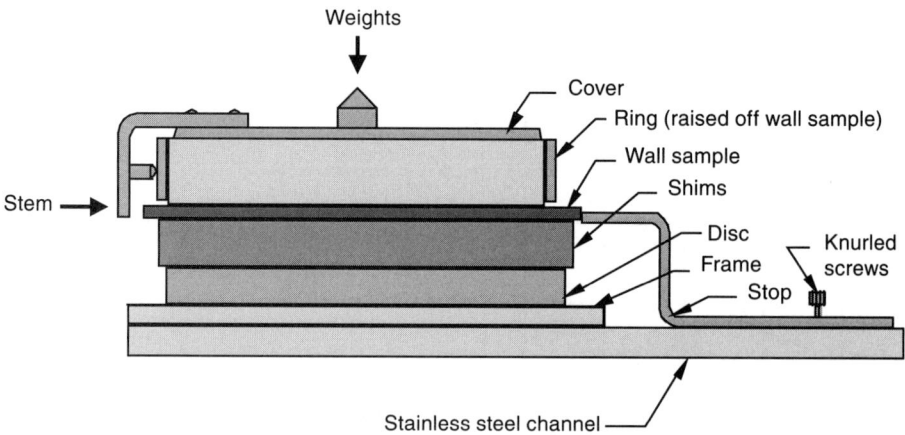

FIGURE 14 Jenike direct shear test, wall friction test set-up.

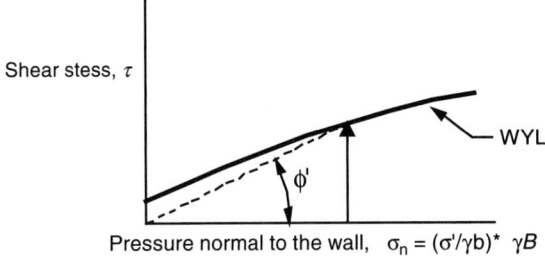

FIGURE 15 Example of wall yield locus generated from wall friction test data.

since the majority of pharmaceutical process utilize bins with a conical hopper, but the methods to calculate the recommended mass hopper angles for a planer hopper (θ_p) with a slotted outlet are similar in approach and are outlined in Ref. 1. It is worth noting that the recommended mass flow angles for planer hopper walls (θ_p) can often be 8° to 12° shallower than (θ_c) for the same sized opening.

An example of such a design chart for a conical hopper is shown in Figure 16. Note that, for illustration, the design chart shown is specifically for a bulk solid with an effective angle of internal friction (δ) of 40° and that the design charts will be different for different values of δ. Hopper angles required for mass flow are a function of δ, since flow along converging hopper walls involves inter-particle motion of the bulk solid (and the effective angle of internal friction is used to characterize the degree of resistance to this motion). For any combination of ϕ' and θ_c that lies in the mass flow region, mass flow is expected to occur. If the combination lies in the funnel flow region, funnel flow is expected. The uncertain region is an area where mass flow is expected to occur based on theory, but represents a 4° margin of safety on the design, to account for inevitable variations in test results and surface finish. As an example of using the design chart, if a hopper with a conical hopper angle (θ_c) of 20° is used and the measured wall friction angle at the outlet size being considered is 35°, the bin would be expected to discharge in funnel flow. In that case, the designer would need to find another wall surface with a lower wall friction angle of 20° to ensure mass flow discharge.

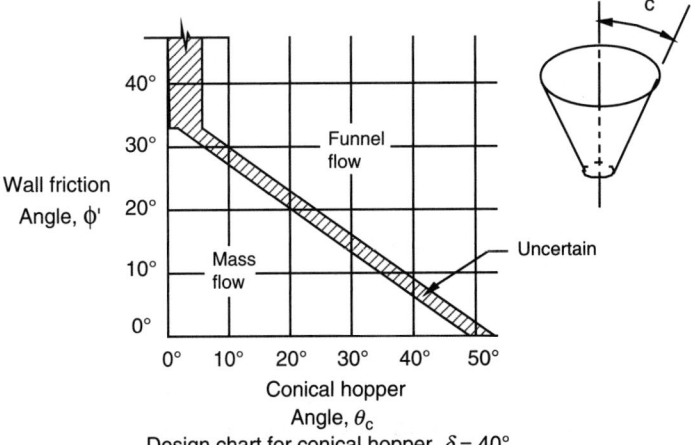

FIGURE 16 Mass flow/funnel flow design chart for conical hopper handling a bulk solid with an effective angle of internal friction (δ) of 40°.

The wall friction angle ϕ' is determined by the wall friction tests described above. With respect to choosing the appropriate value of ϕ' to use for the hopper design charts, it is important to note that ϕ' is a function of the normal pressure (σ_n) against the surface. For many combinations of wall surfaces and powders, the wall friction angle changes depending on the normal pressure. When mass flow develops, the solids pressure normal to the wall surface is given by the following relationship:

$$\sigma_n = (\sigma'/\gamma b)^* \gamma B \tag{4}$$

Ref. 1 provides charts giving values for the ($\sigma'/\gamma b$) term. Assuming ($\sigma'/\gamma b$) and the bulk density γ are constant for a given powder and hopper (a reasonable assumption for a first approximation), the pressure normal to the wall is simply a linear function of the span of the hopper, B, at any given point. Generally, ϕ' increases with decreasing normal pressure (σ_n). Therefore, the critical point is at the outlet of the hopper where the span (B) is smallest, with the correspondingly lowest normal pressure to the wall (σ_n). Therefore, it is at the outlet where the wall friction angle (ϕ') is the highest for a given design, provided the hopper interior surface-finish and angle remain constant above the outlet.

When considering scale effects, the implication of the above analysis is that the hopper angle required for mass flow is principally dependent on the outlet size selected for the hopper under consideration. Note that the hopper angle required for mass flow is not a function of the flow rate, the level of powder within the bin, or the diameter or height of the bin. However, and as previously noted, hopper angles are a function of the effective angle of internal friction (δ) for the powder itself. Since the wall friction angle generally increases with lower normal pressures, a steeper hopper is often required to achieve mass flow for a bin with a smaller outlet. For example, assume that a specific powder discharges in mass flow from a bin with a certain outlet size. A second bin with an equal or larger outlet size will also discharge in a mass flow pattern for this powder, provided that the second bin has an identical hopper angle and surface finish. This is true regardless of the actual size of either bin, since only the outlet size needs to be considered. Conversely, if the same hopper angle was used for a bin with a smaller outlet, it may not necessarily discharge in mass flow. It should also be noted that mass flow is highly dependent upon conditions below the hopper. Therefore, a throttled valve, a lip or other protrusion, or anything which can initiate a zone of stagnant powder can convert any hopper into funnel flow, regardless of the hopper angle or surface finish.

The application of these design parameters (θ_c, θ_p) to design new equipment or develop corrective equipment modifications is further discussed later in this chapter.

Bulk Density

The bulk density of a given powder is not a single or even a dual value, but varies as a function of the consolidating pressure applied to it. There are various methods used in industry to measure bulk density, utilizing different sized containers that are measured for volume after being loosely filled with a known mass of material ("loose" density) and after vibration or tapping (tapped density), such as the USP <616> method (11). While such methods can offer some repeatability with respect to the conditions under which measurements are taken, they do not necessarily represent the actual compaction behavior a bulk solid being handled in a bin, chute or press hopper.

To more fully assess the variation in bulk density, it can be measured as a function of the applied consolidation pressure via a compressibility test (1,12). The results of the compressibility test can often be plotted as a straight line on a log–log plot (Fig. 17). In bulk solids literature, the slope of this line is typically called the "compressibility" of the bulk solid.

The resulting data can be used to determine capacities for storage and transfer equipment and evaluate wall friction and feeder operation requirements. As an example, when estimating the capacity of a bin, the bulk density based upon the average major consolidation pressure in the bin can be used. For the calculation of the arching dimensions (B_c) and recommended mass flow hopper angles (θ_c), the bulk density based for the major consolidation pressure at the bin outlet can be used.

Permeability

The flow problems that can occur due to adverse two-phase (bulk solid and interstitial gas) were reviewed previously. These problems were more likely to occur when the target feed rate (tableting rate) exceeds the "critical flow rate." The results of the permeability test are one of the primary flow properties used to determine the critical flow rate. The permeability of a bulk solid is a measurement of how readily gas can pass through it. The permeability will have a controlling effect on the discharge rate that can be achieved from a bin/hopper with a given outlet size. Sizing the outlet of a piece of equipment, or choosing the diameter of a transfer chute, should take into consideration the target feed rate.

Permeability is measured as a function of bulk density (12). A schematic of the permeability tests is provided in Figure 18. In this test set-up, gas is injected at the bottom of the test cell through a permeable membrane and the pressure drop and flow rate across the bulk solid are measured. The method involves measuring the flow rate of air at a predetermined pressure drop through a sample of known density and height. The permeability is then calculated using Darcy's law. The permeability of a bulk solid typically decreases as the bulk density increases, so the test is conducted over a range of bulk densities. Once permeability/bulk density relationship is determined (an example is shown in Fig. 19), it can be used to calculate the critical flow rates that will be achieved for steady flow conditions though various orifice sizes. The details of calculating critical flow rates (which are dependent upon bin geometry, outlet size, and consolidation

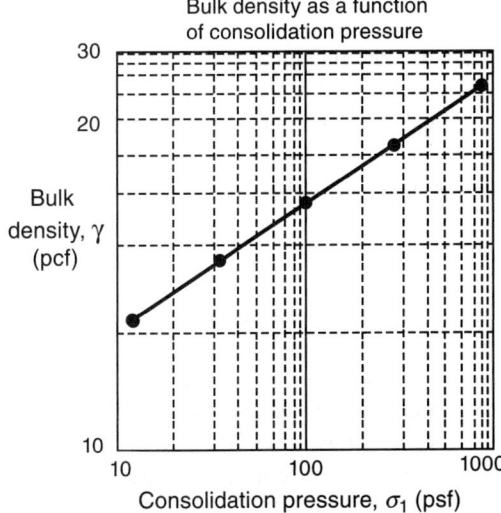

FIGURE 17 Example of bulk density versus consolidation pressure plot from compressibility test data.

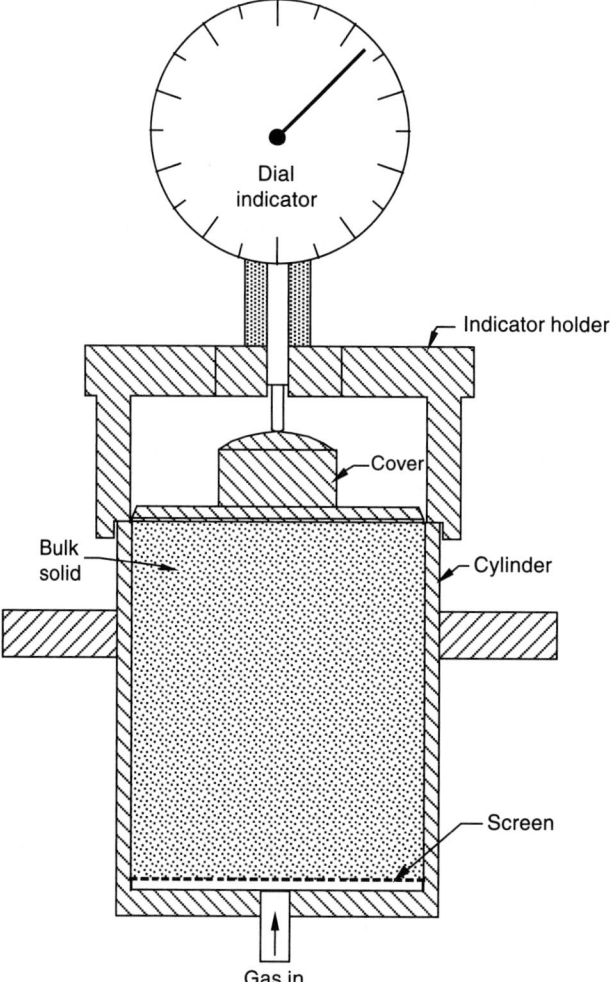

FIGURE 18 Schematic of permeability test set-up.

pressure) are outside the scope of this chapter, but mathematical models have been developed for these calculations.

Higher flow rates than the calculated critical flow rate may occur, but can result in non-steady or erratic feed and the resulting adverse effects. Permeability values can also be used to calculate the time required for fine powders to settle or deaerate in equipment.

Additional Test Methods

There are instances where a *qualitative* test for comparative or quality control (QC) purposes may be desired and the *quantitative* test methods used for equipment design or analysis purposes described in the preceding sections are not essential for the flow concerns being assessed. These non-scalable, qualitative tests may be used to measure certain attributes/characteristics of the bulk solid within a pre-defined range. These attributes may include chemical composition, particle size, color, moisture, and often, flow properties.

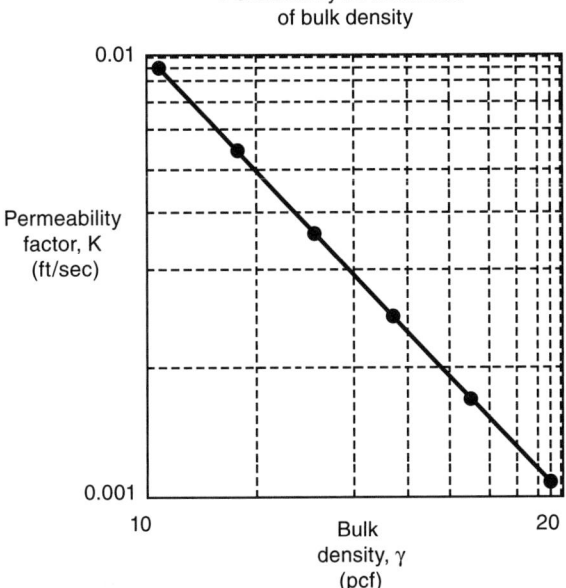

FIGURE 19 Example of permeability versus bulk density plot from permeability test data.

The applicability of the flow property test used is highly dependent on what the user is trying to capture. As an example, if there is concern that a certain batch of material may arch when transferred into a bin, a shear test may be the most comprehensive QC test. However, a quantitative test such as a shear test may require more time/resources to conduct than is practical, so faster test methods are often desired. One option is abbreviated shear cell testing (1).

Commonly conducted qualitative tests are the angle of repose, compressibility index or Hausner ratio, and flow rate through an orifice, all of which are thoroughly reviewed in the literature (17).

Studies have also been conducted comparing the Jenike direct shear test method to other test methods used to measure a powder's "flowability" (3), including the Hosokawa Micron Powder Characteristics Tester (Hosokawa Micron, Osaka, Japan), Peschl® shear tester, and Johanson Hang-up Indicizer (Johanson Innovations, San Luis Obispo, California, U.S.A.). This is not an exhaustive list of all the powder testers available. In general each tester has its own test method, which measures some property of the powder that changes as the "flowability" changes. As stated previously, however, the term flowability must be taken in context.

Any physical characterization related to flow behavior could in principle be used as a QC test, and often the most convenient, fastest test is selected. This is an acceptable practice provided the user is aware of the test's limitations. Since non-scalable, qualitative test methods like angle of repose and flow funnels do not isolate specific attributes of the powder, the results generated and the specified acceptance limits are empirical. Using empirical results typically relies on extensive testing (e.g., a comprehensive database or expert system), experience and/or judgment, as to how to apply these results. In principle, several batches of "good" product must be made (covering the acceptable limits on quality), along with several "bad" batches. Note that determining "good" and "bad" batches without quantitative, scalable flow properties test results, as a baseline, may be challenging and time-consuming.

Another concern with using the various qualitative test methods will be that different test methods may yield significantly different results regarding "good" versus "bad" material/batches, since different physical mechanisms are likely being measured in each test. There have been numerous studies showing that for a group of materials, different test methods give a different ranking of these materials with respect to flow (13–15). With different rankings by each QC test, how does one apply the results? Ultimately, the application and equipment must be considered, and the test method most closely simulating the flow behavior in the actual process should be selected. Therefore, the measuring the flow properties outlined in the proceeding sections is often a critical first step for the designed to obtain the parameters required for consistent, reliable flow through the handling equipment.

FACTORS THAT AFFECT FLOW PROPERTIES

Regardless of what methods of flow property measurement are used, there are a number of external factors that can affect the resulting values. This section will discuss a number of the more common factors that can be encountered in industrial powder handling applications, and relate some typical influences on basic design properties such as wall friction and cohesive strength.

Common Factors

The most common factors that influence bulk flow properties are:

1. moisture content and relative humidity,
2. particle shape and size distribution,
3. temperature,
4. storage time at rest,
5. vibration and overpressures,
6. chemistry and composition.

Each one of these factors is discussed in more detail in the following sections. Other factors that may also affect the flow properties (e.g., electro-static effects, particle hardness) are not discussed in this chapter.

Moisture Content and Relative Humidity

Generally, a powder's cohesive strength increases as moisture content increases, especially when the moisture is concentrated at the surface of the solid particles and not internal, although not in direct proportion. Increases in moisture content will also generally make powders more compressible, due to the lubricating effect of the water on the ability for particles to reorient themselves under a compressive force. Increases in compressibility will influence other properties, such as cohesive strength and wall friction, given the more tightly compacted material at similar pressures. More specific influences on bulk properties can be found when hygroscopic materials, or excess moisture, are considered.

Hygroscopic materials can experience significant increases in moisture content when exposed to humid air. Depending on the nature of this contact, whether it is during transfer and blending versus while a large quantity of material is stored at rest, the extent of the influence of a humid environment can vary greatly. Typically moisture uptake occurs within a relatively thin surface layer of a stored bulk powder in containers such as a drum or a portable bin. This means that during storage, a smaller quantity of material will see the influence of the humid environment, as opposed to when the material was blended in an open container surrounded by humid air. Increases in cohesive strength from moisture uptake can be due to additional liquid bridging between particles, but can also be due to changes in surface properties of the particles themselves, such as softening or swelling.

In extreme cases, where a material can be exposed to excessive and varying amounts of moisture, the question may become where the peak, "worst-case" flow behavior will occur. In this case, the main properties of interest, namely cohesive strength and wall friction have to be considered separately. The worst-case wall friction may occur at any moisture level, particularly when adhesion is factored in as well. To determine this worst case, wall friction tests over a range of different moistures must generally be run, since a determination "by eye" or by qualitative means is often not possible. However, the worst-case cohesive strength will generally be found in the range of 60–90% of saturation. Above this range, there is so much free water present amongst the particles that it tends to act as a lubricant, and allow for easier flowing. Below this range, there is generally not enough moisture present amongst the particles to induce the worst-case behavior.

Particle Shape and Size Distribution

There is no predictive correlation between particle size, shape, and bulk flow properties. However, there are some general trends that can be observed, particularly if other properties are held constant. For instance, as materials get finer, they typically become more cohesive and difficult to handle. In addition, angular or fibrous particle materials are typically more cohesive than those that have rounded particles, since there will be more particle to particle friction, interlocking, and surface contact between the particles in those cases. Uniformly sized particles are generally easier flowing than those with a wide distribution. Friable particle materials can break down and become finer under compressive forces from storage, or due to surface impact from transfer operations. There are more basic particle properties that may be at work affecting the resulting flow properties for friable materials, such as particle hardness, surface characteristics, and inter-particle forces.

Larger particle diameter materials will tend to be more permeable, and hence less prone to the adverse two-phase flow effects discussed previously. Shifts in particular size ranges, such as an increase in the percentage of the finest cut (e.g., d10 value) can have a dramatic and adverse effect on the resulting two-phase flow behaviors even if the mean particle size remains the same. This trend is due to changes in the powder bed packing, and the ability of fines to more effectively fill in the voids around larger particles, thus decreasing the permeability of the powder.

Particle properties can also play a role in wall friction behavior. For instance, one would expect that more spherical particle materials are, in general, less frictional. Other factors that may affect the wall friction behavior include the PSD, particle hardness, and the roughness average (R_a) of the wall surface being used (18). The effect of these parameters upon the wall friction behavior along a given wall surface can vary, so conducting wall friction tests is recommended to fully assess their effect for a given application.

Temperature

For some materials, the effect of temperature on flow properties is a gradual change, while for others it may be a distinct shift at a certain temperature. Some materials undergo softening or crystallizing at elevated temperatures (which can also be affected by relative humidity), which can result in a significant increase in cohesive strength and wall friction. Other behaviors can be the drying of liquid bridges or moisture migration from the interior of particles.

In addition to the mean temperature experienced, the temperature profile over time can have a significant affect on a material's flow properties. For example, a significant increase in cohesive strength was measured in a resin after overnight storage at rest while maintaining elevated temperature. However, if the temperature of the resin was allowed to cool down to room temperature, no significant gain in cohesive strength was noticed (19). Conversely, the particles of some materials will expand with heating and contract with cooling. The cycling of temperature in these cases can cause the particles to reorient themselves and become more compact, leading to high pressures and caking if stored in a fixed container (20).

No matter the cause, the effects of temperature rises or cycles can be directly measured by flow property testing with the temperature profile of interest matched during the tests. These results can provide information for the setting of environmental controls during storage and transport.

Storage Time at Rest

When a powder resides in a storage container for a period of time without moving, it can become more cohesive. Settling and compaction, crystallization, chemical reactions or adhesive bonding can cause such cohesion. These effects can be further influenced by the humidity and temperature of the environment, as discussed previously. The powder may also experience adhesion if allowed to remain at rest against a surface, such as the steel of a container or a plastic bag liner. Adhesion can result in an increase in wall friction between the material and the surface, which can require hopper angles or external forces (e.g., vibration) to overcome the adhesion effects.

Generally these behaviors are unfavorable with respect to material handling, and can be investigated through flow property tests with time at rest described previously in this chapter. The results of these tests may indicate the need for steeper bin walls for unaided flow and/or larger openings to prevent cohesive arching.

Vibration and Overpressures

Vibration of a powder placed within a container can result in additional settling and compaction beyond what would be seen if the powder were simply subjected to consolidation pressures due to its own weight. Vibration can reduce the frictional forces that form between a material and a wall surface, increasing the influence of the weight of material as an added compressive force. Vibration also causes inter-particle motion that can result in a reorienting of particles and additional packing (compression) of the material bed. The results of the compressibility test (uniaxial compaction at relatively low pressures as would be seen from bulk storage) versus the tapped density tests will provide an initial assessment of the sensitivity of the powder to vibration effects. If a moderately higher density is achieved from the tapping as compared to compression, then it could be concluded that the material is susceptible to vibration effects.

Overpressure is a term describing the extra force beyond the weight of the material itself, and can be due to additional factors beyond vibration. These additional factors resulting in overpressure may include impact loads from dropping material into a container from above, additional weight added on top of a powder bed, and fluid or gas pressure changes (note that equilibrated pressures throughout a container and its outlet will not have an effect).

All the behaviors described above have the same effect in varying degrees to result in powder that is compacted more than it would otherwise be. Powders that are particularly susceptible to these influences are ones that are fine and very compressible. Compacted powder can attain higher cohesive strength, and become more difficult to handle. The compacted powder can also become much more prone to adverse two-phase flow behaviors, due to the decrease in permeability that accompanies an increase in density.

Chemistry and Composition

The chemical state of a material or composition of a powder blend can influence its flow behavior. For instance, a change in the hydration level of a crystalline material may result in variations in flow properties. Additives, such as fumed silica, have been used in small quantities as a means of overcoming the poor flow of active ingredients and fillers in powder blends. Lubricants, such as magnesium stearate, are typically used in powder blends destined for tableting in order to provide a non-oil-based glidant for close contacting steel tool surfaces, while aiding in the compaction of the powder itself. These materials are typically "lightly" blended as a final step in a batch preparation process, so that they will remain more readily available to coat tool surface. If over-blended or added in too high a quantity, these materials can contribute to excess compaction within a tablet. Overblending may also result in increased coating of the particles that may reduce dissolution with a hydrophobic material. It is interesting that the flow behavior of additives and lubricants by themselves is often poor, often due to their typically fine PSD, and yet when added in small quantities can beneficial to the final blend flowability. This effect comes from the dispersion of the material within the blend, the particles of which act as a coating and serve to prevent some of the interparticle contacts of the base material that would otherwise lead to cohesion.

BASIC EQUIPMENT DESIGN TECHNIQUES FOR RELIABLE FLOW

The primary objective this section is to review basic design techniques for the bin-to-press feed system to provide consistent, reliable flow for gravity feed. Note that design techniques to minimize segregation are discussed elsewhere in this volume.

In particular, we will review the following basic design techniques:

1. reliable funnel flow design (preventing a rathole);
2. reliable mass flow designs for the bin, chute and press hopper;
3. minimizing adverse two-phase flow effects (e.g., feed/tableting rate limitations, flooding).

For each of these different design concerns, we will review the key equipment parameters and flow properties. Note that these common flow concerns (arching, ratholing, adverse two-phase flow effects) and flow patterns (mass flow vs. funnel flow) were discussed previously in this chapter. Regardless of whether the equipment being designed is a bin, transfer chute or press hopper, a crucial first step in designing a reliable feed system is determining the flow pattern and designing accordingly. The wall friction tests and design charts used to determine if a hopper will discharge in mass flow or funnel flow were discussed previously.

Reliable Funnel Flow Design (Preventing a Rathole)

Funnel flow occurs when the hopper walls are not smooth and/or steep enough to promote flow at the walls, and can be prone to ratholing if the material is cohesive. This section will focus on preventing ratholing in a funnel flow bin handling a final blend, but the design techniques can also be applied to preventing ratholing in a transfer chute with convergence or a press hopper. These techniques can be applied to any powder, including handling an API or major excipients in bins upstream of the final blender.

A funnel flow bin/chute/hopper design can be considered if all of the following design criteria are met:

1. *A final blend is being handled in which segregation is not primary concern.* Since a funnel flow bin will discharge in a first-in-last-out flow sequence, any side-to-side segregation that occurred as the bin was filled will often be exacerbated in funnel flow discharge.
2. *The final blend has relatively low cohesive strength* so the formation of a stable rathole is not a concern. This can be checked by comparing the bin outlet diameter/diagonal length to the *critical rathole diameter* (D_f) for the estimated major consolidation pressure [σ_1, Equation (3)] for the given bin design. If the outlet diameter is less than D_f, ratholing is a concern.
3. *Flooding due to a collapsing rathole is not a primary concern.* Flooding can result in highly aerated (low density) powder being fed from the bin to the press, which may have an adverse effect on the tablet properties (weight, hardness, dissolution variation) and can result in segregation.
4. *A non-uniform feed density is not a primary concern.* Since tablet presses operate as *volumetric* feeders, variation of the feed density into the press feed frame can result in tablet weight variation. A funnel flow bin will typically have a more non-uniform feed density than a mass flow bin, since the blend in the funnel flow bin will be subjected to different consolidation pressures depending upon where in the bin it is discharged from. For instance, the blend located at the bottom of the bin at the hopper walls, which is outside the flow channel, may be more consolidated and have a higher density than the blend within the flow channel.

If all of these design criteria are met, a funnel flow bin design can be considered. If a funnel flow bin design is acceptable, the first concern is checking that the outlet diameter is greater than the critical rathole diameter (D_f) to ensure that a stable rathole will not form. If the diameter of the funnel flow bin is not greater than D_f, the following steps can be considered to reduce the likelihood of ratholing:

1. *Enlarge the bin opening*: This may require using a slotted outlet, which would require a feeder capable of feeding uniformly across the entire outlet (e.g., mass flow screw feeder) or a valve capable of shutting off such an outlet. Simply using a larger outlet diameter may not be a practical/feasible modification, since the opening may need to be increased significantly (beyond that of standard valve or feeder sizes) and would still need mate with downstream equipment.

Flow: General Principles of Bulk Solids Handling

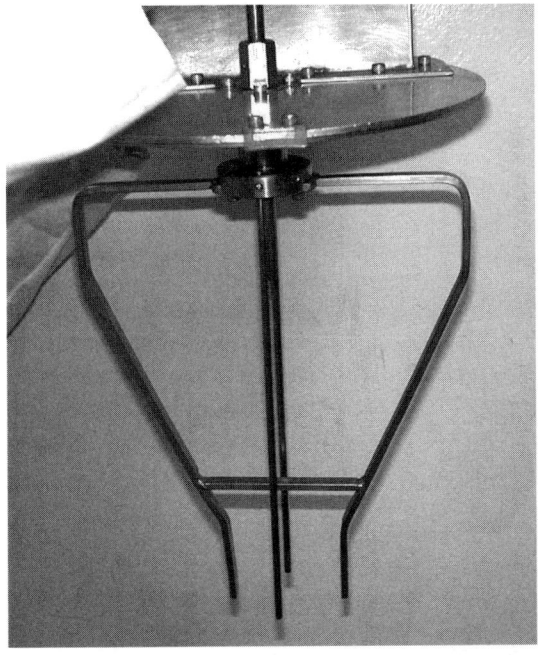

FIGURE 20 Internal agitator.

2. *Reduce the material level in the bin*: Since the critical rathole diameter typically decreases with a reduction in the major consolidation pressure (σ_1), which depends upon the fill height, this could be considered but will then require using multiple smaller bins to handle the bulk solid.
3. *Using an internal, mechanical agitator*: An internal, mechanical agitator, such as an agitator with "arms" that rotate about a central vertical shaft (Fig. 20) may be a practical modification on a small scale for a press hopper, but will likely be less practical for a large scale bin due to the required motor size, cleaning concerns, etc. A bin with a discharge valve (e.g., Matcon discharge valve in Fig. 21) could also be considered as a means of failing a stable rathole, but would need to be assessed via full-scale trials to determine the operating parameters required (valve "stroke" setting, etc.)
4. *Using external vibrators*: The effectiveness of external vibrators to collapse a stable rathole would need to be assessed via full-scale trials prior to installation, since vibration may actually increase the strength on the blend in the bin and the likelihood of ratholing. Trials would be required to assess the optimum vibrator type (high-frequency/low-amplitude vs. low-frequency/high-amplitude), number of vibrators required, location, frequency settings, etc.

Since there are several adverse effects of using an bin that discharges in funnel flow (first-in-last-out flow sequence, non-uniform feed density, exacerbation of segregation) and the potential options to prevent a rathole are often limited or impractical, a common design technique for preventing ratholing is to redesign the bin for mass flow. The design techniques for mass flow are discussed in the following section.

Reliable Mass Flow Designs for the Bin, Chute, and Press Hopper

Mass flow discharge from a bin occurs when the following two design criteria are meet:

1. the bin walls are smooth and/or steep enough to promote flow at the walls;
2. the bin outlet is large enough to prevent an arch (cohesive and/or mechanical).

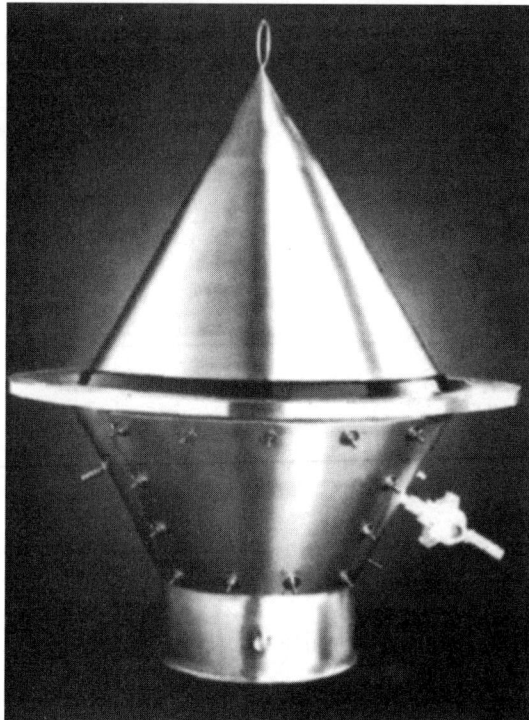

FIGURE 21 Internal agitator (Matcon® discharge valve).

The wall friction tests and design charts used to determine if a bin will discharge in mass flow or funnel flow were discussed previously.

Regardless of whether the equipment being designed for mass flow is a bin, transfer chute or press hopper, the same design criteria apply for obtaining mass flow discharge. Therefore, although this section focus on design techniques for mass flow bins, these techniques may be extended to obtain mass flow in a transfer chute and press hopper as well. These techniques may be applied in designing new equipment or modifying existing equipment to provide mass flow.

When designing the bin to provide mass flow, the following general steps should be taken:

1. *Size the outlet to prevent a cohesive arch* from forming by making the outlet diameter equal to or larger than the minimum required outlet diameter (B_c, Fig. 22). If a slotted outlet is used (maintaining a 3:1 length:width ratio for the outlet), the outlet width should be sized to be equal to or larger than the minimum required outlet width (B_p, Fig. 22). The outlet may also need to be sized based upon feed rate and two-phase flow considerations as discussed in the following section. If the outlet can not be sized to prevent an arch (e.g., press hopper outlet that must mate with a feed frame inlet), an internal mechanical agitator or external vibrator could be considered, as discussed in the proceeding section
2. *Once the outlet is sized, the hopper wall sloped should be designed to be equal to or steeper than the recommended hopper angle for the given outlet size and selected wall surface.* For a conical hopper, the walls should be equal to or steeper than the recommended mass flow angle for a conical hopper (θ_c, Fig. 22). If the bin has a rectangular-to-round hopper, the valley angles should be sloped to be equal

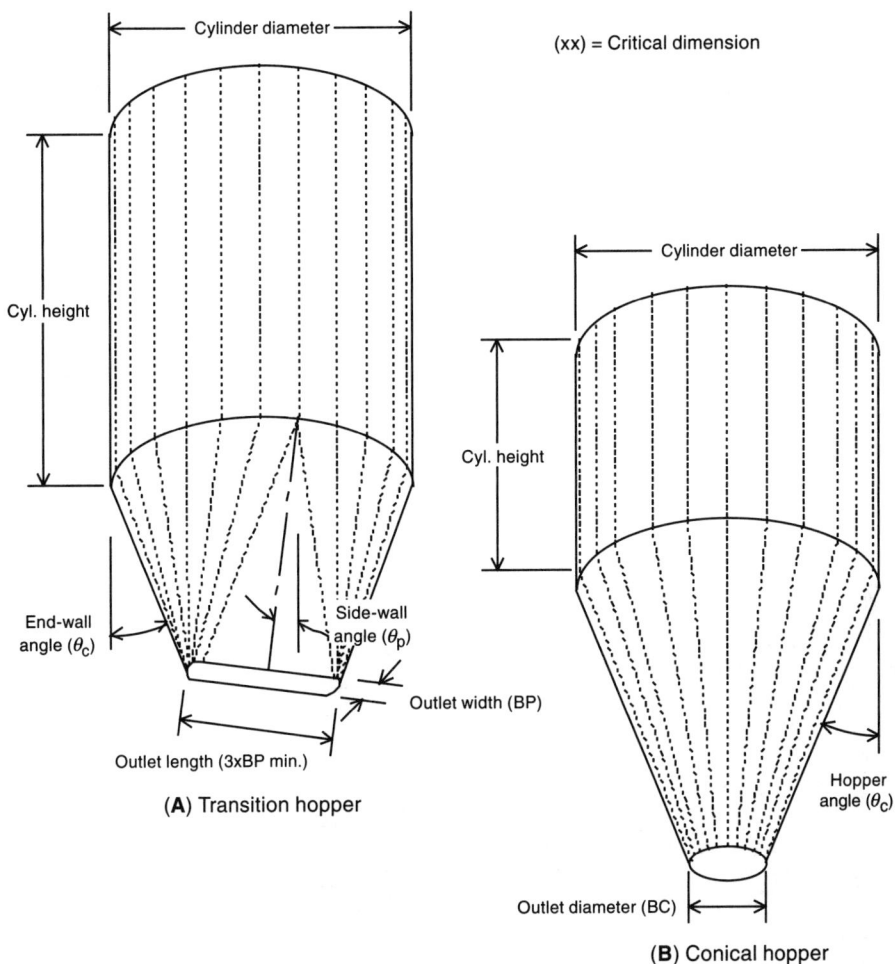

FIGURE 22 Mass flow design parameters (BC, BP, θ_c, θ_p).

to or steeper than θ_c. For planar walls, the walls should be equal to or steeper than the recommended mass flow angle for a planar hopper (θ_p, Fig. 22).

3. *Pay careful attention to the interior wall surface finish.* When conducting the wall friction tests, it is beneficial to conduct tests on several different finishes (e.g., #320 grit finish, #2B cold rolled finish, #2B electro-polished finish, etc.) to have a range of design options and assess the sensitivity of the wall friction results to different finishes. It is not sufficient to simply test a 304 or 316 stainless steel with no regard to the interior finish, since the wall friction of the blend may vary significantly from finish to finish. The orientation of directional finishes such as a mechanical polish is also critical to assess and control during fabrication. In addition, it cannot be assumed that an interior surface finish with a lower average roughness (R_a) will provide the best wall friction properties.

4. *Consider velocity gradients.* Even when a bin is designed for mass flow, there still may be a velocity gradient between the material discharging at the hopper walls (moving slower) versus the center of the hopper (moving faster), assuming a symmetric bin with a single outlet in the center. Depending upon the application, the

bin designer may want to increase the velocity gradient to enhance blending between vertical layers of material in the bin or reduce the velocity gradient to enhance blending on a side-to-side basis. This will be dependent upon the segregation that occurs upon filling the bin and its affect upon content uniformity, which is discussed in another chapter in this book. The velocity gradient is reduced by making the hopper slope steeper with respect to the recommended mass flow hopper angle (θ_c). The velocity gradient is increased by making the hopper slope shallower with respect to the recommended mass flow hopper angle. Changing the interior surface to reduce friction or using an insert (discussed more below) are other methods used to control the velocity gradient. Asymmetric hoppers, which are common for press hoppers, are especially prone to velocity gradients since the material will move faster at the steeper hopper wall. In addition, the velocity gradient cannot be completely eliminated, especially as the material level in the hopper empties. Velocity profiles, and their effect on blending material, can be calculated a priori given the geometry of the bin (θ_c) and measured flow properties that were discussed previously (i.e., ϕ, δ, ϕ).

5. *Avoid upward-facing lips/ledges* due to mismatched flanges (Fig. 23), level probes, view ports, partially opened valves, etc., especially in the hopper section. Ideally, interior protruding devices should be located in the cylinder section of a bin/press

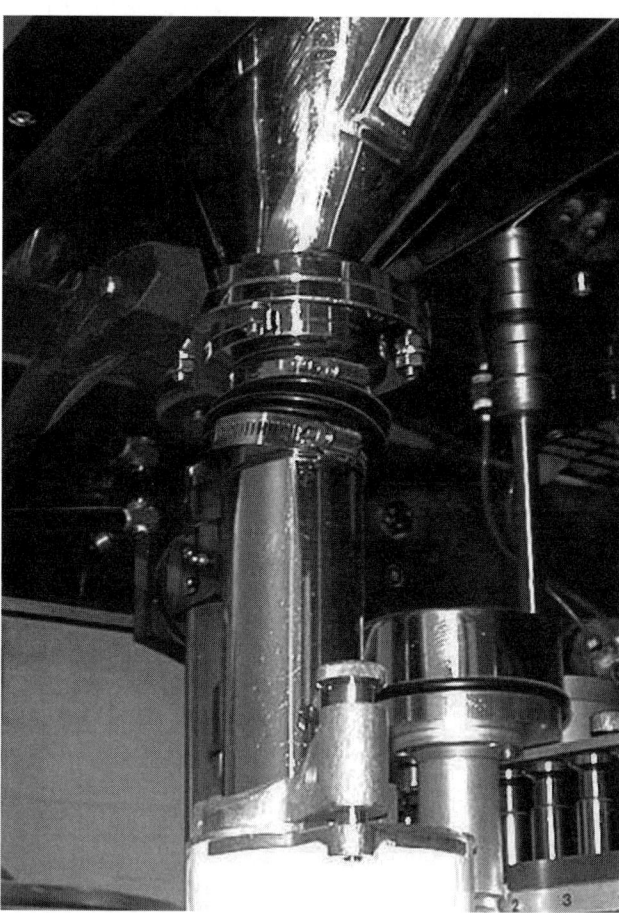

FIGURE 23 Example of an upward-facing ledge at a flange connection.

hopper if possible, where they will be less detrimental in upsetting a mass flow pattern.

If modifying an existing funnel flow bin to provide mass flow, several different options can be considered including:

1. *Use a different interior surface finish* with better wall friction properties (lower friction). Conduct wall friction tests on alternative wall surfaces to assess if changing the surface finish while still using the existing bin geometry (e.g., electro-polishing an exiting #2B finish) will convert the bin from funnel flow to mass flow. This is often one of the most cost-effective modifications to obtain mass flow.
2. *Use a flow-controlling insert* such as a Binsert® (Fig. 24) to obtain mass flow within the same bin. A properly designed insert can change the stresses that develop in the bin during discharge so that mass flow can be obtained at a wall where the material was previously stagnant.

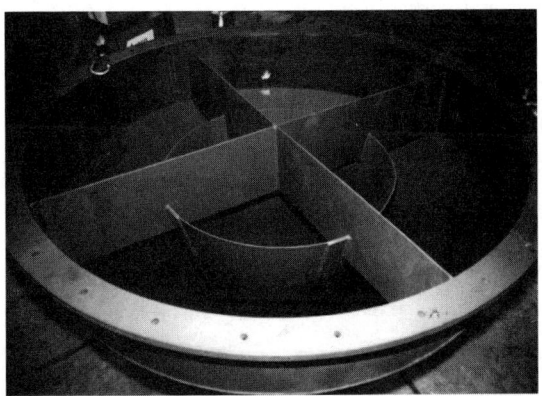

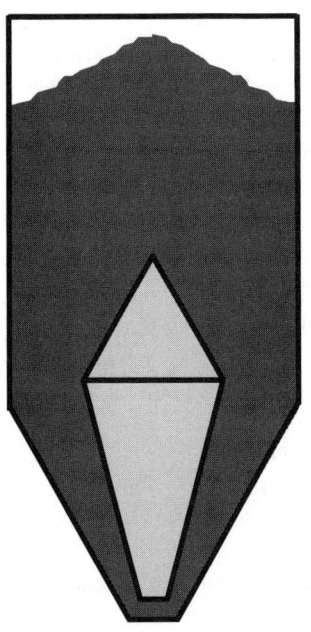

FIGURE 24 Examples of (**A**) an "open" Binsert design and (**B**) a "closed" Binsert design.

3. *Modify the hopper geometry*. Use a different geometry that is more likely to provide mass flow (e.g., conical instead of a rectangular-to-round hopper with shallower valley angles). If the hopper is modified to have a slotted outlet, it is crucial that the feeder the hopper mates to withdraw material across the entire outlet.

In addition to these design techniques for bins, there are several additional design techniques for designing transfer chutes for reliable mass flow including:

1. For *converging* sections that are flood loaded and have a full cross section (i.e., hoppers), use the same design criteria used for mass flow bins discussed above.
2. For *non-converging* sections of the chute, the chute should be sloped to exceed the wall friction angle (ϕ') by a least a 10° margin of safety. As an example, if the measured wall friction angle for the given wall surface from the wall friction test results is 40° from horizontal, the recommended chute angle for the non-converging portion of the chute would be at least 50° from horizontal.
3. If a bifurcated chute is used, then the sloping chute legs should be symmetric to prevent velocity gradients and the possibility of stagnant material in the shallower leg.
4. Use mitered joints between sloping and vertical sections.

Minimizing Adverse Two-Phase Flow Effects

There are three common modes of flow with respect to two-phase (powder: interstitial gas) flow behavior:

1. steady flow,
2. flooding,
3. flow rate limitation.

The primary focus in preventing adverse two-phase flow affects is to ensure that the bulk solids handling equipment is designed so that the critical flow rate through a given outlet, determined from the permeability and compressibility results, is greater than the target feed rate. The target feed rate is often set by the required maximum tableting rate for the process (e.g., 1000 tablets per min $\times$ 100 mg per tablet = 6 kg/hr). Adverse two phase-flow effects are likely to be most pronounced at the press feed hopper, which often has the smallest outlet in the entire press feed system (i.e., bin, transfer chute, etc.) and, therefore, will have the smallest critical flow rate.

When designing the bulk solids handling equipment to minimize adverse two-phase flow effects, the following general design techniques are beneficial:

- *Design the equipment for mass flow*: Mass flow will provide consistent feed and a more uniform consolidation pressure acting on the bulk solids. In addition, having a first-in-first-out flow sequence will allow the material more time to deaerate before being discharged through the outlet, which will reduce the likelihood of flooding. Mass flow will also prevent collapsing ratholes that can result in the powder aerating and flooding as it falls into the central flow channel. It is worth noting that mass flow can result in a lower, but more stable, critical flow rate than funnel flow and therefore may not be the only corrective action required if a flow rate limitation occurs, so other design techniques to address a flow rate limitation are discussed below. However, designing the equipment for mass flow is often the first step in addressing adverse two-phase flow effects.

- *Use larger outlets for the handling equipment*: Since the critical flow rate is a strong function of the cross-sectional area of the outlet, increasing the outlet can often be highly beneficial in reducing two-phase flow effects. The goal would be to increase the outlet size until the critical flow rate for the selected outlet size exceeds the target flow rate. Since this may not be feasible for a press feeder hopper, in which the outlet size is fixed to mate with the press feed frame inlet, additional design techniques are discussed below. Computer software can be used to model the two-phase flow behavior to assess the effect of changing the outlet diameter.
- *Reduce the fill height in the handling equipment*: Since the critical flow rate through a given outlet increases as the major consolidation pressure (σ_1) decreases, reducing the fill height will be beneficial but will be much less effective than increasing the outlet size.
- *Reduce the target feed rate*: If possible, reducing the target feed rate (tableting rate) to be less than the critical flow rate will be beneficial, but is often impractical since it will result in a decreased production rate.
- *Consider gas pressure differentials*: A gas pressure differential can have a beneficial or adverse effect upon two-phase flow effects. A positive gas pressure differential at the outlet (i.e., bin/press hopper/etc. at a higher gas pressure than the equipment downstream) may be beneficial in overcoming a feed rate limitation, as the air pressure is forcing the material in the direction of flow. Conversely, a negative gas pressure differential at the outlet can further reduce the critical flow rate, since the negative gas pressure acts to further retard the flow rate.
- *Add air permeation*: Air permeation may be added to the system actively via an air injection system or passively through a vent. In particular, adding judicious (often very small) amounts of air at the location in the press feed system where the interstitial gas pressure is lowest can often be beneficial in reducing the likelihood of a feed rate limitation.
- *Changing the PSD of the powder*: The permeability of a powder is a strong function of its PSD. Powders with a finer PSD are often less permeable and, therefore, more prone to adverse-two phase flow effects. Even a reduction in the percentage of "fines" (i.e., d10 value of the PSD) can often be beneficial in increasing the permeability of a powder and, thereby, decreasing the likelihood of adverse two phase-flow effects.

The key to implementing any corrective actions designed to reduce adverse flow-effects will be using a mathematical two-phase flow analysis to assess the effects on the bulks solids stresses and interstitial gas pressure. This analysis would need to use inputs such as key flow properties (permeability, compressibility) and equipment/process parameters (tableting rate, bin/hopper geometry, and gas pressure gradients) to assess the effect of the potential corrective actions outlined above.

REFERENCES

1. Jenike AW. Storage and flow of solids, Bulletin 123 of the Utah Engineering Experimental Station, 1964; 53(26) (Revised 1980).
2. Royal TA, Carson JW. Fine powder flow phenomena in bins, hoppers and processing vessels. Presented at Bulk 2000, London, 1991.
3. Schulze D. Measuring powder flowability: A comparison of test methods, Part I. Powder Bulk Eng 1996; 10(4):45–61.
4. Schulze D. Measuring powder flowability: A comparison of test methods, Part II. Powder Bulk Eng 1996; 10(6):17–28.

5. Standard Shear Testing Method for Bulk Solids Using the Jenike Shear Cell, ASTM Standard D6128-06, American Society for Testing and Materials, 2006.
6. Bausch A, Hausmann R, Bongartz C, Zinn T. Measurement of flowability with a ring shear cell, evaluation and adaptation of the method for use in pharmaceutical technology. In: Proceedings of the 2nd World Meeting APGI/APV, Paris, May 1998: 135–6.
7. Hausmann R, Bausch A, Bongartz C, Zinn T. Pharmaceutical applications of a new ring shear tester for flowability measurement of granules and powders. In: Proceedings of the 2nd World Meeting APGI/APV, Paris, May 1998; 137–8.
8. Nyquist H. Measurement of flow properties in large scale tablet production. Int J Pharm Tech Product Manufact 1984; 5(3):21–4.
9. Ramachandruni H, Hoag S. Application of a modified annular shear cell measuring lubrication of pharmaceutical powders. Thesis research directed by School of Pharmacy, University of Maryland, 2000.
10. Prescott JK, Ploof DA, Carson JW. Developing a better understanding of wall friction. Powder Handing Process 1999; 11(1):27–35.
11. USA<616> Bulk and Tapped Density. The United States Pharmacopia, Vol. 28(3). US Pharmacopial Forum, 2002.
12. Carson JW, Marinelli J. Characterize bulk solids to ensure smooth flow. Chem Eng 1994; 101(4):78–90.
13. Ploof DA, Carson JW. Quality control tester to measure relative flowability of powders. Bulk Solids Handling 1994; 14(1):127–32.
14. Bell TA, Ennis, BJ, Grygo RJ, et al. Practical evaluation of the Johanson hang-up indicizer. Bulk Solids Handling 1994; 14(1):117–25.
15. Schwedes J. Testers for measuring flow properties of particulate solids. Presented at Reliable Flow of Particulate Solids III, Posgrunn, Norway, 1999.
16. Janssen HA. Versuche uber Getreidedruck in Silozellen. Verein Deutcher Igenieure, Zeitschrift. 1895; 39:1045–9.
17. USP<1174> Powder Flow. The United States Pharmacopia, Vol. 28(2). US Pharmacopial Forum, 2002.
18. Bumiller M, Carson JW, Prescott JK. A preliminary investigation concerning the effect of particle shape on a powder's flow properties. Presented at the World Congress on Particle Technology IV, Sydney Australia, July 2002.
19. Purutyan H, Carson JW. Understanding the effects of temperature on bulk solids flow. Chem Process 2000; October:45–51.
20. Purutyan H, Pittenger BH, Tardos GI. Prevent caking during solids handling. Chem Eng Prog 2005; May:22–8.

4
Blending and Blend Uniformity

Thomas P. Garcia
Pfizer, Inc., Groton, Connecticut, U.S.A.

James K. Prescott
Jenike & Johanson, Inc., Tyngsboro, Massachusetts, U.S.A.

INTRODUCTION

Solid blending processes are used during the manufacture of products for a wide range of industries. On a daily basis, individuals encounter and use a wide array of blends of granular and powder materials. The shelves of grocery stores are stocked with numerous products consisting of powder blends (cake mix, flavor packets for quick meals, and instant beverages). Vitamins and minerals are blended with grains during the manufacture of breakfast cereals. Powdered laundry and dish detergents, cleansers, and other household cleaning products contain components that are blended to achieve optimal cleaning performance. The construction industry relies on powder blends during the preparation of mortar and cement products. The agriculture industry uses blends of nitrogen, phosphorus, and potassium salts for the preparation of fertilizers. The diversity of materials that may be blended, as demonstrated by the previous examples, present a number of variables that must be addressed to achieve products of acceptable uniformity. These variables include particle size distribution (including aggregates or lumps of material), shape (spheres, rods, cubes, plates, and irregular), the presence of moisture (or other volatile compounds), and the surface properties of the material (roughness, cohesivity). Although the quality of the product is dependent on the adequacy of the blend in each of the above examples, the consequences of not obtaining uniform blends range from minor (a bad tasting meal) to catastrophic (structural collapse due to the incomplete mixing of construction materials).

One of the most critical applications of blending operations occurs in the pharmaceutical industry during the manufacture of solid dosage forms. Producing a uniform mixture of the drug and its excipients and ensuring that it does not segregate post-blending, is paramount in being able to deliver the proper dose of the drug to the patient. Millions of dosage units may be created from a single batch, and each and every dose must be of acceptable composition to ensure the safety and efficacy of the product. For this reason, the homogeneity of pharmaceutical blends and dosage units is highly scrutinized by regulatory bodies throughout the world. Formulation components and process parameters involved with blending operations should be carefully selected and validated to ensure uniform blends and dosage units are produced. Blend and dosage unit content uniformity data is provided in regulatory submissions and often examined during pre-approval inspections, to ensure that blending processes produce homogeneous blends that do not segregate upon further processing into dosage units. Finally, pharmacopeias require an assessment of content uniformity to be performed on every batch of solid dosage forms manufactured.

The scale of blending operations for the preparation of pharmaceutical dosage forms ranges from the extemporaneous compounding of a few capsules by pharmacists, to large-scale production of batches containing millions of dosage units. The complexity of the blending process can vary substantially. When doing extemporaneous compounding, a pharmacist may use basic blending techniques such as spatulation (the mixing of small quantities of powder on a pill tile using a spatula), trituration (the mixing of powders using a porcelain mortar and pestle), or tumbling (the mixing of powders in a partially filled, closed container). Large-scale production batches use equipment capable of blending hundreds of kilograms of material. Depending on the dose and characteristics of the drug substance, commercial scale blending processes can be complex and may require the preparation of preblends or the inclusion of milling operations to achieve acceptable content uniformity. Regardless of the scale of manufacture, the goal remains the same: to prepare a blend that is adequately blended and can be further processed into dosage units that deliver the proper dose of the drug to the patient.

Blending should not be seen as an independent unit operation, but rather as an integral part of the overall manufacturing process. Blending includes producing an adequate blend, maintaining that blend through additional handling steps, and verifying that both the blend and the finished product are sufficiently homogeneous. Therefore, a holistic approach should be used to assess the uniformity of blends and the subsequent dosage forms produced from them.

The following text is intended to provide the reader with an overview of the principles involved in blending operations, and the equipment used to prepare powder blends. This chapter will only focus on solid–solid blending. Liquid–solid mixing, which often uses the same equipment, will be addressed in the wet granulation chapter. Material properties that can impact blending operations will be discussed, as well as mechanisms that can result in segregation of the blend and approaches to minimize its occurrence. When content uniformity issues arise, techniques to identify and troubleshoot the problem for both the blend and dosage forms will be presented.

SOLID–SOLID BLENDING PROCESS

Mixing and blending are two commonly used terms that can be used to describe various processes, including:

- combining two or more powdered or granular components,
- homogenizing the contents of a vessel before discharge,
- contacting, wetting, or dissolving a dry material with a liquid,
- combining liquid components,
- preparing or maintaining a slurry or suspension,
- kneading a dough or paste.

Distinctions between the terms *mixing* and *blending* have been made, sometimes based on the equipment used, the material handled (liquids vs. solids), or whether one is combining streams of different components or simply homogenizing a product. No definition is universally accepted or used for either term. For the purpose of this chapter,

Blending and Blend Uniformity

we will generally use the term *blending* to describe the combination or homogenization of bulk solids, which we will define as granular or powdered materials, composed of discrete particles. Specific terms using the term *mix* will remain, such as premix, demixing, and high shear mixer.

Mechanisms of Blending

Blending is a reshuffling process involving the random movement of individual and groups of particles. Three mechanisms by which blending processes can occur are diffusion, convection, and shear (Fig. 1) (1,2). Diffusion is the redistribution of individual particles by their random movement relative to one another. It is often referred to as micro mixing in the literature, because it addresses the blending process on an individual particle basis. Examples of where diffusion can occur include:

- fluidization caused by the action of a pneumatic blender;
- movement of material parallel to the axis of a tumble blender caused by collisions with other particles, the walls, or internals of the blender.

Convection is the movement of groups of adjacent particles from one place to another within the blend. It is often referred to as macro mixing because large volumes of material are simultaneously moved. This can occur, for example, as a result of:

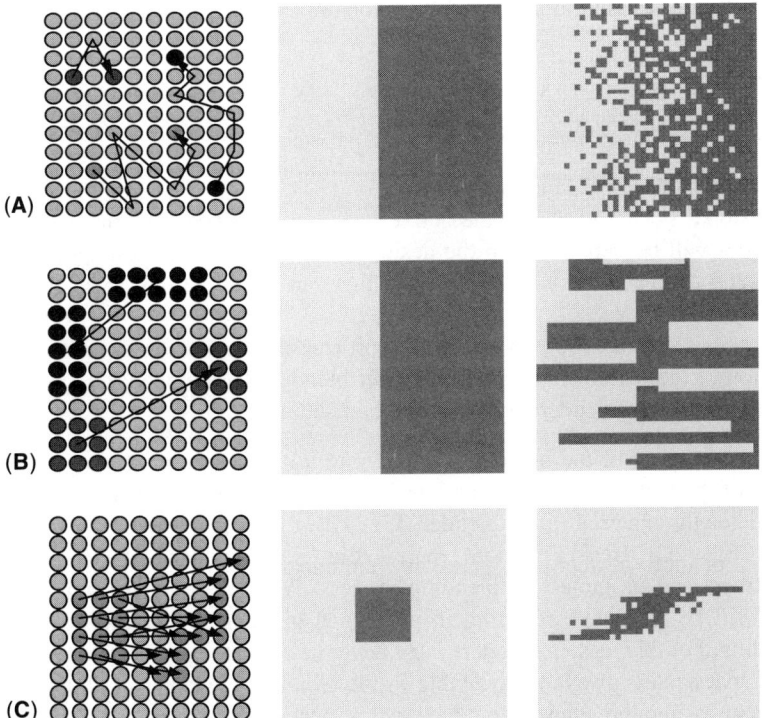

FIGURE 1 Principal mechanisms of blending: (**A**) Diffusion, (**B**) convection, and (**C**) shear. (**A**) Schematic of diffusion: At the particle scale (*left*); At a mesoscale for initial state (*center*) and after diffusion initiates (*right*). (**B**) Schematic of convection: At the particle scale (*left*); at a mesoscale for initial state (*center*) and after convection initiates (*right*). (**C**) Schematic of shear: At the particle scale (*left*); at a mesoscale for initial state (*center*), and after shear initiates (*right*).

- cascading of material within a tumble blender;
- the action of the blade of a ribbon blender;
- material movement resulting from gas pressure gradients in a pneumatic blender.

Shear is the change in the configuration of ingredients through the formation of slip planes or shearing strains within a bed of material. Mechanical force is imparted to the powders by the blending equipment to induce shear blending. According to this definition, one could conclude that material cascading within a tumble blender would be considered shear. However, the degree of shear in tumble blenders is much lower than that observed in high shear mixers, the latter of which are capable of breaking up agglomerates. Therefore, flow in a shear plane can be considered as an example of convection, where the movement of the body of material results from the flow of material, which involves development of one or more slip planes. For our purposes, we will restrict the definition of the blending mechanism of shear as high intensity impact or splitting of the bed of material to break up agglomerates, or overcome cohesion. This can be very effective at producing small-scale uniformity, usually on a localized basis. Examples of equipment that use shear include:

- intensifiers (choppers) in a variety of blenders;
- pin mixers.

The degree to which the above blending mechanisms influence a process depends on the flow properties (such as cohesion) of the materials being blended and the specific equipment selected, as discussed in subsequent sections of this chapter.

Principles of Blending

Blending operations can be separated into four principal steps (3):

1. The bed of solid particles expands.
2. Three-dimensional shear forces become active in the powder bed. The intensity of the shear forces will be dependent on the design of the blender and the application of devices (such as impellers or agitation bars) that can impart further shear to the powder bed.
3. The powder bed is blended long enough to permit true randomization of particles.
4. Randomization of the particles is maintained after blending has stopped (i.e., avoiding segregation once the blender stops and the bed settles).

When the components of the blend are loaded into a blender, compression forces due to the weight of the materials create a static bed (Fig. 2A). The mechanical operation of the blender dilates the material in the blender (Fig. 2B), resulting in the expansion of the powder bed (Fig. 2C). Bed expansion creates void spaces, which enhance interparticulate movement and promotes the blending process. Without bed expansion, particle movement will be restricted, resulting in prolonged blending times and possibly incomplete blending. For this reason, blenders must never be filled to liquid capacity, and a sufficient void space must always be available in the blending container to allow bed expansion to occur. Although unusual characteristics peculiar to specific particulate systems can create complications in the blending process, poor blends usually result from violating one or more of the above principle steps that occur during blending.

Once particle movement is made possible through the expansion of the powder bed, velocity gradients within the material further enhance movement between particles (Fig. 2D). Together, compression, tension, and shear forces result in the application

Blending and Blend Uniformity

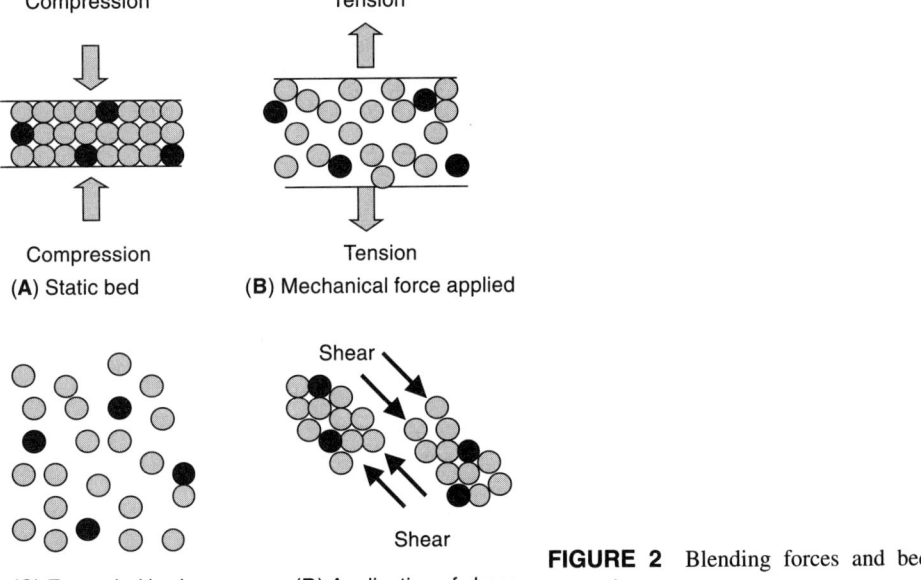

FIGURE 2 Blending forces and bed expansion.

of three-dimensional stress to the material inside the blending container, producing the required random particle movements. If the shear force applied to the powder bed is inadequate to overcome particle-to-particle attraction, agglomerates can form and move together without being dispersed throughout the powder bed, resulting in a poor blend.

Despite temptations to increase the batch size, especially for high-volume products, a general guideline for tumble blenders is to only fill them to approximately 65–75% of their total capacity. The importance of fill volume has been demonstrated Llusa and Muzzio (4) as well as Brone et al. (5). Figure 3 provides an example of the effect of fill level (40%, 60%, and 85% of total blender capacity) on the uniformity of magnesium stearate in the resulting blend after various numbers of revolutions. As the fill level in the blender increased, blending efficiency decreased, and additional revolutions were required to obtain uniformity. The impact of fill level on blending efficiency was greater for shorter blending times. Although longer blending times eventually compensated for higher fill levels, this is typically an impractical solution for the routine manufacture of a commercial product, as there is significant cost in tying up equipment. Conversely, excessively low fill levels (20%) may lead to excessive sliding of the blend as a bed (versus tumbling of particles), which also results in poorer blending (6).

Kinetics of Blending

Blending Model

Blending processes produce a random redistribution of particles. A "perfect" mix is when the ratio of particles in any given sample remains constant regardless of the location that the sample is taken from. For example, a perfect mix resembles a checkerboard (Fig. 4A) such that when two adjacent particles of a 50:50 blend of two components are sampled, the probability of obtaining one particle of each component is 100%. Perfect

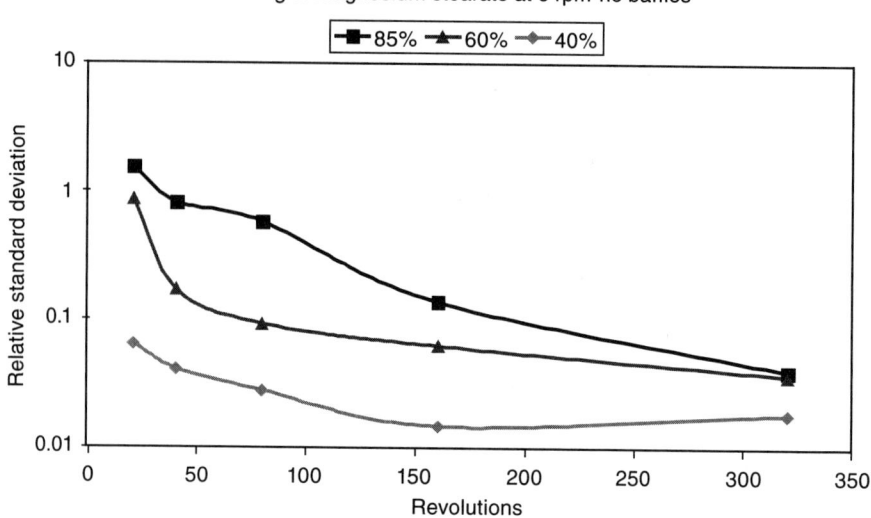

FIGURE 3 Impact of fill level on blending efficiency. *Source*: From Ref. 4.

mixes cannot be achieved as it violates the laws of probability. A random mix (Fig. 4B), which will never be "perfect" but is governed by laws of probability, is the best situation that can be achieved during blending operations. A random mix may be inadequate if the particles are large relative to the dose, whereas if they are small, it may be acceptable. The concept of the scale of uniformity is discussed later. Also, segregation (within the blender and post-discharge) of some degree will always be present in the blend. Therefore, one needs to determine at what point an acceptable blend of all components is achieved, such that the performance or quality of the product will not be adversely affected. This end-point is generally established by setting acceptance criteria for the standard deviation (or a similar statistic, such as relative standard deviation or RSD), which describes the spread in the distribution of a set of data. (This will be discussed in more detail later in this chapter.)

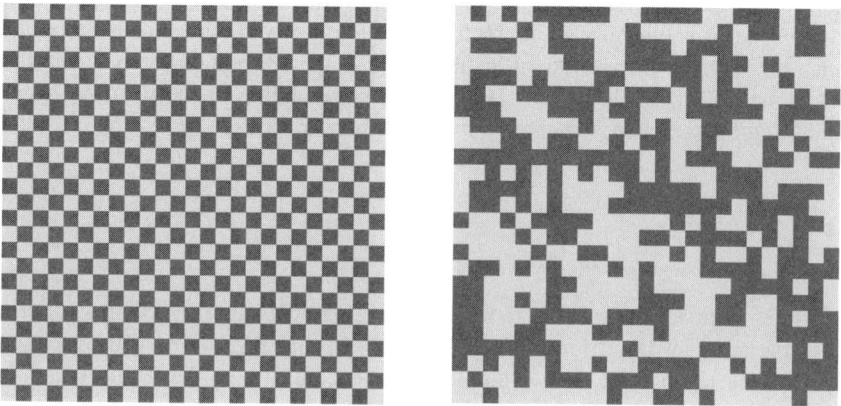

FIGURE 4 Illustration of a perfect mix (**A**) and a binary mixture that is random (**B**).

Blending and Blend Uniformity

Under ideal conditions (such as all particles having the same size, shape and density, and assuming forces that result in cohesion and electrostatic charge have no impact on the blending process), blending processes are dependent on the probability that a particle re-ordering event happens in a given time. They generally obey the following first-order equation, which assumes that the blend is paced by a single mechanism.

$$M = \text{RSD}_\infty + (\text{RSD}_0 - \text{RSD}_\infty)(e^{-kt}) \qquad (1)$$

where M is the degree of blending (RSD at time t), RSD_∞ is the best possible blend state (e.g., a random mix), RSD_0 is the initial blend state, t is the time, and k is the rate constant for blending, in units of 1/time.

The term $(\text{RSD}_0 - \text{RSD}_\infty)$ can be thought of as the initial resistance to blending. Equation (1) demonstrates that the blending process is a function of both time and the application of minimal energy levels to overcome the initial resistance of the materials to be blended resulting from their interparticle forces. If we assign a value of $\text{RSD}_0 = 25\%$, $\text{RSD}_\infty = 3\%$, and $k = 0.15$ min^{-1}, the plot in Figure 5 is obtained. Initially, the rate of blending is very rapid. With further processing time, the rate of blending decreases due to the asymptotic nature of Equation (1). For this particular set of values for the RSDs and k constant, a reasonable blending time that balances producing a mixture of adequate uniformity with the economics associated with the blending operation would be approximately 25–30 min. Further blending beyond 30 minutes is unlikely to contribute any further practical change in the uniformity of the blend, as the asymptotic portion of the curve has been reached.

Demixing

It is also possible that blend uniformity can worsen with further blending time, which is a situation known as demixing (Fig. 6). In such instances, the blend will undergo three stages: the mixing zone, a steady state, and a demixing zone. The first two stages of the

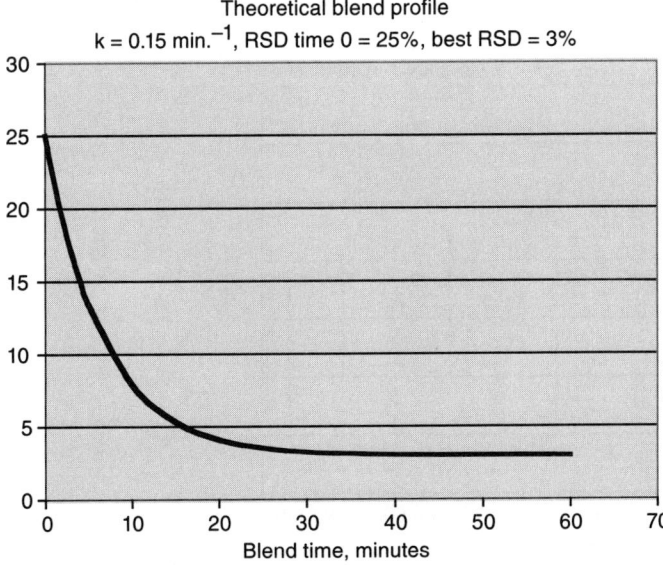

FIGURE 5 First order decay for blending.

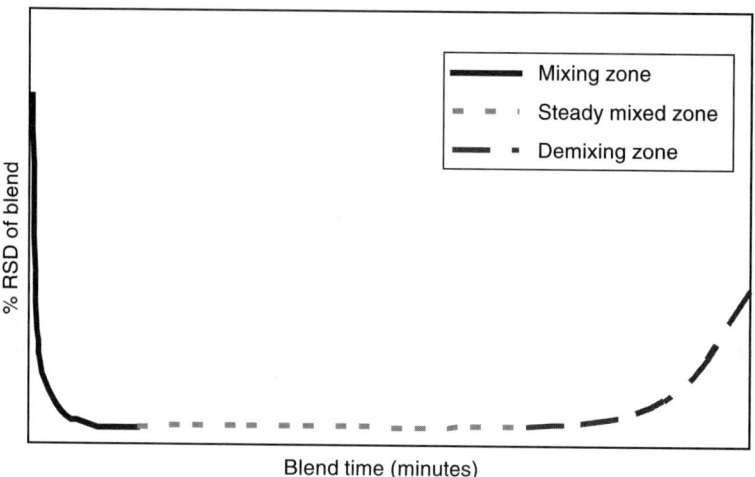

FIGURE 6 Stages of blending processes.

plot describe the first-order behavior of blending processes as previously presented in Equation (1) and Figure 5. In the first stage (mixing zone) there is a rapid decline in the RSD of the blend as it becomes more homogeneous through convective and dispersive blending. In the second stage (steady mixed zone), the blend reaches a dynamic equilibrium, where mixing and de-mixing occur at relatively the same rate, resulting in the homogeneity of the blend remaining relatively constant. In the third stage, segregation mechanisms dominate and the blend begins to become less homogeneous. As a result, the process deviates from the first order model described in Equation (1). Figure 7 contains an illustration of a blend that underwent demixing. The vertical axis is RSD (note the log scale), while the horizontal axis is blend time. The error bars are based on the confidence of the RSD given the limited number of samples.

It is important to note that demixing may not occur for all formulations. However, the potential of a blend to demix should always be investigated during formulation and

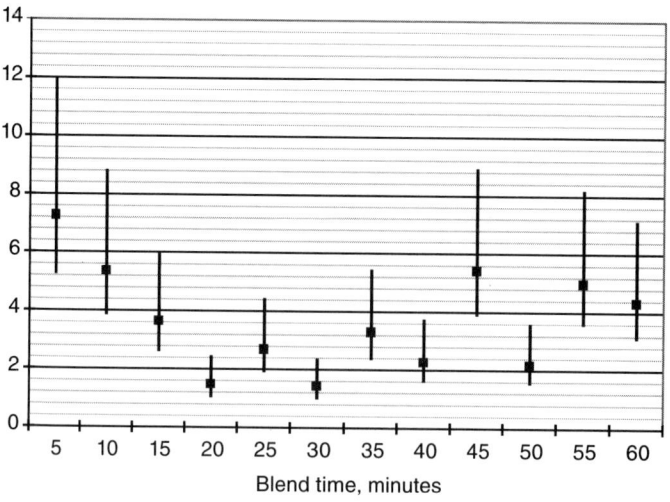

FIGURE 7 Example of a blend that has undergone demixing.

process development. Demixing can occur with both free flowing (i.e., low cohesion) and cohesive powders. For free flowing powders, differences in particle size, shape, or density of the materials being blended can result in decreased homogeneity with further blending. Developing a formulation that uses excipients with similar properties to those of the active ingredient can minimize the potential of this mechanism to occur. Larger particles tend to flow better than smaller ones, which could lead to material segregation and is one of the primary causes of demixing. For cohesive powders, segregation can occur due to agglomeration of the active to itself. Later in this chapter, we will describe how incorporating shear into the blending process can be used to control this problem.

Size induced demixing patterns were demonstated by Tommasson et al. (7) while studying mixing patterns of colored beads of different size (1.6 mm blue and 4 mm red beads) in a 1 quart double cone blender. A segregation pattern appeared within the first few rotations of the blender whereby smaller particles form a contiguous core through the blend that runs parallel to the axis of rotation. Although the above example is vivid illustration of how demixing can occur, it is relatively uncommon for pharmaceutical formulations unless extremely long blend times, or unusual material properties are present.

Identifying Acceptable Blending Times

Acceptable ranges for blending times are determined by performing blend studies. An experimental design or protocol should be drafted prior to the start of the studies, including the sampling plan and acceptance criteria that will be used to demonstrate uniformity of the blend. Batch size, blender speed, and load patterns must be maintained constant over the course of the study, unless the experimental design contains specific trials to investigate the potential impact that these variables may have on the uniformity of the resulting blend. Samples should be taken from a suitable number of locations to adequately map the blender, and target suspected regions where sub- or super-potent material could exist. The samples should be taken and assayed from at least three or four blending times to examine the uniformity of the blend. The range of sampling times should be sufficiently broad, with one or two of the selected times being in the vicinity of the expected edges of failure. However, as the purpose of the study is to identify a range of blending times that will produce a blend of suitable uniformity, at least two of the examined times should produce acceptable results. For at least one time (e.g., the best estimate of the ideal time), stratified samples (discussed later) should be collected to diagnose within- and between-location variations. Error bars (confidence intervals) showing the range of possible RSDs, based on the number of samples collected, should be included to better diagnose true variations from statistical noise. Additionally, sample locations can be grouped and plotted separately (e.g., comparing all samples on the left to all samples on the right side of a blender), to identify areas of super- and sub-potency within the blending container.

Studies to identify lubrication blending times can use the above strategy, but also must consider the impact that prolonged blending times (of often lipophilic excipients) can have on the physical properties of the resulting dosage form, especially hardness and dissolution profiles. The optimal blending time may not necessarily be the time which provides the most uniform dispersion of the lubricant in the blend. For drugs that have poor aqueous solubility, the selected lubricant blending time may be skewed towards the lower end of the identified range, to minimize the risk of over-lubrication of the blend. Acceptable performance of the blend on compression or filling equipment, and the ability of the resulting product to comply with acceptance criteria, should be considered when identifying a range of lubricant blending times.

Once a uniform blend has been obtained, it is essential that the particles in the blend cease movement to allow the system to exist in a state of static equilibrium without segregation occurring. From a practical point of view, this is not possible as subsequent material transfer during the compression or filling operations involves material flow. Therefore, care must be exercised to ensure that the impact each subsequent handling step has on the equilibrium achieved for the blend at the conclusion of the blending operation is minimized. The mechanisms by which powders can segregate, as well as means to control it, will be discussed later in this chapter.

Factors Affecting Blending Processes

Particle Size, Shape, and Density

As previously discussed, differences in the particle sizes of materials being blended can lead to segregation. Therefore, proper formulation development entails the selection of materials that have comparable particle size distributions whenever possible. Many excipients, such as lactose and microcrystalline cellulose, are available in a variety of grades, which are reflective of the particle size, density, or flow characteristics of the respective material. Careful selection of the grade to be used in the formulation enhances the ability of the blending process to prepare uniform blends.

Drug substances are often milled, to increase the number of drug particles (on a per unit weight basis) in a batch, and thereby improves content uniformity of the resulting blend and dosage units. Milling avoids the problem of having just a few "large" particles dictate the uniformity of the dose, where small deviations in the number of particles contained in the dosage form can have a pronounced impact on the amount of drug delivered to the patient. Note that milling is not only applied to break up single particles, but is also used to disperse agglomerates as well. Zhang and Johnson (8) defined a model that predicts the impact of drug substance particle size on content uniformity. This model simulates the number, size, and mass of the drug particles in the batch and distributes them evenly across all unit doses. Such models are very useful tools during development, as they identify preliminary targets for the particle sizes of raw materials used in the formulation. However, the model assumptions include ideal blending and a log-normal function for the particle size distribution. Therefore, the predictive results of the model should be verified through actual content uniformity results. Others (9,10,) have also studied the significance of drug content and drug proportion to the content uniformity of solid dosage forms.

Particle shape can also affect blending processes. Spherical and cubic shaped particles typically exhibit good flow properties and therefore promote blending. However, readily flowing materials may also be more prone to segregation. Plates and needle shaped particles have poor flow properties, are harder to dilate/expand, and are more likely to agglomerate. As a result, it may be more difficult to achieve uniformity when blending plate and needle shaped particles. Conversely, a benefit to this decreased mobility is that once blended, these are more likely to stay blended.

The densities of components in a blend should also be matched, as large differences can lead to segregation. However, differences due to the density of materials alone are less likely to impact the uniformity of the blend, and are typically insignificant below a 4-fold difference. Differences in density are more likely to contribute to segregation when combined with other factors such as different particle sizes (11,12).

Blending and Blend Uniformity

Cohesivity

One definition of a cohesive powder is a situation in which the adhesive forces (mechanical, electrostatic, Van der Waals, surface tension) between particles exceed the particle weight by at least an order of magnitude (13). The magnitude of adhesive forces is greatly influenced by physical properties of the particles, such as size, shape, morphology, and moisture (14,15). Surface moisture has a more pronounced impact on cohesivity than uptake potential. It is possible to handle a very hygroscopic material in a dry environment without issues, but a minimally hygroscopic material with high moisture can be more of a problem. The packing density of the material also affects cohesivity, as it determines the number of interparticle contacts per unit area. Packing can result from pressure (e.g., from the weight of material), as well as vibration that can result in settling of smaller particles as they move through the interstitial void spaces in the powder bed. The cohesive strength of a material as a function of consolidation (packing) can be measured using a variety of shear cells (discussed in Chapter 3).

The flow characteristics of cohesive materials can be variable. Very cohesive materials can be difficult to discharge out of bins, hoppers, and chutes. Flow problems such as ratholing (in funnel flow), bridging/arching, erratic flow, and flooding may result. Poor material flow can also produce excessive weight variability for dosage units due to bulk density variations, and the uneven filling of die cavities on a tablet press.

Although slightly cohesive powders may blend faster than free-flowing materials, and reach a greater degree of homogeneity, highly cohesive powders are more difficult to blend than free-flowing materials. Cohesive powders often require the application of external stress to achieve uniformity. This additional stress is needed both to dilate the bed and to disperse agglomerates. Most problems associated with blending cohesive powders are the result of low shear in the blenders.

A powder will flow when the stresses exceed the cohesive strength of a material. The cohesion number (π_c) is one metric that could be of assistance when scaling up blending processes for cohesive materials (4). This metric is calculated according to the following equation:

$$\pi_c = (\sigma/\rho g R) \qquad (2)$$

where σ is the effective cohesive strength under flow conditions, ρ is the powder density under flow conditions, g is the acceleration of gravity, and R is the vessel size. As the vessel size of the powder under flow conditions increases, the cohesion number decreases. In larger blenders, gravitational forces increase with increasing scale, and can overcome existing cohesive forces. Therefore, cohesive effects are often more significant in smaller scale blenders, and the impact of scaling-up to a larger vessel size often results in successful blending operations despite a limited understanding of the cohesive nature of the materials.

The application of sufficient shear is required when blending cohesive materials. This is especially critical for small-scale tumble blenders, which based on Equation (2) provide little gravitational force and therefore shear during the blending process. High shear mixers are frequently used to prepare premixes of cohesive drug substances, as they impart sufficient shear to both dilate the bed and to break apart loosely bound agglomerates. In addition, by preparing a uniform premix of the drug and diluent, the diluent particles form a physical barrier that impedes the ability of drug particles to come together and form agglomerates. As a result, the rate at which the drug particles reagglomerate during subsequent blending and material handling operations decreases. However, the use of high shear mixers for lubrication processes should be discouraged.

The exposure of lubricants to prolonged shear could reduce their particle size resulting in over-lubrication of the blend that subsequently leads to poorer compression characteristics of the blend and slower rates of dissolution of the dosage form.

For all but very high dose products, the presence of agglomerates is the biggest risk to be overcome when blending cohesive particles, due to their propensity to form super-potent tablets. Breaking up the agglomerates during the blending process is much slower than random mixing of the component itself. As a result, deagglomeration can become the rate determining step in the blending process, especially for the dilution of drugs with low doses (16). For this reason, it is encouraged that all materials are passed through a screen or mill to break-up agglomerates prior to blending operations. Even at concentrations <5% w/w, cohesive drugs can agglomerate during blending processes, resulting in the production of super-potent tablets that are much greater than 100% label claim (e.g., potency much greater than 115%). This phenomenon often occurs only in a very small percentage of dosage units in the batch and as such, is difficult to detect. Even when they are detected, they are often incorrectly dismissed as being anomalies or potential laboratory errors (17).

Subjecting the material to shear either through the use of high-speed choppers, agitation bars, or screening the drug substance prior to charging the blender all help to disperse any agglomerates, and alleviates the potential of manufacturing super-potent dosage units (4). Although milling drug substances increases the number of particles per unit weight, smaller particle sizes may have a greater propensity to form agglomerates, especially if the material is hygroscopic or develops an electrostatic charge. As previously stated, static baffles impart minimal, if any, shear. Once the agglomerates are broken up by the application of shear, care must be taken to insure that they do not reform during subsequent blending or material transfer steps. Ways to help minimize re-agglomeration include minimizing flow of the material (blending time, transfer steps), minimizing holding time (allowing agglomerates to strengthen) and exposure to high humidity. Formulation modifications (e.g., the addition of a glidant such as fume silica) may also be beneficial in minimizing agglomeration tendencies.

The preparation of preblends via high shear blending may not be sufficient in dispersing tightly bound agglomerates. It may be necessary to incorporate a milling step into the manufacturing process, to break-up large rigid agglomerates prior to the preparation of the final blend. Blend–mill–blend operations are useful when blending cohesive materials that form large and strong agglomerates. Conical mills apply high shear rates to materials passed through them, improving the distribution of the drug particles, and minimizing the formation of drug agglomerates. Although they will break up agglomerates, milling operations generally do not produce adequate blends by themselves, and an additional blending step post-milling is typically required to achieve uniformity.

Humidity and Temperature

Humidity also can have a significant impact on cohesivity of the blend (18), and high levels of moisture can accelerate the formation of agglomerates. Surface moisture plays a key role in the formation of agglomerates, and has a greater impact than hygroscopicity on the cohesive nature of materials. For hygroscopic drug substances, optimal blending times must be identified which provide a sufficient time to achieve acceptable uniformity, while minimizing the opportunity for the drug to sequester moisture from the environment, or even from excipients. Powders that pick up ambient moisture may be prone to forming agglomerates. In such situations, as the blending time continues, the uniformity will increase up to a certain point, and then decrease due to formation of agglomerates, loading to demixing.

The temperature of a blend can impact the cohesive and agglomeration tendencies of materials. Although most blending operations take place in typical "room temperature" conditions, heating can occur when sufficient energy is imparted due to flow in the blender. In some cases, heating can cause softening of particles, which can in turn increase cohesion and result in the formation of agglomerates. Softer particles may also be more prone to sticking onto equipment surfaces. Cooling (via jacketing of the blender or other means) may be needed to keep the material temperature below critical softening points.

Blender Rotation Speed

The rotational speed that tumble blenders are operated at can influence blending processes. Ottino (19) described material movement during blending processes as a function of blender rotation speed. At low rotation speeds, the flow comprises discrete avalanches or slumping, in which one stops before the other begins. At higher rotation speeds, a steady flow is obtained with a thin cascading layer at the free surface of the rotating bed (continuous flow, rolling, or cascading regime). At still higher speeds, particle inertia effects become important resulting in centrifuging of the particles to the walls of the blender as the container rotates.

Rotation speed impacts shear rate and therefore blending efficiency, especially when cohesive materials are being blended. However, the relationship between rotation speed and uniformity is affected by the complex nature of the flow of cohesive materials, and the number and size of avalanches per revolution. Blending performance in bench scale tumble blenders demonstrated that the rotation speed did not significantly impact the blending of free-flowing materials (5,20).

Electrostatic Charge

When two surfaces come into contact, the transfer of electrons can occur and upon separation, result in opposite charges on each material's surface. When contact charging between different materials is accompanied by energetic friction, rubbing, sliding, rolling, and impact, the term triboelectrification is used. Therefore, the relative movement of particles and collisions with surfaces during blending and powder transfer operations provide ideal conditions for triboelectrification to occur. The charge distributes itself over the surface at a rate (relaxation time) that is dependent on the permittivity and surface resistivity of the materials. Conductors have rapid (instantaneous) relaxation times, while insulators may have much longer relaxation times (minutes or hours).

When a particle becomes charged by triboelectrification, two types of interactions may contribute to the deposition and adhesion of the particle, namely electrical double layers and Coulombic interactions. Electrical double layers are considered to result from the formation of a shell of oppositely charged electrical layers at the interface upon contact. Coulombic interactions result from the forces of interaction which arise between charged particles and uncharged surfaces.

Electrostatic charging is a complex phenomena and the degree to which it occurs is affected by a number of factors including contact surface properties of both materials coming into contact with each other, particle properties, the contact event (contact pressure, area, time, and frequency), and atmospheric conditions (21,22). Particle size, shape, surface nature, purity, roughness, and the properties of the powder and contact material (particle size and shape, surface roughness) all influence triboelectrification (23–26). The composition of the contact surface (e.g., metal, plastic, glass) and its electrical and mechanical properties, as well as surface contamination can all affect triboelectrification. However, the effects that these factors may impart are often unpredictable. Powders may become positively or negatively charged, depending on the type of surface that they come in contact with (27–29). Careful selection of the materials used to construct equipment and processing conditions can impact the sign and magnitude of the electrostatic charge.

Particle–steel interactions occur in many pharmaceutical unit operations, such as milling, blending, fluid bed drying, material transport, and sieve testing. Particle–plastic interactions can occur during blending or fluid bed drying (in Plexiglas containers), material transport and device filling. Pavey (30) presented typical charge levels seen for powders during various unit operations (Table 1).

Electrostatics can have a pronounced effect, especially for low density materials, and controlling their effects can be challenging (31–33). Furthermore, the effects are often difficult to reproduce. The generation of electrostatic charge can be highly configuration specific, with different effects occurring for different sites, scales, and equipment. This could be a contributing factor for instances where acceptable blends may be obtained on pilot scale using blenders constructed out of Plexiglas, but unacceptable blends result upon scale-up into commercial scale stainless steel blenders.

The propensity of a material to be affected by electrostatics can be evaluated via testing to measure volume resistivity and charge relaxation time. The measurement of electrostatic charge is often conducted using a Faraday pail or well. However, this technique has limitations and exhibits a lot of variability. Atomic force microscopy (34) and a capacitive probe apparatus have also been used (35,36). Various formulation and process remedies have been used to control electrostatic build-up during blending processes, including the addition of a component which may aid in dissipating charge (colloidal silica), increasing the moisture content of the blend or relative humidity of the processing room, avoiding tribocharging via sliding on surfaces, and the use of grounding.

If the relative humidity in processing rooms is very low, electrostatic charges can become more pronounced and result in particles adhering to the walls of the blender. This can result in reduced potency of the subsequent dosage units. This problem can be detected following discharge of the blender, by dislodging any material that may have adhered to its walls and assaying it for potency. If the assay results indicate the material is drug rich, adherence to the walls of the blender could be one of many points in the process where drug is being removed from the blend, causing low potency values for the dosage units. An estimate of the amount of residual material on the equipment can be used to perform a mass balance calculation, to see if the loss in active drug is accounted for solely due to adhesion to equipment.

TABLE 1 Typical Mass Charge Density

Operation	Typical mass charge density (C kg^{-1})
Sieving	10^{-3} to 10^{-5}
Pouring	10^{-1} to 10^{-3}
Scroll feeding	1 to 10^{-2}
Grinding	1 to 10^{-1}
Micronizing	10^2 to 10^{-1}
Pneumatic conveying	10^3 to 10^{-1}
Triboelectric powder coating	10^4 to 10^3

Manufacture of Low Dose Blends

The distribution of a small quantity of drug substance in blends can be challenging to achieve acceptable uniformity. Low dose formulations often require additional blending techniques to incorporate minor components into the bulk of the blend.

Geometric dilution is a technique to aid in the distribution of smaller quantities of active ingredients into the larger bulk of the blend. It involves blending a quantity of the active ingredient (X) with an equal part of diluent (X). Once blended, an additional quantity of diluent equal to the total quantity already blended in the first step (2X) is added to the previous blend and blended. This process is repeated by adding 4X, 8X, 16X, etc. quantities of diluent until the active ingredient is sufficiently diluted to be incorporated into the remainder of the batch. Geometric dilution can be done in a single blender, or may require the use of a larger blender for the combination of larger quantities in the procedure. In its simplest application, geometric dilution is used by pharmacists during the extemporaneous compounding of a prescription, typically using a mortar and pestle to uniformly incorporate the drug into the remaining formulation components. On a large scale, drug manufacturers use geometric dilution during the manufacture of both pilot and large-scale batches of solid dosage forms. The same principle applies in each case, with the only difference being the type of equipment used to accommodate the quantities of materials being processed.

Another technique used to distribute small amounts of drug in a blend is to manufacture a preblend that is subsequently introduced into the bulk of the blend. Preblends can be made in a variety of blenders, although high shear mixers are often used based on their proven efficiency in preparing such blends. This mixing efficiency allows the ratio of excipient to drug to be higher than that used for geometric dilution. The preblend is then added to a larger blender containing the remaining components of the blend.

Wet granulation processes can also be used to homogeneously distribute small quantities of drugs in dosage forms. If the drug is sufficiently soluble, it can be dissolved in the binder solution, which is subsequently used to granulate the remaining powders. The formation of granules can lock the drug product into place and depending on the efficiency and robustness of the resulting granulation, may minimize the potential for the blend to segregate. Similarly, dry granulation also locks particles of the drug substance in the granules that are produced, and therefore is another acceptable means to produce uniform final blends that can be further processed into dosage forms. The ability of dry granulation to produce acceptable blends is dependent the preparation of a uniform preblend that can be fed through the roller compactor to produce the ribbons or slugs of powder that are subsequently milled into granules. Other attributes that must be controlled during the manufacture of low dose products using dry granulation include minimizing the amount of material that by-passes the rollers, and optimizing the friability of the resulting granules.

Dissolving the drug in a suitable solvent and spraying it onto an excipient that is a major component of the formulation can also achieve acceptable content uniformity for low dose products. This technique produces stronger interactions between the drug and carrier particle, and will be further discussed in the section on the preparation of ordered mixtures. Spraying a solution of the drug substance can also be performed in a fluid bed dryer. This process is desirable for drugs that have low aqueous solubility, and therefore would require large volumes of liquid to be sprayed onto the carrier particles, which if performed in a high shear blender would likely produce a thick paste or slurry if wet granulation was pursued. Performing the process in a fluid bed dryer allows the solvent to be simultaneously removed during the process, thereby overcoming the previous issue.

When using fluid bed processors, there is always the risk of fines (in particular of drug substance) being trapped in the filter bags. At the end of fluid bed processing, the filter bags are shaken to release the material in them, which could result in a drug enriched layer collecting on the surface of the material in the equipment's bowl.

Ordered Mixing

Ordered mixing is a process in which particles are created that are a combination of two or more components of a blend. The ordered unit is the smallest entity that constitutes an ordered mixture. Below this size, it would only be possible to sample an incomplete unit or even a single ingredient.

The pharmaceutical industry uses ordered mixing to adhere fine particles of the drug substance onto coarser carrier particles (37,38). This technique offers significant advantages in the manufacture of dosage forms that contain low quantities of potent drug substances by improving the content uniformity of the blend. The ability of the ordered unit to remain intact defines the robustness and life of the ordered mixture. As long as the bond strength cannot be easily broken, ordered mixing can decrease the ability of blends to segregate, thereby maintaining homogeneity standards throughout processing (39). The small particle size of the drug may also result in faster dissolution rates, while the coarse carrier particles provide favorable compression characteristics desired for tablet manufacture.

During the production of an ordered mixture, sufficient energy must be input by the blender to break down agglomerates of the fine cohesive component, which are then adhered to the surface of the carrier particles (40) The formation of ordered mixes can occur by mechanical ordering, adhesional ordering, or the production of coated ordered mixtures.

Mechanical Ordering

Mechanical ordering occurs as a result of particle–particle collisions between the drug substance and carrier particles as they are blended. The ordered units are formed without bonding forces, which causes them to be very unstable and susceptible to segregation during discharging from the blender and subsequent material handling steps.

Adhesional Ordering

Adhesional ordering is based on the fine particles possessing intrinsic cohesional properties that allow them to adhere to larger carrier particles. Mechanical, Van der Waals, electrostatic, surface tensional, and capillary forces can all be responsible for the binding of particles in ordered units. To allow the formation of ordered units, the adhesional force between the drug and carrier must be greater than the cohesional force for either component.

During the blending process, particles of the drug substance adhere to the carrier substrate until an even coating of the fine particles per unit surface area of carrier particles results. For ordered mixes prepared by adhesional forces or coating process (see below), the size of the ordered unit is largely controlled by that of the carrier particle (41). By maintaining a tight particle size distribution of the carrier, the amount of drug substance adsorbed onto the surface of a saturated carrier particle remains fairly constant. This decreases the susceptibility of the ordered mixture to changes in the content uniformity of the blend resulting from particle size induced segregation.

It is possible that the cohesive drug particles could simultaneously form agglomerates with themselves during the ordered blending process. For that reason, adhesional ordering depends on the ability of the larger coarse carrier particles to crush and break down any agglomerates of the drug substance that may form during the process. The degree of size reduction is dependent on a number of factors including the duration of blending, the physical properties of the smaller drug particles, and the particle size and weight of the carrier particles. If the carrier particles cannot break up the agglomerates, mechanical shear must be imparted to the blend (such as agitators or high-speed chopper blades) to break up the agglomerates of the individual constituents. However, caution should be exercised to ensure that shear used to break agglomerates of the drug substance does not also strip the active from the carrier particles, or cause excessive attrition of the carrier particles.

Free drug substance can occur in blends made from ordered mixtures. Decreasing the size of the drug particles enhances blend uniformity in accordance with random mixing theory, and improves the adhesional interaction between drug and carrier particles. However, it is possible that an excessive reduction in the particle size of the drug can result in saturation of the carrier's surface with a lower amount (thinner layer) of drug on a per weight basis. The addition of a third component into the ordered system can preferentially adhere to the carrier particles, thereby displacing the drug substance from their adhesion sites (42). In both of these instances, the free drug substance can agglomerate and reduce the uniformity of the blend.

Coated Ordered Mixtures

Coated ordered mixtures are formed by applying a coating to carrier particles to form the ordered units. Typically, a solution of the drug substance is sprayed onto the carrier particles. In other applications, an excipient coating may be applied to a drug particle for taste masking purposes. In either case, this process results in complete bonding such that segregation of the two constituents cannot occur except under extreme circumstances. The homogeneity of the ordered mixture is dependent on the size of the coated particles. Smaller particles have a greater surface area (on a per unit mass basis) which when coated, results in a higher loading of coating. When large and small particles segregate, differences in potency and therefore content uniformity can result.

The properties of ordered mixtures are directly related to the force that bonds the two constituents together (43). Whether an ordered mixture is formed depends on a number of factors. Sufficient energy must be imparted to the blend to completely break up agglomerates of the cohesive material that may form. The ratio of the drug substance and carrier particles must be balanced to avoid the saturation of the adhesion or adsorption sites on the carrier substrate. Concentrations of drug substance that oversaturate the adsorption sites of the carrier particles result in excessive drug in the blend. This can produce a situation in which a blended random/ordered system exists that can result in the formation of agglomerates and/or segregation. Once saturation is reached, additional active drug remains mobile, and given its significantly smaller particle size relative to the carrier, can be highly prone to segregation. In this case, higher drug loading can result in worse content uniformity, which is the reverse of what is typically expected when one works with a purely random (non-ordered) mix.

One way to test an ordered mixture is to pass the blend through a nest of sieves and assay each particle size fraction. The lesser the variation in potency across the cuts, the better the ordered mix. Note that this test is highly dependent upon how much energy goes into the sieving process. Shaking the sieves by hand would be expected to produce different results than using an ultrasonic method.

Scaling of Blenders

Currently, there are no numerical/computational approaches to assess, a priori, how multiple components of a typical pharmaceutical material will blend in a given blender, without performing experimental work as the basis of understanding flow and blending behaviors (44,45). Typically bench or intermediate scale trials are conducted in a given blender, and then this is scaled to a larger production process. Scaling still remains an art, though as numerical modeling and process monitoring improves, the understanding of blending behaviors will improve. In the meantime, the general approach is to try-it-and-see at a smaller scale, and if this is successful, to use some general rules of thumb to scale the blending process. Due to their limitations, these rules of thumb are not agreed upon. Since tumbling blending is the most common method for final blending, where uniformity is most critical, the scaling of tumble blending is discussed below.

There are three parameters that should be kept similar in scaling tumble blenders. These include geometric, kinematic, and dynamic similarity. This approach is valid for tumble blending without the use of shear (such as an intensifier bar), for low-cohesion materials. Cohesive materials have poor flow and hence blend less efficiently at smaller scales; therefore, this technique may overestimate the blending time for scaling up, and underestimate the time when scaling down.

Geometric similarity is keeping the ratio of all lengths constant between scales. In other words, the shape remains the same, while the size changes. An analogy is photocopying a drawing—when the copy is enlarged the shape stays the same but the copy gets bigger. To maintain geometric similarity, blender angles (such as the cone on a double cone blender, or the angle made by the two legs of a V-blender) stay the same, as does the position of the axis of rotation. Further, the fill level must also remain similar, as does the method and order of filling the blender. Maintaining the initial fill locations is critical as tumble blenders are more efficient in the radial direction (perpendicular to the axis of rotation) than axial (parallel to the axis of rotation); hence top-to-bottom layering provides faster blending than side-by-side layering. Unfortunately, it can be a challenge to match how a blender is filled at a small scale (whereby material may be hand-scooped into the blender) to that at a larger scale (whereby material may be loaded from bins, drums, or conveyors). Unfortunately these scaling procedures do not accommodate modifications to geometric similarity, so if it is violated, the effect is unknown. This is a particular problem when one wants to consider changing equipment, for example, from a V-blender to a bin-blender. In this case one is back to the beginning of conducting initial trials at a small scale.

Dynamic similarity is maintaining constant forces. The Froude number (F), described in Equation (3), is often used for scale-up:

$$F = \text{RPM}^{2} * r/g \tag{3}$$

where RPM is blender rotation speed in revolutions per minute, r is a characteristic radius, and g is the gravitational constant. This approach sets the speed of the blender, but blenders seldom have variable speed drives to allow for fine tuning of the speed. Fortunately blending is not a strong function of speed for "typical" operating speeds of most commercial blending equipment.

Scale-up based on kinematic similarity is performed by maintaining a consistent number of revolutions (RPM × time). For example, consider how to scale from a 20-l V-blender which produced an acceptable blend at 8 RPM for 20 min, to a 200-l scale. What

Blending and Blend Uniformity

should it look like, and what should the blender speed and time be? Following geometric similarity, we need an identical shaped V-blender, with a 10-fold increase in capacity. This requires lengths to increase by $10^{(1/3)}$ or 215%. Angles stay the same, as would the axis of rotation, fill level and fill pattern. Following dynamic similarity, the new RPM would be:

$$\text{RPM}_{(200\,l)} = [\text{RPM}_{(20\,l)}{}^{2*}\, r_{(20\,l)}/r_{(200\,l)}]^{(1/2)} = [8^2/215\%]^{(1/2)} = 5.4 \qquad (4)$$

Generally one accepts the speed that the larger blender is capable of, unless it is far off from these scaling rules. Assuming that 5.4 RPM could be achieved in the larger scale blender, one can calculate the blend time following kinematic similarity, and realize it takes 29.6 minutes to achieve comparable blending as 160 revolutions used at the smaller scale.

SEGREGATION

Introduction

Segregation can be defined as having particles of similar properties (size, composition, density, resiliency, static charge, etc.) preferentially distributed into different zones within given equipment or processes. Segregation most notably affects the localized concentration of the drug substance, resulting in blend and content uniformity problems. In addition to segregation of the drug substance, segregation of other components of the blend can be responsible for variations in properties such as dissolution, stability, lubrication, taste, appearance, and color. Even if the blend remains chemically homogeneous, variations in particle size can affect flowability, bulk density, weight uniformity, tablet hardness, appearance, and dissolution. Additionally, segregation can create concentrations of dust, which can lead to problems with agglomeration, yield, operator exposure, containment, cleanliness, and increased potential for a dust explosion.

Segregation can occur any time there is powder transfer (e.g., from a blender to a bin), or when forces acting on the particles (such as air flow or vibration) are sufficient to induce particle movement. This includes handling steps upstream of a blender (including segregation of raw materials at a supplier's plant or during shipment), movement within the blender, during its discharge, or in downstream equipment. Of these, the most common area for problems is post-blender discharge.

The current state of understanding segregation is limited to having empirical descriptors of segregation mechanisms, and prior experiences with diagnosing and addressing specific segregation behaviors. There are no "first principle" models that describe segregation, whereby one can plug material properties such as particle size and chemical composition, and get back a prediction of segregation potential. At best, computational models such as discrete element modeling are evolving which can be tuned to match specific segregation behaviors that are created in physical models. As these models evolve they will become more powerful and have fewer assumptions and limitations, but for the time being the average pharmaceutical scientist will not be making use of them to predict or solve the segregation problems they will likely encounter. Since the current state involves a combination of art and science, it is critical to utilize as many resources as possible to understand and address segregation problems—real or potential.

Segregation Mechanisms

Three primary segregation mechanisms are of interest in typical pharmaceutical blend handling operations. Other mechanisms exist (46), but are less frequently encountered. The segregation mechanisms of interest are:

- sifting (sometimes called percolation);
- fluidization (sometimes called air entrainment);
- dusting (sometimes called particle entrainment in an air stream).

These terms are not universally defined, so one must use caution when using them. Segregation may occur as a result of just one of these mechanisms, or a combination of several. Whether segregation occurs, to what degree, and which mechanism or mechanisms are involved depend on a combination of the properties of the blend and the process conditions encountered.

Material Properties that Impact Segregation

Several properties of the materials being blended can influence segregation tendencies. Both the mean particle size and particle size distribution should be characterized. Although segregation can occur with blends of any mean size, different mechanisms become more pronounced at different particle sizes. Multi-modal blends are more likely to segregate than uni-modal blends. Relying on the mean particle size to assess segregation potential is risky, as the tails of a distribution can have different segregation tendencies than the mean. Differences in the density and shape of the components in a formulation can lead to segregation. Rounded particles may have increased mobility than irregularly shaped particles, which can allow more segregation. Particle resilience influences collisions between particles and surfaces, which can lead to differences in where components accumulate. As a general rule, more cohesive blends are less likely to segregate. However, if enough energy is added to dilate the blend and/or separate particles from one another, even a very cohesive material can segregate. The ability of components to develop and hold an electrostatic charge, and their affinity for other ingredients or processing surfaces can also contribute to segregation tendencies.

Of all of these, segregation based on particle size is by far the most common (47). In fact, particle size is the most important factor in all of the primary segregation mechanisms considered here.

Processing Conditions that Impact Segregation

Particular care must be taken at points of storage and transfer post-blending, since these present the greatest opportunity for such conditions to occur.

Process conditions that commonly exacerbate segregation generally occur around operations that involve material transfer and handling. This includes interparticle motion within a bed of particles in contact with one another, especially true during pile formation upon filling of a container. Free falling material, especially when dropped from greater heights, and severe changes in the direction of material flow can contribute to segregation (48). Mechanical vibration (especially if sufficient to induce particle motion), fluidization (especially if the gas velocity is lower than that which provides blending) and air currents (specifically if airborne particle are present) can also cause segregation.

Blending and Blend Uniformity

Sifting Segregation

Sifting segregation is the most common form of segregation for many industrial processes. Under appropriate conditions, fine particles tend to sift or percolate through coarse particles. For segregation to occur by this mechanism there must be a range of particle sizes. A minimum difference in mean particle diameters between components of 1.3:1 is often more than sufficient. In addition, the mean particle size of the mixture must be sufficiently large (typically greater than about 100 μm) (49), the mixture must be relatively free-flowing to allow particle mobility, and there must be relative motion between particles. This last requirement is very important, since without it even highly segregating blends of ingredients that meet the first three tests will not segregate. Relative motion can be induced in a variety of ways, such as when a pile is formed when filling a bin, vibration from surrounding equipment (such as a tablet press), or as particles tumble and slide down a chute.

The result of sifting segregation in a bin is usually a side-to-side variation in the particle size distribution. The smaller particles will generally concentrate under the fill point, with the coarse particles concentrating at the perimeter of the pile (Fig. 8).

Fluidization Segregation

Variations in particle size or density often result in vertically segregated material when handling powders that can be fluidized. Finer or lighter particles often will be concentrated above larger or denser particles. This can occur during filling of a bin or other vessel, or within a blending vessel once the blending action has ceased.

Fluidization often results in horizontal gradation of fines and coarse material. A fine powder can remain fluidized for an extended period of time after filling or blending. In this fluidized state, larger and/or denser particles tend to settle to the bottom and fine particles may be carried to the surface with escaping air as the bed of material deaerates. For example, when a bin is being filled quickly, the coarse particles move

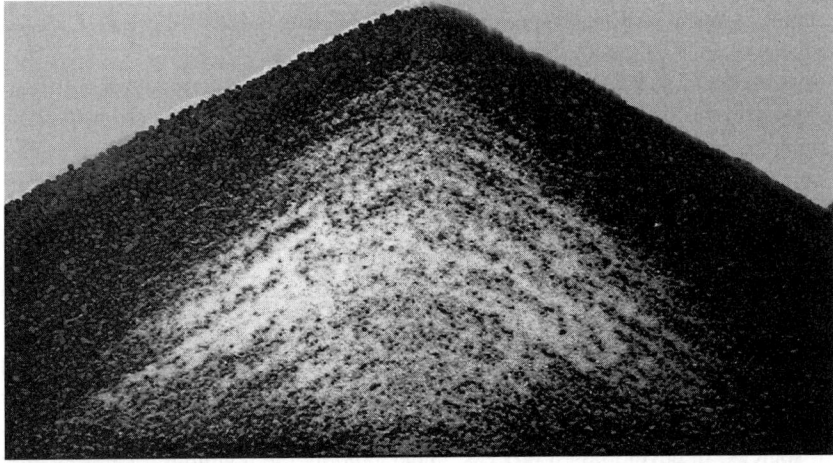

FIGURE 8 Example of sifting segregation in a two-dimensional pile. Note the dark particles are approximately 1200 μm, while the light particles are approximately 350 μm. *Source*: Courtesy of Jenike & Johanson, Inc.

downward through the aerated bed while the fine particles remain fluidized near the surface. This can also occur after blending if the material is fluidized during blending.

Fluidization is common in materials that contain a significant percentage of particles smaller than 100 µm (50). Fluidization segregation is likely to occur when fine materials are pneumatically conveyed, when they are filled or discharged at high rates, or if gas counter-flow occurs. As with most segregation mechanisms, the more cohesive the material, the less likely it will segregate by this mechanism.

Fluidization via gas counter-flow can occur as a result of insufficient venting during material transfer. As an example, consider a tumble blender discharging material to a drum, with an airtight seal between the two. As the blend transfers from the blender to the drum, air in the drum is displaced and a slight vacuum is created in the blender. If both are properly vented, air moves out of the drum and, separately, into the blender, but if not, the air must move from the drum to the blender through the blender discharge. In doing so, the fines may be stripped off of the blend and carried to the surface of the material still within the blender.

Dusting Segregation

Like fluidization segregation, dusting is most likely to be a problem when handling fine, free flowing powders (typically with particles smaller than about 50 µm) (50) that are made up of a range of particle sizes. If, upon filling a bin, the dust is created, air currents created by the falling stream will carry particles away from the fill point. The rate at which the dust settles is governed by the particle's settling velocity. The particle diameter is much more significant than particle density in determining settling velocity.

As an example of this mechanism, consider a mix of fine and large particles that is allowed to fall into the center of a bin. When the stream hits the pile of material in the bin, the column of air moving with it is deflected and sweeps off the pile toward the perimeter of the bin, where it becomes highly disturbed, but generally moves back up the bin walls in a swirling pattern. At this point, the gas velocity is much lower, allowing many particles to fall out of suspension. Because settling velocity is a strong function of particle diameter, the finest particles (with low settling velocities) will be carried to the perimeter of the bin while the larger particles will concentrate closer to the fill point, where the air currents are strong enough to prevent the fine particles from settling.

Dusting segregation can also result in less predictable segregation patterns, depending on how the bin is loaded, venting in the bin, and dust collection use and location.

Segregation Testing

In developing a product or designing a process, it is beneficial to know whether the material will be prone to segregation, and, if so, by which mechanism(s). During formulation development, this information can be used to modify the material properties (such as excipient selection, component particle size distribution, moisture content, or cohesiveness) to minimize the potential for segregation and to refine ingredient specifications or sources. In developing a process, understanding the potential for segregation can alert the equipment or process designer to potential risks that may then be avoided. In some cases, significant process steps, such as granulation, may be required to avoid potential segregation problems.

Blending and Blend Uniformity

There are two ASTM standard practices on segregation test methods (51,52). These testers are designed to isolate specific mechanisms, and test a material's tendency to segregate by that method. A brief description of these test methods follows.

Sifting Segregation Test Method

The sifting segregation test (Fig. 9A) is performed by center-filling a small funnel flow bin and then discharging it while collecting sequential samples. If sifting segregation occurs either during filling or discharge, the fines content of the discharging material will vary from beginning to end. Samples are collected from the various cups (i.e., the beginning, middle, and end of the discharge) and measured for segregation by particle size analyses, assays, or other variables of interest.

The sequence for performing the sifting segregation test is depicted in Figure 9B. The blend is placed in mass flow bin (1) and material is discharged from a fixed height, dropping into a funnel flow bin (2). This transfer of material will promote segregation if the material is prone to segregate due to sifting. Material is discharged from the funnel

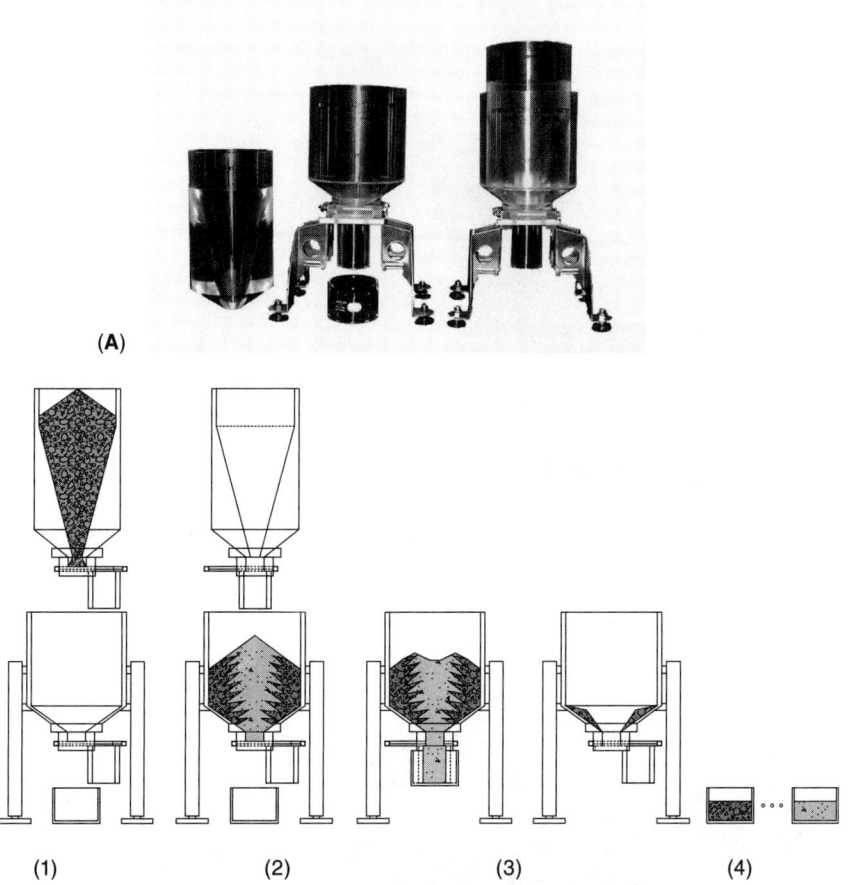

FIGURE 9 Sifting segregation testers (**A**) and sifting segregation test sequence (**B**). *Source*: Courtesy of Jenike & Johanson, Inc.

flow bin (3). The discharge pattern will cause material from the center to discharge first, and material from near the walls to discharge last. The collected samples are then measured for segregation (4).

Fluidization Segregation Test Method

The fluidization segregation test (Fig. 10) is run by first fluidizing a column of material by injecting air at its base. After the column is initially thoroughly fluidized it is held near a minimum fluidization velocity for a pre-determined period of time. The air is then turned off and the material is allowed to deaerate. The column is then split into three equal sections (top, middle, and bottom) and the resulting samples are measured for segregation.

Several other researchers and companies have developed various segregation testers including methods that induce vibration (16,54), shearing in a cell (56), and methods that capture material from a pile after it has formed (55–57). Improvements and variations to the ASTM test methods have also been made. A new fluidization segregation tester that utilizes a different mechanism to fluidize the bed has been developed

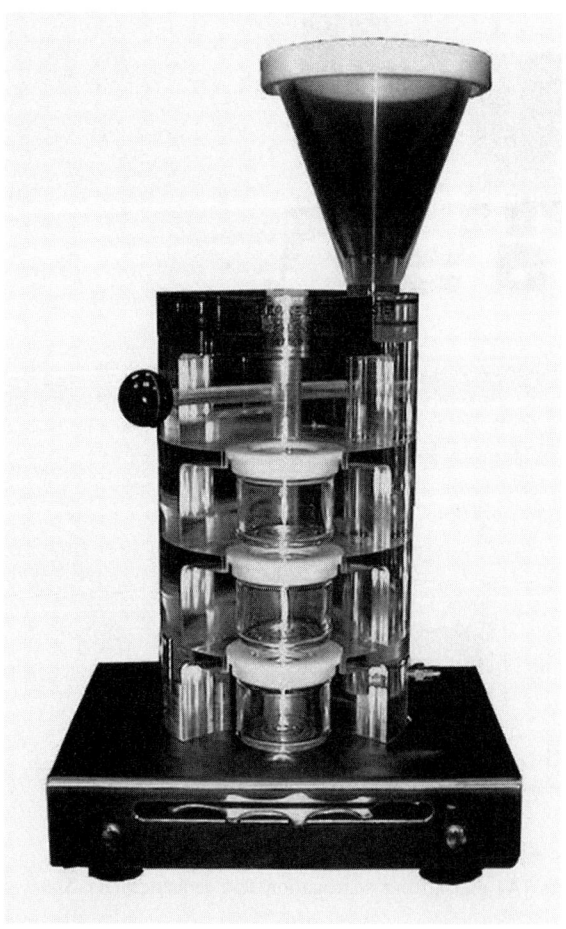

FIGURE 10 Fluidization segregation tester (controls not shown). *Source*: Courtesy of Jenike & Johanson, Inc.

Blending and Blend Uniformity

(58). It uses a smaller test sample, and provides unit–dose samples for analysis. An alternate way to run the sifting segregation test involves cycling the blend multiple times to strengthen the segregation "signal" (59).

Segregation tests are useful for identifying which segregation mechanism(s) might be active for a given blend, the general trend that may be observed in the process, and as a comparator between materials. However, the test results have limitations. Most notably, there is no direct way to use the results as a basis for designing a system that will minimize segregation. The results are not scaleable, and not tied quantifiably to the process. Testing points out, with comparative data, whether a material or blend is prone to segregation by a particular mechanism. However, it does not necessarily mean that a highly segregating material cannot be handled in a manner that prevents content uniformity problems.

Solutions to Segregation Problems

Determining which segregation mechanism or mechanisms are at work, and then correcting a segregation problem is seldom a simple exercise to accomplish. It requires knowledge of the material's physical and chemical characteristics, as well as an understanding of the segregation mechanisms that can be active. One must identify the process conditions that can serve as a driving force to cause segregation. Flow properties measurements (wall friction, cohesive strength, compressibility, and permeability) can help to provide understanding of the behavior of the material in storage and transfer equipment. Consideration should be given to the fill/discharge sequence, including flow pattern and inventory management, which gives rise to the observed segregation. Testing for segregation potential can provide additional insight about the mechanisms that may be causing segregation. Sufficient sampling is required to support the hypothesis of segregation (e.g., blend samples and final product samples, samples from the center vs. periphery of the bin). Finally, one must consider the impact of analytical and sampling errors specific to the blend under consideration, as well as the statistical significance of the results, when drawing conclusions from the data.

From the previous discussion about segregation mechanisms, it can be concluded that certain material properties as well as process conditions must exist for segregation to occur. Elimination of one of these will prevent segregation. It stands to reason then that if segregation is a problem in a process, one should look for opportunities to either change the material or change the process.

Changes to the Material

Often, changing the material is not an option, but the question should always be raised, particularly when developing a new product or process.

Changing the particle size distribution is sometimes the answer. Segregation based on particle size would not be possible if all particles were the same size. In practice, it is seldom practical to achieve this, but reducing the range of particle sizes within the material, or adjusting the mean particle size, may improve the situation significantly. Matching the particle size distributions of the different components is another way to minimize compositional variations due to size-based segregation. This may require purchasing one or more ingredients with a larger size than desired and milling them to achieve the desired size range.

Another possible solution may be to increase the cohesive strength of the material. Particularly in the case of sifting segregation, cohesive materials are much less likely to segregate. The caveat is that the material cannot be too cohesive; otherwise, flow problems may result. In our experience, most pharmaceutical blends that experience segregation problems are "too free flowing," that is, the blends have little or no cohesive strength. In these cases, cohesive strength could be increased without creating flow problems during manufacturing. Some formulators and excipient suppliers have the misconception that the most free-flowing formulation is the best. In selecting a material, the thought may be that the lowest angle of repose, the fastest flow funnel time, or the lowest shear strength is the desired state. While flow problems are avoided, the resulting blend is much more likely to segregate, in addition to possibly having other problems like excessive dust generation. The preferred state is to have a moderately cohesive material, one that is sufficiently free flowing so as not to create flow obstructions or weight variability during manufacturing, yet has ample strength to reduce particle mobility that can give rise to segregation.

In some cases, granulation can be used to bind different components of a blend together to form "unit particles" that are each composed of all of the ingredients of the blend. This is discussed in a previous section.

Changes to the Process and Equipment

Some generalizations can be made when designing equipment to minimize segregation. The complete details on how to implement these changes correctly are beyond the scope of this chapter. However, all equipment must be designed based on the flow properties and segregation potential of the blends being handled. Several courses of action that could be implemented to minimize segregation tendencies, as discussed below.

Whenever possible the number of material transfer steps should be minimized. With each transfer step and movement of the bin or drum, the tendency for segregation increases. Ideally, the material would discharge directly from the blender into the tablet press feed frame with no additional handling. In-bin blending is as close to this as most firms can practically obtain, and is the best one can ask for, as long as a uniform blend can be obtained within the bin blender in the first place. Another way to minimize material transfers is to use continuous blending operations that directly feed material to the compression or filling equipment.

Storage bins, press hoppers, and chutes should be designed to allow mass flow during their discharge. Two flow patterns are possible when discharging a bulk solid from a vessel: mass flow and funnel flow (60). In mass flow, the entire contents of the vessel are in motion during discharge, while in funnel flow, stagnant regions exist. These flow patterns are discussed in more detail in Chapter 3. Minimizing transfer chute volumes reduces the volume of displaced air and the volume of potentially segregated material. However, the chute must remain large enough to provide the required throughput rates. A tall aspect ratio should be used for bins. For a given storage capacity, a mass flow bin with a tall narrow cylinder will minimize the potential for sifting segregation as compared to that of a short, wide bin. A downside is the taller drop height may exacerbate other segregation mechanisms. Bins and blenders should be vented to avoid gas counterflow. Air that is in an otherwise "empty" bin, for example, must be displaced out of the bin as powder fills it. If this air is forced through material in the V-blender, perhaps in the interest of containment, this can induce fluidization segregation within the blender.

Blending and Blend Uniformity

To avoid this, a separate pathway or vent line to allow the air to escape without moving through the bed of material can reduce segregation.

Velocity gradients within bins should also be minimized (60). To achieve this, the hopper must be significantly steeper than the mass flow limit, which may result in an impractically tall bin. Alternate approaches include the use of inserts. However, these must be properly designed and positioned to be effective. Asymmetric bins and hoppers should be avoided, and symmetrical ones should be used whenever possible. Eccentric hoppers should be avoided due to their inherently large velocity gradients.

Dust generation and fluidization of the material should be minimized during material movement. Dust can be controlled by way of socks or sleeves, to contain the material as it drops from the blender to the bin, for example. Some devices are commercially available. An example of this is a solids decelerator shown in Figure 11. Drop heights should be minimal, as they aerate the material, induce dust, and increase momentum of the material as it hits the pile, all of which can increase the tendency for each of the three segregation mechanisms to occur. Valves should be operated correctly. Butterfly valves should be operated in the full open position, not throttled to restrict flow.

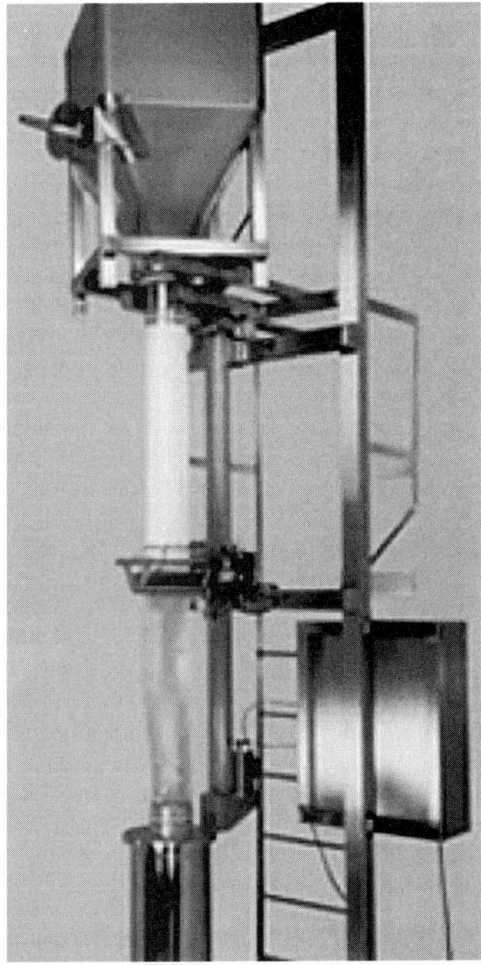

FIGURE 11 Example of a solids deceleration device. *Source*: Courtesy of GEA Process Engineering.

Restricting flow will virtually assure a funnel flow pattern, which is usually detrimental to uniformity.

Whenever a process stream is divided (e.g., a bifurcated chute to feed two sides of a press), a symmetrical split should be maintained to eliminate potential differences in the flow between the two streams (61). Consideration must be given to any potential for segregation upstream of the split. Even "little" details like orientation of a butterfly valve prior to a split can affect segregation. Proper designs should be utilized for hopper, Y-branches (Fig. 12) to avoid stagnant material and air counter flow.

Other specific solutions may be apparent once the segregation mechanism has been identified. For example, if material is segregating by sifting when it is loaded into a bin, an inlet distributor may help. An inlet distributor works by breaking up a single incoming stream into multiple streams and distributing them around the bin so that a single central pile does not form. However, distributors are generally ineffective for dusting or fluidization segregation mechanisms.

Mass flow is usually beneficial when handling segregation-prone materials, especially materials that exhibit a side-to-side (or center-to-periphery) segregation pattern, with overall uniformity in the vertical direction. Sifting and dusting segregation mechanisms fit this description.

It is important to remember that mass flow is not a universal solution; it will not address a top-to-bottom segregation pattern. As an example, consider the situation in a portable bin where fluidization upon filling the bin has caused the fine fraction of a blend to be driven to the top surface. Mass flow discharge of this bin would effectively transfer this segregated material to the downstream process, delivering the coarser blend first, followed by the fines.

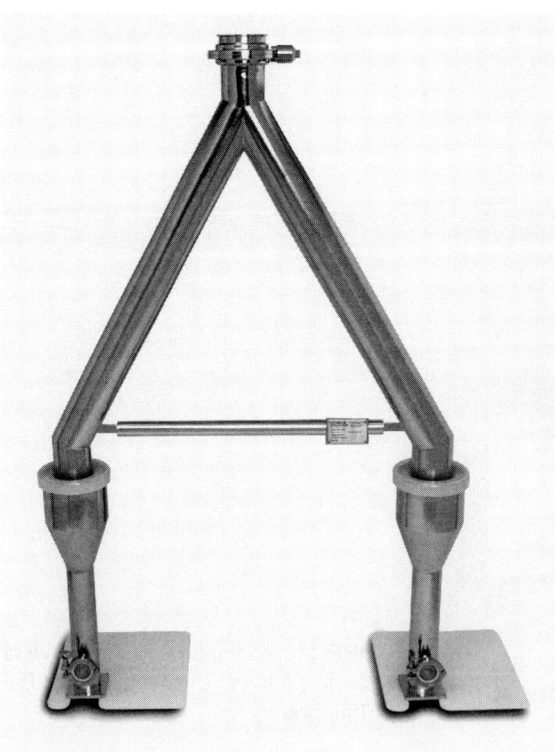

FIGURE 12 Y-Branch design to minimize segregation. *Source*: Courtesy of Jenike & Johanson, Inc.

ASSESSMENT OF UNIFORMITY

Introduction

Current good manufacturing practices (CGMPs) requires the assessment of adequacy of mixing to ensure uniformity and homogeneity [21 CFR 211.110(a)(3)]. However, the history of the application of this requirement is one embroiled in controversy. Blend uniformity analysis is particularly challenging due to difficulties associated with the removal of representative samples from the blend as a result of limitations in the capability of powder sampling technology. As a result, it was not uncommon to encounter situations where failing blend data was obtained, but uniformity of the resulting dosage units was acceptable. In such instances, part of the investigation into the cause of the failure included the testing of reserve samples (also taken from the failed location). Historically, if acceptable results were obtained from these samples, the failing result was often attributed to being due to sampling error. Although this conclusion was frequently correct, such investigations generally did not provide sound scientific explanations for an out of specification result, and ran the risk of prematurely discounting a legitimate failure.

In 1993, the Wolin decision in the *U.S.* v. *Barr Laboratories* case (62) highlighted deficiencies in practices used to assess blend uniformity. The Wolin decision pressed the FDA to reexamine and modify their policies regarding blend uniformity analysis. Interpretation of this decision has been incorporated into the revised policy for assessing blend uniformity that was subsequently issued by the FDA. For example, although sampling material directly from the blender is preferred, samples could also be taken upon their discharge into drums or other transfer containers. The decision also addressed sample weight and discouraged the analysis of bulk samples that were often much larger than the weight of the dosage units. To ensure they were reflective of the uniformity of the product, blend samples were to be within 1–3× the weight of the dosage unit.

Following the Wolin decision, the FDA published a recommendation in the *"Human Drug CGMP Notes"* in May 1993 (63), that included the testing of at least 10 samples (1–3× of the dosage form weight) during blend validation. Each of the 10 blend samples must be between 90% and 110% label claim, with an RSD ≤5%. The policy also discouraged the use of acceptance criteria for the blend similar to that defined for the final product in USP <905> Uniformity of Dosage Units (64) (assay for all samples between 85 and 115%; RSD ≤6.0%). Unfortunately, this policy did not provide a pathway to address legitimate sampling errors.

The Parenteral Drug Association sponsored a committee composed of industrial representatives to examine issues associated with blend uniformity analysis (65). This was the first concerted effort on behalf of industry to introduce science-based approaches when conducting blend uniformity analysis. The group examined blend sample sizes and identified a holistic approach for establishing meaningful acceptance criteria. In addition, the group discussed the use of proper analytical techniques and proposed an approach for conducting investigations into out of specification results. In particular, and method for identifying sampling problems, and isolating their effect from the overall assessment of uniformity, was conceived, which used statistical analyses. The output from the group was presented to the FDA for review and comment. Comments were received from the FDA, but the strategies provided in the paper were not incorporated into regulatory guidance at that time.

In August 1999, the FDA published a draft guidance document *ANDAs: Blend Uniformity Analysis* (66) to address industry concerns regarding the inconsistent application of regulations requiring the assessment of pharmaceutical blends. This guidance recommended that 6–10 blend samples 1–3× the dosage unit weight be taken for each commercial batch. It did allow for sample sizes "usually no more than" 10× to be taken if sampling bias was encountered for smaller weights, with justification. Acceptance criteria were the mean of the blend samples must be between 90.0 and 110.0%, and the RSD ≤6.0%. The pharmaceutical industry raised many concerns over the lack of scientific merit behind the approach defined in this guidance document. This was a strong motivation for the formation of the Product Quality Research Institute (PQRI) and their Blend Uniformity Working Group (BUWG).

The results of a survey of pharmaceutical manufacturers to obtain feedback on practices used to demonstrate blend uniformity were published in 2001 (67). Typically samples 1–3× the dosage unit weight were removed from the blend with conventional sample thieves, and analyzed using wet analytical chemistry methods. Problems with blend sampling were encountered for approximately 10–20% of the products, with most believed to be due to sampling or analytical error. At the time, most companies had not adopted any process analytical technologies (PAT) to aid in the assessment of batch homogeneity. A public workshop was also held (68) to discuss issues involved with blend uniformity analysis, during which it was noted that solids mixing is a poorly understood process. The difficulties associated with taking samples from powder beds with conventional sample thieves (discussed later in this chapter) and the associated sampling errors were also highlighted. As such, attendees felt that blend uniformity testing was not a value-added exercise. Subsequently, the PQRI BUWG highlighted many of the short-comings associated with blend uniformity analysis (69) that lead to the proposal of an alternative science-based approach to assess both blend and dosage unit uniformity (70).

The draft guidance document *ANDAs: Blend Uniformity Analysis* was withdrawn on May 17, 2002, and replaced with a subsequent draft guidance document *The Use of Stratified Sampling of Blend and Dosage Units to Demonstrate Adequacy of Mix for Powder Blends* (71). Although this draft guidance document has not been finalized (as of this writing, it still remains in draft status), it has been embraced by many in the industry and continues to be successfully applied to numerous products by multiple pharmaceutical companies. At approximately the same time the stratified sampling guidance document was issued, PAT became a favorable means to assess blend uniformity (72). PAT offers alternative analytical techniques that has revolutionized the manner in which blend uniformity analysis is performed. They offer many advantages including being noninvasive and having the potential to provide real time data and process control by blending to an end-point.

Assessing Blend Uniformity

Sampling is essential in determining the state of the blend in the blender and in downstream equipment. Collected samples are assayed for active drug(s), but could also be analyzed with respect to other physical or chemical properties of interest (e.g., particle size, excipient concentration, dissolution rate, color), depending on the application. The overall average of the sample results reflects the average composition of the blend, while variations from sample to sample reflect the homogeneity of the blend. Although the variability is often expressed as a RSD, many other "mixing indices" exist (73). However, as discussed later, a single mixing index, including the RSD, does not tell enough about what is happening.

Blending and Blend Uniformity

There are two major concerns with collecting and analyzing samples to assess blend homogeneity. The first is being able to collect a sample that truly represents the state of the blend from where it was sampled. This is a significant challenge due to the potential for sampling error and due to the fact that sampling locations can be difficult to establish. The second concern is being able to process or analyze the data in a meaningful way. Although this chapter is not intended to cover aspects of statistics needed to fully analyze these issues, the message to the reader is that statistical analysis must be considered in greater detail than many companies in the pharmaceutical industry are presently doing.

Sampling Thieves

Sampling from a stationary bed (e.g., within a blender, bin, drum) is usually accomplished with a sampling thief, though other methods like scooping are not uncommon. A sampling thief is a probe that can be inserted into a bed of material to collect a sample from below the surface. Many designs exist, but in their basic form, they are shaped like a rod, or a lance, frequently with a pointed tip and with some type of handle to aid in insertion. Grain (or pocket) and plug thieves are two common types of sample devices that have been widely used in the pharmaceutical industry.

Grain thieves (Fig. 13) extract blend samples by allowing the powders to flow into a sampling chamber that is exposed to the blend at the desired sampling location. Sampling chambers often screw onto the end of the inner rod and are available in various volumes to allow the desired amount of blend to be extracted from the mixer. The thief is inserted into the blend in the closed position. Once at the desired sampling location, the inner sampling chamber is rotated to align it with an opening in the outer sleeve of the thief (open position), thus allowing material to flow into the cavity of the thief. The thief

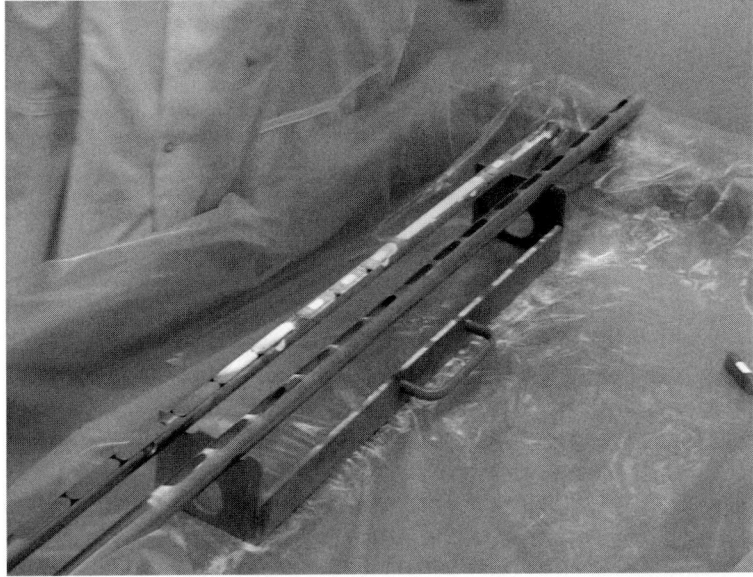

FIGURE 13 Side sampling (grain) thief with removable dies (inner rod is removed from sleeve). *Source*: Courtesy of Jenike & Johanson, Inc.

is returned to the closed position and removed from the blend. To remove the sample from the thief, it is returned to the open position and discharged into a suitable container. The ability for grain thieves to pull samples from a blend is dependent on the flow properties of the material being sampled. The preferential flow of one component of the blend into the sampling chamber over the others could result in sampling bias.

Plug thieves (Fig. 14) are basically a rod within an outer tube (imagine a syringe with its tip cut off). They are inserted into the blend with the inner rod pushed beyond the outer tube (closed position). The inner rod should be rounded to avoid excessive carrying down of powder from upper regions of the blender upon insertion into the blend, yet still allow a plug of powder to remain in the thief when it is extracted from the blender. Once at the targeted sampling location, the inner rod is pulled back to the desired length to extract a volume of the powder of acceptable weight. The thief is then pushed downward to force a plug of powder into the cavity, and subsequently removed from the blend. The sample is removed from the thief by returning the rod to the closed position, which pushes a plug of powder out of the thief. Plug thieves remove samples from the blender in a manner that is independent of material flow. However, the blend being sampled must be sufficiently cohesive to form a plug of material in the thief that will not fall out of it during removal from the blender. Plug thieves require more initial training to use, and inexperienced operators may extract samples with higher weight variation than those removed by seasoned operators. Because they remove a sample in a manner that is independent of material flow, plug thieves may not be as prone to sample bias as their grain counterparts for some formulations (74).

Sampling Error

Sample thieves have severe limitations, which collectively lead to sampling error. The insertion of a thief disturbs and smears the bed, resulting in a sample that may not represent the material that was there prior to the thief being inserted (75). Results from a

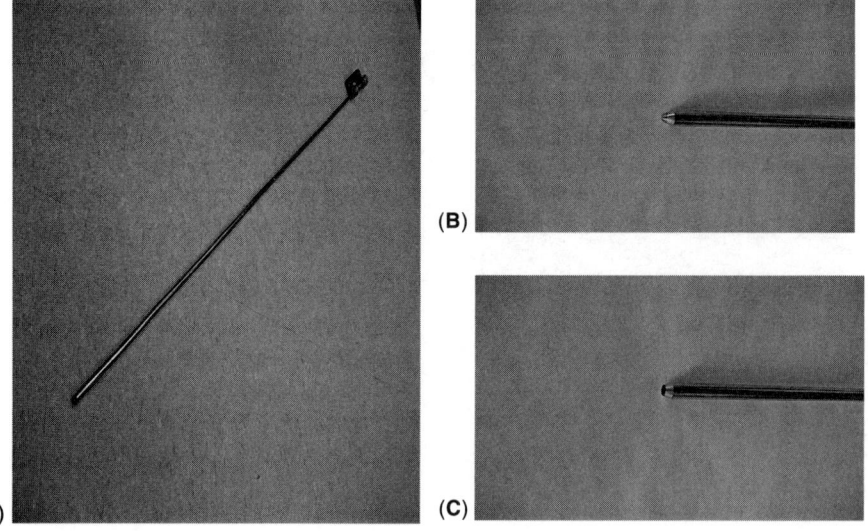

FIGURE 14 Plug thief: (**A**) plug thief, (**B**) insertion/closed position, and (**C**) retraction/open position.

Blending and Blend Uniformity

thief can be highly operator-dependent. Changes in the angle of insertion, insertion rate, twisting or rocking during insertion of the thief or collection of the sample all contribute to variability that can yield significantly different findings (76). In some cases, operators who have pulled "bad" samples have been disallowed from collecting samples in the future, if it was determined (correctly or not) that the operator was somehow responsible for the failing results. Thief results can be a function of its depth of penetration, such that even if the blend were uniform, results would be different from top to bottom of the blend (77). The lack of a standard thief design adds further uncertainty. It has been shown that merely changing the design of a thief can change blend results from unacceptable to passing. In a real application, it would be difficult to know which thief was giving the "correct" results.

There are three basic forms of thief sampling error. One type of error results in increased variability of samples, yielding data indicating that the homogeneity of the blend is worse than it actually is. This shows up as having poor blend uniformity while having good dosage unit content uniformity. As an illustration of this, Figure 15 summarizes the correlation between blend and dosage unit RSD values for 149 batches of tablets obtained from a survey of pharmaceutical companies (69). For this data set, a good correlation existed between the blend and dosage unit RSD values when the blend RSD was < 3%. When the blend RSD was between 3% and 5%, the correlation between blend and dosage unit RSD worsened. When the blend RSD was > 5%, there was no correlation between the blend and dosage unit values. Although this data set may be biased towards problematic products, it still demonstrates the difficulties in extracting representative blend samples from blenders and highlights the issue of sampling error. This "false positive" type of sampling error is very common, and as a result, is often cited as having

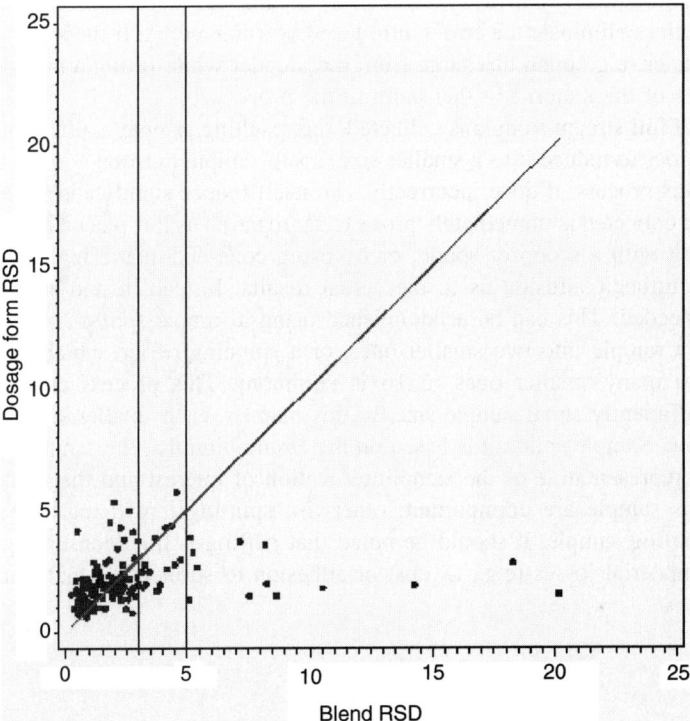

FIGURE 15 Correlation between blend and tablet data. *Source*: Courtesy of PQRI.

occurred when blend results are bad (based on product data looking good). Unfortunately, sometimes this claim is made even without specific data to support it.

A second type of error is an overall shift in the results, whereby the measured average from the samples collected is higher or lower than the anticipated blend composition, possibly without introducing any additional variability in the results. This type of error is often referred to as bias. Bias can result if one component adheres to, or is repelled by, the thief, or due to preferential flow of one component into the thief. Bias can also result if samples are not collected from appropriate locations; for example, if no samples are collected from a dead zone in the blender that is holding the "missing" material. However, a true shift in potency may also be occurring, if raw components were dispensed incorrectly or if preferential material losses have occurred. Therefore, great care must be taken with biased data, and its true cause must be determined.

A third type of error, less common than the other two, is from a sampling device that yields lower variability than is actually present in the blend. This can arise due to smearing of the sample (in effect providing localized blending), or it can also arise due to sampling from locations that are "more uniform" than the blend as a whole. This "false negative" type of error, nicknamed "counterfeiting," is hard to detect, in part because statistical tools do not identify it, and in part because the user is generally reluctant to dismiss data that passes acceptance criteria.

It has been said that, as the name implies, "a thief is not to be trusted." In recognizing these limitations, many industries have been asking for a "perfect" thief for a long time, so attempts have been made to improve upon the design of the thief to give results that are more accurate. The focus has been on how to collect a sample without disturbing it. Unfortunately, any thief violates the two golden rules of sampling and thus will never be perfect. These two "Golden Rules" of sampling are: (*i*) always collect the sample while it is in motion, and (*ii*) always collect a full stream sample for a short-time period (78). These practices eliminate the errors introduced in using a thief. If the sample is collected in this manner (e.g., upon discharge from the blender while filling a bin), it represents the true state of the material at that point in the process.

Unfortunately if a full stream sample is collected, the resulting sample is often too large for analysis. In order to reduce it to a smaller size, a sub-sample must be collected from the larger one. This process, if done incorrectly, can itself induce significant errors (79). The larger sample collected is immediately prone to segregation as it is placed into a container. Sub-sampling with a scoop or spoon, or by using cone-and-quartering techniques, will result in further confusion as to the actual results. Instead, a non-biased splitting technique is needed. This can be accomplished using a sample splitter, which will uniformly divide a sample into two smaller ones, or a spinning riffler, which can separate a sample into many smaller ones (6–16 is common). This process can be repeated to get to a sufficiently small sample size. In this manner, each smaller sample represents the larger one. Sample splitting is based on the assumption that the sample to be split is sufficiently representative of the sampling location of interest and that non-uniformities within this sample are unimportant; otherwise splitting it will mask any variation within the starting sample. It should be noted that riffling is time consuming, and may be prone to material losses (e.g., as dust or adhesion to surfaces), which can affect the results.

Sample Size

Although, to the statistician, the term *sample size* generally means the number of samples collected, in powder sampling this more often refers to the mass (or weight) of the sample collected. The size of the blend sample analyzed needs to reflect that consumed by the patient or customer. This is critical as larger samples may mask micro-nonuniformities, such as those caused by a few agglomerates. Similarly a size below the dosage unit size could exaggerate non-uniformities that are not relevant to the consumer. It has been generally accepted, and cited from the Wolin decision to the draft guidance document *"The Use of Stratified Sampling...,"* that the sample size range should be 1–3× (i.e., one to three times the dosage unit weight).

Unfortunately, sampling errors tend to get more pronounced with decreasing sample size, even for cases where micro mixing appears to be adequate. Therefore, to get around sampling errors, one approach is to use larger sample sizes. The withdrawn draft guidance *ANDAs: Blend Uniformity Analysis* allowed larger samples, generally < 10×, provided their use was justified. The draft guidance document *"The Use of Stratified Sampling...,"* places the burden on the development side to define the effect of sample size, and an appropriate weight of blend to sample.

Once a sample larger than 3× is collected, a question remains as to what to do with that sample prior to assay. The withdrawn draft guidance *ANDAs: Blend Uniformity Analysis* recommends sample sizes 1–3× to be collected, but that the sample weight tested (assayed) should be equivalent to the dosage used. Unfortunately any subdivision of the sample is likely to induce either potency losses or segregation, so the logistics of how to subdivide such a sample remains a challenge.

As discussed later, the uniformity of the product is best assessed by analyzing dosage forms. Micro-nonuniformities can best be caught at this stage, where blend sampling and handling issues are not present. The remaining goal of blend sampling (when called for) is to investigate macro-nonuniformities, such as incomplete blending. Therefore, blend sample size is not overly critical; it should be one where sampling error (within-location variation) is minimized and correlation to the product results is maximized.

Good Blend Sampling Practice

Good sampling practices can improve upon the quality of samples taken from the blender. The sampling technique should be clearly defined, and operators should receive hands-on training prior to having to take blend samples that will be assayed to determine the fate of a batch. This should include cross-shift, cross-product lines, and cross-site training to maintain consistency and best practices corporate wide. Samples from the top layers of the blender should always be taken first, and care should be exercised to avoid disturbing lower regions in the blend prior to sampling those locations. One should never go down the same channel in the blend to pull replicates due to the high probability of knocking powder from the upper areas down into the sampling location. The angle of insertion and movement of the thief to pull samples should be defined (80). Arguments can be made to clean and not to clean the thief between samples. In some cases, priming the thief by inserting it into a blend (away from designated sampling locations) prior to sampling can reduce sampling bias (32). Regardless of whether or not you clean the thief between samples, under no circumstances should residual powder from a previous sample be included in subsequent samples. Finally, to minimize operator-to-operator variability, the same individual should pull samples within a campaign or set of experiments.

Many times, failing blend samples can be attributed to weighing errors or carelessly handling blend samples during their transfer from the processing room to the analytical laboratory. The analytical laboratory should provide pre-labeled and tared containers for each sample to be taken. Special care should be taken to not mix up caps and containers, as this can often lead to failing results. Blend samples should be directly discharged into tared containers, and a second series of sample weights should be recorded in the processing room at the time of sampling. This practice ensures that the sample weight is within the desired target weight. These weights can also serve as back-up values during investigations for out of specification results, by ruling out improper weight as being the cause of the failure. Discharging the blend sample onto paper and then pouring it into the container is discouraged due to the potential for material loss. Samples should be kept in the upright position when transferred from the processing room to the analytical laboratory, to avoid getting powder in the cap that can be spilled when the container is opened.

Sample Locations

In selecting locations for the collection of blend samples, the first question is to ask "what are the blend results intending to tell us?" While the answer seems obvious at first—to determine uniformity—probing this further reveals there is more to consider. As stated previously, the goal of sampling should not be to simply assess a standard deviation, but rather, to challenge possible problem areas. Recall, that patients will consume each and every dose produced; the grand average is not critical but rather possible "outliers" are of most concern. Therefore, possible dead spots (Fig. 16) or other high-risk areas should be assessed. While the uniformity of all regions of the blend must be considered, focusing on high-risk areas adds greater confidence in the assessment of uniformity. If the high-risk areas are challenged and found to be acceptable, generally speaking the rest of the blend will also be acceptable. Presumed in such a statement, however, is that one has the correct evaluation of where the high-risk areas are.

Another consideration in where to collect blend samples is whether to take samples out of the blender, or further downstream in the process. Although sampling following discharge of the blender into drums or intermediate bulk containers (IBC) is allowed, the FDA has articulated a preference for samples taken directly from the blender. While this is the best location to prove that the blend has been optimized within the blender, it does not assure the blend will remain adequately blended throughout the rest of the process, should segregation occur. Therefore, blend samples collected downstream of the blender may be better able to diagnose whether the blend was adequate to begin with, and whether it in fact remains adequate during transfer. In this case, sampling from IBCs, chutes and/or press hoppers may be useful, even if only implemented as a diagnostic tool after uniformity problems are detected in the dosage forms. If sampling from an IBC or other powder handling equipment, again the goal is not to assess an overall uniformity metric, but rather to identify "hot spots" created as a result of segregation. Sampling locations should specifically target those areas where highest/lowest concentrations of

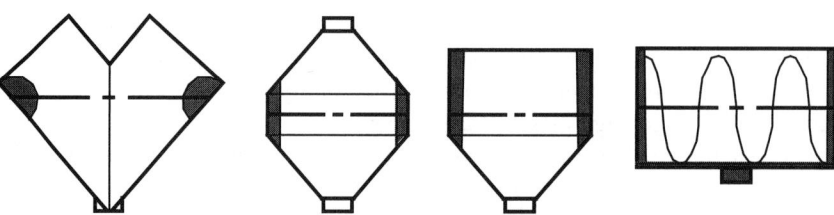

FIGURE 16 Potential areas of weak blending in blenders.

Blending and Blend Uniformity

specific components are suspected. There maybe other advantages to sampling downstream of the blender, including that it may be easier to collect samples (in some cases, sampling from the blender is impossible due to size or space problems), as well as reducing the operator's exposure to the product (which is critical in highly potent/toxic applications or where hazards remain ill-defined).

One must recognize that in making a sampling plan, if the blend variations are not randomly and normally distributed, the sampling locations and number of samples will affect the results. Specifically concentrating samples at problematic locations will yield a higher RSD than if the samples were equally spaced or spaced at random locations. The converse is true as well; if one wanted to reduce the RSD, collect many more samples from areas where uniformity is expected to be good. Obviously, the actual state of the blend is the same, but the results and possible interpretation of the results will vary. This makes the reliance on a simple index such as RSD, while having variable sample locations and number of samples, incompatible with having a universal acceptance criterion. As iterated previously, this is why measuring product uniformity should be given highest consideration; blend uniformity samples may be diagnostic but not proof of adequate uniformity.

Meaningful Analysis of the Data

Interpretation of the results is equally important as obtaining samples. An important consideration is the accuracy of the results, which immediately ties to the often-asked question of how many samples are needed. Certainly there are a minimum number of samples required to meet regulatory guidelines, but additional samples may be needed to diagnose problems or to truly assess whether process changes are beneficial.

In measuring homogeneity (or variability) of a blend, the fundamental estimator is some form of standard deviation. To get a good estimate of the standard deviation, a relatively large number of samples is required, whereas comparatively few are needed to get an estimate of the mean value. The actual number of samples required will depend on the actual variability of the blend (less homogeneous requires more samples) as well as the confidence needed in the result. All of this needs to be balanced by the cost of conducting the tests against the probability and consequences of an improper disposition on the batch. Beyond the need to meet regulatory requirements, there is no universal "right answer," as the number of samples required depends on the application.

Consider the following application where uniformity of the blend is often used to determine blend time, and where standard deviations from two data sets are compared. In this illustrative example, 10 samples were collected from two different time points, one sample set from the blender after 10 minutes blend time, the next set after 14 minutes blend time. The first set yields a mean of 100 and a standard deviation of 1.9. The next set of data coincidentally yields a mean of 100 but a standard deviation of 3.7. Assume both are normally distributed. In this example, one might believe that, based on this data, the blend was segregating with additional blend time, and one may decide that it is essential to keep the blend time to 10 minutes. Our eyes and intuition tell us these are very different data sets. Yet an F-test would show that these values are not different with 95% statistical significance. In this case, additional samples from each time point, in addition to samples collected from other time points, would help address whether the blend has or has not in fact hit an optimum at 10 minutes. All too often, it is assumed that the lowest RSD necessarily came from the best process (or formulation, time point, etc.), when in fact there may be too much statistical noise to truly make such a determination.

Another weakness of relying only on RSD is that it does not describe the distribution of the data. The same RSD can be achieved whether the distribution is near-normal, bi-modal, or even by having a single "outlier", as illustrated in Table 2. In this example, if this were blend uniformity data, the results could be due to either having a complete blend (a), an incomplete blend (b), or an agglomerate (c). In using the RSD of a sample set to estimate the population RSD, it is assumed that the population is normally distributed. Unfortunately this is not always the case. A significant concern is the ability, or lack thereof, to detect agglomerates. These "outliers" fall outside of a normal distribution, and the chance of detecting them can be quite small. The FDA draft guidance document *The Use of Stratified Sampling of Blend and Dosage Units to Demonstrate Adequacy of Mix for Powder Blends* calls for an assessment of normality of the data. It further states, "Indications of trends, bimodal distributions, or other forms of a distribution other than normal should be investigated. If these occurrences significantly affect your ability to ensure batch homogeneity, they should be corrected."

Content uniformity tests, such as USP<905>, utilize the RSD as a metric of uniformity. Additionally, there are upper and lower limits for individual dosage units, in an effort to catch a batch with sub- or super-potent tablets. Bear in mind that even if as many as 1% of the dosage units produced in a batch are super-potent, the odds of having these part of the first 10 units tested are less than 10%, assuming dosage units are selected at random.

There is a risk in selecting dosage units at random (allowed within USP<905>), since trends due to segregation can occur. Such behavior is often confined to significant processing events such as the very beginning or end of a batch, as a bin, chute or press hopper empties, immediately before or after a press shutdown, or during bin changeovers. Since these events may make up only a small percentage of the total batch time, these areas may not be included in a "random" sampling plan. Even if the content uniformity test detected a problem, it would remain unclear what the source of the problem was. For instance, if two tablets were super-potent, were these two tablets produced at the same time? Were they produced during a significant processing event? Did other tablets produced at the same time have these problems? Did other batches experience these problems at the same point in time that these tablets were produced? Did this occur due to

TABLE 2 Comparison of Mean and RSD for Normal, Bimodal, and Outlier Data Sets

	Near normal (a)	Bi-modal (b)	Outlier (c)
	104	102	99.33
	102	102	99.33
	101	102	99.33
	100	102	99.33
	100	102	99.33
	100	98	99.33
	100	98	99.33
	99	98	99.33
	98	98	99.33
	96	98	106.03
Mean	100	100	100
RSD	2.16	2.11	2.12

Blending and Blend Uniformity

poor blending or due to segregation after blending? Could there be other tablets that are worse, which were not sampled? Due to these weaknesses, content uniformity tests should not be relied upon alone during process development and validation, when little processing history exists. As a comprehensive body of data is developed, and uniformity is consistently demonstrated, then content uniformity tests in conjunction with adequate process controls could be sufficient. A more comprehensive approach is to link the uniformity data to the process itself, and to have adequate sampling to separate out the possible root causes of non-uniformities, should they be detected.

Stratified Sampling

CGMPs state that

> To assure batch uniformity and integrity of drug products, written procedures shall be established and followed that describe the in-process controls, and tests, or examinations to be conducted on appropriate samples of in-process materials of each batch. Such control procedures shall be established to monitor the output and to validate the performance of those manufacturing processes that may be responsible for causing variability in the characteristics of in-process material and the drug product. Such control procedures shall include, but are not limited to, the following, where appropriate: . . . Adequacy of mixing to assure uniformity and homogeneity [21CFR 211.110 (a)(3)].

To meet this requirement, the stratified sampling of blends and in-process product is being used by the industry and accepted by FDA (70), which avoids many of the problems of relying on a single RSD. Stratified sampling is the process of selecting multiple units deliberately from various locations within a lot or batch or from various phases or periods of a process (80). By taking replicate samples from each location, (hierarchical or nested sampling plan), variance component analysis (VCA) (81,82), a subset of analysis of variance, can be performed on the data. The results of VCA quantify the variability attributed to uniformity of the process (across locations) as well as any sampling error or small-scale variability (within each location) that may be present. It is important to keep in mind that the purpose of sampling is to uncover hidden blend quality issues, not to mask or overlook suspected problems. Samples should be intentionally collected from suspected "hot spots," or regions where the blend may be less uniform, not just from the middle of the blender (Fig. 17). Such hot spots may include the surface of the material or regions where the material may have been stagnant during blending.

An example of stratified sampling is to collect samples from 10 locations within a blender, in triplicate. All 30 samples are analyzed. In addition to reporting the overall mean for the data, the individual location means should be examined to identify trends throughout the batch. In addition to determining an overall RSD value for the data, VCA should be conducted to separate out the variance between-locations from the within-location variance. High within-location variance, if found, could be attributed to such issues as sampling error, improper sample handling or subdivision, or variability of the analytical method used. It can also be attributed to variability of the blend on a unit dose scale as discussed previously, such as due to agglomerates or other large particles, relative to the sample size. Therefore, high within-location variability of the blend must be investigated relative to the sampling and analytical methods, as well as the formulation itself.

High between-location variance is most likely attributable to poor macro-mixing which can result from incomplete blending or segregation. Additionally, sampling errors

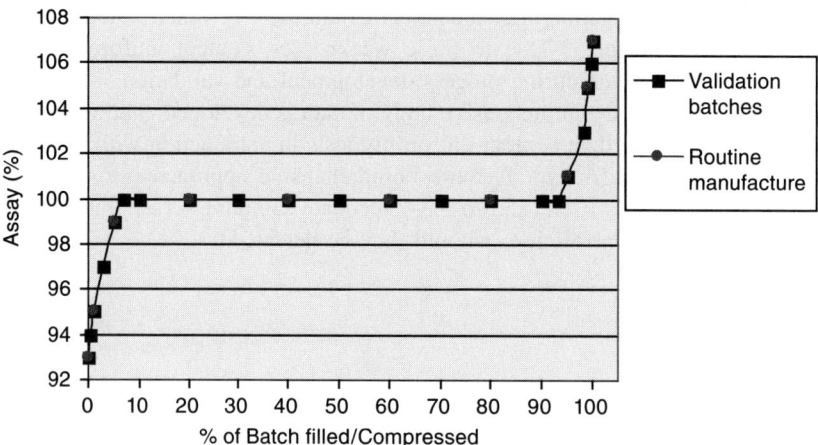

FIGURE 17 Comparison of two stratified sampling plans for a compression process.

(bias as a function of sample location) can yield between-location variations that do not exist within the blend (83).

The concept of stratified sampling is not restricted to the blend. Stratified sampling of the product remains essential in demonstrating product uniformity. For the drug product, the frequency of sampling is increased around potential events in a compression or filling operation that have a higher propensity to produce high or low potency dosage units. For example, a stratified sampling plan would target the very beginning and end of a compression or filling run. If the process relies on multiple bins of blend being discharged onto the compression or filling equipment, intensified sampling around bin change-over would occur (i.e., the end of Bin #1 and the start of Bin #2). Figure 17 contains an example of a stratified sampling plan for a hypothetical product that exhibits low potency at the start of a run and high potency at the end of a run. Figure 17 presents two sampling plans, one with 21 locations (ideal for process validation or larger scale development batches) and the other with 10 sampling locations (suitable for routine manufacture). Both sampling plans are more powerful in identifying high or low potency dosage units than a random sample size of 30 units as recommended by USP<905> Uniformity of Dose.

Comparing the Uniformity of Blend and Product

Powder blend samples are invaluable in determining the state of the blend at various points in the process, and are essential to determine blender and powder handling equipment performance. However, the best way to determine the adequacy of the process as a whole is to sample the product itself, if samples are collected in-process (e.g., at defined time intervals during compression or filling operation, while samples can still be correlated with specific times during the process). Multiple stratified samples of the dosage units should be collected at the tablet press (or encapsulator, etc.) at a given instant, at multiple time points, from the beginning to the end of a batch, or across a meaningful time period if a process is continuous. In-process dosage unit analysis has many positive aspects (70), including:

- It is an accurate and reflective measure of homogeneity of the product.
- It eliminates blend sampling error issues related to thief sampling.

Blending and Blend Uniformity

- It applies resources where they produce reliable, accurate information about the quality of the product given to the patient.
- Weighing errors during blend sample analysis are eliminated.
- It removes the safety issues surrounding blend sampling of toxic or potent drugs manufactured in isolated environments.
- It accounts for potential segregation after blending.

To maximize the knowledge about the content uniformity of the product, a VCA should be performed on the assembled dosage unit data. A comparison of VCA results from the blend and tablet analyses can provided valuable information about the process, as descried in Table 3. As with the approach taken for assessing blend sample data, a stratified sampling plan should be applied throughout the compression or filling process. Sample locations should target suspect areas during the compression or filling process that have a greater propensity to produce dosage units of high or low potency, such as the start and end of the batch and bin change-overs.

Consider a tablet dosage form that has a tendency for low potency at the start of compression run and high potency at the end of the batch (Fig. 17). Although it used fewer samples, the 10 location sampling plan is actually more discriminating than the 21 location sample plan, because it concentrates more samples (6 out of the 10) at points in areas of the process that are more likely to produce high or low potency dosage units. As a result, the RSD value for the 10 location sampling plan will be higher than that for the 21 location plan. This diagram demonstrates the ability of properly designed stratified sampling plans to evaluate the quality of the batch, and emphasizes the

TABLE 3 Comparison of Blend and Tablet Core Variance Components

Observed variances for		
Blend	Tablet cores	Potential implication
High between-location	High between-location	Poor macro mixing; hot/cold spots exist in the blend and tablets
High within-location (> approx. 80% of the total variance), and low or no between-location variance	Low within-location and low between-location	Blend sampling or sample handling errors. Tablets are uniform.
High within-location (> approx. 80% of the total variance), and low or no between-location variance	Low within-location, but higher between-location	Sampling error, and potential segregation of the blend during transfer and/or the compression/filling process
High within-location	High within-location	Poor micro mixing on a unit dose scale. Possible agglomeration
Low between-location variance and low within-location variance	Higher between-location variance (with trending or multiple outliers) and low within-location variance	Blend is uniform but segregates during transfer and/or the compression/filling process
Low between–location variance and low within-location variance	Higher between-location variance (with trending or multiple outliers) and high within-location variance	Blend is uniform but potential agglomeration during transfer and/or the compression/filling process

importance of sample location rather than the number of samples from which dosage units are taken.

Stratified sampling can give insight into what is occurring with the process (such as segregation), as long as other variables are documented at the same time. For example, if there is a surge bin prior to the packaging equipment, it is important to note the level in the bin when each sample was collected. For simplicity, it may be best to initially fill the bin from empty, then let it discharge completely, while samples are collected at regular intervals. As with collecting samples using a thief, additional samples should be taken from potential "hot spots," such as at the beginning or end of the run. In this example, a plot of particle size versus time would likely reveal any trend of segregation induced by the bin and other upstream equipment.

Troubleshooting

Stratified sampling is more likely to reveal uniformity problems than if less discriminating methods were used. A tool was developed and published (84) to aid formulation and process development scientists in troubleshooting content uniformity problems. The approach is that if stratified sample results were available for blend and/or product samples, the data will point the troubleshooter towards potential causes for uniformity problems in rank order of likelihood. Once potential root causes have been identified, areas for further investigation and possible corrective actions are also presented.

Six basic trends commonly observed for product uniformity and blend samples are described, based on stratified nested sampling. The described trends are based on tendencies of the mean, between-location variance, and within-location variance. The six trends are:

1. satisfactory,
2. high within-location variability (based on variance components analysis),
3. high between-location variability (based on variance components analysis),
4. stray value,
5. trending and hot spots,
6. assay shift.

Example plots for each of the above situations are provided in Figures 18–24. Seven common root causes for blend and product content uniformity problems are presented. Each of these possible root causes are:

1. non-optimum blending,
2. thief sampling error,
3. segregation after discharge,
4. weight control,
5. wrong mass or loss of component,
6. analytical error,
7. insufficient particle distribution.

A number of additional points should be considered when interpreting the recommendations from the troubleshooting diagram. The entire history of the product and process should be taken into consideration. Top-level questions one should ask include:

- Is this a new product, or an existing one with a significant body of data?
- Has this problem been seen with this product or one similar to it?
- What is unique or different about this product or process?

Blending and Blend Uniformity

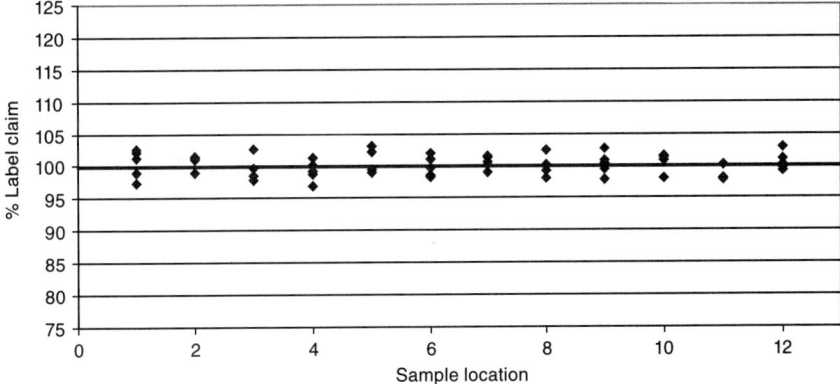

FIGURE 18 Example of satisfactory blend or dosage unit data.

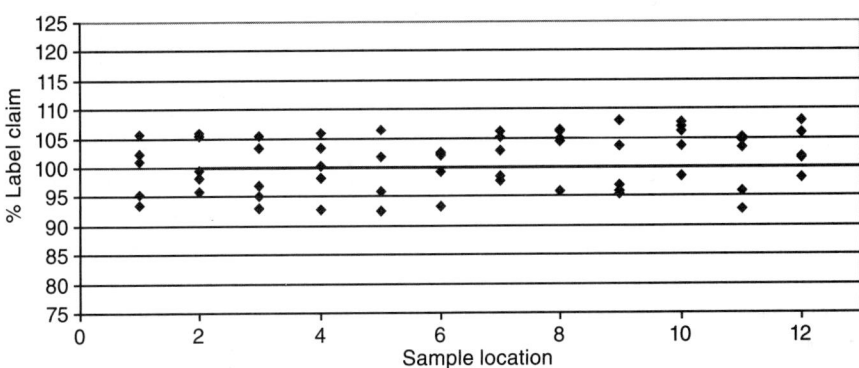

FIGURE 19 Example of high within-location variation for blend or dosage unit data.

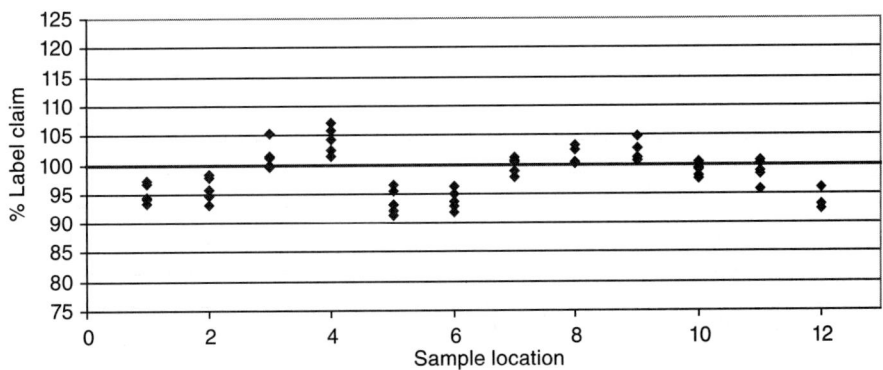

FIGURE 20 Example of high between-location variation for blend or dosage unit data.

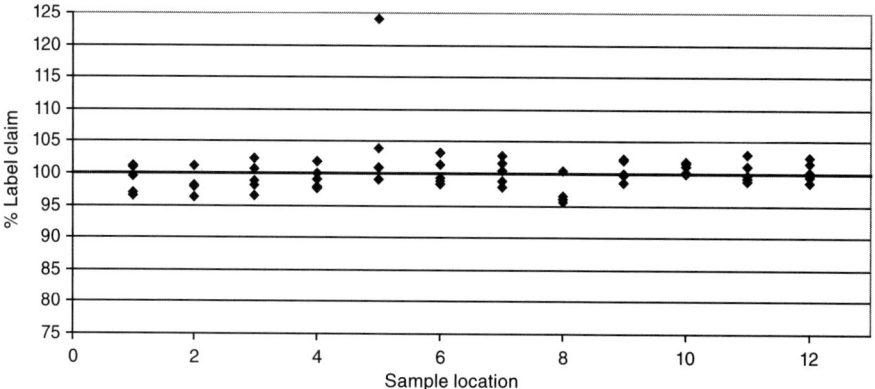

FIGURE 21 Example of stray value for blend or dosage unit data.

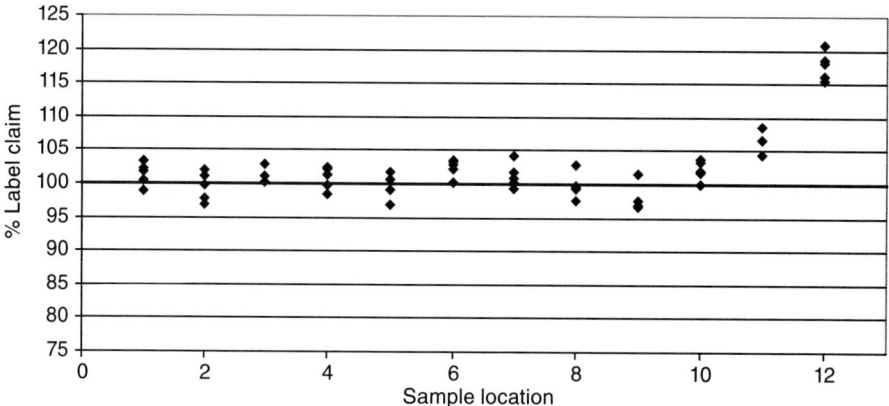

FIGURE 22 Examples of trending for dosage unit data.

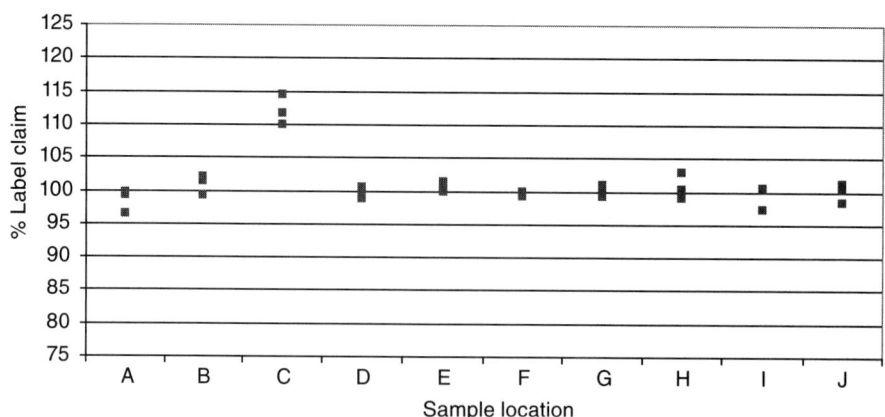

FIGURE 23 Example of "hot" spot in blend data.

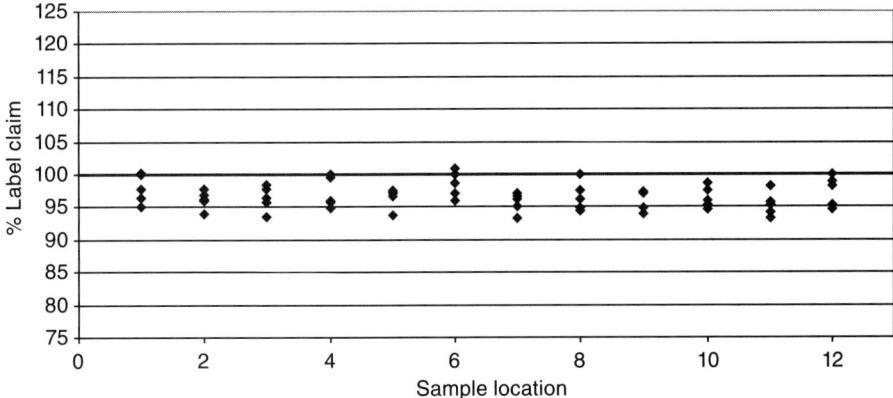

FIGURE 24 Example of an assay shift for blend or dosage unit data.

- Have the materials, processes, operators, equipment, or environmental control changed recently?
- How do the physical characteristics of the materials used for this batch compare to what was intended?
- Is the problem repeatable among multiple batches, or is this an isolated incidence?
- Did the operators observe any anomalies during the manufacture of the batch?
- Were any equipment malfunctions encountered during batch manufacture?
- How do the mean and RSD values for the blend and product compare?
- How do the measured RSDs compare to the theoretical RSD of a randomized blend of particles?

Addressing each of these questions will further assist the scientist in identifying the cause(s) of the problem and its successful resolution. Basic methodologies (e.g., Six-Sigma, Kepner–Tregoe) should be employed to address quality problems; such methodologies are beyond the scope of this chapter. All rely on having meaningful data for analysis, which stratified sampling best provides.

Once possible root causes have been identified, the next step is to perform additional analyses to confirm the primary root cause. Once the primary root cause has been confirmed, corrective actions can be taken.

Process Analytical Technology

PAT has revolutionized the manner in which blend uniformity analysis can be conducted. Near infrared spectroscopy (NIR) is the most widely applied methodology that has been used to assess blend uniformity (85–89), although other techniques such as effusivity (90) have also been advocated for this purpose. PAT offers a number of advantages over traditional blend sampling and testing. PAT measures the uniformity of the blend in a dynamic (vs. static) state, and therefore complies with the golden rule to sample powder in motion. As such, it eliminates many of the problems associated with blend sampling error and bias. Analysis is fast and less labor intensive than traditional wet-chemistry, thereby resulting in the ability to analyze more samples at a significant cost savings. Its on-line capability allows PAT to produce real time data that can be used for process control, and the identification of process variables such as an acceptable endpoint for the blending operation. The technology is non-intrusive, thereby decreasing operator exposure to drug substances during blend sampling. This also makes the technology attractive for use in high containment production suites used for the manufacture of potent drug products. While traditional sampling and analysis focused primarily on the drug substance, PAT also has the potential to provide information about excipient uniformity. These techniques need not be confined to the blender, but could also be expanded to include measuring the uniformity of the blend during material transfer onto the compression or filling equipment, to detect any potential segregation. Further, PAT can be added directly to tablet presses to measure the potency and content uniformity of the dosage units at the press, resulting in a much more complete and holistic approach to assessing content uniformity.

There are some downsides to PAT techniques. The results are highly dependent upon having properly placed sensors at key points in the manufacturing process to fully capture the state of the blend. Typically in a blending application, PAT probes are mounted on the exterior of a blender to assess the composition of material that passes in front of quartz windows built into the sides of the blender. Material at the walls of a blender may not be the same as what is at its core, so sensors located only at the periphery of the blender may not effectively detect such differences in blend uniformity. Multiple sensors at strategic locations (including corners and other known areas of reduced material movement) can minimize the risk associated with this problem. In having multiple sensors, and the ability to collect results at many time intervals, there is a wealth of data generated which can aid in detecting potential problems, that thief sampling would be unable to resolve. Another potential issue is not all APIs can be detected by a given sensor technology, either at all or within the resolution required, to assess blend uniformity.

One area that needs to be addressed when using PAT for content uniformity analysis is the definition of appropriate acceptance criteria. Traditional limits in pharmacopeia content uniformity tests are based on sample sizes of 30, and define how many tablets can be outside of certain ranges (typically 85–115% and 75–125% label claim). Although the ability of PAT to analyze a much greater number of samples increases the confidence in the quality of the batch, higher sample numbers also increases the probability of encountering an out of specification value. Furthermore, using traditional pharmacopeia limits to the results obtained from testing 100–200 or more samples could result in the rejection of a greater number of batches of the same or even higher quality as the current industry standards. Pharmaceutical scientists and statisticians are working together to identify appropriate acceptance criteria, which can adapt the data from large sample sizes to the quality standards established in the various pharmacopeias (91).

BLENDING EQUIPMENT

Defining Equipment Requirements to Achieve a Uniform Blend

Selecting an appropriate blender depends on many factors, including material and logistical considerations, and imposed constraints such as whether existing equipment must be selected or new equipment can be purchased. Recognize that achieving a blend in the blender is only the first step; proper blend transfer is also essential to minimize segregation. Bin and chute designs are covered in Chapter 3.

Prior to evaluating any specific blender, the nature of the material, as well as the required logistics of the process, must be established. If these are ill-defined, a poor choice of blenders can result.

Blending and Blend Uniformity

Material Considerations

Ultimately the purpose of a blender is to homogenize the material to a sufficient level of uniformity to subsequently produce product of acceptable quality. The requirements for uniformity of the blend and product were discussed earlier in this chapter. The ability of a given blender to achieve these requirements depends on the nature of the materials being blended. This includes cohesiveness of the material, potential for agglomerates to be present or to form, and segregation both during blending and upon discharge.

When selecting blending equipment the physical characteristics of the materials that will be blended in it should be considered. Table 4 contains information that should be considered when selecting a blender. The cohesivity of the individual drug particles and their tendency to form agglomerates must be considered in order to select an appropriate blender. This assessment will determine whether or not, and to what extent, shear must be applied to break up agglomerates that may form and grow during the blending process. Shear can also cause attrition of primary particles, so the friability of the material, and its consequences with respect to product performance, must also be considered. For low dose products, the need to incorporate geometric dilution or prepare premixes to ensure adequate dispersion of the drug into the final blend should also be assessed.

Alternately, instead of using shear in the blender, deagglomeration can be achieved outside the blender, such as milling and/or screening of the blend. Although this requires additional transfer steps and equipment, it may be the only option if blenders with high shear are not available.

Some blenders have dead spots, specific regions in the blender where material does not move, or movement is minimal. As a result, materials in these regions are not well blended. Figure 17 contains such regions for some commonly used blender configurations. The location of these dead spots is blender dependent. Dead spots are also affected by the loading (percentage fill) of the blender, operational speed, and the material properties such as cohesive strength and friction against surfaces. Dead spots are more likely for highly cohesive materials or materials that stick to surfaces.

The choice of a blender also depends on the segregation characteristics of the material. This includes segregation during blending as well as segregation upon discharge of the blender both of which have been previously discussed in this chapter.

The final blend must discharge from the blender reliably and completely. Cohesive materials may require large outlets, special operation of the blender during discharge (e.g., jogging a blending screw), manual intervention (poking), or a flow aid device to maintain flow. Erratic flow can aerate materials, which in turn can lead to segregation of the material.

Logistical Considerations

Once the formulation requirements are understood, knowledge of the processing requirements (logistical considerations) are still needed to then select the appropriate equipment to perform the blending operation.

The blender may need to fit within an existing plant, so layout considerations often come into play. This includes not only the height and footprint consumed by the blender, but also additional operations such as fitting an IBC underneath a blender to receive the blend, and methods to load the blender initially. The headroom available beneath a blender may affect the choice of IBC (e.g., drums, steep conical hopper, shallow pyramidal hopper), which can ultimately affect segregation and content uniformity. Having a layout that allows ease of peripheral operations such as cleaning, inspection, and

TABLE 4 Advantages and Disadvantages of Blending Equipment

Blender type and examples	Mechanism	Advantages	Disadvantages
Tumble blenders V-blenders Bin blenders Double cone blenders Slant cone blenders Horizontal/vertical/drum blenders	Diffusion, convection	Lower shear forces decrease the extent of particle size reduction. Blending container may be used to transfer blend (and enhance product containment and uniformity) Useful for blending friable materials Easy to clean Intensifier can be added	May not be suitable for blending cohesive materials, as they are incapable of breaking up agglomerates without the addition of shear Baffles may be needed to overcome slow axial blending rates Can take up significant space
High shear blenders Horizontal high intensity mixers (side driven) Vertical high intensity mixers (top or bottom driven)	Convection and shear	Very efficient in producing uniform blends; often used for the manufacture of preblends and ordered mixes Good for blending cohesive powders as they break-up agglomerates	Potential to over-lubricate a blend Generate heat Typically need to be discharged into an intermediate bulk container Potential to reduce particle size
Screw/paddle blenders Ribbon blenders Orbiting screw blenders Planetary blenders	Convection and shear	Rapidly produce blends that are less prone to segregation than those produced by tumble blenders Material needs to be discharged into an intermediate bulk container to transfer to the next processing step Good for cohesive materials	Potential dead spots in corners and on the immediate bottom of the blender Can be difficult to clean.
Pneumatic Fluid bed processors	Diffusion; Air passed through the blender to move and blend the material	Can perform multiple operations in a single piece of equipment (blending, granulation, drying, lubrication) Can be contained systems Blending can be rapid	Segregation of fines on top layer following shut down Not well suited for cohesive materials More difficult to clean than bins.
Continuous blenders Modified ribbon and V-blenders	Diffusion and convection	Capable of high through-put Same advantages as listed for their non-continuous counterparts	Same disadvantages as listed for their non-continuous counterparts

Blending and Blend Uniformity

sampling is often an afterthought. In the absence of PAT, consideration must be given early on, on how to insert a sampling thief into all regions of a blender; which often necessitates headroom above the blender equal to its depth.

A blender is typically not dedicated to a single product but rather must be used for a wide range of products. Therefore versatility, in terms of ability to handle a range of blending requirements, is also an important consideration. This also includes an ability to handle a wide range of batch sizes. It can be challenging to accurately assess what materials a given site may handle even in the near future.

The scalability of the blender is a factor to consider (scaling methodologies for tumble blending were previously discussed). Vendors of blenders offer their products over a wide range of capacities to cover the manufacture of small development and pilot scale batches through commercial scale production. If possible, blending equipment available in development facilities should match that available in production plants. This situation allows blenders of the same design and operating principle to be used throughout the development and commercialization of a product, which could facilitate the accrual of better process knowledge and understanding for blending operations over the entire course of the product lifecycle. However, frequently development scientists are limited in their choice of blenders to equipment that is currently available in the development and/or commercial manufacturing facilities. This could result in the development of a blending process that is not robust and produces blends of poorer quality. For example, if the available equipment is not capable of delivering the necessary shear forces to break up agglomerates of cohesive materials, difficulties will be encountered in obtaining a uniform blend. This can lead to the rejection of batches due to content uniformity failures, which over time could be much more costly than the price associated with the purchase of a proper blender. Since it is easier to acquire lab-scale equipment that matches production (rather than vice-versa), the burden is on development organizations to obtain appropriate blenders based on proper scaling-down of those that will be used in production.

Many blenders can also serve as processing vessels, allowing for drying and/or granulation steps. Prior to purchasing a blender, consideration should be given to whether such processing may be needed in the future. For example, blenders can be purchased with appropriate jacketing (for heating/cooling), vacuum/pressure capabilities, and means for liquid addition.

Production efficiency is another factor that should be considered when selecting a blender. The total cycle time from batch-to-batch must be considered, which includes time for loading, blending, sampling (if required), discharge, and cleaning (as required).

Cleanability is another factor to consider, for both between batches of the same formulation as well as for different products. Blenders with easy access to all surfaces are easier to clean. The inclusion of internal components (such as baffles, ribbons, augers, or I-bars) can make it more difficult to clean the blender compared to simple rotating shells.

Containment of the material during loading, blending, and discharge is also important, especially for highly potent compounds, to protect the operators from exposure to the drug substance. Ideally, the blending container should also be used for material transfer. With any contained system, the impact that counter-current airflow during material movement has on the segregation potential of the blend must be identified. Sampling the blend, if required, is a particular challenge for contained processes. Such equipment utilize more complex valves to minimize dust during material transfer out of the bin, which often inhibit the ability to reach all areas of the blending containers.

For this reason and in the interest of operator safety, it is the authors' preference that for highly potent/toxic compounds, non-intrusive techniques such as PAT should be used to assess blend uniformity. If PAT is not available, then sampling of the final product should be an acceptable alternative to blend sampling. Sampling requirements are discussed elsewhere in this chapter.

Although the capital cost of a new blender (if required) must always be justified, once one realizes the financial implications of having a blender that does not perform adequately, total cost becomes a better means of comparison. Therefore, capital cost should only be considered in comparing two identical blenders.

Classification of Blending Equipment

Blending may be accomplished on a batch or continuous basis. Batch blending processes consist of three sequential steps: weighing and loading the components, blending, and discharging. Unlike a continuous blender, the retention time in a batch blender is rigidly defined and controlled, and is the same for all of the particles.

Batch blenders come in many different designs and sizes, and make use of a wide range of blending mechanisms. In the pharmaceutical industry, batch blenders are used almost exclusively. The primary reason for this is that batch blending has historically provided tighter quality control in terms of better uniformity and batch integrity, as compared to continuous blending. Continuous mixers are discussed later on in this section.

All blending equipment use one or more of the following mechanisms to induce powder blending: convective blending, shear blending, and diffusive blending. These mechanisms form the basis of one classification system that categorizes equipment into diffusion blenders, convection blenders, and pneumatic blenders (92). Subsets of these classifications are also routinely used. Although they are a subclass of convection blenders, the term high shear mixers is often applied to a number of very efficient blenders that impart significant shear to the materials being blended through the use of both rotating impellers and high-speed chopper blades. The term high shear mixers distinguishes them from other convection blenders that may impart lower levels of shear to the materials during the blending process.

Another classification system for blenders is based on their design. This system categorizes blenders into two categories, those that achieve blending within a moving vessel, and those with fixed vessels that rely on internal paddles or blades to move the materials. The later category could also include fluid bed processors, which use air to move the materials to be blended (53).

As a result of the multiple classification systems, a number of terms have evolved throughout the industry to describe families of blenders. Regardless of the terminology used to classify the blender, the important thing is for the pharmaceutical scientist to understand the capabilities and limitations of the equipment when selecting an appropriate blender for a particular product. This is especially important during process transfer or scale-up, when equipment of different design and operating principle may need to be used. Table 4 contains the advantages and disadvantages for various classifications of blenders.

Tumble Blenders

Tumble blenders are commonly used in the pharmaceutical industry. Their principle of operation is based on particles being reoriented in relation to one another when they are

Blending and Blend Uniformity

placed in motion. As the blending chamber is rotated, the angle of inclination of the material overcomes its angle of repose and the powder tumbles, subsequently leading to expansion of the bed. As the material avalanches, the particles migrate from layer to layer, providing diffusion. As the vessel rotates, the shape of the container, and how it changes as perceived by the bed of powder, provides convection. Because the uniformity of the blend is paced by diffusion of the particles, the manufacturing equipment addendum for SUPAC IR/MR classifies tumble blenders as diffusion blenders (92). Their geometric shape and the positioning of their axis of rotation generally distinguish subclasses of tumble blenders. Figures 25–28 contain pictures of a V-, double-cone, and bin blenders.

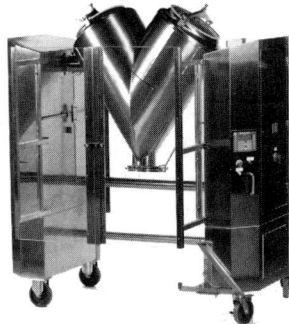
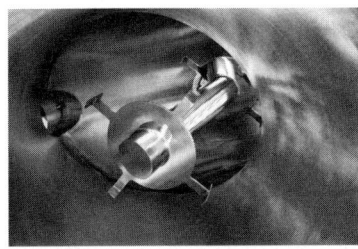

FIGURE 25 V-Blender and intensifier bar. *Source*: Courtesy of Patterson-Kelley.

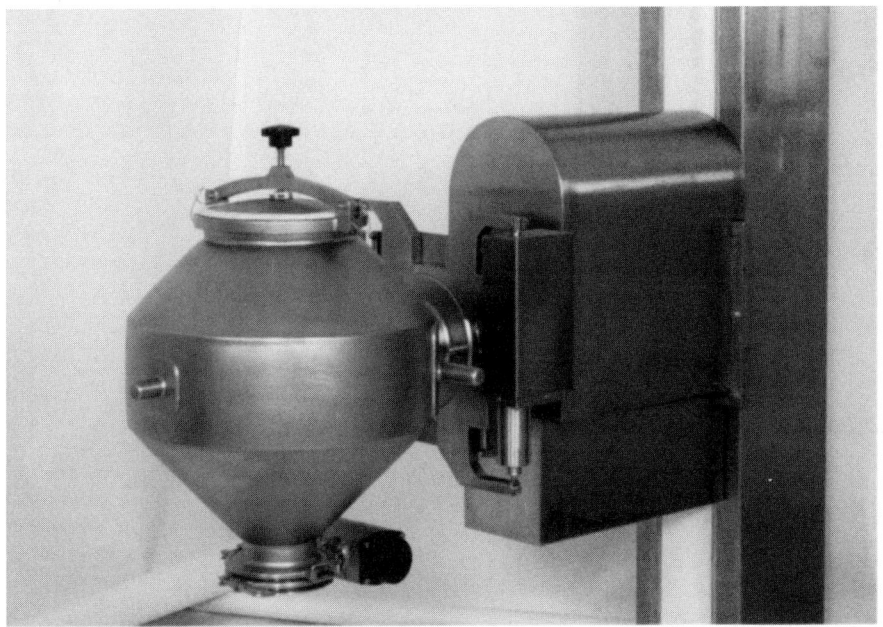

FIGURE 26 Double cone blender. *Source*: Courtesy of Patterson-Kelley.

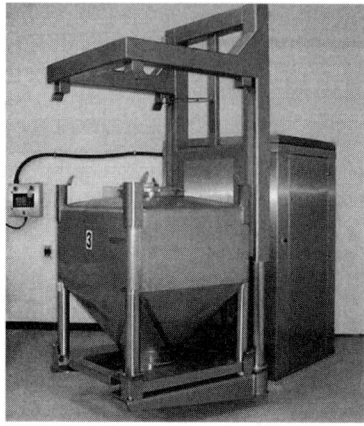 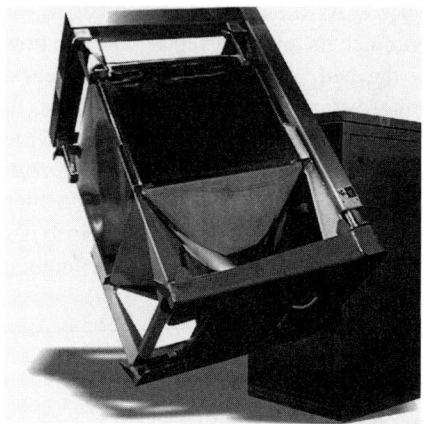

FIGURE 27 Matcon S series 1500-l IBCs and blender. *Source*: Courtesy of Matcon, U.S.A.

Tumble blenders also impart shear forces to the powders being blended, as slip planes form between the walls of the blender and layers of the blend. The amount of shear force is often low for small-scale blenders, but can increase with increasing scale of the blending container. Because they tend to provide gentler blending and have less of an affect on the particle size of the materials being blended (compared to high shear mixers),

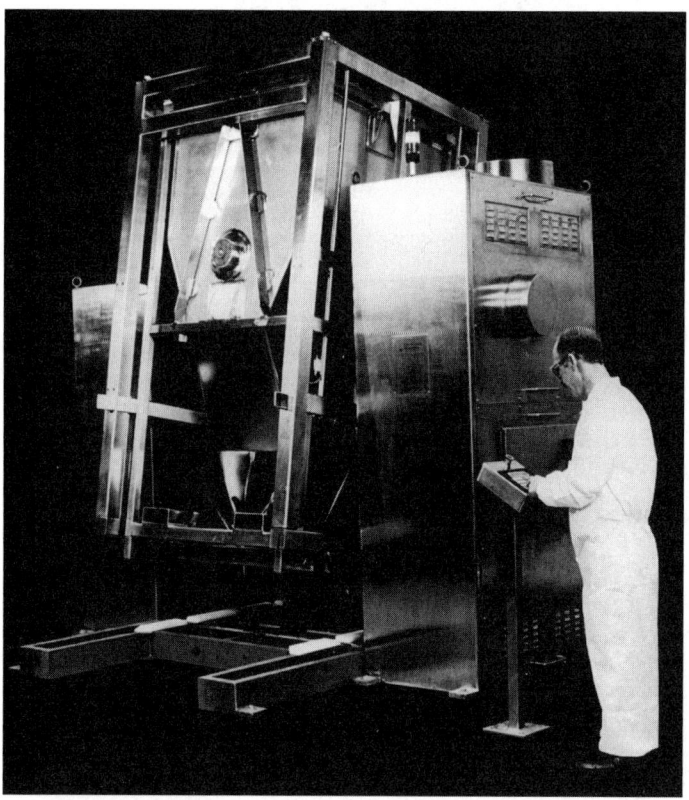

FIGURE 28 In-bin tumble blender with I-bar for cohesive, agglomerating material. *Source*: Courtesy of Jenike & Johanson, Inc.

Blending and Blend Uniformity

tumble blenders have also been described as being low shear blenders. As such, they are commonly used to lubricate formulations. This is particularly important for drugs with low solubility that are prone to over-lubrication. High shear mixers can reduce the particle size of the lubricant during the blending process, which can lead to greater coverage of particle surfaces and increased hydrophobicity of the blend. This could result in slower dissolution rates (and negatively affect the bioavailability of the drug product) and reduce the compressibility of the blend.

Some subtypes of tumble blenders (such as bin blenders) serve a dual purpose. In addition to providing the container in which blending is accomplished, bin blenders can also be used to transfer the powder blend to the next unit operation. This is of particular value when manufacturing blends that have the tendency to segregate when discharging the blend onto the compression or filling equipment. This also makes the use of bin blenders desirable during the manufacture of potent drug products that must be processed in high containment facilities. Additionally, by decoupling the blending bin from the drive mechanism, the bin filling, discharge and cleaning takes place at a separate time and location, which increases the efficiency and utilization of equipment.

Tumble blenders do have limitations associated with their use. The lower magnitude of shear forces imparted to the materials being blended may not be sufficient to break up agglomerates or disperse cohesive materials, which could result in poor micromixing. Passing the drug and excipients through either a vibratory screen or mill prior to charging them into tumble blenders will break up any existing agglomerates of the raw materials. If agglomerates form during the blending process, additional shear forces may be imparted to the blend through the installation of intensifier or agitation bars in some tumble blenders (Fig. 25 and Fig. 28). The use of blend–mill–blend processes can also be used to break up agglomerates and improve content uniformity.

The rate at which radial blending (perpendicular to the axis of blender rotation) occurs is more than one order of magnitude faster than the rate at which axial blending (parallel to the axis of blender rotation) occurs in tumble blenders (Fig. 29). This also implies that convective blending occurs at a much greater rate than diffusion, which is the primary mechanism influencing axial blending in tumble blenders (4,5,7). This observation demonstrates the importance of loading blenders using a layering technique, and avoiding the addition of an entire quantity of a minor component of the formulation to

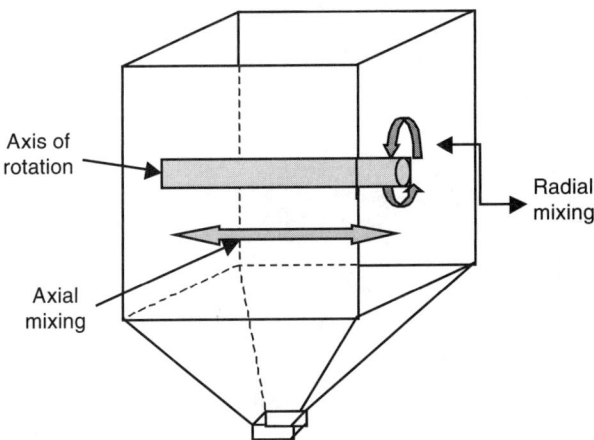

FIGURE 29 Axial and radial blending in a bin blender.

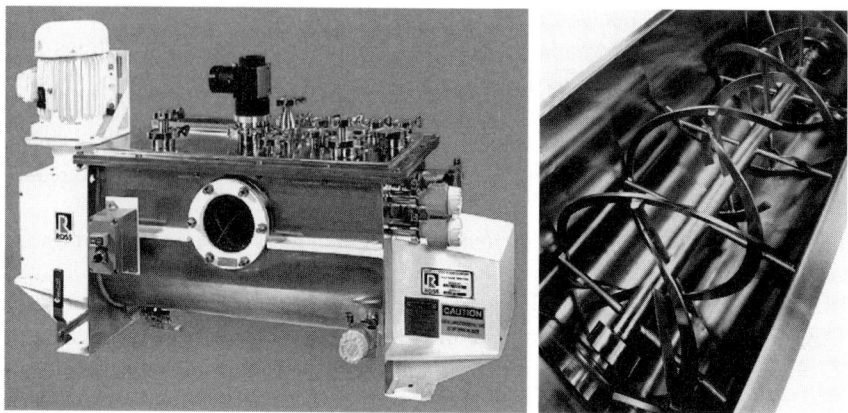

FIGURE 30 Ross sanitary ribbon blender model 42N-05 and mixing blades. *Source*: Courtesy of Charles Ross & Sons Company.

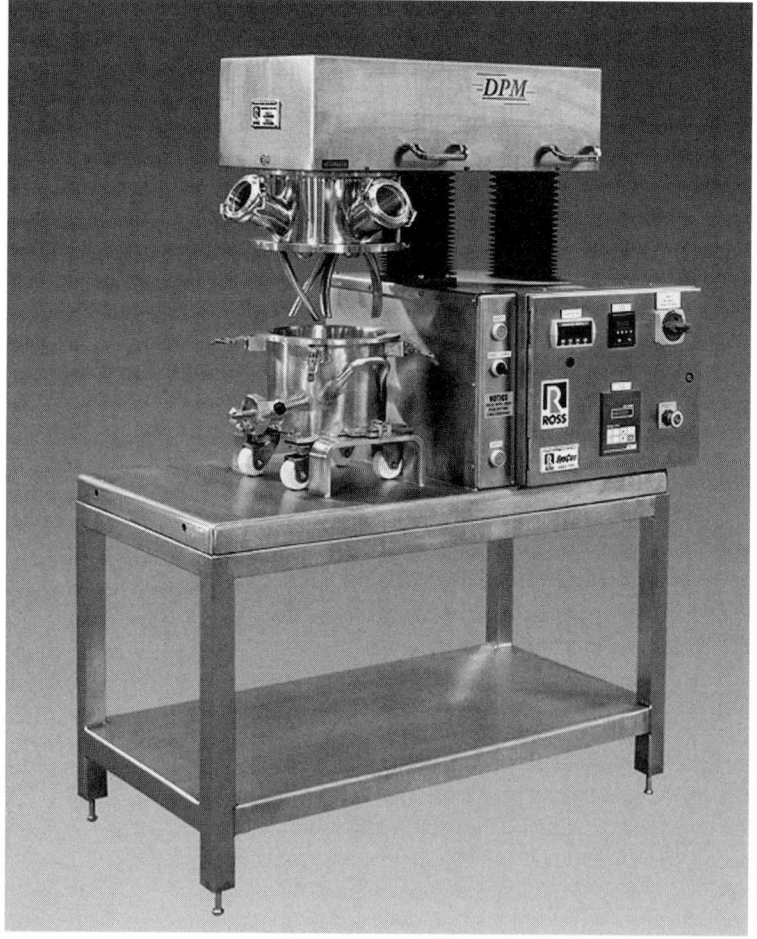

FIGURE 31 Ross 2-gallon sanitary double planetary blender. *Source*: Courtesy of Charles Ross & Sons Company.

Blending and Blend Uniformity

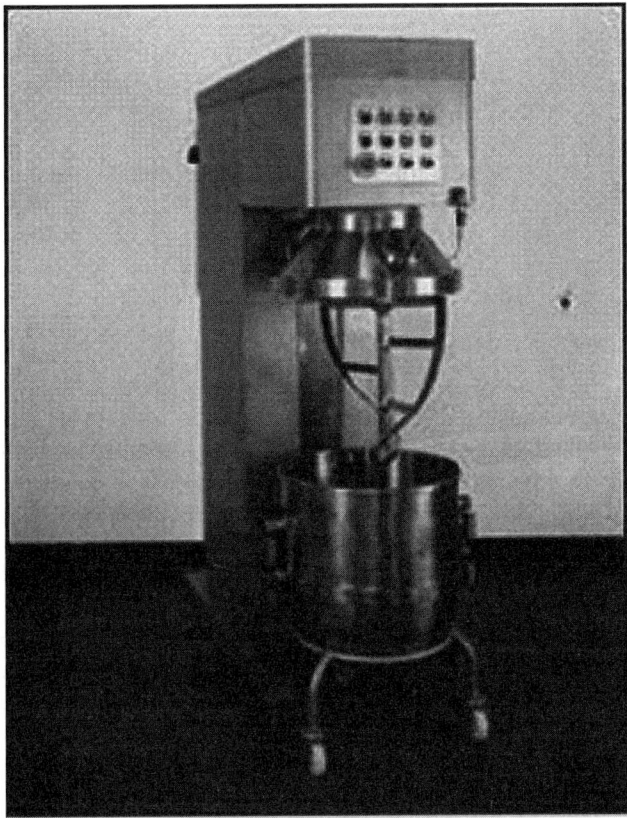

FIGURE 32 Planetary blender. *Source*: Courtesy of GEA Collette NV.

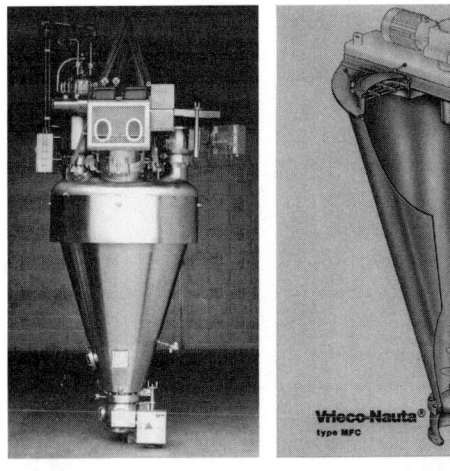

FIGURE 33 Vrieco-Nauta model 1.2 VDC-41 orbiting screw blender. *Source*: Courtesy of Hosokawa Micron Powder Systems.

one side of the blending container. Internal baffles can be used in tumble blenders to increase the rate of axial blending. However, baffles will not affect the shear rate substantially, nor will they improve the homogeneity of cohesive powders by breaking up agglomerates. Particles on the surface of the dynamic bed move at greater velocity than those in the center of the bed. Because material velocity is slower around the axis of rotation, areas in the center of the blend also have the potential to be problematic. Corners and areas above discharge valves are additional locations that may have restricted movement of material, which could result in areas of non-uniformity, especially when blending cohesive materials. For these reasons, sampling plans should target each of these areas when developing and validating blending operations.

Convection Blenders

Convection blenders reorient groups of particles in relation to one another as the result of mechanical movement, for example, caused by a paddle or a plow. As a result, circulation patterns result in this type of blenders. Subclasses of convection blenders are typically defined by vessel shape and impeller geometry. Ribbon blenders (Fig. 30), planetary blenders (Figs. 31 and 32), orbiting screw blenders (Fig. 33) are examples of convection blenders. High shear mixers comprise another sub-class of convection blenders that will be discussed separately.

Convection blenders have some drawbacks associated with their use. Many of the older designs have dead spots due to limited movement of materials in these areas. Problem locations include the corners of the blending vessel and the clearances

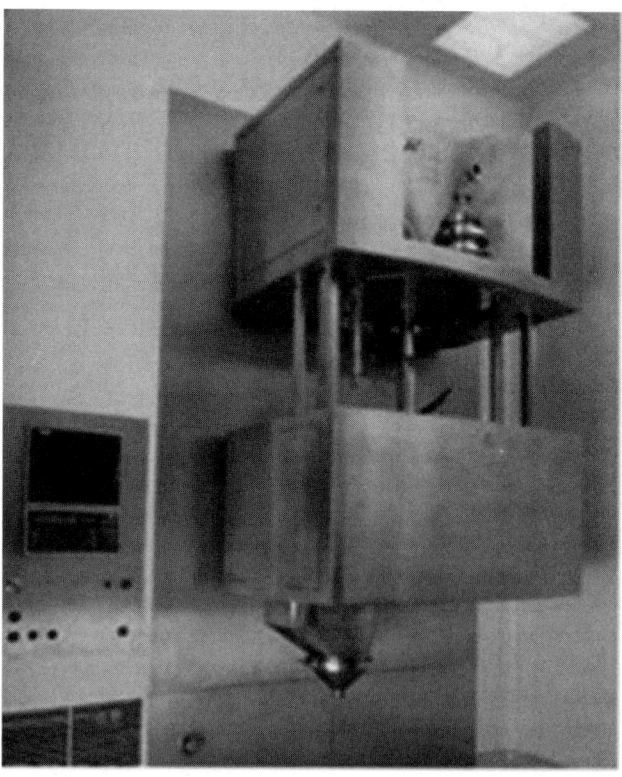

FIGURE 34 ULTIMAGRAL™ – 300 high shear mixer. *Source*: Courtesy of GEA Collette NV.

Blending and Blend Uniformity

between the ribbons or plows and walls of the blending container. For this reason, convection blenders should be extensively sampled during process development and validation exercises to ensure the blend is uniform, particularly in known problematic areas (70). Convection blenders must be discharged into an intermediate container to transfer it to the next unit operation, which as previously noted can lead to segregation of the blend.

High Shear Mixers/Granulators

Although they are often associated with the manufacture of wet granulations, high shear mixer/granulators can also be used for the manufacture of dry powder blends. They are a type of convection blenders that impart high mechanical energy to the materials being blended, resulting in the formation of slip planes. Circulation patterns predominate in these blenders and are influenced by the bowl geometry, the shape of the main impeller, and the location of the high-speed chopper. Figures 34 and 35 are two examples of high shear mixers commonly used in the pharmaceutical industry.

High shear mixers are very efficient and particularly useful for blending highly cohesive products that require the application of a significant amount of shear to uniformly distribute particles and break up agglomerates. They are often used to prepare

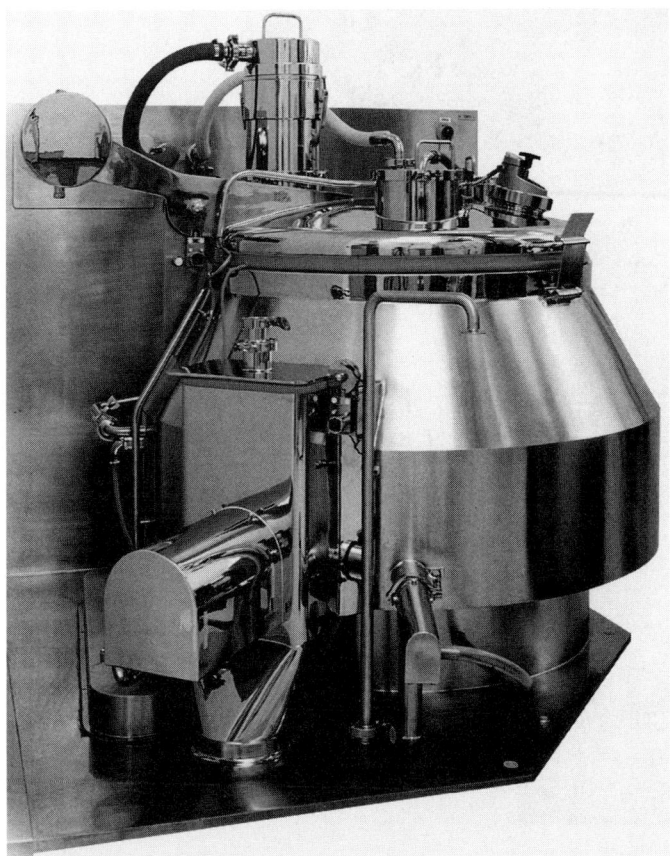

FIGURE 35 PharmaMatrix (PMA 600) high shear mixer. *Source*: Courtesy of Niro Inc.

premixes for blends containing a small quantity of active ingredient. The preblends may be directly added to the remaining components of the batch, or diluted in a stepwise fashion (i.e., geometric dilution) to further enhance the ability to prepare a uniform product. High shear mixers are also very effective in the production of ordered mixes.

High shear mixers do have some drawbacks associated with their use. They impart a considerable amount of energy into the blend, which can result in a slight increase in the temperature of the powder bed. [Some high shear mixers can be equipped with jacketed vessels that allow heating or cooling of the bowl to control this potential problem.] The shear applied to the blend can also break down particles, which could affect the physical properties of the blend and subsequent operations such as compression. Because

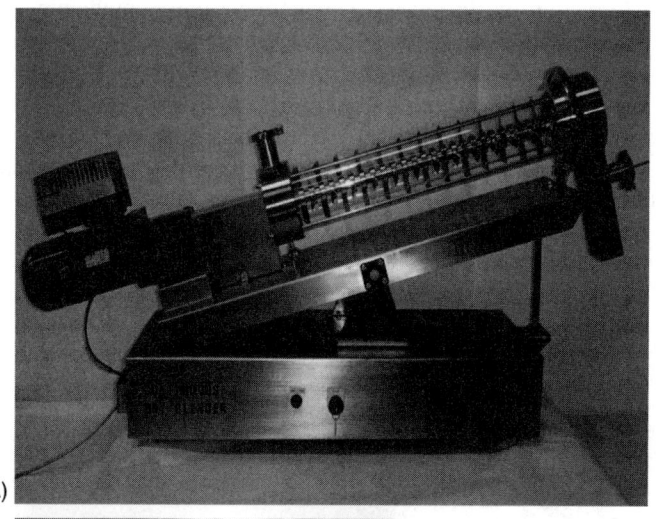

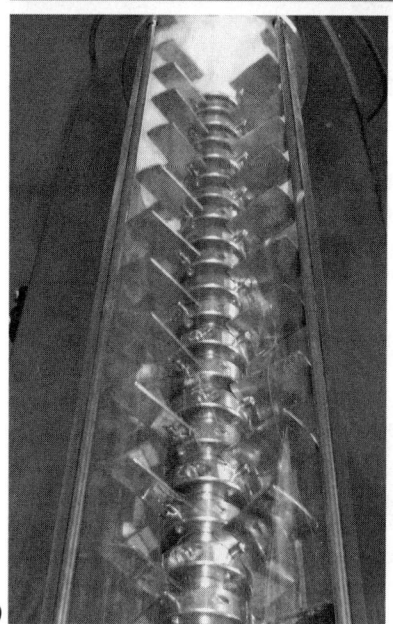

FIGURE 36 Continuous blender (**A**) and mixing paddles (**B**). *Source*: Courtesy of Buck Systems Ltd.

Blending and Blend Uniformity

they are such rapid blenders and can reduce the particle size of materials being blended, one must exercise caution when lubricating blends in high shear mixers. As previously discussed, this is especially important for blends containing drug substances having low aqueous solubility, where over-lubrication could suppress dissolution and therefore bioavailability.

Other Types of Blenders

Pneumatic blenders: Pneumatic blenders use a gas to expand the powder bed and reorient particles in relation to one another. Fluid bed processors are an example of blenders in this category, as they pass air through a powder bed resulting in fluidization and circulation patterns of the material within the expansion chamber. Fluid bed processors are typically only used for blending when another operation (such as wet granulation) is subsequently performed in the equipment. When the fluid bed processor is shut off, fine particles will remain suspended in the headspace of the expansion chamber, which will eventually settle out as a thin layer on the surface of the powder bed. Similarly, shaking the filter bags at the conclusion of processing will contribute to the layer of fines on top of the bed. If the fines are off-potency (typically drug enriched, but could also be sub-potent), the material should undergo a subsequent blending operation (perhaps in conjunction with lubrication) to ensure this off-potency layer is uniformly distributed throughout the remainder of the blend. Because the material must be transferred into an intermediate bulk container at the conclusion of processing, segregation upon discharging should be of concern. If pneumatic conveying is used to discharge the fluid bed processor, the segregation could be exacerbated.

Extruders: Extruders can also be used to blend powders, but usually only in conjunction with a subsequent melting operation. They consist of parallel screws that are constructed of individual sections that are specifically designed to move or mix the material as it passes through the extruder. The configuration of the screws affects the residence time of the material in the extruder, which can affect the degree of blending achieved.

Continuous blenders: Figures 36 and 37 contain pictures of two types of continuous blenders, which have been developed for the manufacture of large volume products. They are designed to continuously accept raw materials (input) and provide a uniform blend (output) that can be constantly fed to filling equipment over a sustained period of time. The defined "batch size" when using such blenders may be determined by

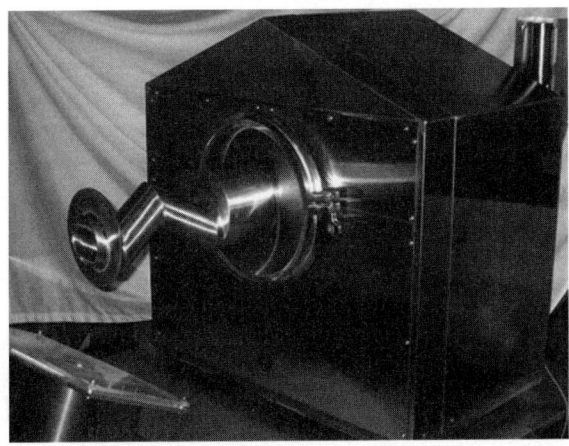

FIGURE 37 Continuous blender.
Source: Courtesy of Patterson-Kelley.

the amount of material produced over a standard period of time. In a continuous blending process, the weighing, loading, blending, and discharge steps occur continuously and simultaneously. Product motion is on average directed from the feed point toward the outlet. The blend quality for a particular continuous blender is a function of the retention time. Retention time is influenced rather than controlled, with some particles remaining in the blender longer than others, based on the design and operation of the blender, and material input rates.

Though continuous blending has been used by other industries for many years, it is just beginning to be more widely investigated by the pharmaceutical industry. This is due in part to advances in the ability to monitor the uniformity of the blend (e.g., via NIR), and improved abilities to accurately monitor and control feed rates of incoming materials. The advantage to continuous blending, if done correctly, includes the ability to monitor and control the blend at the point where it is most critical, for example, just prior to the compression or filling operations. Continuous blending eliminates transfer steps that can lead to segregation. Also, these blenders take up significantly less space than batch blenders that provide the same total throughput capacity. Further, once a "steady-state" is achieved, the state of blend uniformity should remain relatively constant, eliminating "tails" that can occur with batch blending.

REFERENCES

1. Rippie E. Powders. In: Osol A, Chase G, Gennaro A, Gibson, M, Granberg C, eds. Remington's Pharmaceutical Sciences, 16th ed. Easton, PA: Mack Publishing Company, 1980:1535–52.
2. Venables H, Wells J, Powder mixing. Drug Dev Ind Pharm 2001; 27(7):599–612.
3. Train D. Pharmaceutical aspects of mixing solids. Pharm J 1960; 185:129–34.
4. Llusa M, Muzzio F. The effect of shear mixing on the blending of cohesive lubricants and drugs. Pharm Tech 2005; 29(12):s36–s45.
5. Brone D, Alexander A, Muzzio F. Quantitative characterization of mixing of dry powders in v-blenders. AIChE J 1998; 44(2):271–8.
6. Alexander A, Arratia P, Goodridge, et al. Characterization of the performance of bin blenders, Part 1 of 3. Pharm Tech 2004; 28(5):70–86.
7. Tomassone M, Chaudhuri B, Faquh A, et al. Discrete element simulations for fundamental process understanding, Pharm Tech 2005; 29(12):s28–s35, s46.
8. Zhang Y, Johnson K. Effect of drug particle size on content uniformity of low-dose solid dosage forms. Int J Pharm 1997; 154(20):179–83.
9. Yalkowski S, Bolton S. Particle size and content uniformity. Pharm Res 1990; 7(9):962–6.
10. Egermann H, et al. Significance of drug content and of drug proportion to the content uniformity of solid dosage forms. Acta Pharm Jugosl 1988; 38(4):279–86.
11. Rippie E, Faiman F, Pramoda M. Segregation kinetics of particulate solids systems IV. Effect of particle shape on energy requirements. J Pharm Sci 1967; 56:1523–5.
12. Lloyd P, Yeung P, Freshwater D. The mixing and blending of powders. J Soc Cosmetic Chem 1970; 21:205–20.
13. Antequera, M, Ruiz, A, Perales, et al. Evaluation of an adequate method of estimating flowability according to powder characteristics. Int J Pharm 1994; 103(2): 155–161.
14. Sudah, O Arratia, P, Coffin-Beach, D, et al. Mixing of cohesive pharmaceutical formulations in Tote (bin) blenders. Drug Dev Ind Pharm 2002; 28(8):905–18.
15. Orr N, Pharm B, Shotton E. The mixing of cohesive powders. Chem Eng London 1973; 12–8.
16. Ahmed H, Shah N. Formulation of low dose medicines—Theory and practice. Am Pharm Rev 2000; 3(3):9–15.
17. Garcia, T, Carella A, Pansa V. Identification of factors decreasing the homogeneity of blend and tablet uniformity. Pharm Tech 2004; 28(3):110–22.

18. Abouzeid A, Fuerstenau D. Effect of humidity on mixing of particulate solids. Ind Eng Chem Proc Des Dev 1972; 11: 296–301.
19. Ottino J, Khakhar D. Mixing and segregation of granular materials. Annu Rev Fluid Mech 2000; 32:55–91.
20. Brone D, Muzzio F. Enhanced mixing in double-cone blenders. Powder Technol 2000; 110(3): 179–89.
21. Rowley G. Quantifying electrostatic interactions in pharmaceutical solid system. Int J Pharm 2001; 227:47–55.
22. Cross J. Electrostatics: Principles, Problems and Applications. Bristol: Adam Hilger, 1987.
23. Cartwright P, Singh P, Bailey A, et al. Electrostatic charging characteristics of polyethylene powder during pneumatic conveying. IEEE Trans Ind Appl 1985; 1(A-21):541–6.
24. Coste J, Pechery P. 3rd International Congress on Static Electricity, Grenoble, 1977: 4a–4f.
25. Homewood K. Do dirty surfaces matter in contact electrification. J Electrostat 1981; 10: 299–304.
26. Lowell J. Charge accumulation by repeated contacts of metals to insulators. J Phys D 1984; 17: 1859–70.
27. Peart J. Powder electrostatics: Theory, techniques and applications. KONA: Powder Particle 2001; 19:34–45.
28. Staniforth J, Rees J. Short communication. Powder mixing by triboelectrification. Powder Technol 1981; 30(2):255–6.
29. Staniforth J, Rees J. Investigation of triboelectric and ionization methods for electrostatic charging of powder particles. Int J Pharm Tech Prod Mfr 1982; 3(3):69–72.
30. Pavey I. CENELEC document CLC/TR 50404:2003 (also issued by BSI as PD CLC/TR 50404:2003), Electrostatics: Code of practice for the avoidance of hazards due to static electricity.
31. Eilbeck J, Rowley G, Carter P, et al. Effect of materials of construction of pharmaceutical processing equipment and drug delivery devices on the triboelectrification of size-fractionated lactose. Pharm Pharmacol Commun 1999; 5(7):429–33.
32. Eilbeck J, Rowley G, Carter P, et al. Effect of contamination of pharmaceutical equipment on powder triboelectrification. Int J Pharm 2000; 195(1–2):7–11.
33. Carter P, Rowley G, Fletcher E, et al. Measurement of electrostatic charge decay in pharmaceutical powders and polymer materials used in dry powder inhaler devices. Drug Dev Ind Pharm 1998; 24:1083–8.
34. Pollock H, Burnham N, Colton R. In Rimai D, Sharpe L, eds. Advances in Particle Adhesion. Amsterdam: Gordon and Breach, 1996; 71–86.
35. Carter P, Rowley G, Fletcher E, et al. An apparatus to measure charge distributions in particulate systems. J Aerosol Sci 1992; 23(S1):S397–400.
36. Singh S, Hearn G. Development and application of an electrostatic microprobe. J Electrostat 1985; 16:353–61.
37. Hersey J. Preparation and properties of ordered mixtures. Aust J Pharm Sci 1977; 6(1): 29–31.
38. Stephenson P, Thiel W. The mechanical stability of ordered mixtures when fluidized and their pharmaceutical application. Powder Technol 1980; 26:225–7.
39. Bryan L, Rungvejhavuttivittaya Y, Steward P. Mixing and demixing of microdose quantities of sodium salicylate in a direct compression vehicle. Powder Technol 1979; 22: 147–51.
40. Poux M, Fayolle P, Bertrand J, et al. Powder mixing: Some practical rules applied to agitated systems. Powder Technol 1991: 68:213–34.
41. Theil W, Lai F, Hersey J. Comments on suggestions on the nomenclature of powder mixtures. Powder Technol 1981; 28:117–8.
42. Lai F, Hersey J. A cautionary note on the use of ordered powder mixtures in pharmaceutical dosage forms. J Pharm Pharmacol 1979; 31:800.
43. Hersey J. The development and applicability of powder mixing theory. Int J Phar Tech Pro Mfr 1979; 1(1):6–13.

44. Alexander A, Muzzio F. Batch size increase in dry blending and mixing: Pharmaceutical process scale-up. In: Levin E, ed. Drugs and the Pharmaceutical Sciences, 1st ed, Vol 118. New York: Marcel Dekker Inc., 2002.
45. Wang R, Fan L. Methods for scaling up tumbling mixers. Chem Eng 1974; 8(11):88–94.
46. Bates L. User Guide to Segregation. London, U.K.: British Materials Handling Board, 1997.
47. Williams J. The segregation of particulate materials: A review. Powder Technol 1976; 15: 245–51.
48. Liss D, Conway S, Zega J, et al. Segregation of powders during gravity flow through vertical pipes. Pharm Tech 2004; 28(2):78–96.
49. Williams J, Khan M. The mixing and segregation of particulate solids of different particle size. Chem Eng 1973; 7(1):19–25.
50. Pittenger B, Purutyan H, Barnum R. Reducing/eliminating segregation problems in powdered metal processing. Part I: Segregation mechanisms. P/M Sci Tech Briefs 2000; 2(1):5–9.
51. Anonymous. Standard Practice/Guide for Measuring Sifting Segregation Tendencies of Bulk Solids. ASTM International 2003; D6940-03.
52. Anonymous. Standard Practice for Measuring Fluidization Segregation Tendencies of Powders. ASTM International 2003; D6941–03.
53. Williams J. The mixing of dry powders. Powder Technol 1968; 2:13–20.
54. Globepharma's Powdertest™ http://www.globepharma.com/html/powertest.html (accessed September 2006).
55. Massol-Chaudeur S, Berthiaux H, Doggs J. The development and use of a static segregation test to evaluate the robustness of various types of powder mixtures. Trans IchemE June 2003; 81(Part c):106–18.
56. Johanson K, Eckert C, Ghose D, et al. Quantitative measurement of particle segregation mechanisms. Powder Technol 2005; 159(11):1–12.
57. De Silva S, Dyroy A, Enstad G. Segregation mechanisms and their quantification using segregation testers. In Solids Mechanics and Its Applications, Vol. 81. IUTAM Symposium on Segregation in Granular Flows, 1999; 11–29.
58. Hedden D, Brone D, Clement S, et al. Development of an improved fluidization segregation tester for use with pharmaceutical powders. Pharm Tech 2006; 30(12):54–64.
59. Alexander B, Roddy M, Brone D, et al. A method to quantitatively describe powder segregation during discharge from vessels. Pharm Tech Yearbook 2000; 6–21.
60. Jenike A. Storage and flow of solids. University of Utah Engineering Experiment Station, Bulletin No. 123, Nov. 1964 (Rev 1980), 16th Printing, July 1994.
61. Carson J, Royal T, Goodwill D. Understanding and eliminating particle segregation problems. Bulk Solids Handling 1986; 6:139–44.
62. Anonymous, united state of America, plaintiff V. Barr Laboratories, Inc. et. al., Defendants, united states District court for the District of New Jersey, Ciuil Action No. 92-1744 opinion, February 1993.
63. Motise P, Crabbs W, Lord T. Solid oral dosage forms: blend uniformity acceptance criteria. Human Drug CGMP Notes 1993; 1(2):5–6.
64. The United States Pharmacopeia, 29th Revision, <905> Uniformity of Dosage Units, The United States Pharmacopeial Convention, Rockville, MD, 2006; 2778–9.
65. Berman J, Elinski D, Gonzales C, et al. Blend uniformity analysis: Validation and in-process testing. J Pharm Sci Tech 1997; 51(6): Technical Report No. 25.
66. Anonymous. Guidance for Industry: ANDAs: Blend Uniformity Analysis. U.S. Department of Health and Human Services, Food and Drug Administration, Center for Drug Evaluation and Research, Office of Generic Drugs, 1999.
67. Workshop on Blend Uniformity, September 2000. Arlington, VA: Product Quality Research Institute.
68. Boehm G, Clark J, Dietrick J, et al. Report on the industry blend uniformity practices survey. Pharm Tech 2001; 25(8):20–6.

69. Boehm G, Clark J, Dietrick J, et al. Results of statistical analysis of blend and dosage unit content uniformity data obtained from the Product Quality Research Institute Blend Uniformity Working Group data-mining effort. J Pharm Sci Tech 2004; 58(2):62–74.
70. Boehm G, Clark J, Dietrick J, et al. The use of stratified sampling of blend and dosage units to demonstrate adequacy of mix for powder blends. J Pharm Sci Tech 2003; 57(2):64–74.
71. Anonymous. Guidance for Industry, Powder Blends and Finished Dosage Unites – Stratified In-Process Dosage Unit Sampling and Assessment. U.S. Department of Health and Human Services, Food and Drug Administration, Center for Drug Evaluation and Research, Pharmaceutical CGMPs, 2003.
72. Anonymous. Guidance for Industry, PAT–A Framework for Innovative Pharmaceutical Development, Manufacturing, and Quality Assurance. U.S. Department of Health and Human Services, Food and Drug Administration, Center for Drug Evaluation and Research, Center for Veterinary Medicine, Office of Regulatory Affairs, Pharmaceutical CGMPs, 2004.
73. Boss J. Evaluation of the homogeneity degree of a mixture. Bulk Solids Handling 1986; 6(6): 1207–15.
74. Garcia T, Taylor M, Pande G. Comparison of the performance of two sample thieves for the determination of the content uniformity of a powder blend. Pharm Dev Tech 1998; 3(1):7–12.
75. Harwood C, Ripley T. Errors associated with the thief probe for bulk powder sampling. J Powder Bulk Solids Tech 1977; 1(2):20–29.
76. Berman J, Planchard J. Blend uniformity and unit dose sampling. Drug Dev Ind Pharm 1995; 2(11):1257–83.
77. Berman J, Schoeneman A, Shelton J. Unit dose sampling: A tale of two thieves. Drug Dev Ind Pharm 1996; 22(11):1121–32.
78. Allan T. Particle Size Measurement. 2nd ed. London: Chapman & Hall Ltd., 1975.
79. Allan T, Khan A. Critical evaluation of powder sampling procedures. Chem Eng 1970; May: 108–12.
80. Glossary and Tables for Statistical Quality Control. Milwaukee, Wisconsin: ASQC Quality Press, 1983.
81. Davies O, ed. Design and Analysis of Industrial Experiments. New York: Hafner (Macmillan), 1960.
82. Box G, Hunter W, Hunter J. Statistics for Experimenters, An Introduction to Design, Data Analysis, and Model Building. New York: John Wiley and Sons, Inc., 1978; 556–83.
83. Prescott J, Ramsey P, Gladysz K, et al. Bench-scale segregation tests as a predictor of blend sampling error. AAPS Annual Meeting, Indianapolis, IN, 2000.
84. Prescott J, Garcia T. A solid dosage and blend content uniformity troubleshooting diagram. Pharm Tech 2001; 25(3):68–88.
85. Hailey P, Doherty P, Tapsell P, et al. Automated system for the on-line monitoring of powder blending processes using near-infrared spectroscopy Part 1. System development and control. J Pharm Biomed Anal 1996; 14:551–9.
86. Sekulic S, Ward H, Brannegan D, et al. On-line monitoring of powder blend homogeneity by near-infrared spectroscopy. Anal Chem 1996; 68:509–13.
87. Cho J, Gemperline P, Aldridge P, et al. Effective mass sampled by NIR fiber-optic reflectance probes in blending processes, Analytica Chimica Acta 1997; 348:303–10.
88. Sekulic S, Wakeman J, Doherty P, et al. Automated system for the on-line monitoring of powder blending processes using near-infrared spectroscopy Part II. Qualitative approaches to blend evaluation. J Pharm Biomed Anal 1998; 17:1285–309.
89. Kaushik D, Madan K, Dureja H. Near-infrared spectroscopy: Applications in solid dosage form analysis. Tablets & Capsules 2006; 4(7):22–8.
90. Roy Y, Mathis N, Closs S, et al. Online thermal effusivity monitoring: A promising technique for determining when to conclude blending of magnesium stearate. Tablets & Capsules 2005; 3(2):38–47.

91. Sandell D, Vukovinsky K, Diener M, et al. Development of a content uniformity test suitable for large sample sizes. Drug Info J 2006; 40(3):337–44.
92. Anonymous. Guidance for Industry, SUPAC-IR/MR: Immediate Release and Modified Release Solid Oral Dosage Forms, Manufacturing Equipment Addendum, U.S. Department of Health and Human Services, Food and Drug Administration, Center for Drug Evaluation and Research, 1999.

5
Milling

Benjamin Murugesu
Quadro Engineering Corp., Waterloo, Ontario, Canada

INTRODUCTION

Modern medicine and pharmaceutics have far surpassed the days of tonics and teas, plasters, and compresses. Since the advent of the tablet, the solid dosage form has remained the most popular drug delivery system, comprising over 80% of all ethical and generic preparations produced today. As it is rare for pre-blended and sized material to be available in the ideal form for tableting, the introduction of solid dose forms placed a demand upon industry for the design and development of new size reduction technology. This in turn motivated the research into the science of size reduction and powder behavior. Progress has been made towards understanding fracture mechanics, static energy, and agglomeration of particles. There are still areas of size reduction that are not fully understood due to the dynamic nature of crystals and powder blends.

SIZE REDUCTION OVERVIEW

Key applications of milling in the manufacture of solid dosage forms is in the size reduction of a wet granulation prior to drying and sizing dried particles prior to tableting. However, the equipment discussed in this chapter are also widely used in the pharmaceutical industry for many other applications including pre-conditioning, calibrating product and raw material, dispersion, blending and mixing of formulations, deagglomeration, densification and reclaim of off-spec tablets and capsules. The benefits derived from the use of size reduction equipment continue to reinforce the critical role of milling in the industry, despite the progress of directly compressible of materials.

The benefits associated with size reduction are listed below.

- Wet dispersion prior to drying:
  - provide homogeneous and uniformly sized wet particles for drying
  - optimize dryers efficiency due to uniformly sized product with high surface area for evaporation and even drying
  - eliminates moist centers
  - eliminates hard, over dried particles
  - reduced drying time
  - reduced fines when sizing dried mass

- Dry sizing:
  - particle size calibration for uniformity
  - final sizing of dry product to better suit the final process (i.e., Compaction/packaging/mixing, etc.)
  - enhance fluidity and achieve narrow particle size distribution curve
  - bulk density refinement
  - particle size to affect optimum reactivity, dissolution, and drug release as a finished product
  - increase surface area

Size reduction involves the decrease in size of a particle or granule by fracturing the material using, generally, one of the four forces: shear, compression, impact, and tension. Single or combination of forces being applied to the material affect the level of size reduction that will be achieved, but also the magnitude and duration of the applied force(s) will help determine the overall resultant particle size distribution.

The process begins by placing the material under stress through interaction with the moving parts of the size-reduction equipment (Fig. 1). Initially the material will absorb this stress as a form of strain energy however if the stress is carried past the critical limit (determined by the characteristics of the material being size reduced), the particle or granule will cleave along its weakest point(s), resulting in fracture. For a dried granule, these points can be either the binder–particle interface, the binder bridge between individual particles, a flaw within the particle itself or a combination of these faults. Alternately for a wet granule, fracture will normally occur by exceeding the surface tension of the granulated mass and capillary forces.

Efficiency of the size reduction process can be realized if the minimum energy required to fracture the granule to create new surfaces can be applied by the system. In fact most methods of size reduction are relatively inefficient in terms of energy when its considered that only a percentile of the energy supplied by the equipment achieves the desired particle rupture. This could partially be attributed to the lack of knowledge of surface energies, mechanisms and design attributes, therefore leading to gross miscalculations in terms of the minimum energy required. The bulk of the energy involved with size reduction is translated into other physical and mechanical variables such as:

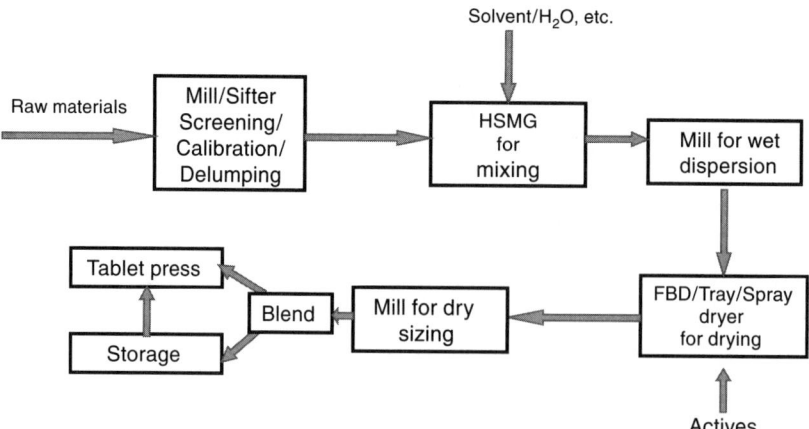

FIGURE 1 Typical solid dosage manufacturing process layout.

Milling

- heat,
- noise,
- friction,
- vibration,
- strain energy of unfractured granules,
- efficiency of drive mechanism and general mechanical design of the equipment.

Energy requirements related to size reduction may seem unreasonable, however, the overall power requirements dedicated to this process is generally outweighed by the benefits gained in achieving the final product.

OVERVIEW OF MILLING TECHNOLOGIES

The evolution of milling technology up until the last century had been relatively mundane. The stone grinder was originally called upon for the milling of grains and seeds and was essentially a large scale mortar and pestle. Working with the principles of compression and tension, the stone grinder was effective for the agricultural industry but eventually did not meet the more refined particle size distributions required for pharmaceuticals.

Soon to follow the stone grinder were the roll crusher and lump breaker. While still in use today, the roll crusher is more apt to be found size reducing rocks and other aggregates in a more industrial setting. The lump breaker similarly is also commonly used in the food industry although it is still occasionally used in the pharmaceutical industry for size reducing agglomerates. The pharmaceutical industry demanded a more refined approach to repeatability led to the invention of the hammermill, oscillator, and conical screen mill.

Hammermills

Hammermills are still in use in the pharmaceutical industry. There are two common design configurations for the hammermill: a vertical rotor shaft and the horizontal rotor shaft. The more common of the two—the horizontal hammermill—introduces the feed material perpendicularly to the rotating shaft where size reduction is achieved through direct impact with vertically suspended steel bars (Fig. 2). These bars have either blunt edges for hammering of the material, or knife edges for shearing, and can be fixed or swinging from the centre shaft.

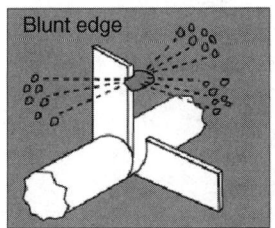
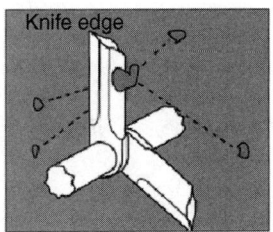
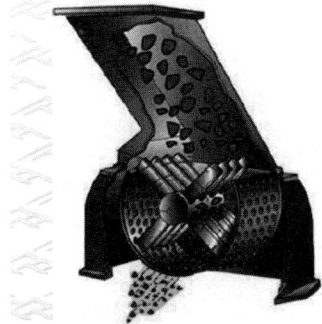

FIGURE 2 Cross sectional views of typical hammermill. *Source*: From Ref. 6.

Once impacted the material is, theoretically, directed towards the discharge screen at the bottom of the drum. The material within the milling zone is repeatedly impacted by the rotating hammers, until the particles are size reduced small enough to pass through the screen opening. The capacity of a hammermill and the final product characteristics are determined by the number of hammers rotating about the shaft (i.e., offset angles from neighboring hammers), size, sharpness, speed, screen opening, and gap between hammer tips and milling drum (Fig. 3).

Hammermills are designed for milling with a controlled feedrate, inlet, and discharge connections can be designed to mate with up and down stream equipment if desired. Scale-up of a hammermill is possible and is heavily dependent on maintaining the rotor rpm; and also note that the scale-up between the horizontal rotor and the vertical configuration is more complicated as the vertical design allows for a diametrical discharge of product (as opposed to the 180° with horizontal shafts) and marginally increasing the capacity of the equipment over the horizontal design. In addition to this, the hammermill does offer a range of screens and meshes to fit the discharge as well as blade types.

The performance of a hammermill is greatly affected by the feedrate and the moisture content (Table 1). Not suited for wet granulations, hammermills must be control fed to avoid equipment overloading and product resistance to discharge from the milling zone in a timely manner thus producing more fines, higher amperage draw and a reduced output. The efficiency of a hammermill is also reduced when the infeed product enters the milling zone on the upstroke of the hammers. Product introduced in the wrong direction will lead to inefficient dissipation of the hammer's energy, and the product will tend to bounce back out of the milling zone (blow back).

Oscillating Granulators

Oscillators have played a significant role in the pharmaceutical industry by providing low shear size reduction through the use of oscillating bars (Fig. 4). Size reduction is accomplished by direct pressure of the material between the oscillating bars and the wire mesh screen.

By varying the speed, oscillating motion, and the mesh size of the screen, the particle size distribution curve can be altered according to the end users specifications.

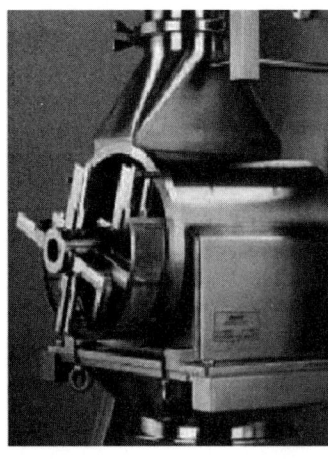
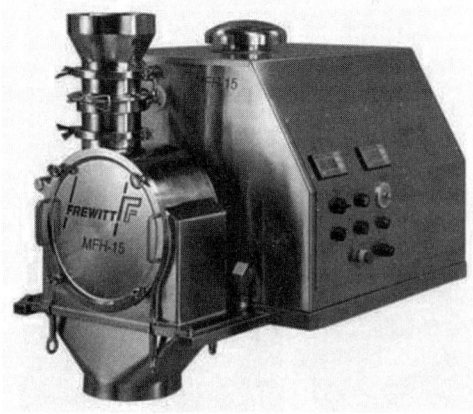

FIGURE 3 Frewitt hammermill. *Source*: From Ref. 7.

Milling

TABLE 1 Fitzmill Models and Scale-Up

Model	Chamber			Rotor			Machine limits	
	Capacity factor	Nominal width (in/cm)	Screen area (in²/cm²)	Diameter (in/cm)	Number of blades	Tip speed factor	Maximum rpm	Maximum horse power
Homoloid	0.4	2.5 6.3	43 277	6.625 16.8	12	1.73	7200	10.0
M5A	0.7	4.5 11.4	76 490	8.0 20.32	16	2.09	4600	3.0
D6A	1.0	6 15.24	109 703	10.5 26.67	16	2.75	4600	5.0
DAS06	1.0	6 15.24	109 703	10.5 26.67	16	2.75	7200	15

These variables and the low shear action make the oscillator well suited to size reduce more difficult to mill products (i.e., waxy and/or heat sensitive) however oscillators are not high capacity mills and the potential for metal contamination due to tooling wear is higher than other alternatives. Process integration is generally cumbersome and has a large foot print. Cleaning and maintenance cost are relatively high.

Conical Screen Mill

The operating principle of the conical screen mill is relatively simple. Material is introduced into the milling chamber either by gravity feed or by vacuum transfer. In the milling chamber the particles will encounter a rotating impeller and a stationary conical screen. The rotation of the impeller imparts a vortex flow pattern to the product. Centrifugal acceleration forces the product outwards to the surface of the screen where the particles are impinged between the edge of the impeller and the screen. Tangential action fractures the particles and the material is instantaneously discharged through the screen opening diametrically. This action dramatically reduces retention time of product in the milling chamber and improves power benefits.

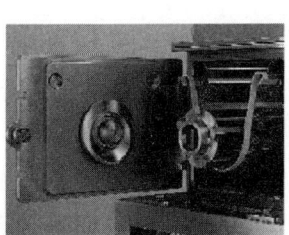
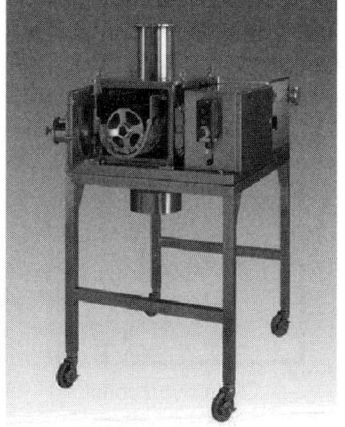
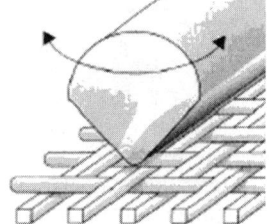

FIGURE 4 Frewitt oscillator. *Source*: From Ref. 7.

Conical Mill Concept

Trigonometric attributes support in the design of screens and mathematically expanding diameter for various models to support capacity requirements. This is done without loss of base attributes of scale-up value. The conical design contributes to various benefits in the development and fabrication of the screens (Fig. 5).

Understanding the various forces acting about the cone facilitates in the design criteria for strength and tangential deviations.

There are two designs concepts for the cone mill: the overdriven and the underdriven designs. The over drive cone mill is belt driven with the spindle assembly for the impeller entering the milling chamber from above. The under drive mill has a direct driven gearbox which introduces the spindle assembly into mill housing from below (Fig. 6). The main design differences between the two can be summed up as follows:

- infeed path—angled vs. straight through,
- overall height—feed to discharge,
- infeed and discharge diameter,
- total Surface Area—the underdriven is more efficient,
- integration flexibility, and
- footprint.

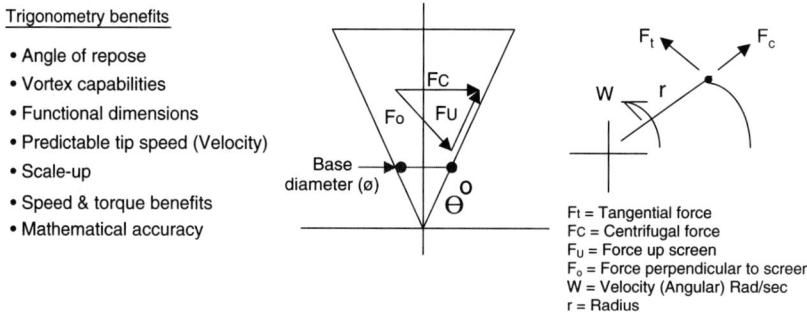

FIGURE 5 Conical concept trigonometry.

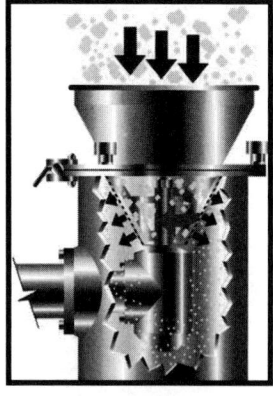
Underdriven comil
(Invented 1990)

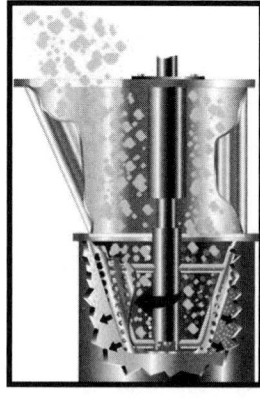
Overdriven comil
(Invented 1976)

FIGURE 6 Quadro Comil: underdriven and overdriven designs.

Milling

The underdriven cone mill is ideal for integrated inline applications, providing for higher capacity, while offering a smaller footprint than the more traditional overdriven unit. Both design variations will yield similar PSD and are interchangeable (Fig. 7).

The conical screen mill provides many benefits over some of the other equipment designs including (Fig. 8):

- low speed,
- 360° gravity discharge,
- low noise,
- high capacity,
- easy clean design,
- low energy (power),
- choke/plug feed,
- low dust,
- tight uniform particle size distribution, and
- no metal-to-metal contact.

The cone mill also lends itself well to integration into existing systems (small footprint), inert milling, containment milling, ATEX/XP design, and ASME pressure vessels (Fig. 9).

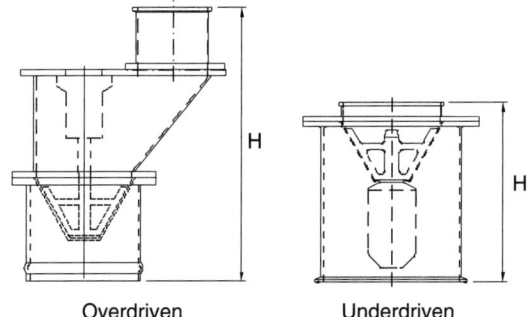

FIGURE 7 Overdriven and underdriven design schematics.

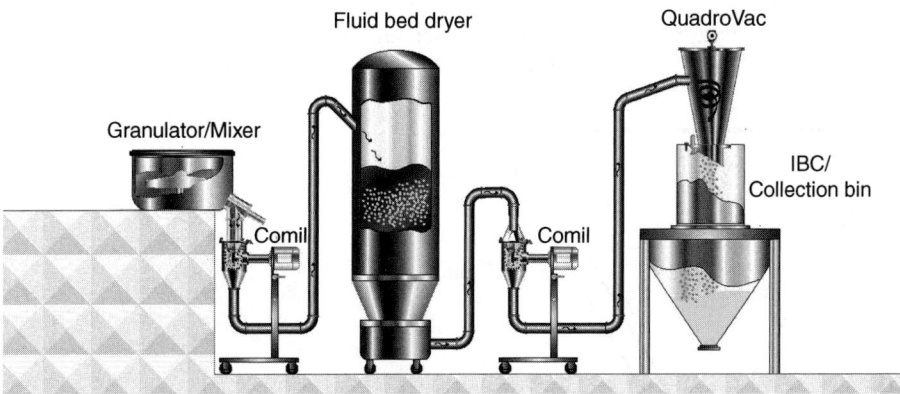

FIGURE 8 Typical pharmaceutical system layout.

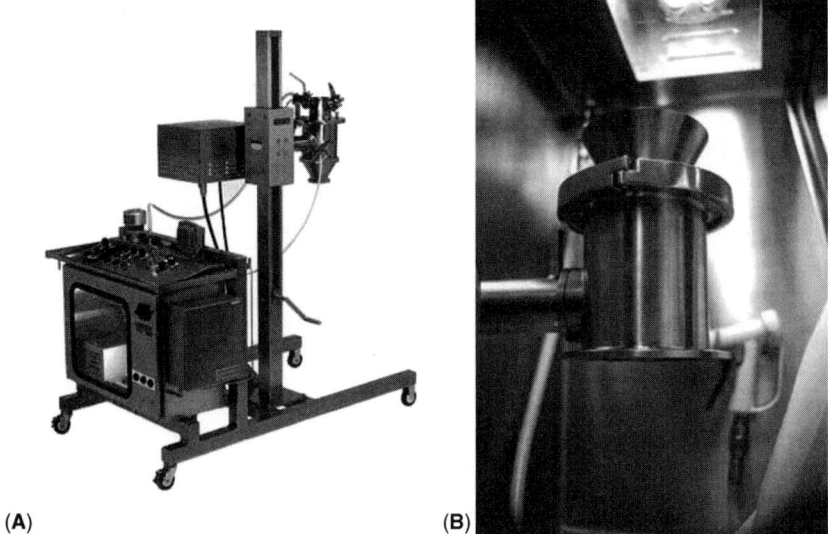

FIGURE 9 (**A**) Quadro Comil U10 with nitrogen purge system; (**B**) Quadro Comil U5 mounted inside of a glovebox.

Critical Milling Factors

The critical factors involved with obtaining the desired grind with the cone mill are:

1. Close impeller/screen gap
2. Proper tooling selection:
   - impeller type
   - screen type
3. Tip velocity (ft/min, m/sec)
4. Feed condition (plug feed)
5. Discharge condition/downstream equipment

Impeller/Screen Gap

A close impeller/screen gap to ensure lower residence time of product in the milling zone to increase capacity due to rapid discharge of product through the mill and avoiding product slippage between the impeller and screen. With reduced residence time the product will experience less friction resulting in low-heat generation and fines (Fig. 10).

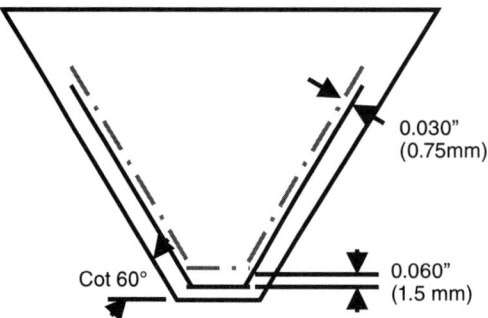

FIGURE 10 Impeller/screen gap.

Milling

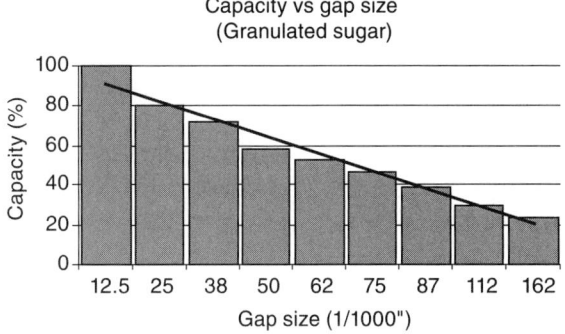

FIGURE 11 Capacity vs. gap size for granulated sugar in conical screen mill.

Maintaining a close gap is also necessary to ensure process repeatability and optimum milling efficiency and tool life (Figs. 11 and 12).

Impellers

The choice of impeller can also greatly affect the overall particle size distribution curve. The use of a round bar impeller results in a compressive force at the screen surface, impinging the material more aggressively thus making it more suited to dry granulations. Alternatively a square arm impeller shape induces low shear and functions well as a universal tool, working well for both wet granulation and most dry granulations (Fig. 13).

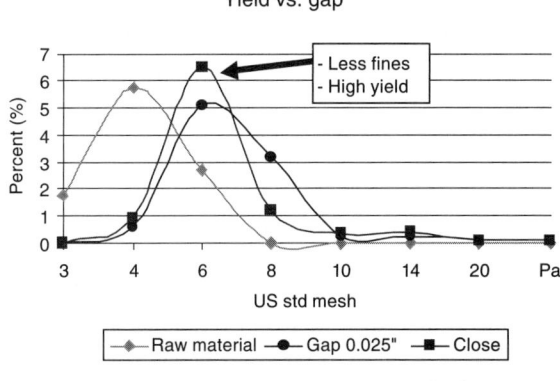

FIGURE 12 Yield vs. gap setting for granulated sugar in conical screen mill.

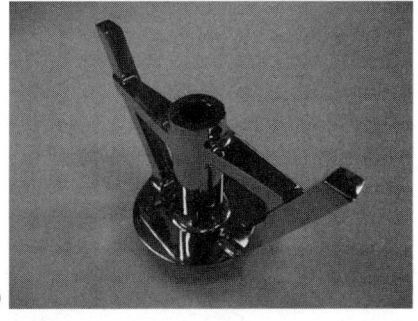
(A)

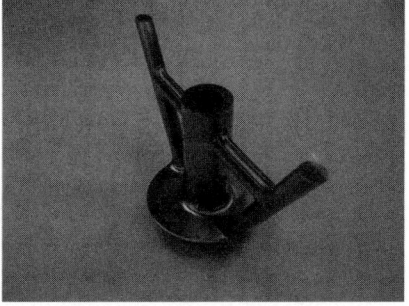
(B)

FIGURE 13 Typical conical screen mill impellers (1609): (**A**) square arm design, (**B**) round arm design.

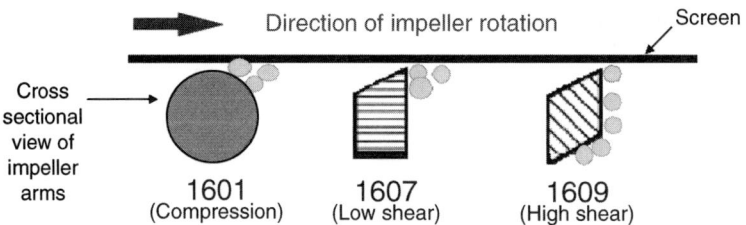

FIGURE 14 Impeller geometries.

The basic geometry of impellers can be altered to provide flexibility for specific applications. As an example, a square arm impeller with a positive leading edge (Fig. 13) applies higher shear action to size reduce, but unlike the standard square arm design, results in higher fines, increased product retention time and lower capacities (Fig. 14).

Screens

The type of screen chosen for an application is also an important factor. Variety of hole geometries have been developed to provide flexibility in the desired PSD. The most common hole geometry is a round hole which is used mainly to size reduce or delump dry material. Ranging in hole diameter size from 0.006 in (0.15 mm) to 0.250 in (6.35 mm) the round hole screen remains one of the more versatile options in tooling. For wet granulations the more common screen geometry is a square hole, although the square hole also functions well for basic delumping of bulk material; alternatively rectangular opening is more suitable for milling pseudo-elastic material. For brittle products requiring a more aggressive grind, the grater hole screen (rasp) is applied. Based on a round hole screen design the impact edge of the hole is dimpled (up set) to raise the geometry of the hole for shear action. From these four basic geometries a multitude of screens are available through combinations of designs (i.e., Slotted grater hole) and methods of manufacture (i.e., perforated, punched, or etched).

When selecting a screen the characteristics of the material must be taken into consideration but also the final PSD desired and the capacity required. The general approach when selecting a hole size is to choose a hole diameter two steps larger than the desired particle size target zone. This is based on established effects of centrifugal velocity (ft/min, m/sec) and apparent hole size. It must be kept in mind as the particle approaches the screen hole tangentially, resulting in the diameter of opening seen by the particle is actually less than the actual hole diameter (Fig. 15). Screen hole size can also

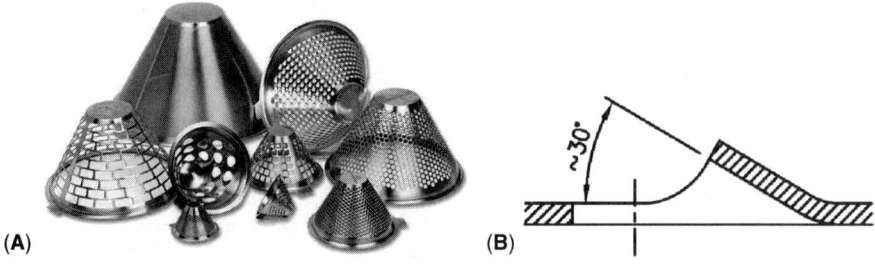

FIGURE 15 (A) Examples of various conical screens available, (B) profile of a grater screen hole.

Milling

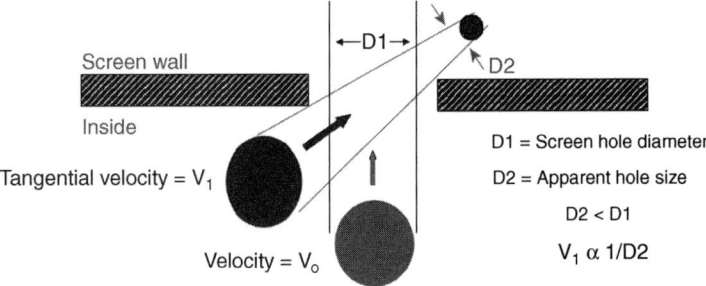

FIGURE 16 Apparent hole size of screens.

affect capacity as a smaller hole diameter will constrict the flow of product. A coarser screen will tend to result in a higher capacity due to percentage open area (Fig. 16).

Tip Velocity

The ability of comminuting mills to scale-up from lab to production scale is one of the most important characteristics size reduction equipment must offer. Scale-up in conical screen mills is achieved through the maintaining of the tip velocity of the tooling as applied in the pilot scale (Fig. 17).

Table 2 illustrates typical scale-up for conical screen applications and facilitates flexibility to meet various product characteristics.

Based on scalability, speed, torque and capacity curves are linearly expressed (Fig. 18). Base scale-up data and milling results can be transferred accurately from R&D and pilot scale plants to full scale production with relative ease. Essential to the success of maximizing milling attributes and yield, tip speed (ft/min), and product consistency must always be taken into consideration.

Feed Conditions

Typical conical screen mill applications will best function when flood fed (plug), providing an uniform head pressure to the material in the milling zone thus forcing product to the screen surface and for uniform discharge. However some products will not respond well to this type of set-up (i.e., waxy, heat sensitive) and at times it can be recommended that the unit be controlled fed instead.

MILL SELECTION CRITERIA

When selecting milling equipment various conditions must be considered to ensure that the equipment not only meets the current demand at hand but also is flexible for future requirements.

The properties of the feed material should be well known when specifying a mill. The size, shape, moisture content, physical and chemical reactivity, and temperature sensitivity of the material need to be considered in order to determine how best to size reduce, be it

Tip speed = $\dfrac{\pi DN}{12}$ (Ft/min), $\dfrac{\pi DN \times .0254}{60}$ (M/sec)

FIGURE 17 Equation for tip speed calculation. *Abbreviations*: D, diameter of the impeller; N, rotational speed of impeller.

TABLE 2 Scale-Up Chart: Underdriven/Overdriven

Comil model	Power kW (hp)	Standard impeller speed	Capacity scale-up factor	Tip speed m/sec (Ft/min)	Screen diameter	Capacity lb/hr (kg/hr)
U5	0.375 (0.5)	3450 rpm	0.5 ×	14.2 (2800)	3.25" (83 mm)	425(195)
197/U10	1.1 or 1.5 (1.5 or 2.0)	2400 rpm	1 ×	14.2 (2800)	4.84" (123 mm)	800–850 (360–390)
194/U20	4 (5.4)	1400 rpm	5 ×	14.2 (2800)	8.2" (208 mm)	3900–4250 (1750–1950)
196/U30	7.5 or 11 (10 or 14.7)	900 rpm	10 ×	14.2 (2800)	12.17" (309 mm)	7800–8500 (3500–3900)
198	15 (20.1)	450 rpm	20 ×	14.2 (2800)	24" (609 mm)	15,000–20,000 (7000)
199	22 (29.5)	360 rpm	40 ×	14.2 (2800)	30" (761 mm)	Over 20,000

through impact, shear, attrition, or compression. Knowledge of the product to be processed is the first step in achieving successful size reduction. Final particle size distribution must also be understood prior to selecting mill type and model. The desired particle size distribution and shape of the particles will also dictate the range of options and capabilities of a mill necessary to successfully achieve the process requirements and specifications.

The equipment selection must be versatile to allow for flexibility and expansion or alterations in process trains. Some key functions to note is the ability of the equipment to mill both wet and dry masses, variable tip speeds and tooling selection including safety and environmental requirements. The equipment must also be able to scale-up in terms of capacity and PSD, from formulation labs to production, is a key requirement. Additional point to consider is whether the process is batch or continuous type.

Consideration must also be given to ancillary requirements that will be necessary to support the milling process. Such equipment could include cooling systems, dust collectors, special electrics and conveying mechanisms which will affect capital requirements and day to day operating costs. Dust-free manufacturing capability is a very important requirement in current industry standards.

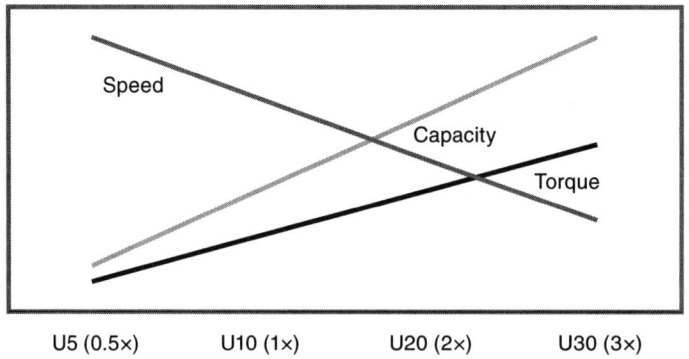

FIGURE 18 Speed/torque/capacity correlation for conical screen mills.

Milling

Other attributes that must also be considered during the selection of milling device including power consumption, metallurgy, noise, cleanability, ergonomics, suitability for integration, and containment.

COMPARATIVE ANALYSIS

Conical Screen Mill and Hammermill

In industry there are many applications where the hammermill and the conical screen mill will overlap, however, in recent years there has been an increased demand for the conical screen mill as they are amore efficient and predictable technology. Developed in 1965, the hammermill has been replaced by conical screen mills particularly in the pharmaceutical industry. The main benefits of the conical screen mill includes low noise, low dust, a tighter particle size distribution, flexibility to mill both wet and dry material, ability to be flood fed and generally a higher capacity due to the 360° discharge available with the conical design.

INERT MILLING

For some applications there is a need to further protect the operators and the facility due to the explosive and/or combustible nature of the product being milled. For those products with a minimum ignition energy (MIE) of 10 mJ or less (without inductance; other constraints may be required depending on level of MIE) inerting with nitrogen gas is generally recommended. In the past manufacturers have relied on a "control of ignition sources" method of protection, however, this is not always the safest method to apply. This is due to the fact that it is impossible to fully guarantee the removal of all sources of ignition within the mill and/or reduction of the generated dust concentration to a safe level (Fig. 19).

The inerted mills can range from a very simple design to a more intricate controlled loop system. The selection between an open loop system (with or without oxygen monitoring) or a closed loop system is determined by the end-user (Fig. 20).

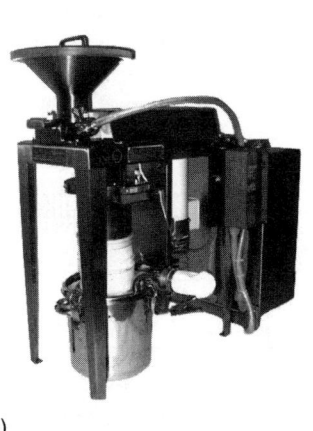
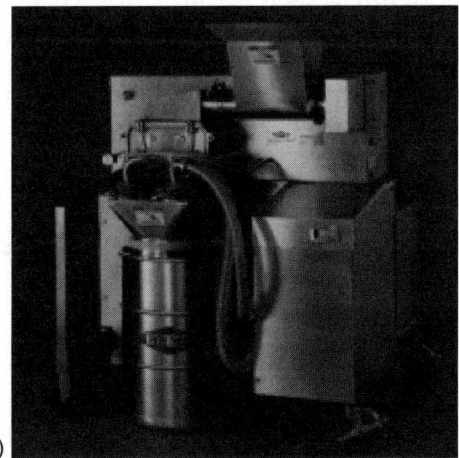

FIGURE 19 (**A**) Quadro Comil Lab unit with inert control system, (**B**) FitzMill D6A with product containment and inert processing. *Source*: From Ref. 6.

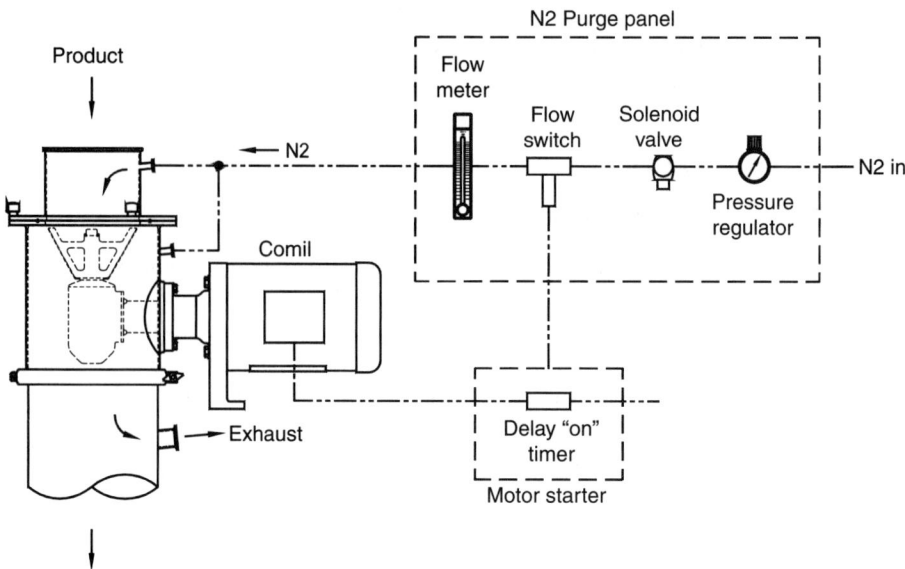

FIGURE 20 Inert control system—open loop with oxygen monitoring.

FINE MILLING/MICRONIZATION

The generally accepted definition of micronization is the size reduction of particles down to 1–30 μm in diameter. Although it is possible to use some of the previously discussed equipment to reduce the particle size distribution of a product down to this range they are not ideally suited to the application as the distribution curve can be fairly wide spread and possibly even bimodal where as a tight PSD and single node curve is the goal of most manufacturers (Fig. 21). The equipment commonly used are: pin mills, hammermills, fine grind, and jet mills.

Fine Grind F10

The Fine Grind F10 unit was initially developed to produce a mill with a sanitary GMP design, with minimal number of parts for easy cleaning and maintenance and to produce a particle distribution between 5 and 150 μm. Operating as a mobile stand alone system, the benefits of the Fine Grind F10 in comparison to its peers include low noise, dust, heat, and energy consumption (Fig. 22).

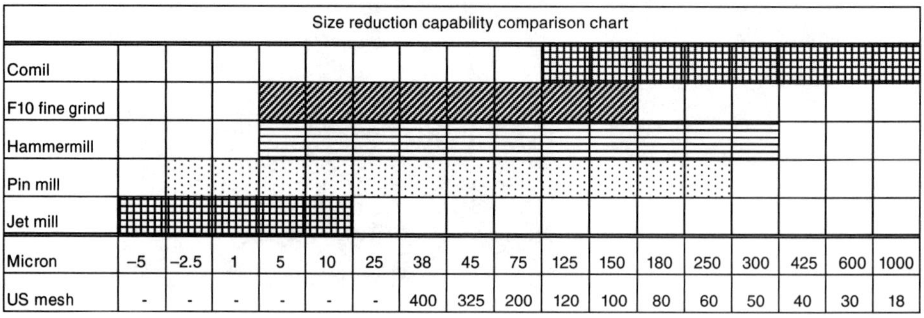

Size reduction capability comparison chart																
Comil																
F10 fine grind																
Hammermill																
Pin mill																
Jet mill																
Micron	−5	−2.5	1	5	10	25	38	45	75	125	150	180	250	300	425	600	1000
US mesh	-	-	-	-	-	-	400	325	200	120	100	80	60	50	40	30	18

FIGURE 21 Size reduction capability comparison chart.

Milling

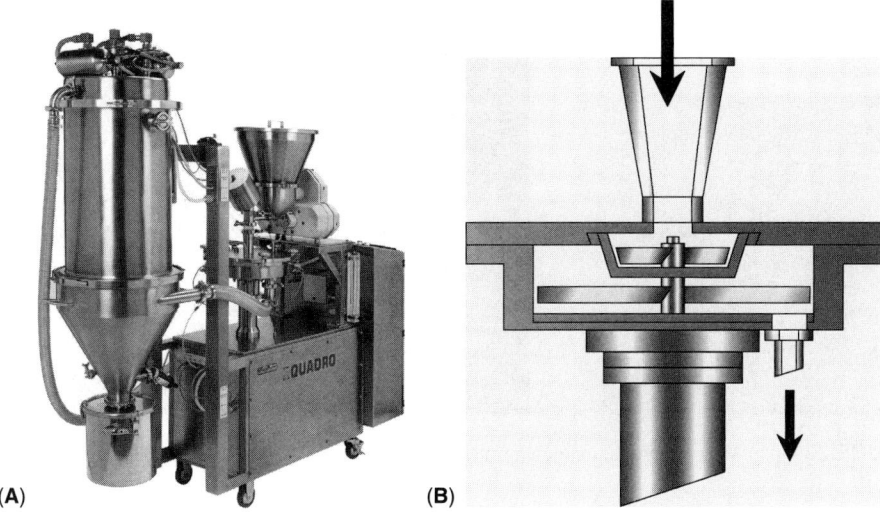

FIGURE 22 Quadro fine grind unit; (**A**) turnkey unit, (**B**) cross-sectional view of milling chambers.

The basic operation of the Fine Grind F10 begin with the control feeding of product into a conical screen chamber where a rotating impeller imparts a vortex flow pattern to the incoming material. From there the product passes through to the lower chamber with a second impeller. During this second stage of the size reduction, the majority of size reduction occurs through inter-particulate attrition. The product remains fluidized in the air stream and discharges efficiently through the bottom of the milling chamber and into the collection system.

PSD target ranges can be controlled to yield higher or lower averages (while retaining same tight bell curve profiles) by adjusting the speed, product feed rates and exhaust blower's vacuum. Other variables, which allow further fine tuning of PSD, include screen size, impeller geometry and exhaust port size. The F10 fine grind mill provides repeatable and tight particle size distribution bell curves, with good capacity throughput and minimal product retention—even when testing samples in small batches.

Micronizing Fluid Energy Mills

The principle behind micronizing fluid energy mills (also known as jet mills or spiral mills) is the size reduction of particles through interparticulate collisions combined with surface collisions due to acceleration of product. These mills use accelerated fluid streams (normally compressed air) to generate a high speed vortex which the particles are introduced into. The vacuum created by a venturi-nozzle propel the product throughout the milling chamber, forcing particles to collide with themselves as well as the chamber walls. One of the more unique characteristics of this grouping is the lack of moving parts within the mill itself.

Within this grouping of mills are several different designs including the pancake jet mill (horizontal milling chamber), the loop jet mill (also known as oval mills), spiral jet mill, opposed-jet mills (opposed jet streams), and classifier mills (Fig. 23).

Key components and attributes that affect micronization are:

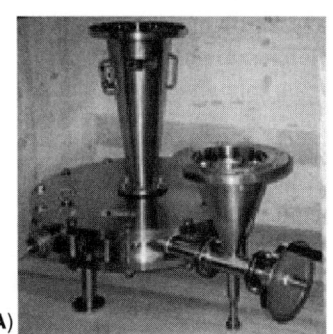 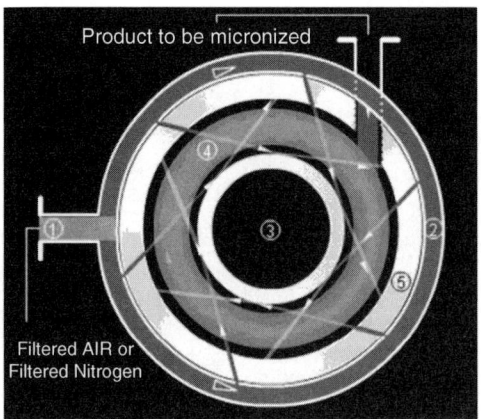

FIGURE 23 (**A**) Micro-macinazione chispro jet-mill, (**B**) typical air jet orientation. *Source*: From Ref. 10.

- nozzle design and direction of air jets;
- efficiency of air compressors;
- efficiency of filters and separators.

CRYOGENIC AND DRY ICE MILLING

It is, at times, necessary to cool or freeze a product before milling, in order to enhance the milling process and/or to protect a sensitive product from heat created during the milling process.

The amount and method of cooling/freezing a product requires, before or during milling, is determined by the size and nature of the product to be milled and the size that is desired after milling.

Cryogenic Milling

Cryogens, such as liquid nitrogen or carbon dioxide, can be used to cool a product before and during milling. Depending on the degree of cooling applied, the products can be frozen solid and embrittled or simply kept below their critical temperature during milling.

It is important that the cryogenic liquid be applied in such a manner as to limit its consumption while efficiently cooling the product. It takes a certain weight of cryogen to cool a certain amount of product to a desired temperature. The cost associated with this depends on the type and amount of cryogen required and is directly dependent on the characteristics of the product to be chilled and the method in which the cryogen is applied. Strict safety measures are required when applying cryogens during milling; proper ventilation must be in place as well as proper apparel must be worn.

Soft or Elastic Products

At room temperature, many products are soft and do not shatter easily into smaller particles. These products tend to distort during grinding, and if forced through a fine mesh, may extrude instead of break (e.g., waxes, fats, etc.).

Milling

Elastic materials tend to return to their original shape after a force is applied (e.g., rubber, gums, etc.). Grinding these products at room temperature will be difficult and, since they do not disintegrate, a large amount of work is required and resulting in excessive heat generation. Generally, elastic products respond better to cutting forces.

Soft, or elastic products, when frozen, become brittle and can be shattered. Freezing these materials greatly simplifies the milling process and fine particle size can be achieved. Extrusion and excessive heat are thereby avoided.

Heat Sensitive Products

The temperature at which a product will melt, deteriorate, or otherwise adversely change is a critical temperature. For many products, particularly in the pharmaceutical industry, it is very important that this critical temperature be avoided.

Heat generation during the milling process and can build up over time. When the temperature inside the milling chamber exceeds the critical temperature of the product it may melt, change color, burn, or otherwise change adversely (e.g., degradation of active properties). This change can affect the product's quality or cause extrusion and smearing.

Cryogens

There are many types of cryogenic liquids available. Some examples of these would be liquid oxygen, nitrogen, carbon dioxide, hydrogen, and Freon® (E. I. du Pont de Nemours and Company, Wilmington, Deleware, U.S.A.). The type of cryogen used for milling applications is often decided on the basis of safety and price. Two cryogens of choice for most food, pharmaceutical and chemical milling applications are liquid nitrogen and carbon dioxide. Some solid carbon dioxide (dry ice) "snow" is used for smaller scale batch applications.

Liquid Nitrogen

Nitrogen itself is a relatively inert substance with no toxic effects except that it can displace air and cause suffocation without proper venting. Liquid nitrogen has a temperature of minus 320°F (-196°C). Its appearance is that of water, however, it is extremely cold and requires special safety equipment and precautions to be handled correctly.

Liquid nitrogen is stored and shipped at minus 320°F at essentially atmospheric pressure in an insulated tank. When introduced into a product, the large temperature differential between the nitrogen and the product results in a very rapid product cooling/freezing. The only way to determine the costs of freezing a specific product so that it is suitable for milling is through testing and metering.

Carbon Dioxide

Liquid carbon dioxide is commonly used although it is generally the number two choice for most manufacturers. Shipped and stored under a pressure of 300 psig and a temperature of 2°F, the liquid flashes into approximately one half gas and one half snow when released into a milling chamber. Both the snow and the gas have an initial

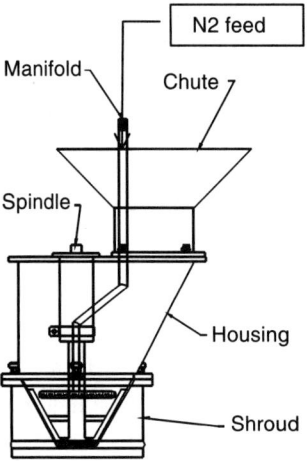

FIGURE 24 Typical cryogenic manifold for introducing liquid nitrogen into the milling chamber.

temperature of –109°F. Carbon dioxide will produce a dry ice snow on a continual basis and its this snow that can build up on surfaces, making it not as practical as liquid nitrogen.

The allowable level of carbon dioxide in a work area is less than 0.5%. Care must be taken so that excessive carbon dioxide gas is not released from the milling system into the work place.

Dry Ice

Solid carbon dioxide, commonly called dry ice, can be used as a coolant during the milling process. Dry ice can be purchased in blocks, snow or pellets. Generally the dry ice is added to the product within a mixer then passed though the mill once the desired product temperature is reached.

Cryogen Application and Usage

In order to freeze a product, the cryogen must come in contact with the product. It must retain in contact long enough to bring the entire particle or piece of product to the desired temperature. The time to cool a product is highly dependent on the surface area to volume ratio (Fig. 24).

When choosing the method of introduction of the cryogen to a milling system the size of the product to be cooled or frozen plays a major part, as well as the temperature to which a product is to be cooled. Proper method of cryogen introduction to a product will help control the costs. Added benefit of the cooling of the mill components with the introduction of the cryogen will assist the displacement of oxygen in the chamber, effectively protecting a product from oxidization and/or reducing the risk of an explosion.

ACKNOWLEDGMENTS

The author would like to thank Mr. Charles Phillot of Groupe Frewitt, Mr. Scott Wennerstrum of the Fitzpatrick Company, and Dr. Luca Bolzani of Micro-Macinazione

SA for providing photographs and diagrams for this chapter. In addition thanks are owed to Dilip M. Parikh of Atlantic Pharmaceutical Services Inc. for his guidance.

BIBLIOGRAPHY

Earle RL. Unit Operations in Food Processing <http://www.nzifst.org.nz/unitoperations/sizereduction1.htm/> NZIFST Inc., 1983.
Fitzmill Website (www.fitzmill.com), The Fitzpatrick Company, Elmhurst, IL.
Frewitt Website (www.frewitt.com), Groupe Frewitt, Fribourg, Switzerland.
Galanty HE. Size Reduction Paradox. Livingston, NJ: Franklin Miller Inc 1963.
Hixon L, Prior M, Prem H, Van Cleef J. Sizing Materials by Crushing and Grinding. Chem Eng 1990; 97(11):94.
Hutton S. Quadro Engineering Corp., Waterloo, Ontario.
Larran JM. Micronisation of Pharmaceutical Powders for Use in Inhalation. Pharmaceutical Manufacturing and Packing Sourcer. Spring 2005.
Micro-Macinazione Website (www.micro-macinazione.com), Micro-Macinazione S.A., Switzerland.
Rekhi GS Vuppala MK. Sizing of Granulation. In: Parikh DM, ed. Handbook of Pharmaceutical Granulation Technology. New York: Marcel Dekker, Inc., 1997: 389.
Skilling J. Size Reduction <http://www.chemeng.ed.ac.uk/~jennifer/solids2001/prod/node2.html/> (29 October 2001).
Skilling J. Types of Size Reduction Equipment <http://www.chemeng.ed.ac.uk/~jennifer/solids2001/prod/node2.html/> (29 October 2001).

6
Drying

Cecil Propst
SPI Pharma, Grand Haven, Michigan, U.S.A.

Thomas S. Chirkot
Patterson-Kelley, Division of Harsco Corp., East Stroudsburg, Pennsylvania, U.S.A.

INTRODUCTION

In the manufacture of tablets it is often necessary to include a wet granulation step. Wet granulation serves several purposes, including increasing particle size, supplying a binder to the formulation, improving flow and compression characteristics, and improving content uniformity (2–10). In the context of drying wet granulations, drying is usually understood to mean the removal of water (or other liquid) from a solid or semi-solid mass by evaporative processes. Some drying processes may be abetted by mechanical removal of liquid prior to the drying step. Mechanical removal of the liquid is generally not feasible for wet granulation but could offer economic advantages as a pre-drying step for other pharmaceutical drying processes that are not concerned with maintaining a particular particle size.

The moisture content of a dried substance varies from product to product. It must be kept in mind that drying is a relative term, and means simply that the moisture content has been reduced from some initial value to some acceptable final value. This final value depends on the material being dried. For example, a stable hydrate may be considered dry after all free, or chemically unbound water has been removed. An acceptable final value does not necessarily imply the lowest possible value achievable with the drying equipment. Overly zealous drying could lead to final product that is susceptible to static charge and issues with product segregation.

In describing equipment that may be used for drying pharmaceutical granulations, there are several classifications that may be used. One such classification is whether or not the process is a batch process or a continuous process. Batch equipment is usually favored when production rates are low (as they are in the production of pharmaceuticals, compared to bulk chemicals), when residence time in the unit is long, or when many different products are to be dried in the same unit. This is not meant to imply that continuous processes are inferior to batch processes; indeed, the converse may be true. A continuous process, if designed properly, is a steady state process. This can lead to greater product uniformity, control improvements due to reduced transients in process conditions, higher throughput, and possibly reduced labor costs. However, due to the relatively low batch size of most pharmaceuticals, there are relatively few continuous drying operations in the pharmaceutical industry (11). It is common to see pseudo-continuous processes, such as granulation followed by drying in fluidized bed equipment. Product containment issues for highly potent compounds may direct pseudo-continuous processes into a combination granulator/dryer known generally as a single pot processor (SPP).

Another useful classification is whether or not a dryer is a direct or indirect dryer. A direct contact dryer is one in which the material is dried by exposure to a hot gas, whereas in an indirect contact dryer, the heat required for evaporation is transferred from a heating medium through a metal wall to the material. Generally, direct heat dryers are more efficient. Dryer efficiency is defined by the fraction of energy supplied to the drying equipment which actually causes the evaporation of the liquid. As we shall see later in the chapter, heating is not always necessary to achieve drying.

One further classification is the dynamic state of the granulation bed in the dryer. A static or stagnant bed is defined when the particles are positioned on top of one another and experience no relative motion with respect to each other. A moving bed is one in which the particles flow over others, and where the volume of the bed is only slightly expanded. Particle motion is induced by either gravity or mechanical agitation. A fluidized bed is obtained when the particles are supported in an expanded state by gases moving up through the bed. The velocity of the gas must be less than the entrainment velocity, or conveyance will occur. The solids and gases are mixed together more or less uniformly, and when considered as a whole the system behaves like a boiling fluid.

The nature of the product also influences the choice of the dryer. It must be kept in mind that drying of granulations requires the handling of solids or semisolids. It is important to consider the capability of the equipment in this regard. Obviously, fragile crystals or friable granulations must not be subjected to severe mechanical stress while being loaded, dried, or unloaded from a dryer.

Another consideration in choosing equipment is cost. Examples of cost analyses of drying processes may be found in the engineering literature (12,13).

There is no single theory of drying that covers all materials and dryer designs. Differences in the method of supplying the heat required for vaporization, the mechanism of the flow of moisture through the solid, and moisture equilibria make it impossible to present a single unified treatment. Therefore, some of the more important components of drying will be discussed individually, while some may be presented together.

Drying of solids involves two fundamental processes. Heat is transferred to the granule to evaporate liquid, and mass is transferred as a liquid or vapor within the solid and as a vapor into the surrounding gas phase. The factors that influence the rates of these processes determine the drying rates. Since drying involves both mass and heat transfer, it must be kept in mind that these two phenomena may influence one another. For example, the vaporization of solvent will cool the granulation. Therefore, provision must be made for the addition of heat energy to provide for the enthalpy of evaporation (latent heat) in addition to heating bulk solid and liquid (sensible heat) in the material being dried.

A final consideration with drying, particularly in the context of wet granulation, is endpoint determination and process control. Regulatory initiatives (14) encompassed within the general term of process analytical technology (PAT) offer opportunities to provide deep process understanding and real time analysis during the drying step.

MODES OF HEAT TRANSFER

In general terms, discrete quantities of matter possess thermodynamic properties that render this matter as hot or cold in relation to one another. Heat transfer describes the

Drying

means by which any exchange occurs between the relative hot and the relative cold. When the heat transfer is part of a mechanism to drive some unit operation, then it can be more adequately described as process heat transfer; drying being one such unit operation.

There are three means of heat transfer that apply to drying processes. These are conduction, convection, and radiation. Conduction is the transfer of heat from one body to another part of the same body, or from one body to another body in direct physical contact with it. This transfer of heat must occur without significant displacement of particles of the body other than atomic or molecular vibrations. Conductive heat transfer is analogous to electrical flow and can be described by similar terms such as potential and resistance. Some examples of conduction would include heating of metal pipes by a hot liquid inside of them, or heat supplied to a solids bed via a metal shelf.

Convection is the transfer of heat from one point to another within a fluid by the mixing of one portion of the fluid with another. In natural convection, the motion of the fluid is caused by gradients of temperature and gravity. In forced convection, the motion is caused by mechanical means that enhance the rate of heat transfer over natural convection. An example of convection drying would include the use of hot air in tray dryers and fluid bed dryers.

Radiation is the transfer of heat energy (or any other kind of radiant energy) between two separate bodies not in contact with each other by means of electromagnetic waves moving through space. Examples of this may be infrared or microwave drying, depending upon which part of the electromagnetic spectrum is being used to influence the character of heating. Infrared wavelengths induce surface heating while microwave may preferentially heat the interior of the granule.

All three types of heat transfer may occur at the same time or in various combinations. For example, in convection drying, there is a flow of hot gases past the wet surface of a granule. However, at the immediate surface of the granule, there is a relatively quiet layer of gas known as the film, or stagnant layer. Heat is transferred from the bulk gas through the film to the granule via molecular conduction. The resistance of this stagnant layer or film to heat flow depends primarily on its thickness. This is one of the reasons why increasing the velocity of the drying air will increase the heat transfer coefficient. As the velocity of the drying air increases, the stagnant layer becomes thinner. However, under the conditions used in the convective drying of granulations, there will always be a thin film of stagnant air surrounding each granule.

In summary, when discussing modes of drying, one predominant mode is usually associated with a particular drying design for the sake of simplicity.

PSYCHROMETRY

Psychrometry can be defined as the study of the relationships between the material and energy balances of water vapor/air mixtures. If a system other than air and water is involved, then psychrometry is concerned with the mass and energy balances for the particular liquid(s) and gas(es) at hand. The air/water vapor system is the most common system encountered in the drying of pharmaceutical granulations, but the air/ethanol or air/ethanol–water systems are also frequently encountered.

Before going any further, it is important to emphasize the fact that drying is largely a mass transfer problem; mass transfer considerations are usually more important than heat or other energy transfer phenomena in drying processes. The evaporation of water or other solvents is dominated by the concentration gradient which must exist between the moist granule and the surrounding atmosphere. For drying to occur, there must be a difference between the vapor pressure of the particular solvent(s) at the evaporating surfaces of the granule and the vapor pressure of the solvent(s) in the drying gas or vacuum. In other words, before drying can begin, the moist solid must be heated to a temperature at which the vapor pressure of the liquid to be evaporated exceeds the partial pressure of the liquid (in vapor form) in the surrounding gas. Obviously, under vacuum conditions the vapor pressure may be exceeded at room temperature.

The reader must be aware that in a general discussion of vapor pressures, concentration gradients, and the effects that changing temperatures can have on these phenomena, the individual components of the system must be kept in mind. For example, if one is drying a granulation made with a hydroalcoholic solution, a change in the humidity may have a dramatic effect on how fast the water dries, but will have little to no effect on how fast the alcohol dries. In other words, increasing the temperature of an air stream will change the relative humidity and the drying rate of water (because of changes in the concentration driving force, not the temperature). However, because the original concentration of organic solvent in the air was probably zero and remains zero, there will be less of an effect on the drying rate of the alcohol. The practical significance of this is that the manner in which the solvents come off of the granulation can change the structure of the resultant particle.

The concentration of water vapor in air is called the humidity of the air. However, humidity may be expressed in several ways. To understand the interrelationships among temperature, vapor pressure, heat energy, and humidity, one may consult psychrometric charts that are found in most chemical engineering handbooks (15–17). Charts may be differentiated for certain conditions of temperature and pressure. For example, charts are designated for low, medium and high temperature as well as for conditions of pressure. A particularly lucid discussion of the use of the psychrometric chart may be found in Ref. 18.

Since there are several definitions of humidity that may be considered in a discussion on drying, it will be helpful to define some of them. The term dry air is used frequently (but loosely). Very rarely would an air sample contain 0% moisture, particularly on the scale required for an industrial drying process. Therefore, there must be some means of specifying the actual amount of water vapor (or other vapor) in a given quantity of air. The absolute humidity (ω) is defined as the mass of water vapor per unit mass of air. Since the driving force for the transfer of water from the wet surface of the granulation to its surrounding air is dominated by the vapor pressure gradient, it follows that the lower the vapor pressure (partial pressure) of water in the air, the greater the rate and extent of evaporation, all other things being equal.

The saturation humidity (μ_{sat}) is the absolute humidity at which the partial pressure of water vapor in the air is equal to the vapor pressure of pure bulk water at a particular temperature. Since there would be no difference in vapor pressure, there would be no concentration gradient and hence no evaporation at the saturation humidity.

The dew point (T_{dp}) is the temperature to which a particular mixture of air and water vapor must be cooled to become saturated with respect to water vapor. If the mixture is cooled below the dew point, then the system becomes supersaturated and it will separate into a two-phase system of saturated air and liquid water. Many of the best humidity meters are actually dew point detectors.

The relative humidity (φ) may be expressed as the ratio of the actual concentration of water vapor in the air to the saturation concentration of water vapor in the air under the

Drying

same conditions of temperature and atmospheric pressure. Relative humidity may be defined as:

$$\phi = \frac{p_{\text{partial}}}{p_{\text{saturation}}} \times 100 \tag{1}$$

Relative humidity is probably the most familiar expression of moisture content in the air.

Two other quantities of interest are the wet-bulb temperature (T_{wb}) and the dry-bulb temperature (T_{db}) of a thermometer. The dry-bulb temperature is simply the equilibrium temperature measured by an ordinary thermometer. The wet-bulb temperature is read from a thermometer whose tip containing the temperature indicating medium (e.g., mercury) is wrapped in a material which may be soaked in water. If there is a difference between the vapor pressure of the water surrounding the tip of the thermometer and the vapor pressure of water in the surrounding atmosphere, some of the water will evaporate. This (to an extent governed by the latent heat of vaporization) will cool the evaporating surface to a point below that of air. As the tip of the thermometer cools, heat will flow from the surrounding into the cooler region. Eventually, the rate of heat transfer to the surface will equal the rate of heat loss by evaporation. Once this equilibrium is established, one may determine the relative humidity by recording the temperatures on the two thermometers and consulting a psychrometric chart. This principle is utilized in the sling psychrometer, which is a simple device used to obtain the relative humidity.

The psychrometric chart can be used for a number of other purposes since it is really just a graphical means of presenting the mathematical relationships between the material and energy balances in the air/water vapor systems. It may be pointed out that psychrometric charts exist for systems other than air/water vapor. The charts may be drawn in different ways, but they usually include a basic temperature (dry bulb) and humidity (absolute humidity) set of coordinates (Fig. 1). Additional lines or parameters that are usually included are:

1. constant relative humidity lines;
2. constant moist volume (humid lines);
3. adiabatic cooling lines which are the same as wet-bulb lines for water, but not for other solvents;
4. the 100 % relative humidity, or saturated air curves;
5. enthalpy values.

With any two values known, the chart can be used to determine any other value of interest.

In an air sample, the partial pressures of the various gases and water vapor add up to some total pressure, which is usually one atmosphere. The amount of water and of air can be estimated by employing a form of the ideal gas law; $PV = nRT$,

$$n_{\text{water}} = \frac{p_{\text{water}} V}{RT} \tag{2}$$

where n denotes the number of moles, V the volume (in liters), R is the universal gas constant (0.083 l-atm/moles/degree K[1]), and T is temperature in degrees Kelvin. It follows that if the total pressure is one atmosphere, then $p_{\text{air}} = 1 - p_{\text{water}}$, so that

$$n_{\text{air}} = \frac{(1 - p_{\text{water}}) V}{RT} \tag{3}$$

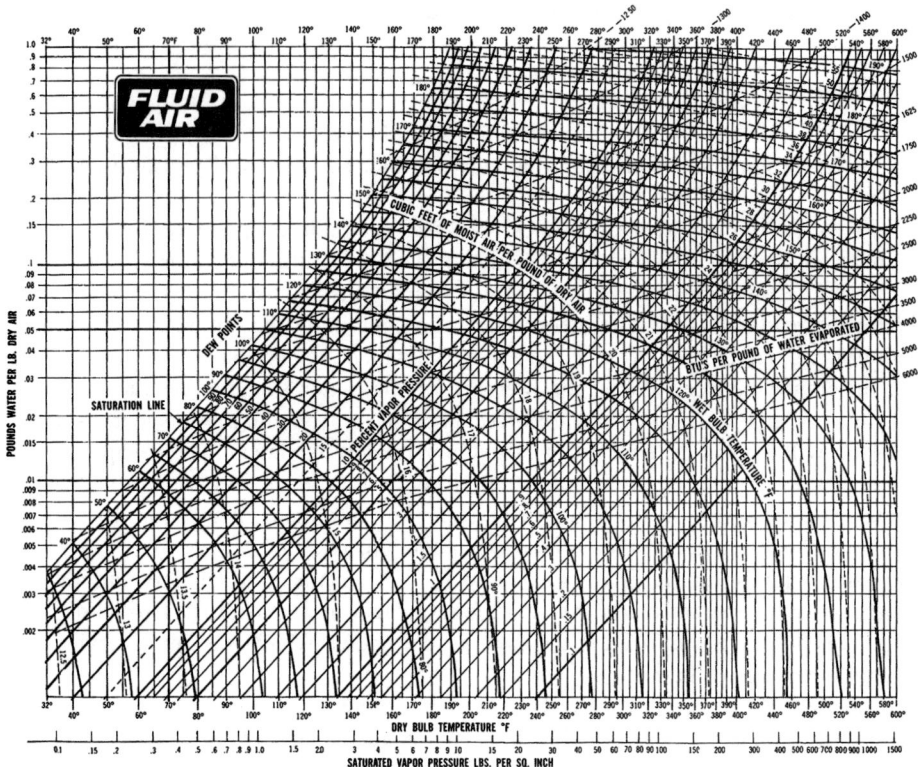

FIGURE 1 Psychrometric chart. *Source*: Courtesy Fluid Air Inc.

It is therefore possible to calculate the amount of each component in a particular volume of moist air, simply by knowing the water vapor pressure. For instance, in saturated air at 50°C, given that p_{water} is 0.1217 atm, it follows that p_{air} is $1 - p_{water}$ or 0.8783 atm. The molecular weight of water is 0.018 kg/mol, and that of air is 0.029 kg/mol. The masses (m) of water and of air in a $1\,m^3$ (10^3 L) sample of saturated air at 50°C are, therefore:

$$m_{water} = \frac{0.1217\ \text{atm} \times 10^3\,\text{l} \times 0.018\ \text{kg/mole}}{0.0831 - \text{atm} - \text{mole}^{-1}{}^\circ\text{K}^{-1} \times 323.15°\text{K}} = 0.0817\ \text{kg} \quad (4)$$

$$m_{air} = \frac{0.8783\ \text{atm} \times 10^3\,\text{l} \times 0.029\ \text{kg/mole}}{0.0831 - \text{atm} - \text{mole}^{-1}{}^\circ\text{K}^{-1} \times 323.15°\text{K}} = 0.9496\ \text{kg} \quad (5)$$

The absolute humidity (ω) is therefore $0.0817/0.9496 = 0.086$ kg water per kg of dry air.

One would like to assume that for 50% relative humidity that the absolute humidity would be one-half of that found above. This is not quite correct, as a quick calculation would show:

$$p_{water} = 0.5 \times 0.1217\,\text{atm} = 0.06085 \quad (6)$$

So, $p_{air} = 1 - 0.06085 = 0.93915$ atm.

$$m_{water} = \frac{0.06085\ \text{atm} \times 10^3\,\text{l} \times 0.018\ \text{kg/mole}}{0.0831\ \text{atm} - \text{mole}^{-1}{}^\circ\text{K}^{-1} \times 323.15°\text{K}} = 0.0408\ \text{kg} \quad (7)$$

$$m_{air} = \frac{0.93915 \text{ atm} \times 10^3 1 \times 0.029 \text{ kg/mole}}{0.0831 \text{ atm} - \text{mole}^{-1 \circ}\text{K}^{-1} \times 323.15^{\circ}\text{K}} = 1.0154 \text{ kg} \qquad (8)$$

The absolute humidity is therefore $0.0408/1.10154 = 0.0402$ kg H_2O/kg dry air.

As we can see 0.0402 is close to $0.5(0.086) = 0.043$, but it is not the same.

One can approximate the results of these calculations by using a psychrometric chart (Fig. 1). Actually, a psychrometric chart is created from these kinds of calculations. To use the chart to obtain the same results as above, first locate the dry-bulb temperature on the abscissa (50°C or 120°F). Follow the vertical line up until it intersects with the curve labeled "50% humidity." At the intersection, follow the horizontal line to the left, which ends at the absolute humidity of 0.04.

Drying of a granulation is actually evaporation of water (or other solvent) which is accomplished by providing heat energy, Q (in joules) to the granulation. If the heat of vaporization of water is h_{fg} joules per kilogram, then the amount of water than can be evaporated is Q/h_{fg} kilograms. If one knows the heat content (the enthalpy h in joules/kg) of the incoming dry, it is possible to calculate the heat Q given off to the granulation as the difference in the enthalpy between the incoming (h_i) and the outgoing (h_o) air. The heat content of air samples can be determined by the use of the psychrometric chart.

In the actual drying operation there is a certain rate of air going into the dryer. On a dry basis, the same amount of air leaves the dryer as entered it. However, on a moist basis a larger amount of air leaves the dryer than entered it, because the outgoing air contains the mass of water it evaporated during its residence time in the dryer. By means of the psychrometric chart and by measuring the flow rate of air and the drying time, it is possible to calculate the theoretical mass of water m_1 that can be evaporated. This should equal the amount of moisture (m_2) lost by the granulation as determined by moisture assay or weight loss before and after drying. In reality, m_2 will never equal m_1, and the ration of m_2 to m_1 is a measure of the efficiency of the dryer.

DRYING MECHANISMS AND PERIODS OF DRYING

Since it is generally difficult to study liquid and vapor movement within a granulation, the drying process is more readily modeled and studied by determining the drying rates as the material progresses from its initial solvent concentration to the final level of acceptable solvent.

Before discussing the drying processes, it may be helpful to define a number of terms often used in chemical engineering and drying technology reference books.

Bound moisture is water (or other solvents in nonaqueous systems) held by a material in such a manner that it exerts a lower vapor pressure than that of the pure liquid at the same temperature. Water may be chemically or physically bound. Unbound moisture is therefore moisture in association with a solid that exerts the same vapor pressure as the pure liquid. In a discussion of bound versus unbound water, it should be pointed out that are not only different equilibria to be considered, but that the binding energies and kinetics are different.

The free moisture content of a substance is the amount of moisture that can be removed from the material by drying at a specified temperature and humidity. The amount of moisture that remains associated with the material under the drying conditions specified is called the EMC. One should note that the EMC can be altered in a transfer step from a dryer to subsequent processing. This exposure to the ambient conditions of humidity and temperature can be particularly significant for a material that is dried to a very low solvent level.

Drying Profiles

Drying behavior of a granulation may be conveniently studied by starting with experimental drying profiles. In this case, the moisture content of the solid is expressed on a dry basis; that is, as mass of liquid per mass of dry solid. Moisture content W (kg water/kg dry solid) determinations may be made on samples of the granulation at pre-selected time points. If W is plotted versus time, a graph such as shown in Figure 2A may be obtained. The slope of the curve dW/dt at any particular time is denoted the drying rate at that time.

Since the drying rate may be subject to variation with respect to time and moisture content, it may be more informative to plot dW/dt versus W, or dW/dt versus t. dW/dt may be determined graphically or by numerical differentiation of the curve in the W versus t graph. Figure 2B and 2C shows the respective plots of the data in Figure 2A after determination of dW/dt values. As can be seen in these graphs, there are a number of portions of the curves that may be identified as different drying periods. One particular feature of Figure 2C is that a plot of this sort shows how long each drying period lasts.

Segment A–B on each curve is a warming-up or initial induction period in which the wet material is heated to the drying temperature. Segment B–C represents the constant rate (or steady state) period during which the drying rate per unit surface area is constant. At point C, the granulation reaches the point that is commonly called the critical moisture content. The portion C–D of the curve is termed the falling rate period (of which there may be more than one if different moisture transport mechanisms apply). Each of

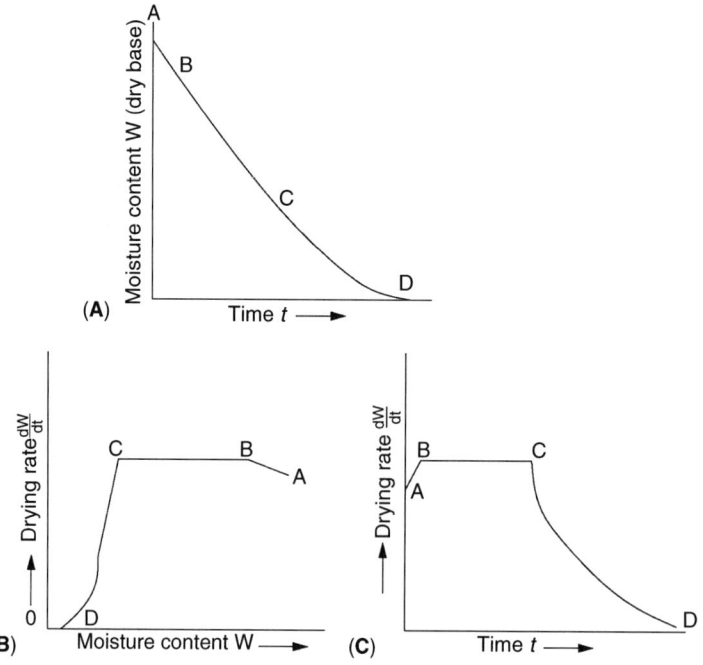

FIGURE 2 Drying profiles. *Source*: From Ref. 15.

Drying

these drying periods will be discussed in more detail in the next few paragraphs. It should be pointed out now that in drying profiles, some of the periods may not be observed. For example, if the initial moisture content of a granulation is below the critical moisture content, then a constant rate drying period will not be observed.

Constant Rate (Steady State) Period

In the constant rate period, the granulation behaves as if there is a free liquid surface of constant composition and vapor pressure. Moisture movement to the surface is rapid enough to provide sufficient bulk liquid to ensure that the evaporation is essentially independent of the granule's structure. The rate of drying is governed by the rate of heat transfer to the evaporating surface. Water (or other solvent) diffuses from the saturated surface, through the stagnant diffusion layer, and into the surrounding atmosphere. This atmosphere may be the drying gas (convection) or a vacuum (conduction and radiation). The rate of mass transfer balances the rate of heat transfer and while the steady state period is maintained, the temperature of the saturated surface remains constant.

If heat is transferred solely by convection from a hot gas, the surface temperature of the granulation will approach or reach the wet-bulb temperature. If conduction and/or radiation contribute to heat transfer, the surface temperature of the material will reach a temperature between the wet-bulb temperature and the boiling point of the liquid. Thus, combining convection with conduction and/or radiation may allow an increase in the rate of heat transfer (with a resultant higher drying rate) provided that the vapor pressure gradients can be maintained.

If conduction or radiation is the predominant mode of heat transfer, the surface (and possibly the interior) moisture may literally boil regardless of the temperature or the humidity of the environment. This may be readily demonstrated by microwave drying. Thus, if control of granulation temperature is important, direct heat (convection) dryers usually offer greater control and product safety since the material's surface does not exceed the wet-bulb temperature during the steady state period. However, it will be shown later in this chapter that properly controlled dielectric drying may also be used to dry heat sensitive materials.

The simultaneous heat and mass transfer balances occurring during constant rate drying may be expressed in the steady state equation:

$$-\frac{dW}{dt} = \frac{h_t A(T - T_s)}{\lambda_s} = k_a A(p_s - p) \tag{9}$$

where dW/dt is the drying rate, kg H_2O/sec, h_t is the heat transfer coefficient, W/m^2·°C, A is the surface area for heat transfer and vaporization, m^2, T is the average source temperature of all heat transfer components, T_S is the liquid surface temperature, °C, λ_S is the latent heat of vaporization at T_S, J/kg H_2O, k_a is the mass transfer coefficient, kg/sec-meter^2-kPa, p_s is the liquid vapor pressure at T_S, kPa, and p is the partial pressure of vapor in the gas environment, kPa.

The magnitude of the constant rate drying depends on the following five factors:

1. the heat transfer coefficient;
2. the mass transfer coefficient;
3. the surface area exposed to the drying medium;
4. the temperature gradient between the wet surface of the solid and the gas stream;
5. the vapor pressure gradient between the wet surface of the solid and the gas stream.

The latent heat of vaporization is in the constant rate drying is typically associated with the heat transfer portion of Equation (9).

For convenience, Equation (9) may be rewritten in terms of the decrease in moisture content rather than the mass of solvent evaporated. If we consider the case of evaporation from a stationary bed of granulation on trays:

$$-\frac{dW}{dt} = \frac{h_t a}{\rho_m d_m \lambda_s}(T - T_s) \qquad (10)$$

where dW/dt now has units of kg H_2O/kg dry material-sec, ρ_m is the dry material bulk density, kg/m^3, d_m is the thickness of the bed of granulation, m, and a is the heat transfer area per unit bed volume, m^{-1}. ρ_m can be measured, but the quantity h_t is usually calculated by inserting experimentally obtained data in Equation (10).

Critical Moisture Content

When discussing drying processes, the critical moisture content may be defined as the moisture content of the granulation at the end of the constant drying rate period. The critical moisture content is reached when the reduced amount of available moisture prevents a completely wetted surface from being maintained on the exterior of the granule. This moisture content is a function of the chemical nature of the material being dried (as well as porosity and other physical properties), the constant drying rate, and the particle size. It must be pointed out that the critical moisture content may be of little use for standardization of drying operations unless the drying method and conditions are carefully specified. For example, particle size distribution determines surface area to mass ratios. The smaller the particles, the shorter the distance the internal moisture must travel to reach the surface. Therefore, large particles usually have higher critical moisture contents than small particles.

Another phenomenon that may affect the critical moisture content is known as case-hardening. In this instance, the surface of the material is dried so rapidly that a layer of dry, non-porous material forms. This over-dried surface acts as a barrier to moisture diffusion, since diffusivity decreases with moisture concentration. This may occur in vacuum drying, which will be discussed later in the chapter. To reduce the risk of case-hardening, the relative humidity of the drying gas may be increased to assist in maintaining a higher surface EMC until the internal moisture has diffused to the surface.

The Falling Rate Period

After the constant rate period ends, the falling rate period begins. This period may be seen as one or more of the terminal segments of the drying profile. The falling rate period begins when the rates of heat and mass transfer are no longer balanced, usually when internal moisture cannot move to the surface quickly enough to maintain the saturated character encountered in the steady state period. The drying front retreats from the primary surface involvement to deeper regions of the granule. The internal mass transfer mechanisms that control falling rate include: (*i*) capillarity in porous and fine granular material; (*ii*) liquid diffusion and surface tension in continuous materials, in which the liquid is soluble (e.g., gelatin/water systems); and (*iii*) pressure-induced flow of liquid and vapor when material is heated on one side (or in the interior by dielectric heating) and vapor escapes from the opposite surface.

Drying

Even though one mass transfer mechanism can usually be invoked to approximate the drying kinetics at any particular time, in reality several mechanisms may occur simultaneously. For this reason it may be difficult or impossible to accurately model drying kinetics in the falling rate period.

In many, if not most of all pharmaceutical drying operations, the drying profiles are or may appear to be in the falling rate period, i.e., corresponding to segment C–D in (Figure 2A). In this case the slope k (Fig. 2B) is linear in W, so that the drying equation will be of the type $\ln W = \ln W_O - kt$, where W_O is the moisture content at the critical point.

A presentation for a theoretical model of constant rate and falling rate drying is available in work by Yang et al. (19) in a study of a vibro-separator. Major factors discussed include the role of vacuum level, air bleeding rate, the critical moisture content, vibratory energy transfer, and particle size. The modeled drying rates are compared to experimental values.

PHARMACEUTICAL GRANULATION DRYING METHODS

Common drying methods for pharmaceutical granulations include tray drying, fluid bed drying, vacuum drying, microwave drying, and various combinations of the above. Many of these technologies incorporate the ability to granulate as well as dry in the same vessel.

Tray Drying

Although tray drying is slow and relatively inefficient, it is still a commonly used method of drying and has been widely reported in the literature (20–22). In tray drying, wet granulation or wet product is placed on trays that are then placed in a drying oven (Fig. 3). The trays are usually made of metal and often are lined with paper. The trays themselves may be placed onto racks in the oven, or may be placed on a large rack with wheels called a truck. This truck is then wheeled into a large oven or room for drying. This particular arrangement is known as truck drying. Since any agitation is minimized, friable granules can be more readily dried in trays than in a more aggressive environment.

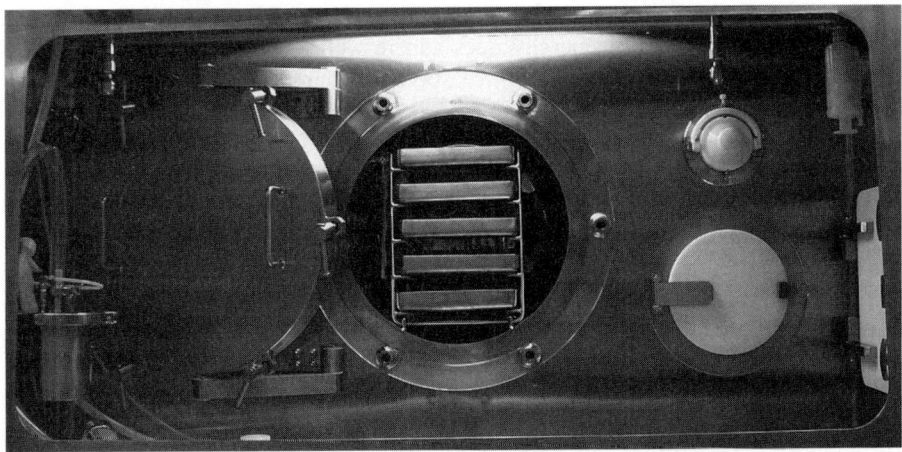

FIGURE 3 Tray drying isolator. *Source*: Courtesy Powder Systems Ltd., Liverpool, UK.

The bed itself is generally shallow allowing for a favorable heated surface to bed volume ratio.

Tray drying and truck drying are obviously batch procedures, and are labor intensive. Most tray dryers are direct dryers, in that hot gas or air is circulated over (or through) the granulation bed. Most tray drying operations do not employ trays with fine wire mesh on the bottom, so drying takes place only from the upper surface of the bed. Tray dryers can be used to dry most materials. Drying by circulation of air over the stationary top layers of granulation is slow, and drying cycles may be as long as 48 hour per batch. Drying in a through circulation unit, in which the drying air is forced through the solids bed in a perpendicular direction, is much more rapid than in a conventional cross-circulation unit. However, through circulation is usually neither economical nor necessary in a batch dryer, because shortening the drying cycle does not reduce the amount of labor required for each batch.

Tray and truck dryers are not limited to the drying of granulations. One application in which this mode is particularly useful is in the drying of soft shell capsules. A typical processing temperature might be 37°C with a relative humidity of 10%. The air can be dried by either passing it over a silica gel or through a column with a saturated solution of lithium chloride. In the former case, the unit that dries the air consists of two or more drying towers. One tower contains dry desiccant and the air to be dried passes through this unit. The other tower contains spent desiccant that is regenerated by passing hot gases through it. This way, when the desiccant in one tower becomes exhausted, the air stream can be switched to the other tower with dry desiccant, while the exhausted desiccant is regenerated. The drying of soft shell capsules is a diffusion process, in which a model of diffusion out of a cylinder can be used. In this case the drying equation is:

$$\ln(c - c_\infty) = \frac{-t}{\alpha} + \ln(c_0 - c_\infty) \tag{11}$$

where

$$\alpha = \frac{h^2}{5.8D} \tag{12}$$

In these equations, c is the moisture content at time t, c_0 is the initial moisture concentration, and c_∞ the EMC of the capsule, h is the thickness of the gelatin film, and D the diffusion coefficient of the gelatin film. One must make the simplifying assumption that D is independent of the moisture content of the gelatin. α is defined in Equation (12). Drying of soft shell capsules generally does adhere well to a drying equation such as Equation (11). The drying endpoint is critical, because overdrying causes the capsules to become brittle, and insufficient drying imparts an excessive plasticity to the capsules so that they will adhere to each other and deform on storage.

The above equations can be used to calculate capsule drying time. Suppose a soft shell capsule reaches the required moisture level after 24 h of drying. If the capsule shell wall thickness is increased 20%, how long will it take to dry the new capsules to the same moisture content c? Solution: Using Equations (11) and (12), it is seen that if h is increased by 20% to 1.2 h, then α increases by a factor of $(1.2)^2 = 1.44$. For $(c - c_\infty)/(c_0 - c_\infty)$ to have the same value as for the thinner capsule shell, t must also be increased by a factor of 1.44 (i.e., increased so that t/α remains the same). The drying time for the thicker shell, therefore is $1.44(24 \, \text{hr}) = 35 \, \text{hr}$.

It has been shown (20,21) that the mechanism of drying in a stationary bed appears to be evaporation from the surface of the bed, with movement of liquid water up through the bed to maintain a water concentration gradient. This was supported by the fact that

Drying

calculated diffusion coefficients were on the order of those expected for liquid water diffusion rather than vapor diffusion. The temperature dependence of the calculated diffusion coefficients were also in agreement with what would be expected for liquid water diffusion. This leads to the following drying equation:

$$\ln(M - M') = -kt + \ln(M_0 - M') \tag{13}$$

where M is the mass of the wet granulation at time t, M' is the mass of the dry granulation, and M_o is the mass of the wet granulation at time zero. In casual interpretation, Equation (13) corresponds to the falling rate period.

These findings are also supported by the fact that a water soluble material (dyes for example) may migrate in a stationary bed as heat energy is supplied (22). In the case of tray drying by convection from air passed over the surface, the solute tended to concentrate in the surface layer of the bed. In the same study, infrared radiation, microwave radiation, and vacuum drying were also used to study migration in a stationary granulation bed. The greatest migration occurred when infrared radiation was used, with solute concentrating near the middle of the bed. The granules dried in a vacuum and by microwave radiation experienced very little migration of solute.

To illustrate the processes occurring in tray drying in a more quantitative fashion, we will assume that a tray is filled with a wet granulation to a depth of **a** meters and that the rate limiting step in drying is the transfer of moisture from the bed to the airstream. The rate of moisture loss will follow the equation:

$$-D\left(\frac{\partial C}{\partial x}\right) = \alpha(C_0 - C_s) \tag{14}$$

where D is the diffusion coefficient (m²/sec) of water vapor, C is the concentration of water vapor in the void space of the bed (kg/m³), $\partial C/\partial x$ is the moisture vapor gradient over the interface between the bed and the airstream (kg/m⁴), α is the proportionality constant, and subscripts o and s indicate bed and airstream, respectively.

The airstream is assumed to be perfectly dry, so that $C_s = 0$; therefore C_0 may be denoted simply as C in the following treatment. Initially, when the granules contain surface moisture, the vapor in the void space is at saturation pressure P_{sat} (N/m²):

$$C = \frac{P_{sat}}{RT} 0.018 \text{ kg} \cdot \text{m}^{-3} \tag{15}$$

where R is the gas constant in units of 8.3143 Nm mol⁻¹ deg⁻¹. At this point C is constant and application of Fick's Law gives the drying rate, dM/dt (kg/sec), as

$$-\frac{1}{\varepsilon A}\frac{dM}{dt} = -D\left(\frac{\partial C}{\partial x}\right) = \alpha C \tag{16}$$

where A is the surface of the tray and ε is bed porosity (i.e., $A\varepsilon$ is the cross section through which diffusion occurs). Combining Equations (14)–(16) then gives the zero-order rate of evaporation as:

$$-\frac{dM}{dt} = A\alpha\varepsilon \frac{P_{sat}}{RT} 0.018 \tag{17}$$

It is possible to calculate α from the slope of the initial drying curve if the granules contain surface moisture.

As drying proceeds, the surface moisture of the granules will eventually be exhausted and the vapor pressure in the void space of the granules will drop below P_{sat}.

Now, if in this period, both evaporation from the granules and the internal equilibrium of water vapor in the bed are rapid compared to the transfer of moisture over the bed-stream interface, then the diffusion equation can be solved (23). Using the dimensionless parameter

$$J = \frac{a\xi}{D} \tag{18}$$

The first-order approximation of the solution can be written as

$$\ln\left[1 - \left(\frac{c_t}{c_\infty}\right)\right] = -\left(\frac{\beta^2 D}{a^2}\right)t + \ln\left[\frac{2J^2}{\beta^2(\beta^2 + J^2 + J)}\right] = Gt + \ln K \tag{19}$$

Here, $-G$ and $\ln K$ represent slope and intercept, respectively, β is the smallest possible root of

$$J = \beta \tan \beta \tag{20}$$

where c_t denotes the mass (kg) of water in the granulation at any particular time, and c_∞ is the equilibrium amount of moisture left in the granulation, usually that obtained by proper drying of the product.

Equation (11) shows that the amount of moisture left in the granulation less the equilibrium moisture c_∞, is log linear in time. Also, β^2 can be calculated from the negative slope $(-G)$:

$$\beta^2 = \frac{Ga^2}{D} \tag{21}$$

Figure 4 shows a typical example of tray drying data, with a bed depth of $a = 2.5$ cm, treated according to Equation (19) (24). The least squares fitting slope is $-0.102\,\text{h}^{-1}$ and the intercept is -0.021.

Equations for constant rate drying in trays can be handled similarly to the constant rate in Equation (9). As noted in that discussion, the temperature rate equation is more easily applied.

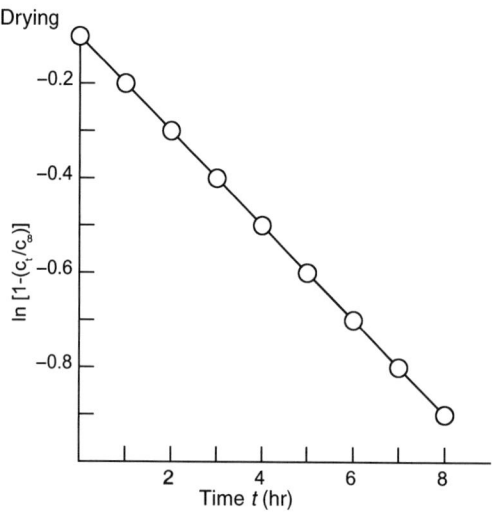

FIGURE 4 Tray drying data. *Source*: From Ref. 1.

Drying

Yang et al. (19) also show a treatment for constant rate drying in a tray-like device. Another treatment for tray drying simulation, albeit for the grain industry, models drying time with respect to moisture content, bed depth, and other factors (25).

Countercurrent Drying

Countercurrent drying is carried out in rotary dryers. These are long cylinders with internal baffles (sometimes helical) that direct the product in the direction opposite to that of the air flow. Because of the rotation, the granules continuously cascade down through the airstream. Because of the countercurrent nature of the product flow, the drier the product, the drier the air it encounters. Countercurrent drying is usually applied to large volume products, and only in automated and semi-automated processes. Pitkin and Carstensen (26) have shown that in countercurrent drying the rate limiting step is the moisture movement within the granule. They showed this in the case

$$\frac{c - c_\infty}{c_0 - c_\infty} = \frac{6}{\pi^2} \sum_{j=1}^{\infty} \exp \frac{1}{2} \left(\frac{-j^2 t}{K} \right) \tag{22}$$

where

$$K = \frac{a^2}{4\pi^2 D} \tag{23}$$

where j is a running index, a is the diameter of the granule, t is time, and D is the diffusion coefficient of water in the granule. D is temperature dependent by the relation:

$$D = D_0 \exp \left(\frac{-E'}{RT} \right) \tag{24}$$

where E' is the activation energy for diffusion, T the absolute temperature, and R the gas constant. Where a range of different particle sizes emerge from the dryer, keep in mind that the moisture content will depend on the particle diameter, since from Equation (22) the drying time t is the same for all particles. When t is of a realistic magnitude, the terms in Equation (22) with j larger than 1 become negligible, and we may write:

$$\ln \frac{c - c_\infty}{c_0 - c_\infty} = -\frac{t 4\pi^2 D}{a^2} \ln \frac{6}{\pi^2} \tag{25}$$

That is $\ln (c - c_\infty)/(c_0 - c_\infty)$ should be linear in $1/a^2$, with an intercept of $\ln (6/\pi^2) = -0.5$.

Since the rate of diffusion of liquid water within a granule is influenced by the porosity (ε) of the granule, we can use the above equation to show how drying times can change with changes in granule porosity brought about by changes in kneading times. For example, if it is assumed that D is proportional to ε, what effect will long kneading have on the drying rate for a wet granulated product? If a granulation is kneaded for 5 minutes and has a porosity of 0.3 after drying, and if after 10 minutes of kneading it would have a porosity of 0.2 after drying, what is the difference in drying time of the two granulations? Solution: Increased kneading time causes a decrease in porosity, and hence an increase in drying time because of the decrease in the diffusion coefficient. In the following, subscripts denote kneading time [Equations (22) and (24)]. For $(c - c_\infty)/(c_0 - c_\infty)$ to be the same, t/K must be the same (i.e., t_{10}/t_5 must equal K_{10}/K_5). Since $D_5 = (0.3/0.2) D_{10}$, it follows that $K = (0.2/0.3)K_{10}$ [Equation (23)]. Hence $t_{10}/t_5 = K_{10}/K_5 = 1.5$, so that the drying time increases by 50%.

Since prolonged kneading is a squeezing process, suppose that a decrease in ε from 0.3 to 0.2 is a result of a decrease by 10% in the diameter of the granules. What is the new drying time? Solution: Using Equation (23),

$$K_{10} = \frac{a_{10}^2}{4\pi^2 D_{10}}, \quad K_5 = \frac{a_5^2}{4\pi^2}D_5 = \frac{1.11^2 a_{10}^2}{4\pi^2 1.5 D_{10}} = 0.82 \qquad (26)$$

so the drying time increases by a factor of $1/0.82 = 1.22$, or by 22 %.

Fluidized Bed Drying

Fluid bed drying (an R&D model is shown in Fig. 5) is suited for drying powders, granules, agglomerates, and pellets with an average particle size normally between 50

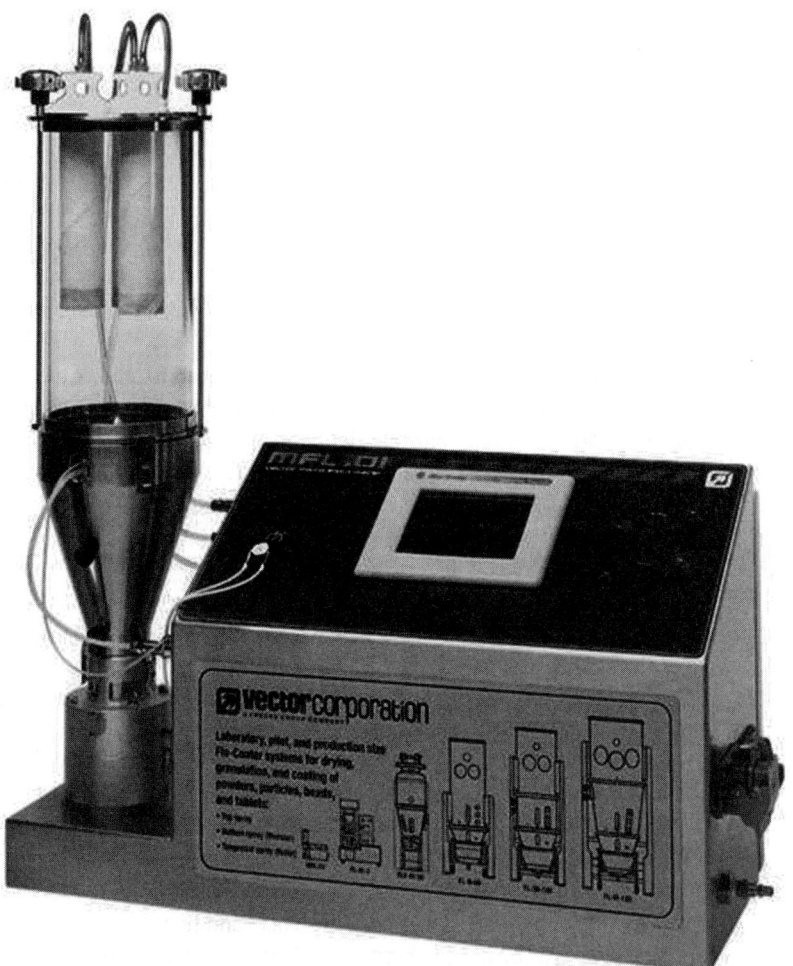

FIGURE 5 An R&D model fluid bed dryer. *Source*: Photo courtesy of Vector Corporation.

and 5000 μm. Very fine powders, less than 50 μm, or highly elongated particles may require added vibration for successful fluidization.

Fluidization is achieved when the bed appears to be fluid-like (27). Like a fluid, denser objects will sink and lighter objects float on the surface of a fluidizing bed.

The fluid bed dryer was designed for rapid drying (28). When running optimally, fluid beds dry in minutes versus hours required for tray dryers. Both temperature uniformity and drying speed is achieved through intimate mixing of drying gas with particles suspended in the gas. The gas is rising in the bed separating particles as well as in rising bubbles.

Fluidization begins just after the bed is lifted. The lift occurs at some point when the air velocity generates a total drag on the particles that equals the total weight of the bed. At that inlet velocity the bed is lifted and the particles are barely fluidized. As more air is added, the particles separate. Thus the bed is expanding more so than being lifted. The lack of entrainment is due to particles in the bed grouping together in dense phases losing some of their air separation and falling back as a group. The extra air is present in the form of bubbles, and in the dense phase air separates particles.

Zoglio et al. (29) found the drying rate constant was more closely related to the linear air velocity (air diffusion) than to water diffusion from the interior of the particle to surface. They also found fine particles are dried faster, and become less dense and larger particles have higher moisture content than smaller particles.

As the bed dries, the weight of the bed decreases as a result of the loss of moisture. Thus higher air velocities are needed early in drying to lift the heavier bed. The fluid bed operates with a powerful exhaust fan able to generate a high volume of air flow at a high head pressure. A typical fan performance curve is shown in Figure 6. Discharge from a wet granulator is the wettest, densest, and most lumpy condition for most products. As the bed is packed, extra inlet air pressure is needed to initiate bed separation and lift.

Discharge of wet granulation through a mill to reduce the size of chunks and drying as soon as possible after discharge is helpful in initiating fluidization. Also helpful is running the built-in fluid bed agitators during initial drying which are present in some fluid bed dryers.

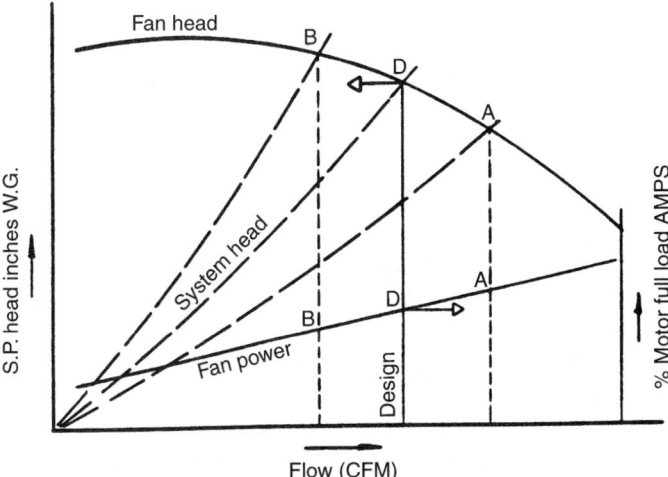

FIGURE 6 Fan performance curve. *Source*: Courtesy of Fluid Air Incorporated.

The maximum achievable fan head pressure directly relates to the maximum weight of the wet bed the dryer can handle. Once drying starts, the weight and density of the bed is reduced, lumps and clusters are broken up, mixing becomes easier and head pressure is reduced. Inlet air velocity is usually set faster initially and then decreased to reduce particle attrition. Too much product in the container can create more back pressure than the fan can handle and prevent fluidization. Also too little product in the bed, or adding more air velocity can create air pierced regions through the bed in channels or spouts. The bed, due to too low depth for the velocity in the channel or too high a cohesion in the bed, will not collapse into the created channels. If the bed collapses into the formed channels the fluidization cycle will begin. Channels form/collapse, and the bed becomes loose enough to begin to bubble randomly. If the initial channels remain, the bed will remain a spouting bed and drying will become uneven. Gao et al. (30) found the rapid rise in the exhaust air temperature (19 min) is an indication of extremely high air velocity and poor fluidization in the fluid bed. As a result, the material swayed from side to side within the dryer, instead of fluidizing. The excess air was not used for heat transfer. They showed sample port moistures at 1.2% with top, middle and bottom bed moistures of 3.2%, 2.7% and 1.9% for a spouting bed wet granulated product.

The overlap gill plate, introduced in 1990, vectors air more horizontally across the bed. It also allows larger opening and less pressure drop and has virtually eliminated the sandwich distributor plate (31).

The air distributor must be maintained clean and unplugged, not only to reduce the fan load but also to prevent air channeling.

Vacuum Drying

In the evaporation of solvent from any moist solid (which is what thermal drying is), the drying potential is the difference between the vapor pressure of the solvent in or at the surface of the wet granule, and the vapor pressure of the solvent in the surrounding gas. The drying (at least in the constant rate period) is also a function of A, the liquid surface area (or the surface area of the granules), and is inversely proportional to the heat of evaporation of the liquid, λ (J/kg). Thus, the drying rate may be written

$$\mathrm{RATE} = N \frac{A}{\lambda}(p_0 - p_1) \tag{27}$$

where p_0 is the solvent vapor pressure at the wet granule surface and p_1 is the solvent vapor pressure in the surrounding gas. The proportionality constant N is a transfer coefficient that is dependent on both heat and mass transfer. It depends, for example, on the interfacial energy between the liquid and the gas.

Pure water at 25°C has a vapor pressure of about 25 torr. If the pressure of the atmosphere surrounding a wet granule is reduced to less than 25 torr, the water will boil. If the water contains dissolved material, then its vapor pressure will, of course, be less than 25 torr. When the solvent boils, the bubbles which form greatly increase the surface area A. Therefore, it stands to reason that subjecting a wet granulation to a sufficiently low pressure should result in rapid drying at a low temperature (33).

Vacuum drying may be a separate unit operation of processing wet granules or it may be one of several unit operations in a single processing machine if the vessel has the capability of acting as a SPP (Fig. 7). Generally, an SPP has an agitator device to facilitate mixing of the solid formulation components as well as liquid addition capability for addition of binder. Once an acceptable granule size has been achieved,

Drying

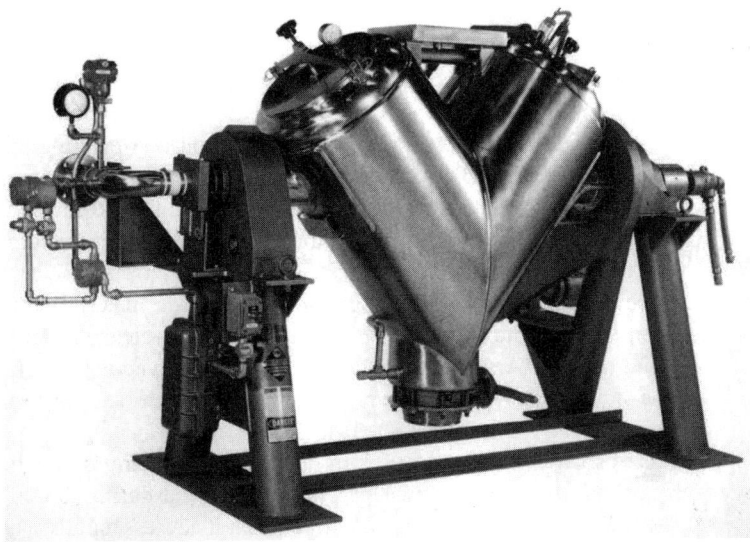

FIGURE 7 Single pot processor. *Source:* Courtesy of Patterson-Kelley.

vacuum drying is initiated. Some additional sizing of granules is possible with judicious use of the agitator bar or control of the rotation speed of the vessel. A study relating particle attrition to the kinetic friction force of blade interaction, pitch angle, angle of repose and bed depth in several drying technologies may be useful in selecting drying conditions (34).

Most SPPs can also engage a cooling loop to reduce the granule temperature after drying and then offer the potential for lubricating the granules prior to discharge.

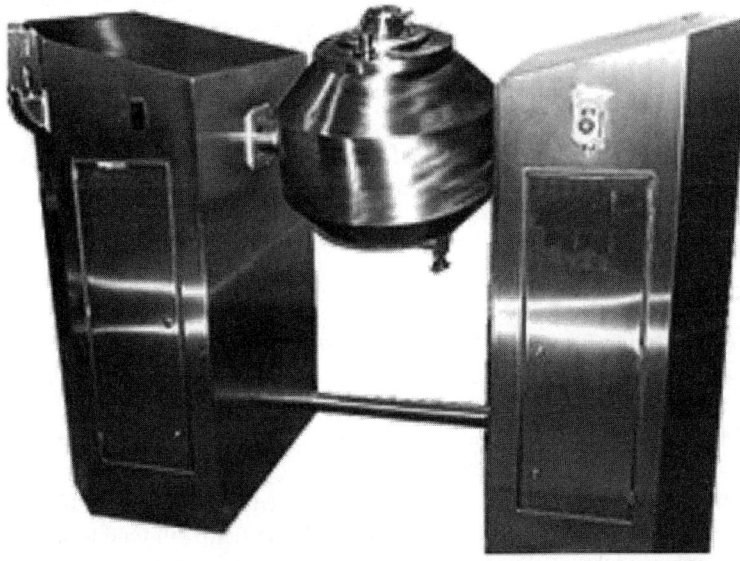

FIGURE 8 Double cone dryer. *Source*: Courtesy of Patterson-Kelley.

When engaging the vacuum drying step, one chooses an appropriate jacket temperature that is safe for the formulation constituents and then reduces the absolute pressure in the vessel with a vacuum pump. Maintaining a vapor atmosphere for as long as possible in the drying vessel is conducive to speeding up the drying process and this requires the specific knowledge rendered in the psychrometric section for selecting the optimum absolute pressure of operation. The vapor atmosphere offers a measure of convective heating to the process since the heat transfer coefficient in the vapor atmosphere may be 10–15 times as large as the heat transfer coefficient gained by point contact of the granule with the heated jacket (35).

Vacuum dryers are equipped with filter devices that prevent fine material from leaving the vessel and entering the pump. The filter may be periodically cleaned with a blowback of inert gas during drying. A condenser accepts the effluent vapor from the vessel and returns it to the liquid state where it may then be collected for disposal or recycling.

When very low levels of solvent are necessary, introduction of a carrier gas may be beneficial. A dry carrier gas can improve the vapor pressure differential during the diffusional drying period. The drawback to the gas introduction is that it acts essentially as a leak on the system and may have a negative impact on the vacuum pump performance.

Scale-up with vacuum dryers is relatively easy and straightforward. Each vessel has a characteristic surface to volume ratio that identifies the quantity of heated surface available and the working volume of the granules in the vessel. The drying time in a laboratory vessel may be used to determine drying time in a larger vessel through use of Equation (28):

$$t_{su} = \frac{t_1 V_{su} A_1}{V_1 A_{su}} \quad (28)$$

where t is time, A is the heated surface area, V is the working volume and the subscripts l and su refer to the laboratory and scale-up vessels, respectively (35).

The shape of the vessel influences the amount of heated surface available and this factor can be a point of choice for selecting a dryer. For example, a typical double cone dryer (Fig. 8) has a surface/volume advantage over a V-shape dryer up to about 300 l of working volume. At working volumes exceeding 300 l, the V-shape gains the surface/volume advantage.

A prime attribute of vacuum drying is its capability of drying substances at low temperature. Theoretically, vacuum drying should be more rapid than tray, truck or countercurrent drying, but not as rapid as fluid bed drying. Other advantages of vacuum drying include the ability to reduce oxidation, contain dust and reduce energy costs.

Dielectric or Microwave Drying

Dielectric or microwave drying is a method of drying in which electromagnetic radiation is applied to the material to be dried. Microwaves at the 915 and 2450 MHz frequencies do not interfere with communication frequencies and thus may be allocated to drying applications. The 2450 MHz frequency is the more useful as it has advantages when used in a dual vacuum/microwave system. A variable output magnetron that generates the mutually perpendicular electric and magnetic fields is the source for MW power. If polar solvent molecules such as water are present, the electromagnetic field will tend to induce orientation of the dipoles in the molecules. As the field oscillates, the polar solvent molecules will attempt to oscillate with the field, resulting in increased kinetic energy

Drying

from the dipolar molecules and their collisions with other molecules. This increase in kinetic energy is manifested as thermal or heat energy. Thus, the energy from the magnetron is converted to an instantaneous potential energy in the dipole alignment and then to kinetic energy as the field oscillates. At 2450 MHz this sequence occurs 2450 million times per second.

Since microwave radiation is able to penetrate the entire granules or bed of granules (depending on field strength and dielectric properties of the solid being dried), heating and vaporization of solvent can occur evenly throughout the mass (Fig. 9). Rapid heat generation within the granule or the bed, with subsequent solvent vaporization results in the vapor pressure gradient which is required for drying. If the vaporization is too rapid or the granule porosity structure lacks a favorable pathway for the vapor, the granule may disassociate due to internal pressure build-up. Since drying rates are proportional to the rate of vapor diffusion rather than liquid diffusion, dissolved solute transfer from the interior to the granule surface is not a problem.

Microwave or dielectric drying has been reported in the pharmaceutical literature as being comparable or superior in terms of efficiency, energy consumption, and cost

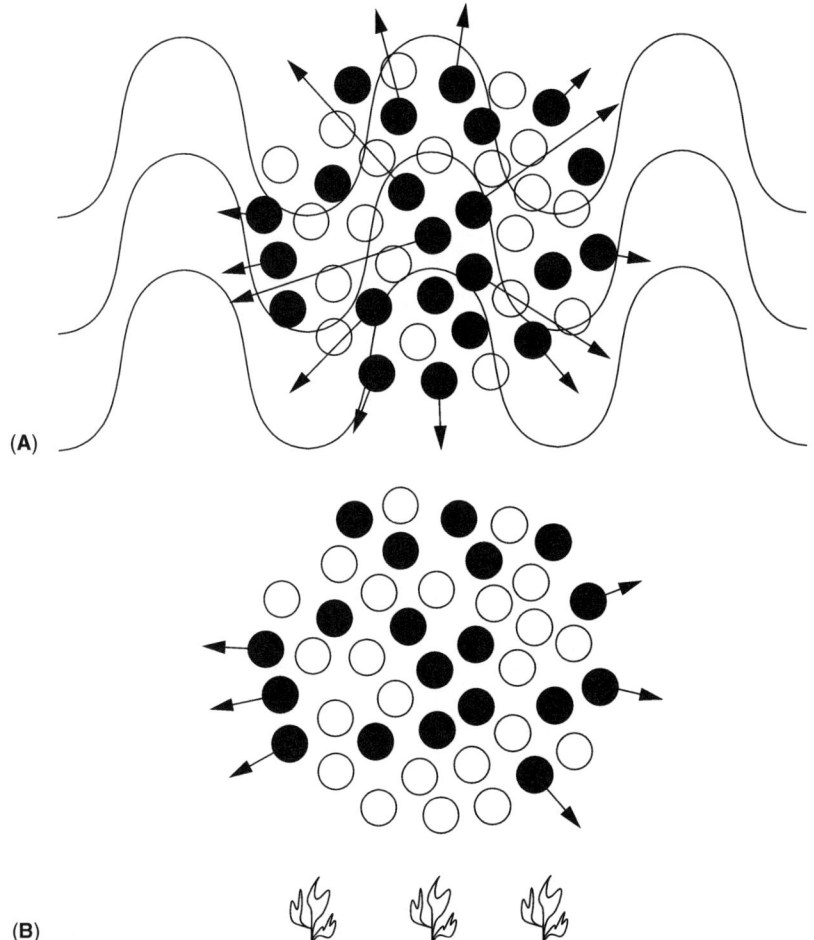

FIGURE 9 Microwave penetration of powder. *Source*: Courtesy of Fitzpatrick Co., Elmhurst, IL.

compared to conventional batch or continuous fluid bed drying methods (36). Energy savings of as much as 70% in industrial settings have been reported (18). Microwave drying may be conducted in a batch or continuous manner, with or without fluidization. It has been shown (36) that a dielectric, vibrating, fluidized bed produced drying rates at low temperatures that were superior to tray drying at 105°C (Fig. 10). It was found that by using dielectric radiation with the proper combinations of bed thickness and airflow, even thermally unstable materials could be dried safely and rapidly. The microwave drying process has not been associated with any deleterious effect to stability or physiochemical properties of granules when compared to other drying methods.

In dielectric drying, the rate of heating is proportional to the dielectric constant of the materials placed in the energy field. If there are large differences between the dielectric constants of the materials in the granules, then rapid and fairly selective drying is possible. For example, since water has a dielectric constant of 70, if the dielectric constant of the granule itself is around 10, then water will be heated much more rapidly than the other components of the granule. This may be shown in Equation (29).

$$P = 2\pi f v^2 E_o E_r \tan \delta \tag{29}$$

where P is the power density of the material, W/m^3, f is the frequency of the applied field, Hz, V is the voltage gradient, V/m, E_o is the dielectric permittivity of free space

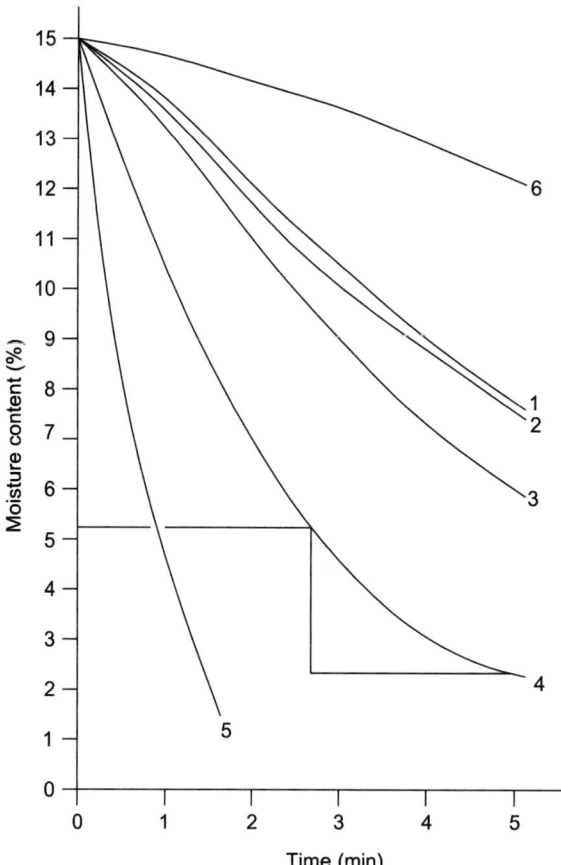

FIGURE 10 Drying rate comparison. *Source*: From Ref. 1.

(8.85×10^{-12} F/m), E_r is the relative dielectric constant of the material, and tan δ is the loss tangent or dissipation factor of the material.

Microwave drying may be used in combination with vacuum drying. A balance is required between the two technologies to avoid adverse internal pressure build-up in individual granules caused by too rapid heating. This concern generally restricts the operating vacuum level to between 30 and 100 mbar (22.5–75 mmHg).

These combination units offer many advantages in the drying of solids. With the production of very low vapor pressures combined with the molecule-selective energy-coupling of microwaves, polar solvents may be evaporated at low temperatures. For example, at a typical process pressure of 45 mbar (about 35 mmHg), water based granulations can be dried at 31°C (37). Another advantage of combining vacuum and microwaves is that the process is practically independent of ambient atmospheric conditions such as relative humidity and temperature, which can have such dramatic effects on conventional drying techniques. Installation of the equipment is fairly straightforward, since elaborate air ducts and explosion relief vents are not necessary. These units are very efficient at their containment of product, which is important in the processing of hazardous or highly potent drugs. A further advantage is the recovery of solvents when organic solvents have been used in the granulation step.

A specific example of granulation properties in the combination vacuum/microwave technology versus forced air drying is reviewed in Ref. 38. The article describes the influence of these drying methods on attributes such as specific surface area, porosity, friability, hardness and morphology.

Combination microwave/vacuum technology does not suffer the scale-up inefficiencies of vacuum drying alone. One study (39) shows that despite a 40-fold increase in batch size, the actual drying time remained similar in the laboratory and scale-up vessels.

ENDPOINT DETERMINATION

Whether the application is drying a slurry, powder or granulation, the ultimate goal is achievement of some solvent level appropriate for transfer of the dried material to a subsequent process step. Thus, a method of endpoint determination is crucial to the economic success of the drying step as well as to the endowment of the proper physical characteristics on the dried material. For example, over-drying may result in unwanted static charge or reduced particle size due abradement of particles.

Perhaps the best known method of endpoint determination is thermogravimetric analysis or loss on drying analysis. This method requires an operator to stop the process and gather a representative sample for analysis. The drying process resumes while the sample is analyzed posing the possibility that the material may exceed the acceptable endpoint while the analysis is made. Loss on drying is not specific to a particular component as all volatile components are driven off in the analysis.

Karl Fischer titrimetry is another endpoint determination method requiring collection of samples from the dryer. This analytical method is more sophisticated than simple loss on drying. It is also more costly, more time consuming and exposes employees to dangerous chemicals. Expenditures are also necessary for the chemical reagents and the safe disposal of these reagents.

High performance liquid chromatography may be used to evaluate samples for specific solvents such as methanol. This method for determination is typically lengthy and requires frequent calibration runs.

The following endpoint determination methods do not generally require a physical sampling to be taken from the dryer and could be termed non-destructive methods.

Near infrared (NIR) spectroscopy relies on the delivery of electromagnetic energy in the NIR band and then analyzing the transmittance or reflectance of this energy. The chemical specificity of the individual solvents can be determined, and by building calibration curves, the level of the solvent in the dryer mass can also be determined.

Effusivity is based on the thermal conductivity, density, and heat capacity of the substance being monitored. Each component in the dryer has a specific effusivity signature and if the solvent in question has a signature distinctly different from the remainder of the formulation, it becomes possible to discern the level of solvent during drying.

Mass spectrometry does not directly monitor the drying bed but monitors the off-gases for solvent traces. It has good specificity for individual solvent entities and can sense to very low levels.

Microwave drying may be monitored by sensing the reflected power. Free solvent couples with the microwave energy and as the amount of solvent is reduced, the measured electric field increases as does the batch temperature. These factors can be calibrated to detect an endpoint.

PROCESS ANALYTICAL TECHNOLOGY

Pharmaceutical processing exists in a highly regulated environment seeking validation of the process steps and then rigidly adhering to the validated protocol. The basis for validation of specific unit operations is encompassed within FDAs current Good Manufacturing Practices. The rigidity to repetitive process steps has hindered continuous improvement in pharmaceutical processing. Many other industries have implemented continuous improvement methods and reaped the benefits. Recognizing this, FDA has embraced a risk-based approach to pharmaceutical manufacturing that includes the topic of PAT. The earlier section discussed methods of determining endpoint. In this section, the appropriateness of transforming these methods into deeper process understanding will be elucidated.

PAT is much more than making a measurement with sophisticated analytical equipment, although the sophistication, miniaturization and enhanced information gathering ability of modern devices are driving PAT. Regarding drying and PAT, sensing the drying endpoint in real time will obviously prevent over-drying with resulting loss of time and energy. In addition to sensing the solvent level, the endpoint determination may be built into a feedback algorithm that takes into consideration and learns the impact of particle size, rotational speed of dryers, fluidization conditions, bed temperature, etc. on drying. This will build a true process knowledge base for the unit operation and promote continuous process improvement and optimization with this knowledge. Considering the lack of human intervention with automated PAT devices, the process will also become more reliable as the dryer remains unopened, the bed is undisturbed and there is no exposure to ambient conditions.

Thermogravimetric and titrimetric methods do not fit readily in the PAT scheme primarily due to the length of analysis. The devices may be situated at the drying area although this does little to improve the speed of analysis.

A prominent method associated with PAT, not only in drying, but also in association with blend uniformity and wet granulation, is near NIR. Fundamental absorption bands occur in the mid-IR region but these absorbances require dilution to bring them into the linear region. Overtones, which are weaker, can be measured without sample preparation. Second derivative spectra are often used to remove baseline scattering and enhance peaks. Other mathematical treatments to the spectra may include standard normal variate, detrend and multiplicative scatter correction.

Establishing a regression equation is usually the first step in developing a quantitative model. A training set of calibration samples is used to derive the regression equation. This calibration or training set shows the expected range of variation. A second set of samples is used to challenge the regression equations. Eventually a spectral library is built with the collected spectra of multiple lots to determine averages and variability. Another quality to consider with NIR analysis is the ability to transfer the library or knowledge set. Transferability is useful when analyzing multiple process lines so that repeated calibration is unnecessary.

Sample analysis with NIR is possible in near real time with a probe situated in the dryer wall. Local differences in density or particle size near the probe window caused by turbulence in the dryer may be problematic. Multivariate treatment methods can usually overcome these issues. Sample collection may be made in a glass vial in order to reduce the turbulence effect without sacrificing an inordinate amount of analysis time. Fouling of the probe windows is also a concern with cohesive powder or granules. Wiping devices or a burst from an inert gas source may be helpful in overcoming the fouling. Another possibility is to monitor the effluent gas with NIR. This method is less complex in that the solid components in the dryer do not interfere. Parris et al. (40) show such an approach in monitoring dichloromethane and n-heptane in a tray dryer and an agitated dryer.

Mass spectrometry has been similarly used in real time analysis of effluent gas (41). It has the advantages of greater sensitivity than optical methods, it can deal easily with multiple solvents and it has excellent concentration linearity in a wide range.

PAT related endpoint control is also feasible in combination microwave/vacuum dryers. When drying begins, there is usually free solvent present, which will couple with the microwave energy. Thus, low electric field strength will be measured in the drying chamber. Low field strength will continue to be measured as the bulk of free solvent is evaporated. This portion of the drying cycle will amount to a steady state phase. It should be noted that water of crystallization does not couple with microwave energy in the same manner as free or unbound water due to the presence of the crystal lattice.

The measured electric field will rise sharply as free solvent becomes exhausted and the microwaves attempt to couple with the ever-decreasing solvent load (or product load). At this time, the temperature may also sharply rise. Therefore, it is imperative to cut back on the amount of microwave energy going into the chamber when the end of the steady state phase is reached. By proper instrumentation of the dryer, careful monitoring of the drying process should allow the operator to prevent overheating of the product. The relationship between the electric field and temperature can be determined experimentally on small batches and ultimately be used to control the drying process.

TROUBLESHOOTING THE DRYING STEP

Problems in drying are often formulation specific, non-quantitative, and difficult to categorize. Drying problems are usually formulation based with formulations often specifically designed for the production equipment to be used (42). Once the formulation is set, adjustments for issues caused by drying are limited to adjustments in process. Thus formulation based issues must be considered in both formulation design as well as taken into consideration in creating a robust production method.

Formulation Issues in Drying

Changes caused by formulation can be classified into two categories, chemical (Table 1) and physical changes (Table 2).

Chemical changes usually can be quantified. They are formulation specific reactions/decomposition of ingredients and/or actives. Most often ingredient compatibility studies point out these problems early in formulation design. If not found in pre-formulation, final tablet stability studies develop quantitative estimates of decomposition/ reaction products and information needed to allow removal of these factors. Often structure change such as hydration states of a compound can change the structure of a tablet. Hausman et al. (43) showed hydrated risedronate sodium (RS) crystal lattice contained channels occupied by water. During the drying process this water is removed. As drying process decreased the final moisture content, the amount of dehydrated RS increased. The lower final moisture showed a greater increase in tablet thickness change during tablet accelerated aging. The expanded tablets softened with age and the amount of hydrated RS increased.

Physical changes are less case specific, tend to be less studied, thus more overlooked in the development phase, and thus result in troubleshooting issues in the mature processes (Table 2.)

Drying, by definition, is a process in which liquid is lost by evaporation. The liquid involved is usually water. At the end of the drying process almost always some moisture remains. At issue in process design is how much moisture should remain, also what migrates with the moisture, and where in the formulation the residual moisture should be located.

Three examples illustrate the complexity of moisture loss.

An insoluble system is the first example—water placed on/in microcrystalline cellulose. Water present with insoluble materials is solute free. It behaves as associated liquid close to the solid surface. As more layers of water are added less and less surface association occurs until at the outer layers water behaves as unassociated free water. Water in capillaries can be considered bound with more heat needed than even associated water to remove water from capillaries. Water thus remains in location after drying in a very predictable manner based on drying temperature and drying duration. As moisture remains solute free, the mass transferring during drying is water only.

A hydrophilic colloid is the second example—water placed on/in plasdone (PVP). PVP is both soluble and hydrates in water. On drying, PVP forms a hydrated film with 15–20% water present in the film.

In the drying step PVP can migrate. Rubinstein and Ridgeway (44) showed PVP concentration on the surface of 12 mm magnesium carbonate granules at the completion of drying varied with the drying temperature. Starting with a 5% PVP in formula and drying at 59.8°C the particle surface content of PVP reached 13%. Dried at 44°C, the surface concentration was closer to 6% PVP and drying at 19.6°C the surface concentration was less than 3%. It is anticipated that the surface concentration of PVP would affect the compactability of the finished granulation.

TABLE 1 Chemical Changes

Reaction/decomposition of ingredients/active	Usually eliminated in pre-formulation stability studies and confirmed with formulation and tablet stability data

Drying

TABLE 2 Physical Changes

Moisture range of hydrophilic colloids	Narrow range of water permitted to develop a plastic deformation and compaction
Moisture range of water soluble carbohydrates	Moisture range is drier for brittle fracture (less than 1.0%). Excess moisture causes stickiness/film formation
Moisture and long term tablet hardness stability	High moisture content (>1%) of water soluble carbohydrates will lead to hardening of the tablets over time. Too low moisture (<0.4%)these same water soluble carbohydrate will soften over time
Migration of binder/active	Higher drying temperature cause greater migration. Binder moves to surface. Movement of soluble active to surface can be eroded during processing and created highly active fines

Hydrophillic colloids are dried to within a narrow range of moisture content. This level leaves the polymer sufficiently wet to plastically deform, yet not too wet allowing a strong bond to form.

The third example is a water soluble sugar system-water placed on dextrose anhydrous. Armstrong et al. (45) studied water addition to both anhydrous dextrose as well as dextrose monohydrate. Water on dextrose anhydrous has a very complex relationship. Tablet tensile strength achievable increased from 0% water present to 8.6%. Above 9.2%, tensile strength achievable falls dramatically as dextrose monohydrate forms and the water is considered in excess. Excess water, above 9.2%, is reported by Armstrong et al., to be a physical barrier that prevents interparticulate bonding. Hydrodynamic resistance to compression is suggested. Greonwold et al. (46) also suggested excess water in sucrose granulation opposes formation of strong bonds. Lerk et al. (47) also showed that bounding strength in tablets made with glucose monohydrate increased with the level of dehydration temperature used to process the monohydrate. Water soluble carbohydrates are usually dried "bone dry." Some residual water still remains but always for most mono and disaccharides less than 1% water remaining is the target for chewable tablets. This low level of moisture is needed to setup a stable amorphous transition in the material. Brittle fracture occurs at these transitions in tabletting at low pressure, creating clean surfaces to allow, at higher pressure, the close contact and crystal bond formation creating tablet hardness in the process.

What happens when a granulation formulation has both a hydrophilic colloid and a water soluble sugar? Even more complex an example is when the soluble sugar is a hydrate. LOD testing of dextrose monohydrate will show total water loss at test temperatures above 80°C. In process drying temperatures above 52°C will show water loss from the hydrate. If the plan is to leave the water in the hydrate and keep the hydrophilic colloid polymer wet enough to plastically deform, then the residual water content needs to be high enough to allow both the hydrate to form and the polymer to contain its appropriate residual moisture. If, however, we want to establish a brittlely fracturing sugar based formulation, then we effectively dehydrate the polymer and dry the dextrose to the anhydrous form maintaining minimal residual moisture and setup up a brittle fracturing granulation.

Migration of Ingredients

Drug solubility in the granulation solvent can effect its distribution in different granule size fractions, thus the granules can come into the drying process as wet granules that are already segregated. This segregation is based on the liquid distribution and the drug dissolved in the liquid. Drugs with high solubility in the granulation solvent have a higher tendency to migrate during drying, creating a drug rich surface on the drying particle. Attrition or abrasion during subsequent handling leads to formation of highly drug concentrated fines relative to the larger particles (48).

Armstrong et al. (49) found if the dye, FDC blue #1 is insoluble in the fluid, migration and hence mottling will be reduced.

Viscosity has a significant effect on drug migration. Drug migration increased from the pendular state being dried to the funicular state being dried. Kapsidou et al. (50) showed drug migration increased with drug solubility and was projected to be a problem above a target range per granulation system. Kiekens et al. (51) showed a minimum liquid viscosity of 100 mPa sec was needed to stop the migration of riboflavin in alpha lactose using PVP K-90 as the wet binder.

When drying is completed larger particles tend to contain more moisture than smaller ones. Once drying is completed, milling, of course, can liberate moisture and cause issues with condensation and caking.

Importance of Cooling After Drying

Before storage, dried material should be brought to within 10°C of the projected storage condition. Stored dried material has a tendency to be warmer than the outside air. Warm air rises slowly from the center, when this air contacts colder particles near the top, it increases in relative humidity causing the top particles to gain moisture. Sometimes the temperature gradient is large enough to cause condensation on the surface particles. Air and dried particles close to cold walls and floors can drop in temperature also causing condensation (52).

OTHER ISSUES

It must be noted that the stringent guidelines associated with the manufacture of pharmaceutical products put constraints on the kinds of drying equipment that can be used. Since few pharmaceuticals are produced in such quantity that drying equipment is dedicated to only one product, the equipment must allow thorough cleaning and validation of the cleaning process. Surfaces that contact the product are usually polished stainless steel, which increases cost. Not only is stock stainless steel more expensive as a starting material, it requires special expertise to fabricate and weld. The welds should be polished to increase cleaning efficiency and decrease pores and crevices in which chemical contaminants or microorganisms may reside. Validated clean-in-place systems are available to automate the cleaning step.

Finally, innovations in engineering and technology have created production scale equipment in which several steps such as mixing, granulating, and drying may be combined. These kinds of multifunction units more commonly called SPP, when appropriate, should be considered for their potential time and energy-saving qualities. A good review of this type of equipment is presented in Ref. 53. In any event, when the purchase of equipment for use in the drying of granulations is being considered, the basic principles of drying and the specific limitations of the equipment must be kept in mind. The pharmaceutical scientist may seek the advice of a competent chemical engineer to develop the best process possible.

REFERENCES

1. Van Scoik K, Zoglio M, Carstensen J. Drying. In: Lieberman H, Lachman L, Schwartz J, eds. Pharmaceutical Dosage Forms: Tablets, 2nd ed; Vol. 2.New York: Marcel Dekker, 1989: 73–105.
2. Carstensen JT. Pharmaceutics of Solids and Solid Dosage Forms. New York: Wiley, 1977: 210–3.
3. Jones TM, Pilpel N. Some physical properties of lactose and magnesia. J Pharm Pharmacol 1965; 17:440–8.
4. Jones TM, Pilpel Nl. The flow properties of granular magnesia. J Pharm Pharmacol 1966; 18: 81–93.
5. Jones TM, Pilpel N. Some angular properties of magnesia and their relevance to material handling. J Pharm Pharmacol 1966; 18:182S–9S.
6. Jones TM, Pilpel N. Effect of grain size distribution and the diameter of the aperture. J Pharm Pharmacol 1966; 18:429–42.
7. Ridgway K, Rupp R. The effect of particle shape on powder properties. J Pharm Pharmacol 1969; 21:30S–9S.
8. Shesky PJ, Williams DM. Comparison of low-shear and high-shear wet granulation techniques and the Influence of percent water addition in the preparation of a controlled-release matrix tablet containing HPMC and a high-dose, highly water-soluble drug. Pharm Tech 1996; 19(3):80–92.
9. Lipps D, Sakr AM. Characterization of wet granulation process parameters using response surface methodology. J Pharm Sci 1994; 83:937–47.
10. Vojnovic D, Moneghini M, Rubesa F, et al. A simultaneous optimization of several response variables in a granulation process. Drug Dev Ind Pharm 1993; 19:1479–96.
11. Koblitz T, Erhardt L. Pharm Tech 1985; 9(4):62.
12. Sapakie SF, Mihalik DR, Hallstrom DH. Drying in the food industry. Chem Eng Progr 1979; 75(4):44–9.
13. Peters MS, Timmerhaus KD. Plant Design and Economics for Chemical Engineers, 2nd ed. New York: McGraw-Hill, 1968.
14. Draft Guidance for Industry: PAT-A Framework for Innovative Pharmaceutical Manufacturing and Quality Assurance: U.S. Department of Health and Human Services, Food and Drug Administration, 08/25/2003.
15. Porter HF, Schurr GA, Wells DF, Semrau KT. Solids drying and gas–solids systems. In: Perry RH, Green D, eds. Perry's Chemical Engineer's Handbook, 6th ed. New York: McGraw-Hill, 1984: Chap. 20.
16. McCabe WL, Smith JC, Harriot P. Unit Operations of Chemical Engineering, 4th ed. New York: McGraw-Hill, 1985.
17. Himmelbau DM. Basic Principles and Calculations of Chemical Engineering, 3rd ed. Englewood Cliffs, NJ: Prentice-Hall, 1974.
18. Rankell RS, Lieberman HA, Schiffman RF. Drying. In: Lachman L, Lieberman HA, Kanig JL, eds. The Theory and Practice of Industrial Pharmacy, 3rd ed. Philadelphia, PA: Lea & Feabiger, 1986.
19. Yang Y, Gerner FM, Hazarati AM. Study of the drying process of a product cake in a vibro-separator. Pharm Eng 1999; 19(5):1–6.
20. Carstensen JT, Zoglio MA. Tray drying of pharmaceutical wet granulations. J Pharm Sci 1982; 71:35.
21. Samaha MW, El Gindy NA. El Maradny, The mixing performance of the fluidized-bed for a. multicomponent system. Pharm. Ind.; 1986; 48:193
22. Travers DN. A comparison of solute migration in a test granulation dried by fluidization and other methods. J Pharm Pharmacol 1975; 27:516–22.
23. Crank J. The Mathematics of Diffusion, 4th ed. Oxford: Oxford (Clarendon) Press, 1970: 56.
24. Carstensen JT, Zoglio MA. Abstracts "Drying" American Pharmaceutical Society Meeting, Kansas City, Missouri, 1979: 10.

25. Wang D-C, Fon, D-S, Fang W. Development of SAPGD - A simulation software regarding grain drying. Drying Tech 2004; 22(3):609–25.
26. Pitkin C, Carstensen JT. Moisture content of granulations. J Pharm Sci 1973; 62(7):1215.
27. Kunii D, Levenspiel O. Fluidization Engineering, 2nd ed. Boston, MA: Butterworth-Heinemann, 1991.
28. Schepky G. Die Wirbelschichtgranulierung. Acta Pharm Technol 1978; 24(3):185–212.
29. Zoglio MA, Streng WH, Carstesen JT. Diffusion model for fluidized-bed drying. J Pharm Sci 1975; 64(11):1869–73.
30. Gao JZH, Gray DB, Motheram R, Hussain MA. Importance of inlet air velocity in fluid bed drying of a granulation prepared in a high shear granulator. AAPS Pharm Sci Tech 2000; 1(4) www.aapspharmscitech.org
31. US Patent 5392531 (1991).
32. Kiekens F, Zelko R, Remon JP. a comparison of the inter- and intragranular drug migration in tray- and freeze-dried granules and compacts. Pharm Devlop Technol 1999; 4(3):415–20.
33. Cooper M, Schwartz CJ, Suydam W Jr. Drying of tablet granulations. J Pharm Sci 1961; 50(1):67–75.
34. Lee T, Lee J. Particle attrition by particle-surface friction in dryers. Pharm Tech 2003; May: 64–72,
35. Fischer JF. Low temperature drying in vacuum tumblers. Ind Eng Chem 1963; 55(2):18–24.
36. Koblitz T, Korblein G, Erhardt L. Pharm Tech 1986; 10:32.
37. Waldron MS. Microwave vacuum drying of pharmaceuticals: The development of a process. Pharm Eng 1988; 8(1):9–13.
38. Killeen MJ. Comparison of granular and tablet properties for products produced by forced air and microwave/vacuum drying. Pharm Eng 1999; 19(2):48–58.
39. Pearlswig DM, Robin P, Lucisano LJ. Simulation modeling applied to the development of single pot processing using microwave drying. Pharm Technol 1994; 18:44–60.
40. Parris J, Airiau C, Escott R, et al. Monitoring API drying operations with NIR. Spectroscopy 2005; 20(2):34–41.
41. De Palma A. PAT provides new insights into drying.PharmaManufacturing.com, http://www.pharmamanufacturing.com/articles/2004/163.html (accessed 11/10/2006).
42. Giry K, Genty M, Viana M, et al. Multiphase versus single pot granulation process: Influence of process and granulation parameters on granules properties. Drug Dev Ind Pharm 2006; 32(5):509–30.
43. Hausman DS, Cambron RT, Sakr A. Application of on-line Raman spectroscopy for characterizing relationships between drug hydration state and tablet physical stability. Int J Pharm 2005; 299(1–2):19–33.
44. Ridgeway K, Rubenstein MH. Solute migration during granule drying. J Pharm Pharmacol 1974; 26(Suppl): 24S–29S.
45. Armstrong N, Patel A, Jones T. The compression properties of dextrose monohydrate and anhydrous dextrose of varying water content. Drug Dev Ind Pharm 1986; 12:1885–901.
46. Greonwold H, Lerk CF, Mulder RJ. Some aspects of the failure of sucrose tablets. J Pharm Pharmacol 1972; 24:352–6.
47. Lerk CF, Zuurman K, Kussendrager K. Effect of dehydration on the binding capacity of particulate hydrates. J Pharm Pharmacol 1984; 36:399.
48. van der Dries K, Vromans H. Relationship between inhomogeneity phenomena and granule growth mechanisms in a high-shear mixer. Int J Pharm 2002; 247:167–77.
49. Armstrong NA, March GA. Colored granules for compression. Drug Dev Ind Pharm 1978; 4(5):511–4.
50. Kapsidou T, Nikolakkis I, Malamataris S. Agglomeration state and migration of drugs in wet granulations during drying. Int J Pharm 2001; 227(1–2):97–112.

51. Kiekens F, Zelko R, Remon JP. Influence of drying temperature and granulation liquid viscosity on the inter- and intragranular drug migration in tray-dried granules and compacts. Pharm Dev Technol 2000; 5:131–7.
52. Kemp I, Gardiner S. An outline method for troubleshooting and problem-solving in dryers. Drying Technol 2001; 19:1875–90.
53. Parikh D. Handbook of Pharmaceutical Granulation Technology, 2nd ed. New York: Taylor & Francis, 2005.

7

Spray Drying: Theory and Pharmaceutical Applications

Herm E. Snyder
Nektar Therapeutics, San Carlos, California, U.S.A.

David Lechuga-Ballesteros
Aridis Pharmaceuticals, San Jose, California, U.S.A.

INTRODUCTION

Spray drying unit operations are used for the production of dried powder across a wide range of material processing applications from food to fertilizer to pharmaceuticals (1). This one-step, continuous process converts a bulk liquid into powder and has been shown to be both robust and scaleable, with the appropriate hardware and process modifications. Materials previously thought not suitable for spray drying such as proteins, have been successfully processed with appropriate formulation and process design. In addition, the ability to rapidly form individual particles enables a level of particle engineering well suited to producing pharmaceutical powders, in particular for inhalation drug delivery.

Spray drying applications in the pharmaceutical industry date to almost 50 years ago. It was first applied as an intermediate processing step in the production of solid dosage forms. Spray dried lactose was used as an excipient for direct compression (2), for compression ready granulations (3), solid dispersions (4,5), and more recently to manufacture dry powders for inhalation (6–11). The first spray dried powder for inhalation (Exubera®, Pfizer Inc., Groton, Connectiot, U.S.A.) which contains insulin for the treatment of diabetes has been recently commercialized (12). The oral delivery of proteins through the lung is one of the technological breakthroughs of 20th century (13).

Spray drying has also become a mainstream process to stabilize proteins by rendering them into the dry state in the presence of stabilizers as an alternative to freeze-drying (14). Other pharmaceutical applications of spray drying include the production of active pharmaceutical ingredient (API) when control of particle properties such as crystallinity, particle size, residual moisture content, bulk density, and morphology is desired (15,16) Additional spray drying applications in drug delivery include the production of rapidly dissolving tablets (17,18), microspheres (19), nanoparticles (20), and liposomes (21,22). Spray drying applications are discussed in more detail following the theory section.

Innovations in particle engineering have been complemented with advances in the understanding of the particle formation process, which has motivated research into the physical and chemical mechanisms that control the drying kinetics and particle formation and many aspects of the drying of droplets in an air stream in small scale spray dryers have been investigated. The importance of the ratio between evaporation rate and diffusion of the solutes within the drying droplet and the solubility of the solute has been highlighted. The concept of the Peclet number, a dimensionless parameter that represents the ratio of evaporation rate and solute diffusion has been used to explain the formation of low density particles (20,23) and the role of solute solubility in determining the particle morphology and surface composition has been determined (23). The role of solute diffusivity, which is inversely proportional to the molecular weight, in determining surface composition of a spray dried particle has also been studied (24–26). In addition, the role of solubility and its effect on the precipitation kinetics has been highlighted studying the formation process of polymer nanoparticles (27). The solubility and propensity to form a crystalline phase of formulation components can also affect the particle density (28) as well as the solid state properties of spray dried particles (11,29). The solute with lowest solubility in a mixture is an important factor in determining the surface composition of spray dried particles (23,26). It has also been found that the solubility and the surface tension of the components affect the composition of the air–water interface of the drying droplet which in turn affect the composition and the cohesiveness of the surface layer of the dry particles (23).

Spray drying has been found suitable in particle engineering applications such as manufacturing hollow, low-density particles for inhalation with controlled surface properties and morphology (9,23,30). In this regard, spray drying has enabled the production of a new generation of dry powders for inhalation which avoids the requirements of mixing with a large crystalline carrier enabling the stabilization of proteins and delivering of higher doses (up to tens of milligrams) in a single inhalation as is the case of inhaled antibiotics (9). The particle formation mechanism is further discussed in the following sections.

SPRAY DRYING PROCESS THEORY

The spray drying process is conceptually simple; a solution is pumped through an atomizer, a plume of liquid droplets containing solid components is created and subsequently exposed to a suitable gas stream to promote rapid evaporative mass transfer of the liquid carrier into the gas. When sufficient liquid mass has been transformed to vapor, the remaining solid material in the droplet forms an individual dried particle which is then separated from the gas stream.

Typical droplet lifetimes and hence particle formation rates can occur over a range of timescales from milliseconds to minutes. Particle formation time is controlled by both the initial liquid droplet size and evaporation rate. The latter is dictated by the heat transfer to the droplet, mass transfer of the vapor away from the droplet into the process gas stream and the specific formulation components. The rate of particle formation is a key parameter which dictates the size of the drying chamber, and hence the scale of equipment required to produce a desired particle size at the target production rate.

Spray drying typically produces particles with favorable flow characteristics conducive to subsequent downstream handling and packaging. The concept has been implemented over a range of equipment scales from bench units to large multi-story commercial drying towers. Powder production rates for a typical bench spray dryer are on the order of grams per hour, while the commercial systems process tons per year. Regardless of the size of the machine, four fundamental sub-processes must occur for successful spray drying (Fig. 1): Feedstock preparation, feedstock atomization, droplet

Spray Drying: Theory and Pharmaceutical Applications

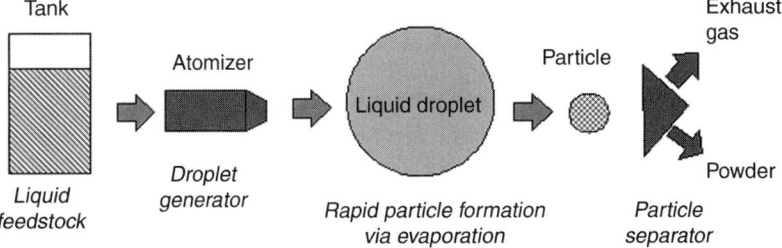

FIGURE 1 Schematic of the spray drying process.

drying or particle formation, and particle separation from the process stream. A clinical spray drying facility is shown in Figure 2 along with the representative atomization, drying, and collection hardware.

Feedstock Preparation

A broad range of feedstock rheological properties have been utilized in spray drying, from low-viscosity solutions, emulsions and suspensions to high-viscosity slurries.

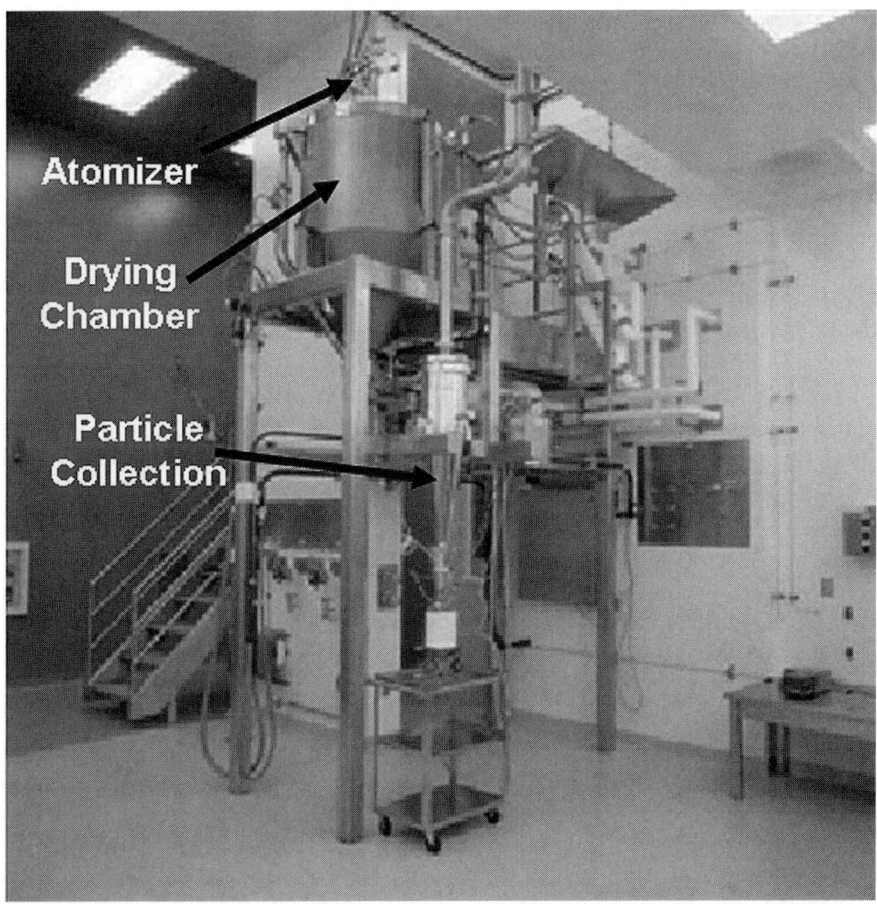

FIGURE 2 Clinical spray drying facility. *Source*: Courtesy of Nektar Therapeutics.

The feedstock design is driven by target product characteristics and stability considerations as well as formulation dictated properties such as solubility, surface tension, viscosity, etc.

The simplest batch preparation utilizes a low viscosity aqueous-based solution with soluble constituents mixed in a tank and pumped to the spray dryer. The carrier is commonly aqueous but organic solvent systems are also used with appropriate equipment safeguards. The processing of highly viscous solutions, emulsion, or suspension systems can add both processing complexity as well as physical stability constraints which require additional process development. For formulations with suitable thermal stability, high-viscosity solutions can often be spray dried by heating the feed lines to reduce solution viscosity and improve pumping and atomization performance. Emulsion or suspension feedstock systems can be effectively processed when the dispersed phase component; emulsion droplets or suspended particles, is significantly smaller than the atomizer nozzle restricting orifices to avoid clogging and provide for stable dryer operation. In addition, the dispersed phase components should be approximately one order of magnitude smaller in size compared to the atomized droplet size in order to assure consistent composition across the final spray dried particle population.

The batch preparation process must be capable of presenting a consistent feedstock with suitable rheological properties to the atomization nozzle, in order to obtain the target droplet size and subsequent powder properties. For any formulation system being delivered to a spray dryer, consistency of the feedstock during the required processing time is crucial to maintaining product quality throughout the batch. Both the formulation design and feedstock handling equipment must work in concert to achieve this goal.

Atomization

The bulk feedstock is delivered to the spray dryer where is it converted to a field of droplets using an atomizing nozzle. A key performance parameter for nozzle design is the resulting liquid droplet size distribution. Both the mean and width parameters of the distribution play a role in determining final product size as well as process yield. Ideally a narrow droplet size distribution, with a geometric standard deviation below two, should be targeted to enable a more uniform drying event and prevent product loss to the dryer sidewalls due to incomplete drying of the larger droplets. Controlling the droplet size distribution is essential for the consistent and efficient production of spray dried particles utilized for inhalation drug delivery in which the output is directly packaged into the final product form. However, if the spray dried product is an intermediate, which is further processed via roller compaction, granulation, tableting, etc., tight control on droplet size may not be a major process control variable.

The atomizer breaks the bulk fluid into a spray field of individual droplets. This initial partitioning of the bulk solution is the primary factor in determining the size distribution of the final dried particles. In addition, the final product size can be impacted by selective wall losses which tend to reduce the portion of large particles in the final product, reducing the mean product size and lowering process yields. The method of particle extraction from the process stream can also alter the resulting powder size distribution. For example, inertial cyclone separators are less efficient at extracting the smaller particle sizes, called fines, which reduces collection efficiency and acts to increase the size of the final captured product. Due to the geometric relationship of particle mass and diameter: Partical Mass $= \rho_{particle} \frac{\pi d_{particle}^3}{6}$, the mass weighted size distributions will be greatly altered by the loss or addition of the larger particles which contain the majority of the population's mass.

Spray Drying: Theory and Pharmaceutical Applications

The final product particle size can be estimated, to the first order, for a solution feedstock, assuming the powder loss to the system and the residual carrier solvent in the powder are minimal, by equating the mass of dissolved solids to the mass of the dried particle yielding the following relation:

$$d_{\text{particle}} = \sqrt[3]{\left(\frac{C \rho_{\text{solution}}}{\rho_{\text{particle}}}\right)} d_{\text{droplet}},$$

where d_{particle} is the particle diameter, μm; d_{droplet} is the Droplet diameter, μm; C is the solution concentration or total solids, g solute/g solution; ρ_{particle} is the particle density, g/cm^3; and ρ_{solution} is the solution density, g/cm^3. Hence the final product particle size is controlled predominantly by the initial liquid droplet size and to a lesser degree by the feedstock concentration along with the solution to particle density ratio.

Measurement of the liquid droplet size can be performed optically within the spray field using several techniques. To obtain a representative droplet size that will be reflective of the powder generated, the entire droplet size distribution must be measured throughput the spray field and appropriately weighted. Laser diffraction instruments generate droplet size information in the line-of-sight across the spray plume. These systems are user friendly and rapidly produce an average distribution along the optical path. Converting this line-of-sight data to a representative weighted averaged for the entire spray can be challenging as these instruments do not directly measure the amount of mass in the line of sight. High speed imaging systems have been modified with software to discern and count individual droplets within an image field. Depending upon the available lens, this approach is generally limited to droplet sizes above 10 μm in diameter.

Phase Doppler velocimetry is a technique capable of simultaneously measuring the droplet size, velocity, and mass flux through a point within the spray field where multiple laser beams intersect. The technique operates over wide ranges of droplet sizes, <1 μm to 1 mm, and droplet velocities from near quiescent to supersonic flows. The advantage of this approach is the high spatial resolution enables the spray mass flux to be mapped out and appropriate weighted average droplet sizes to be calculated. One such automated system in which the spray nozzle is traversed through the measurement location and average droplet size of the spray plume determined is shown in Figure 3.

For applications requiring tight control of the final product distribution, this process must start with the appropriate atomizer nozzle selection. The impact of nozzle performance is illustrated in the scanning electron micrographs shown in Figure 4 for a spray dried protein formulation using two different types of custom atomizing nozzles. Both powders were processed under similar conditions, however due to differences in the liquid droplet sizes produced from the two atomizers, the feedstock concentration for the twin-fluid atomizer was approximately 10 times greater than the ultrasonic nozzle solution. This change as dictated by the larger mean droplet sizes produced from the ultrasonic nozzle and the desire to target particle sizes <5 μm in diameter for pulmonary applications. An improvement in particle size uniformity is evident with the use of the ultrasonic atomizer. The measured particle size distribution using a laser diffraction instrument indicates a significant narrowing of the size distribution with a reduction in the relative span value from 1.9 to 1.0. However, due to the larger mean droplet size produced from the ultrasonic atomizer, a reduced feedstock concentration was required which in turn caused a 10-fold decrease in powder production rate and would negatively impact the processing economics in a commercial powder production system.

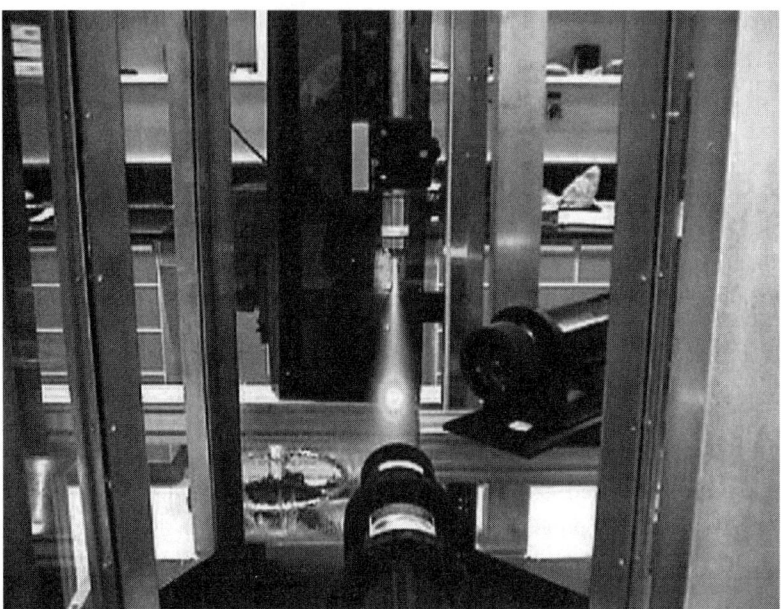

FIGURE 3 Phase Doppler laser instrument probing spray field.

Atomizer Selection

Twin-fluid atomizer. Liquid atomization nozzles provided by commercial spray drying manufacturers for pharmaceutical applications typically fall into two categories: twin-fluid or rotary. Twin-fluid nozzles produce smaller droplets with a broader distribution when compared to rotary atomizers and are therefore preferred for applications targeting smaller particle size, such as pharmaceuticals for pulmonary delivery. These nozzles utilize a high speed gas stream, typically air, to blast the liquid into droplets as illustrated in Figure 5. The atomization is achieved by using the kinetic energy of the gas stream provided by a compressed source with typical pressures operating up to 100 psi (689 kPa). A variety of twin-fluid designs exist with the distinction being the geometry which controls the gas and liquid interaction, and subsequent droplet size performance.

For all atomizer designs, the feedstock rheological properties will impact nozzle performance with the twin-fluid designs generally being less susceptible to a droplet size

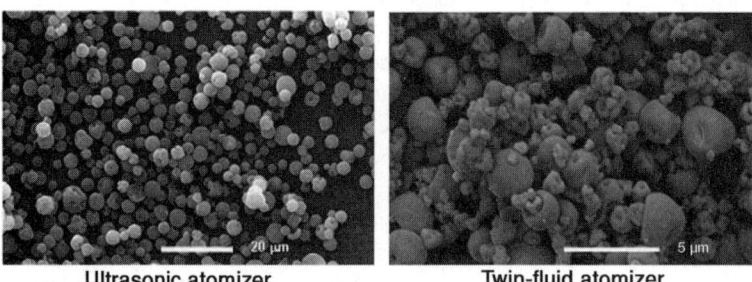

FIGURE 4 Impact of atomization on spray dried particle size and distribution: (**A**) ultrasonic atomizer, span = 1.0; (**B**) twin-fluid atomizer, span = 1.9.

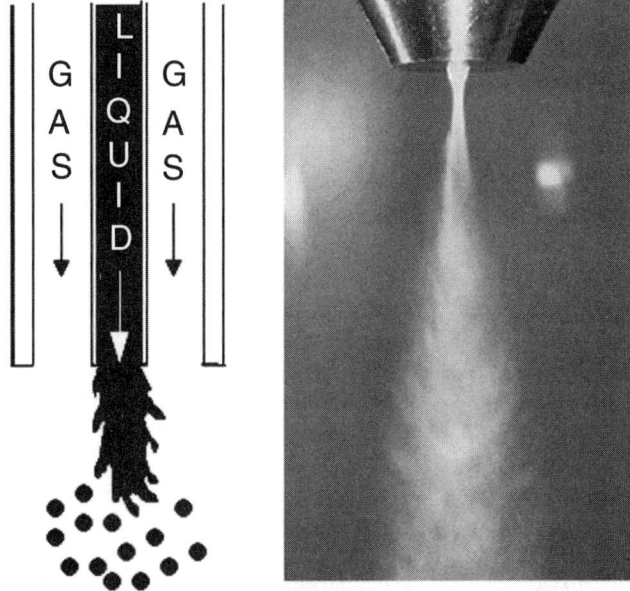

FIGURE 5 Schematic and image of a twin-fluid, air-assist atomizer.

increase as the solution viscosity is elevated. Twin-fluid gas-assist nozzles, extract energy from a high speed gas stream to disrupt the liquid surface. With this approach, the atomization energy per unit mass of liquid can be elevated as the feed viscosity or surface tension increase, performance will still decline, but to a lesser degree, compared to other nozzle types.

A high-speed, high-magnification image at the tip of a twin-fluid gas-assist atomizer, shown in Figure 6, visually captures the impact of the liquid disintegration process for both a low- and a high-viscosity solution. At identical spray conditions, the more viscous fluid displays a delayed droplet formation with thicker ligaments projecting later into the atomization process and larger resulting droplet sizes. Therefore to maintain product quality, rheological properties must be maintained throughout a process batch for applications requiring precise powders size control.

The quantitative effect of the solution viscosity on measured, spray-averaged droplet size performance is shown in Figure 7 for a twin-fluid, gas-assisted nozzle (31).

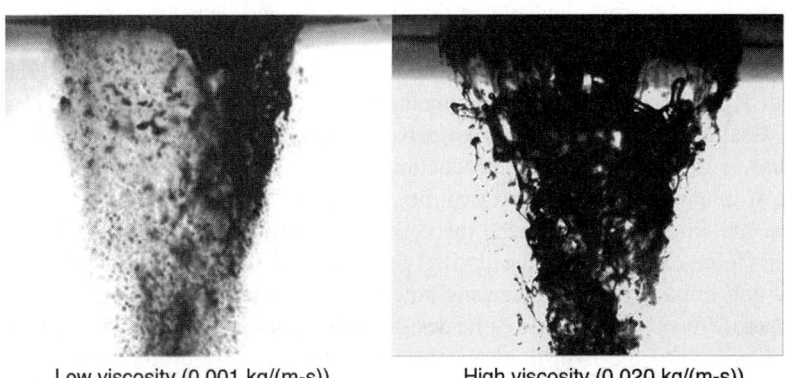

Low viscosity (0.001 kg/(m-s))   High viscosity (0.020 kg/(m-s))

FIGURE 6 Nozzle tip images, twin-fluid atomizer, showing impact of feed rheology.

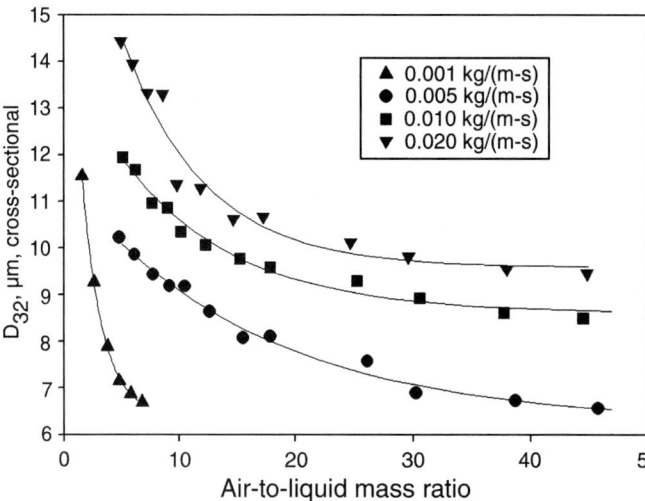

FIGURE 7 Impact of twin-fluid atomizer ALR and feed viscosity on droplet size. *Abbreviation*: ALR, air-to-liquid.

The Sauter mean diameter droplet size (D_{32}) is plotted versus the air-to-liquid (ALR) mass ratio for a range of solution viscosities from water (0.001 kg/m/sec) up to 0.002 kg/m/sec. The more viscous solutions produce both an elevated droplet size compared to water as well as a reduced sensitivity to atomization energy or ALR, with the highest viscosity solutions showing little improvement in droplet size above ALR = 20.

Using a multivariate regression approach based upon a modified El-Shanawany and Lefebvre equation (32) yields for following predictive relation of Sauter mean droplet size (SMD) for a twin-fluid type atomizer (33) utilizing the non-dimensional parameters of ALR, We_{Dp} and Oh_{DP}:

$$D_{32} = D_h \left(1 + \frac{1}{ALR}\right) \left[0.11 \left(\frac{1}{We_{D_p}}\right)^{0.36} + 0.099 Oh_{D_p}\right]$$

where D_{32} is the predicted droplet diameter (SMD); D_h is the hydraulic diameter; ALR is the atomization air (or gas) to liquid feed mass flow ratio; We_{Dp} is the Weber number $= \frac{\rho_{gas} U_{relative}^2 D_h}{\sigma}$; where ρ_{gas} is the gas density, $U_{relative}$ is the relative velocity between the gas and liquid, and σ is the liquid surface tension; Oh_{Dp} is the Onesorge number $= \frac{\mu_L}{\sqrt{(\rho_L \sigma D_h)}}$; where μ_L and ρ_L are liquid viscosity and density, respectively.

Rotary atomizer. Rotary atomizers operate by flinging the liquid from a high speed rotating disk or wheel into a gas environment. The motive force can be a gas driven turbine for the smaller units or electric motor driven wheels for large scale production. The radial nature of this type of droplet production creates a wide spray angle near the atomizer as the droplet trajectories form a two-dimensional sheet radiating outward from the wheel. Once the droplets have escaped the near wheel region they are susceptible to the aerodynamic forces imposed by the drying gas flow and their trajectories will be altered, or they will impact a sidewall causing potential loss of product yield. The spray geometry imposes different constraints on the design of the dryer body shape and air flow pattern when compared to the twin-fluid nozzle. For both cases the droplets need sufficient drying time prior to contacting the chamber side walls in order to assure complete particle formation and minimize film deposition losses to the chamber.

Spray Drying: Theory and Pharmaceutical Applications

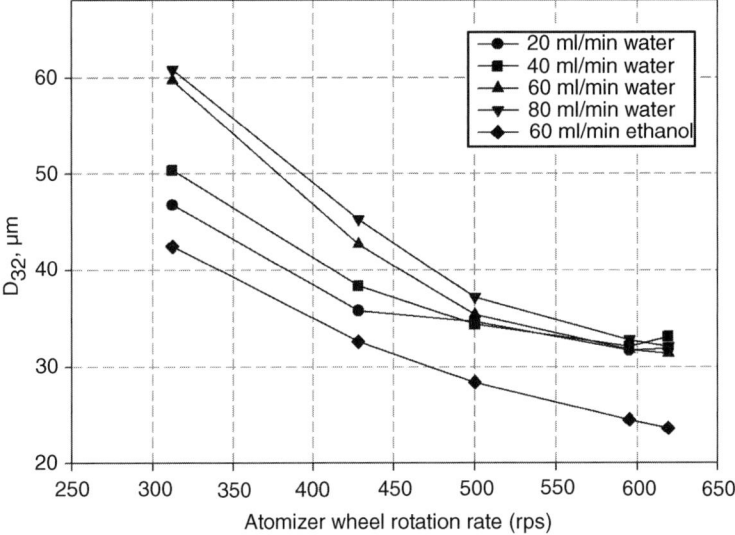

FIGURE 8 Impact of rotary atomizer rotation rate and feed rate on droplet size.

Rotary atomizer produce larger, more uniform droplet size sprays in comparison to the twin-fluid nozzle. The atomization energy is provided by the rotation speed of the wheel and the droplet size will decrease with increased wheel rotation. Results from a series of optical measurements using an air turbine driven rotary atomizer over a range of liquid flow rates are illustrated in Figure 8, indicating that for water, consistent droplet size distribution can be obtained at elevated wheel rotational speed over a range of liquid feed rates. The reference dimension locations for this design are shown in Figure 9. Using a multivariate regression analysis and a modified Frasier equation (32), a predictive correlation was developed for mean droplet size as shown by (31)

$$D_{32} = 0.59 N^{-0.8} \rho_L^{-0.5} \left(\frac{\mu_L m_L}{d}\right)^{0.1} \left(\frac{\sigma}{nh}\right)^{0.3}$$

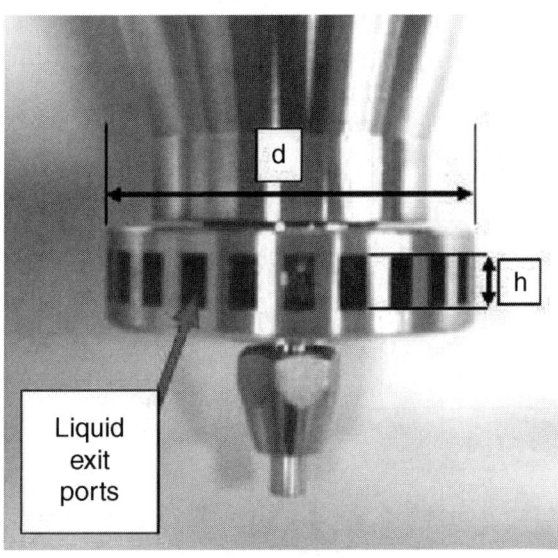

FIGURE 9 Rotary atomizer wheel.

where N is the wheel rotation speed, revolutions per second; ρ_L is the liquid density, kg/m^3; μ_L is the liquid viscosity, Pa-s; $m_L =$ liquid flow, kg/s; d is the wheel diameter, m; σ is the liquid surface tension, N/m; n is the number of vanes on atomizer wheel; and h is the height of atomizer wheel vane, m.

The impact of nozzle selection propagates into the drying environment by dictating the initial droplet size and trajectory. These initial conditions set the stage for the evaporation process within the drying chamber. Therefore, atomizer design and performance parameters should be considered when developing a spray drying process to assure target powder properties such as size, density and thermal exposure are maintained.

Particle Formation

The particle formation process involves the conversion of the atomized spray droplets into solid particles and includes multiple steps as the droplets are exposed to the drying gas medium. First, the droplet must adjust to the temperature of the environment near the nozzle. During this period, the type of atomizer will play a role in the local droplet environment and hence impact the early droplet temperature. For twin-fluid nozzles using air, the expansion of the high pressure atomization gas will decrease the local temperature due to the Joule–Thomson throttling effect (34). The droplet temperature subsequently rises as the atomized droplets and drying gases mix. This physical delay in the mass transfer process can occur very quickly, in less than one millisecond, for droplet diameters of 10 μm or less. Rotary atomized droplets are exposed to the high temperature gas stream immediately upon formation and are therefore only subjected to the physical delay of the droplet heat-up.

The second stage occurs when the liquid droplet has established equilibrium evaporation of the carrier solvent into the surrounding gas stream. This constant rate evaporation process is commonly modeled using the d^2 law methodology, which states that droplet size decreases linearly with respect to the square of the droplet diameter (35,36). The results of these droplet lifetime calculations applied to water droplets with initial diameters of 5–50 μm and surrounding gas temperatures from 40 to 60°C are shown if Figure 10. These calculations assume 0% relative humidity in the gas stream

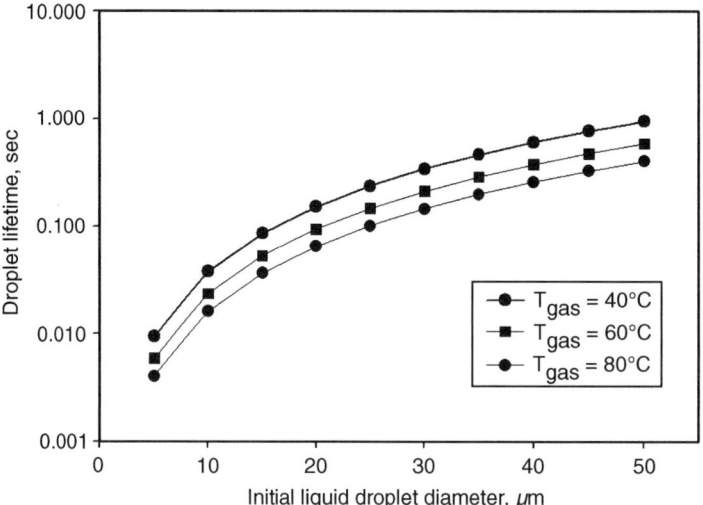

FIGURE 10 Calculated water droplet lifetime using d^2 law, relative humidity $=0\%$. *Source*: From Ref. 36.

and evaporation of the droplet as a pure carrier solvent, ignoring any diffusion limiting effect of solids in the droplet. Therefore, Figure 10 represents the fastest particle formation times theoretically possible for these conditions. During the constant rate drying period, the evaporation rate will be driven by the heat transfer to the droplet which must balance the energy removed due to the evaporative cooling effect as the liquid is vaporized (1). While in this constant rate period, the liquid droplet will experience a temperature close to the thermodynamic wet bulb value which will be significantly below the local drying gas temperature (36). For example, the liquid droplet experiences only 40°C under steady-state evaporation when the internal dryer chamber contains hot air at 80°C and 10% relative humidity (Fig. 11). Increased relative humidity acts to slow the concentration dependent mass transfer into the gas phase, slowing the particle formation rate along with the evaporative cooling of the droplet and elevating the wet bulb equilibrium droplet temperature.

The relative humidity in the spray drying chamber is defined as the partial vapor pressure of water divided by the saturation vapor pressure, at a target temperature (1), that is $RH = 100 \cdot p/p_o$. For particles in mass transfer equilibrium with the process gas stream, the target exit humidity will control the final product moisture level, which can be calculated using the relative humidity value and the product specific sorption isotherms. In addition, for products in which low particle moisture is key, the outlet RH will effectively determine the powder production rate for a given dryer outlet temperature. The non-linear relationship between dryer outlet temperature and RH is displayed in Figure 12. This plot illustrates that higher dryer outlet temperatures are advantageous for producing low moisture product as well as maximizing feed flow and hence powder production. For low feedstock pharmaceutical concentrations, <10% (m/v), the vast majority of the volatile mass which impacts the RH will be delivered to the process gas stream by the conclusion of the constant rate drying period.

The third stage of particle formation occurs after a portion of the solvent carrier has been evaporated and the solid content within the droplet influences the evaporation rate into the gas medium. Typically this reduces the mass transfer rate for the remaining solvent hence this stage is commonly referred to as the "falling rate period." At this point in time, as the solute concentration reaches its solubility, the droplet surface has started to

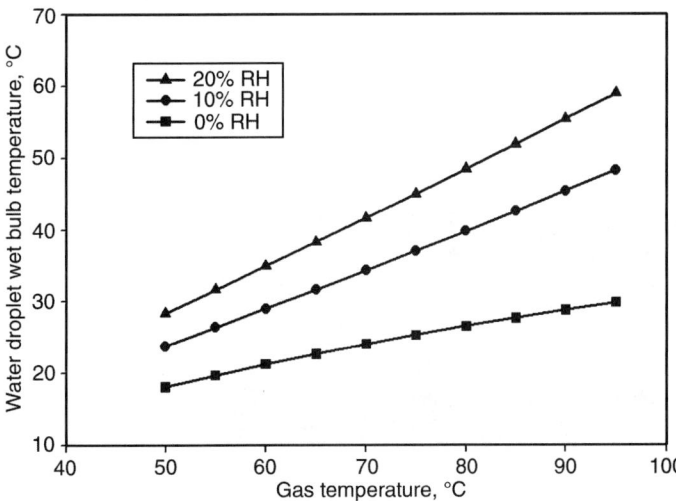

FIGURE 11 Calculated water droplet wet bulb temperatures.

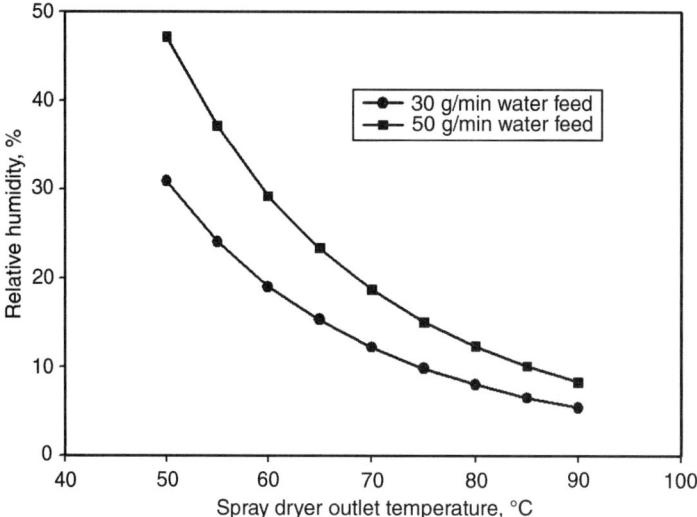

FIGURE 12 Calculated dryer outlet relative humidity, total gas flow = 0.023 kg/sec.

solidify forming a shell. This creates an internal droplet diffusion controlled mass transfer process slowing the rate of solvent escape from the inner core to the surface prior to evaporation into the gas medium. It should be noted that some early surface formation events within spray drying have been found to enhance mass transfer due to a capillary wicking mechanism (1).

For non-suspension, solution based feed stocks the particle morphology is set in this third drying stage. The particle formation kinetics, controlled by the evaporation rate in conjunction with the rising droplet viscosity, imposes stresses on the forming surface which control the morphology of the spray dried particles. The impact of altering one aspect, the drying rate, is shown in Figure 13 for a spray dried protein. Identical formulation composition, concentration and initial droplet size were used in both cases. The particles produced from the higher drying rate displayed a dimpled or first-order shell collapse mode while the lower drying rate particles tended to be more spherical, with smaller surface wrinkles.

The detailed physics of the entire droplet to particle formation process is highly complex and dependent upon the coupled interplay between the process variables such as initial droplet size, feedstock concentration, and evaporation rate, along with the

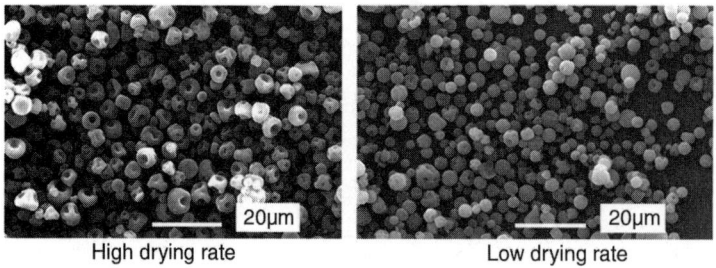

FIGURE 13 Impact of drying rate on particle morphology; increased particle wrinkling at elevated drying rate.

formulation physicochemical properties such as solubility, surface tension, viscosity, and the solid mechanical properties of the forming particle shell. Certain aspects of this process can be simulated using computational methods. A computational fluid dynamic (CFD) model was use to simulate a bench scale spray dryer with multi-phase heat and mass transfer through the constant rate period with a total solids concentration of 1.5% m/v, as shown in Figure 14. For such low-feedstock concentrations, the falling rate portion of the drying event can be ignored. The model simulated the turbulent mixing inside the drying chamber between the hot drying gas and the cool, expanded atomization gas along with an injected water droplet field. The gas flow or continuous phase mass, momentum and energy equations were calculated and then the droplets or dispersed phased impact was simulated utilizing a coupled Lagrangian approach. The atomization process was not modeled; instead measured droplet size data were included as a boundary condition.

The continuous phase velocity contour field extracted from the dryer volume midplane is shown in the first image of Figure 14. The lighter contours indicate higher velocities demonstrating the atomizer plume maintains a narrow spray angle which penetrates deep into the drying chamber, for the hardware and process conditions simulated. This jet-like plume acts to drive the global mixing within the drying environment. In the corresponding temperature map with the lighter contours indicating lower temperatures, there exists a field asymmetry within the drying chamber as the high speed center spray plume, combined with the side chamber discharge causes unbalanced recirculation and a stratified dryer exit temperature profile. Examination of the dispersed phase water spray enables the evaporation rate profile map shown in the third image of Figure 14 to be generated. The lighter contours display the region of maximum evaporation suggesting the mass transfer process is completed at a location roughly half the distance down the chamber. These short droplet lifetimes and corresponding rapid particle formation rates are a result of the operating conditions, internal dryer mixing field and the initial droplet sizes. For this case, the mean size of the initial droplet distribution was 8 μm.

The impact of fluid mechanics on the drying and particle formation process is further illustrated by the range of calculated droplet pathways generated in the simulation. A particle can follow significantly different paths inside the drying chamber,

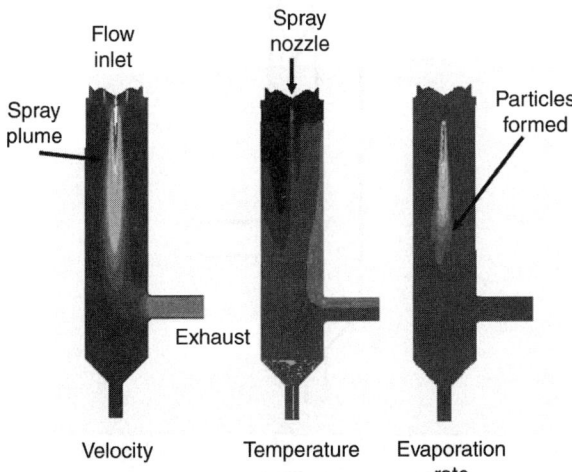

FIGURE 14 Computer simulation of bench scale spray drying process; 3D, turbulent flow with multi-phase heat and mass transfer simulation.

depending upon which streamline it is launched into near the spray nozzle, as shown in Figure 15. The particle formed near the spray centerline will directly exit the drying chamber and experience a residence time of ~42 milliseconds. The particles which get entrained within a recirculation eddy will experience much greater residence times and potentially expose thermally sensitive particles to the inlet drying gas temperature, without the protective shield of evaporation to insulate them.

Performing a series of droplet tracking calculations using the results from the CFD simulation, a representative droplet drying experience can be developed from the example shown in Figure 15. The early droplet temperature profile with time is shown in Figure 16 in which the initial decline, warm-up and constant rate equilibrium are evident. The falling rate period was not modeled hence the particle temperature is seen to rise to the local gas field temperature once evaporation has ceased. Note the time scale for this series of events is less then 6 milliseconds.

While predicting the mixing and evaporation in a realistic dryer setting is currently within the capability of modern computation tools, the approach is currently not suitable for accurately predicting particle morphology. For that challenge, the details of the falling rate drying period would be required along with the time varying solid mechanic properties of the shell and core structures in the evolving particle.

Some empirical observations can help to understand how the feedstock physical state (i.e., suspension, emulsion, solution) and the physicochemical properties of the formulation components relate to the morphology and surface characteristics of the spray dried particles. As mentioned above shell formation will occur when one of the formulation components reaches its solubility and precipitates leading to the formation of a solid shell that may be either amorphous or crystalline. Low aqueous solubility components tend to precipitate early in the drying process and tend to form corrugated

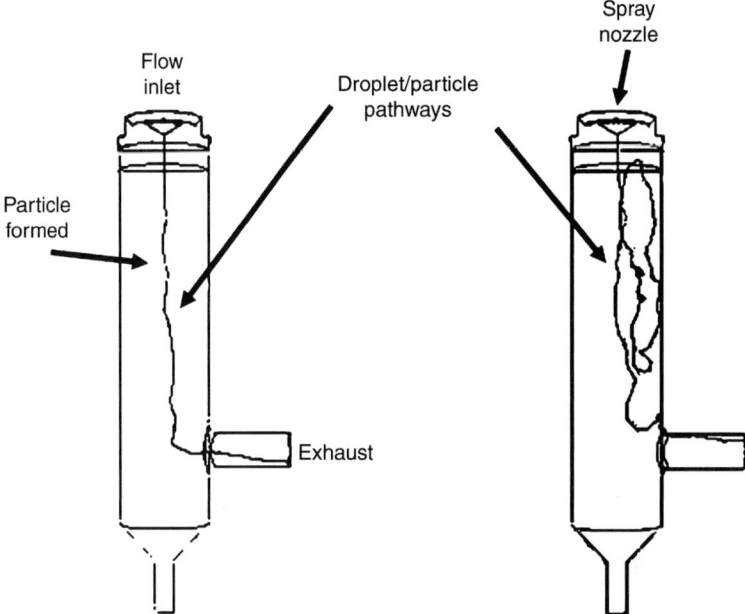

FIGURE 15 Computer simulation indicates multiple particle formation paths exist in bench scale spray dryer; particle formation rate and residence time dependent upon flow streamline.

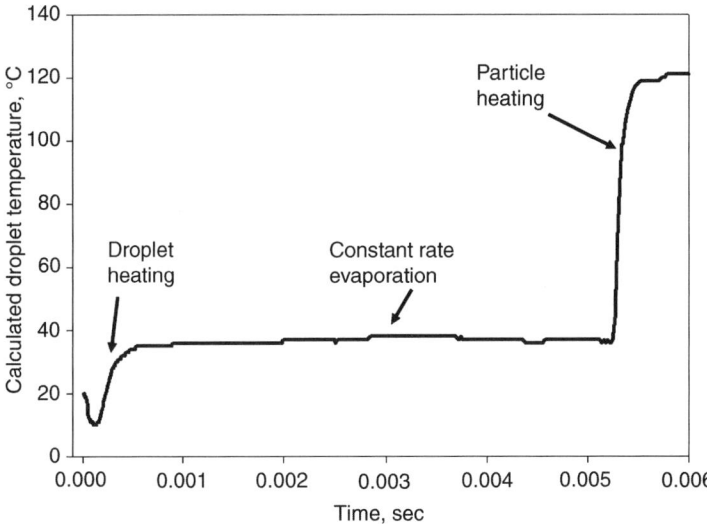

FIGURE 16 Calculated liquid droplet temperature based upon computer simulation of multiphase drying process, $d_0 = 8\,\mu m$, solids $= 1.5\%$ (m/v) (note that falling rate period is not modeled).

particles. In contrast, highly water-soluble components continuously recede as the liquid droplet dries, resulting in a smooth, spherical particle (23). Besides reaching the solubility limit, the ability to form a supersaturated solution will determine the state of the solid particle. For example, formulation components such as mannitol will tend to crystallize, in spite of its high solubility, whereas sugars, such as sucrose, raffinose, trehalose, lactose, will tend to recede with the droplet to finally remain as an amorphous solid. In the case of an amorphous solid, a high glass transition temperature (T_g) is desired to ensure acceptable physical stability. The T_g of the amorphous solid increases rapidly as the moisture content is reduced often exceeding the outlet temperature and thus minimizing the risk of physical instability in the collector.

For example, spray drying of an aqueous solution containing netilmicin, small molecule water-soluble antibiotic, renders smooth spherical particles while addition of trileucine, small molecule of low aqueous solubility, produces corrugated particles (Fig. 17) (23).

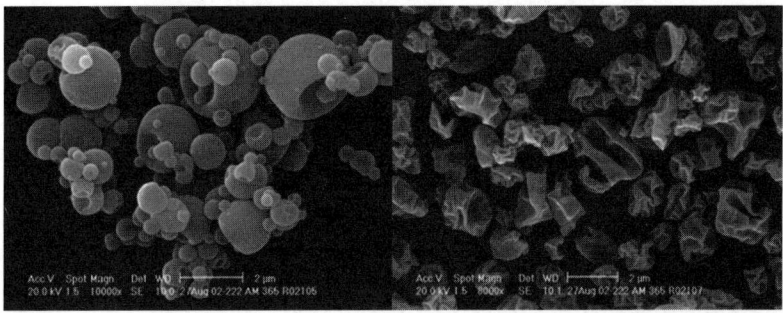

FIGURE 17 Addition of less soluble excipient promotes formation of corrugated particles. *Source*: From Ref. 23.

An alternative approach to modify the particle morphology and therefore particle density is based on the manipulation of the feedstock physical state. This is illustrated in the production of porous particles through spray drying an emulsion, in which the API may be dissolved or suspended in the aqueous phase and the pore forming organic phase is comprised of a nonsolvent liquid with higher boiling than water, such as perfluorooctyl bromide. The immiscible liquids form an emulsion stabilized with a natural surfactant such as dipalmitoylphosphatidylcholine (Fig. 18). Pulmonary applications of these low-density particles have already been demonstrated and are currently in clinical development (9). Other pore forming agents that have been used include volatile salts such as ammonium bicarbonate and other ammonium salts (37). Advantages of porous particles include low particle density which is advantageous to produce aerodynamically small particles for inhalation applications as well as for the parenteral or oral delivery of hydrophobic molecules as they are dispersed in the amorphous state and are presented to the biological fluid in a particle with increased surface area therefore promoting increased dissolution rate (Fig. 19).

In pharmaceutical dry powder applications, ability of the particles to disperse into individual particles is crucial. In general, as particle size is reduced, particle cohesiveness increases. It has been shown that the cohesiveness of spray dried particles, measured as its ability to disperse back into individual particles, can be improved by reducing particle density and inter-particle forces (38). Particle density is largely determined by the particle morphology and it has been shown that corrugated particles disperse better than smooth particles (39). In addition to being affected by particle morphology, particle dispersion is influenced by the particle cohesiveness which is largely determined by surface composition (23). In this regard it has been determined that the surface of spray dried particles may have a different composition than that of the bulk. The surface enrichment observed is owed to a molecular segregation which occurs during the drying process. Such molecular segregation is a function of the diffusivity, solubility, and surface tension of the formulation components in solution. In spray dried mixtures, molecules with large molecular weight or lower diffusivity and surface active components tend to accumulate on the surface (23,24,40–42). For example, spray drying protein solutions in the presence of water-soluble small molecule excipients result in particles with increased protein concentration at the surface with respect to the bulk (or nominal concentration) (24). The observed enrichment of protein on the surface is due to the protein slow diffusivity, which is proportional to the molecular weight of the solution components, compared to the small molecule excipients. The low-diffusing components preferentially enrich the

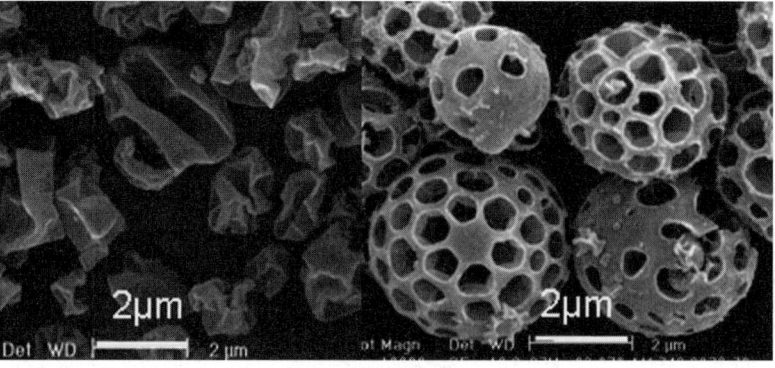

FIGURE 18 Spray dried particles using NEKTAR Technology (www.nektar.com).

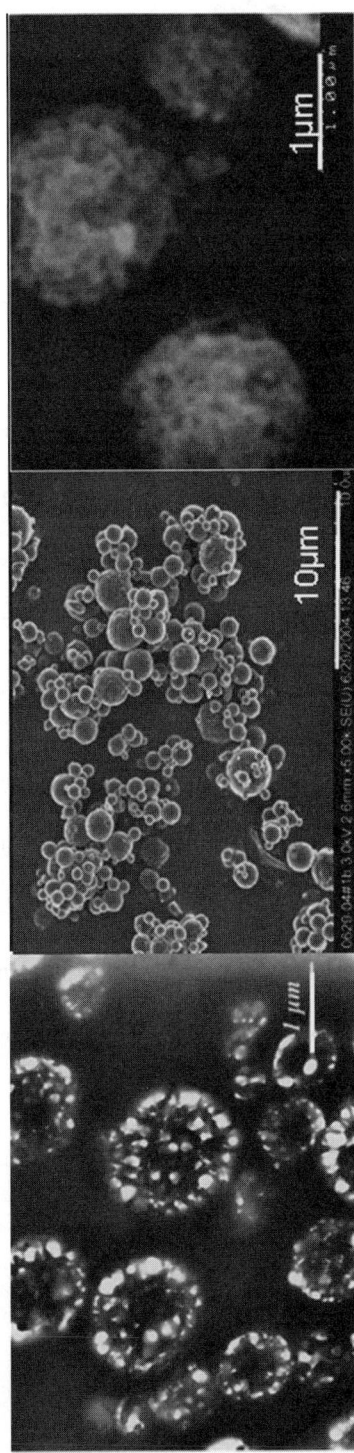

FIGURE 19 Porous particles loaded with hydrophobic molecule increased bioavailability, TEM (left), dry (center) after reconstitution (right).
Source: From Ref. 37.

surface of the receding droplet. Surface enrichment is also a function of the surface tension of the components as the surface active components rapidly compete for the interface (23,40). The effect of solute solubility on surface enrichment has been demonstrated in binary mixtures of trileucine with water soluble APIs such as antibiotics (23).

Particle Collection

Completion of the particle formation process in the spray dryer creates a dispersed particulate aerosol in which the high value solid material must be separated from the process stream. For inhalation drug delivery applications, this task is especially challenging as the particles are designed to be aerodynamically "light" with small Stokes number characteristics such as low terminal velocity and the ability to readily follow gas flow streams (43). Such particle performance attributes are highly desired for dry powder inhalation products which target the deep lung to enable efficient particle dispersion and drug transport past the upper airway constrictions. These same characteristics can work against efficient collection of the pharmaceutical product during spray drying as the particle do not readily settle out of the gas stream.

One of two different methods is typically used for product capture in a pharmaceutical spray drying process, cyclone separation or baghouse filtration. Both approaches have evolved out of the dust pollution control and chemical processing industries in which particle abatement was the primary goal. Each approach offers distinct advantages and disadvantages for efficient recovery of high value pharmaceuticals from a spray drying process. In addition to efficient collection, the selection of the appropriate collection system will be influenced by the required powder characteristics as well as its chemical and physical stability, and how they impact the desired product performance.

The cyclone, or inertial separation method, is a common industrial approach for segregating a dispersed phase from a continuous medium based upon the difference in density between the phases. The concept takes advantage of the velocity lag which occurs for dense particles with respect to a lower density medium when both phases are subject to an accelerating flow field, such as within a rotating vortex. The larger the acceleration, the smaller the particle which fails to follow the continuous phase streamlines and will migrate to the outer wall of the cyclone for collection.

Refinements to the traditional reverse flow Stairmand design have produced designs capable of high efficiency collection of particles as small as $2\,\mu m$ in diameter (43). A flow schematic of a typical reverse flow cyclone is shown in Figure 20 along with a CFD generated velocity contour field. The particle laden stream is fed tangentially into the top of the unit creating a hybrid vortex flow inside the cyclone. Along the outer wall the flow spirals downward and feeds a high tangential velocity central vortex which flows upward, illustrated by the light contour shown in Figure 21. Note for this case the model predicts the center vortex will extend to the bottom of the cyclone dust collector. For applications requiring high collection efficiency of $<5\,\mu m$ diameter particles, understanding the impact of cyclone design and operating conditions of the vortex flow field is crucial for the obtainment of high process yields.

Cyclone separation efficiency is dependent upon the cyclone design, operating conditions, and the particle size distribution of the incoming material. In addition, the particle solid mechanics will play a role in determining yield; ductile, or high surface charge materials may tend to deposit within the collection system as a layer and not produce free-flowing powders which readily migrate to the dust collector region.

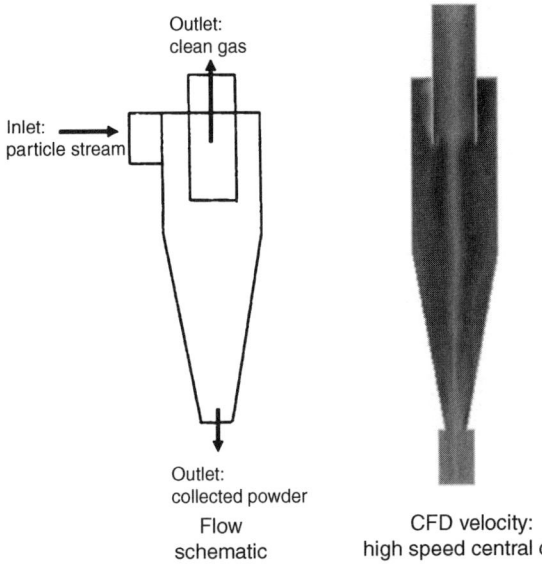

FIGURE 20 Schematic of reverse flow cyclone flow configuration.

Highly friable particles may fracture and malleable particles may deform when thrown onto the cyclone wall. The nature of inertial separation based technologies impose the limitation that larger and more dense particles will be more readily separated from the continuum and therefore obtain higher collection yields compared to smaller less dense particles. Various analytical, semi-empirical and CFD-based methods exist for predicting cyclone fractional collection efficiency and yield (44). However, the ability to a priori predict full cyclone performance from first principles for applications involving inhalation particles is still a considerable challenge.

Cyclones separators have advantages for particle collection in a pharmaceutical spray drying process; including mechanical simplicity with no moving parts, high recovery efficiency, and amenable to being cleaned in place. One such example is shown in Figure 21. Disadvantages can include both hardware scale and particle size dependent capture efficiency which must be addressed during process transfer and scale-up.

Baghouse particle capture systems operate by extracting the particles from the gas stream via either a tortuous path depth filter or a size exclusion membrane filter. The gas phase flows through the filter while the powder forms a layer on the filter media. The filters are typically cylindrical geometries mounted in a parallel array within the containment housing as shown in Figure 22. Final product collection occurs at the bottom of the unit after the powder has been blown off the filter media via a back-pulsing event. With the appropriate filter material and design, higher collection efficiency is possible compared with cyclone collection systems. Powder removal from the filter is a challenge and cleaning and quality concerns must be addressed.

During operation, the powder forms a layer on the filer media, commonly referred to as a "cake." This layer is formed by particle agglomerates which have been compacted together as a result of the pressure differential across the filter and powder layer. The system pressure into the baghouse builds with time as more powder is collected and then reduced through the use of a high pressure air back-pulse mechanism to momentarily knock the cake off the filter. The pressure response across the filters will be a function of the packed powder porosity and adhesives forces acts to hold the powder on the filters.

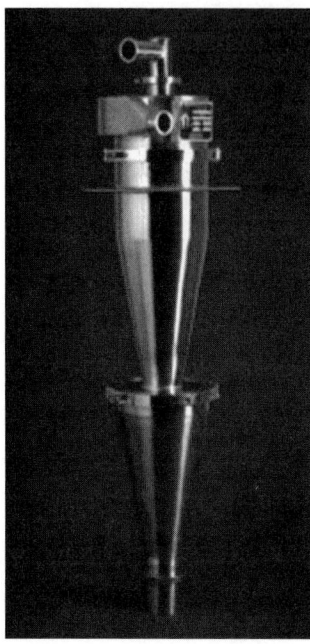

FIGURE 21 Example of high efficiency cyclone for pharmaceutical product collection. *Source*: Courtesy of Fisher-Klosterman.

The more porous the compacted powder cake, the lower the frequency of back-pulsing required and the less likely that filter "blinding" will occur in which the pressure cannot be reduced with back-pulsing. Back-pulsing is used to sever the cake from the filter media and provide sufficient time for the now large agglomerates to settle away from the face of the filter. If the particles are simply re-aerosolized, they will migrate back to the filter and not fall into the collection area, resulting in a gradual increase in system back pressure with time and reduce system operational efficiency.

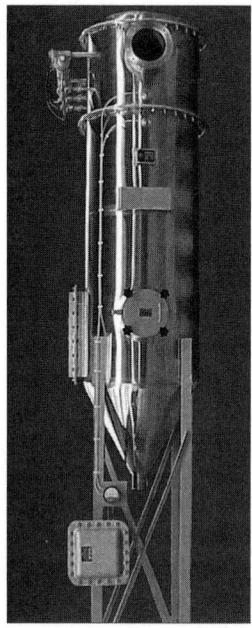

FIGURE 22 Example of pharmaceutical baghouse powder collection hardware. *Source*: Courtesy of Fisher-Klosterman.

The advantage of a baghouse collection system for pharmaceutical spray drying product recovery is the potential for high collection efficiency, even with micron-sized particles. Consistent collection performance over a range of manufacturing scales is possible with reduced scale dependent performance compared to cyclone systems. The disadvantages include: powder compaction, hardware complexity, pulsatile system pressure variations, possible filter media shedding into the product, and cleaning challenges to enable a validated process.

PHARMACEUTICAL SPRAY DRYING APPLICATIONS

Spray Dried Powders for Inhalation

The first pharmaceutical product targeting systemic treatment through the pulmonary drug delivery route was inhaled insulin, Exubera, approved by the FDA on Jaunary 27th, 2006 (12). This dry powder based delivery system utilized the spray drying process to create homogeneous particles containing precise amounts of drug and excipients which were engineered to perform in a predictable manner with a handheld delivery device. In order to make a successful powder for inhalation numerous physicochemical attributes are required such as particle size, both geometric and aerodynamic, physical and chemical stability as well as aerosol dispersibility, the ability to aerosolize.

Systemic drug delivery using the pulmonary approach must target the deep lung region. The alveolus sacks, located deep within the lung and a few tenths of a micron from the capillary walls act as the gatekeeper to the bloodstream. Once the drug has reached the alveoli carried by a single aerosol particle, it must quickly dissolve in the fluid layer on the surface of the deep lung where molecules are solubilized. The dissolved molecules can then pass through the thin single cellular layer of the alveoli into the bloodstream. In order to reach the deep lung a drug must be delivered in tiny particles sized from 1 to 3 μm (Fig. 23), with a slow, deep inhalation. If the particles are too large, they will deposit in the upper airway were absorption is poor. If they are too small, they will stay suspended in the air and be exhaled. Therefore, a tight control on the particle size distribution is crucial to achieve an efficient delivery and reproducible pulmonary deposition (45).

Various approaches have been developed to produce particles with adequate aerodynamic properties, such as nebulization, metered-dose inhalers, and more recently dry

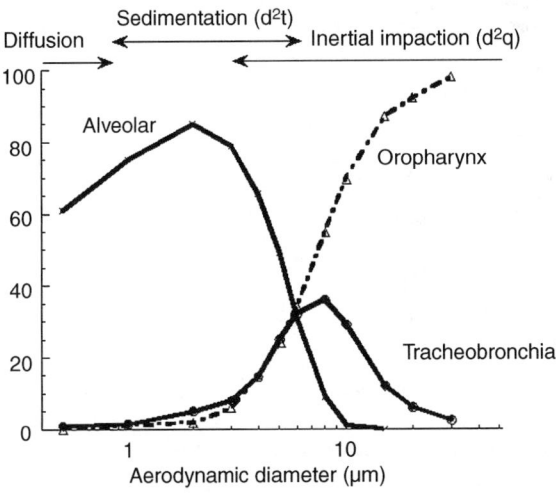

FIGURE 23 Pulmonary deposition as a function of aerodynamic diameter. Aleveolar deposition is optimized by delivering particles with an aerodynamic diameter of 1–3 μm. *Source*: Adapted from Ref. 45.

powder inhalers (DPI) (46). DPI systems offer an efficient and environment-friendly delivery system, especially for large biomolecules. Dry powder formulations of a given protein or peptide have several advantages over a solution or suspension. The low moisture levels and high drug concentrations enable them to be room-temperature stable and resist microbial growth, while also enabling more drug to be delivered per puff inhaled. Typically, DPI formulations consist of either drug alone or drug and one or more excipients such as stabilizers, wetting agents, bulking agents, or carriers. A successful DPI product is a system which combines a stable formulation with the correct particle size distribution and a device to facilitate the delivery to the patient. Spray drying has been shown to be a scaleable, robust, and pharmaceutically viable process for fine powder production.

To obtain appropriately sized particles for inhalation, some type of size reduction has historically been required. Common techniques used in the pharmaceutical industry are crystallization (or precipitation) from solution, milling and more, recently, spray drying. Small particles are cohesive in nature, which leads to agglomeration, poor flowability, and hygrosocopicity, the latter owed to the fact that an amorphous solid phase is invariably produced as a result of the typical milling-based particle reduction methods. Particle size and solid state control, along with recovery of very fine particulates from protein crystallization processes remains a technological challenge. Freeze drying and subsequent milling is one of the available methods of size reduction used to produce biopharmaceuticals for respiratory delivery. One of the most common milling techniques, jetmilling, involves impacting particles against each other or against hard surfaces when accelerated with gas jets. This approach has been used successfully for carrier-based systems, where only the drug component is milled and then blended with a larger sized excipient particle, such as lactose, to act as a carrier or flow aid (Fig. 24).

Such systems are advantageous because of their inherent ability to reduce agglomeration and the ability to dose microgram to milligram quantities of drug. For peptides and protein processing, this method is considered disadvantageous as it usually requires a multi-step process to produce an aerosol powder, since a solid protein or

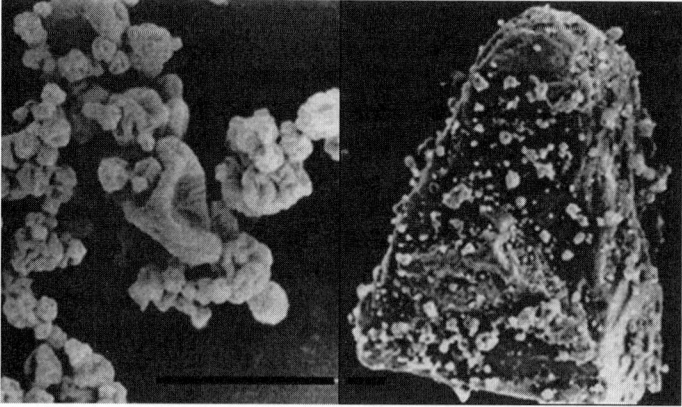

FIGURE 24 Spray dried bovine serum albumin by itself and mixed with crystalline lactose. Bar corresponds to 10 μm. Spray drying has enabled the production of a new generation of dry powder inhalers which avoid the requirement of mixing with a large crystalline carrier, through allowing the intimate mixing of excipients with active drug and facilitates the administration of higher doses in a single inhalation. Source: Adapted from Ref. 90.

peptide has to be obtained from freeze drying, milled, and mixed with a carrier before it is filled into capsules. It is also established that jetmilling processes may induce protein degradation due to localized heating and processing at sub-ambient temperatures may be necessary (47). Finally, in the case of small molecules, jetmilling of crystalline particles leads to the formation of amorphous regions which often result in a stability concern.

A clear advantage of spray drying processes is that they are readily scalable for clinical and commercial manufacturing. Dry particles produced from spray drying are single particles comprised of drug alone or drug and excipients with low levels of residual solvent. Particle properties such as particle size, morphology, and composition can be readily manipulated to obtain highly dispersible particles, avoiding the use of a secondary processing, such as blending with a larger particle size carrier. It has been demonstrated that spray drying is suitable for the production of dry powders containing proteins and peptides since they can be processed from a stable solution and biological activity is kept intact upon reconstitution (7).

Spray dried powders for inhalation aerosol particles can carry up to 100% drug (compared to only 1–2% carried by liquid aerosol particles). As a result, larger therapeutic doses can be delivered to the alveolar epithelium through dry powder system. An additional advantage of dry powder formulations is the low-microbial growth, thereby minimizing the potential to cause serious lung infection (48). Some disadvantages of using spray drying to produce aerosol particles include the fact that yield is dependent on the formulation and that in the case of proteins heat inactivation and surface denaturation are possible. These issues can be addressed through both formulation and process design and reduce the effective shear and thermal exposure during processing.

Protein Stabilization via Spray Drying

Therapeutic peptides and proteins are far more stable in the solid state compared to the liquid state. Delicate proteins often significantly degrade within hours when held at room temperature in the liquid state. All FDA approved therapeutic proteins for human use are injectable products, except Exubera the first inhaleable insulin. A recent survey has shown that 12 of the 30 commercial products are available only as dry powder and 28 of the 30 require refrigeration (49). Not having to refrigerate a pharmaceutical product greatly increases convenience and significantly reduces transportation and distribution costs, this is particularly true for vaccines, where an alternative to break the so called distribution cold chain is badly needed in third world countries.

Improved chemical stability may be obtained by removing water from the formulations (50). Upon water removal, the protein or peptide are molecularly dispersed in non crystalline solid, also known as glassy solid. The molecular mobility of the therapeutic protein or peptide is greatly reduced compared to the liquid state and thus chemical stability is improved. Extent of molecular mobility depends on the glass transition temperature which should be maintained well above the storage temperature the powder formulation will be exposed to during shipping, storage, and use. Usually, drying proteins and peptides requires the use of low-molecular weight excipients (i.e., non-reducing sugars such as sucrose, trehalose, raffinose, and polyols such as glycerol and mannitol) which offer protection against denaturation. However, the use of these low-molecular weight excipients will result in the formation of a hygroscopic and thus noncrystalline powder formulations may require special packaging conditions (51,52).

Freeze drying or lyophilization has been the method of choice to process therapeutic proteins and peptides into dry powder formulations, in spite of its high energy consumption and low throughput. The dosing of a sterile solution into glass vials which can be hermetically sealed after the drying process is a great advantage in the manufacture of sterile products for injection. However, when bulk production of protein dry powders is needed or when particle size control is a must, like in the case of dry powders for inhalation, spray drying has been demonstrated to be a suitable process to stabilize proteins in the glassy state (53,54).

Because of the importance of controlling the solid-state properties a great deal of interest has been generated around understanding the role of water in the formulation since water can act as a plasticizer that will deteriorate both chemical (i.e., protein degradation) and physical (i.e., particle fusion, cake collapse, crystallization) stability. How dry this formulation needs to be depends on the glass transition of the formulation relative to the storage conditions and the so called zero temperature (55).

In the case of spray dried powders for inhalation, residual moisture can also have an effect on powder dispersion and powder flow characteristics (56). Efficient and reproducible particle deaggregation is essential for the generation of a respirable powder aerosol. The presence of moisture may influence the cohesive nature of the powder and lead to the formation of aggregates. Long-term stability can be achieved by using individual (unit dose) packaging, which also enables very precise dosing and the ability to deliver blister-packed doses of different strengths, important for certain drugs such as inhaled insulin. Even though low moisture content is desired for improved stability, too low a moisture content may lead to increased oxidation of amorphous formulations and may encourage the undesired electrostatic charging during powder handling.

Effect of Drying Temperature on Protein Stability

Protein denaturation has been observed during spray drying due to the dehydration process and the use of excipients to replace hydrogen bonded water is often needed (e.g., sugars, polyols, amino acids) in the protein formulation (3,57,58).

Even though the drying air temperature may exceed 100°C in normal spray drying conditions, thermal denaturation of proteins is not generally observed mainly because the temperature of the droplet containing a dilute protein solution hardly exceeds the wet bulb temperature of water ($\approx 40°C$), as previously discussed under the theory section. The protein denaturation temperature is a function of water content (or protein concentration in the dilute solution) and increases sharply with decreasing water content. Dry proteins are relatively stable with denaturation temperatures usually exceeding 100°C (59). However, while the majority of the drying process last only a fraction to a few seconds, prolonged particle exposure to high temperatures (>100°C) later in the process system may cause chemical degradation. In the case of spray dried insulin powders, a correlation between an increase of high molecular weight proteins (a measure of irreversible protein aggregation, dimers and higher oligomers) as a function of outlet temperature is observed (Fig. 25) (60). Control of the particle thermal history after the initial drying event to mitigate possible degradation can be addressed with appropriate process hardware design.

An alternative process for biopharmaceutical powder preparation that avoids exposure to hot air is spray freeze drying. In this process the dilute protein solution is atomized into a cryogenic medium such as liquid nitrogen causing the droplets to rapidly quench, the frozen droplets are then dried by lyophilization. Changes in the drying method can dramatically alter the particle morphology and particle density as it has been shown for rhDNAse and IgE antibody (61). In this case spray freeze dried produced large porous particles with large surface area suitable to pulmonary delivery.

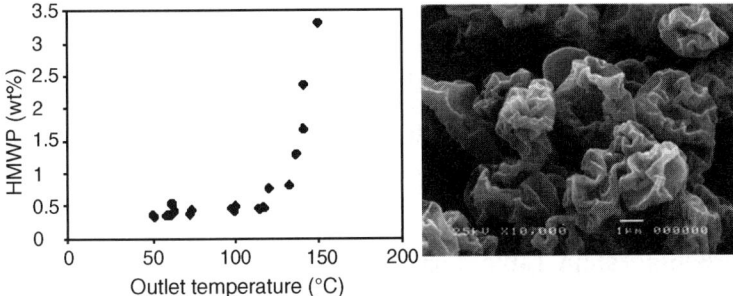

FIGURE 25 Spray dried insulin degradation to high molecular weight protein aggregates as a function of outlet air temperature. *Source*: Adapted from Ref. 10.

Effect of Atomization and Air–Liquid Interface on Protein Stability

Besides the stress caused by thermal dehydration, the protein is subjected to shear stress and exposed to an increased air–water interface during the atomization event. It has been shown that proteins can withstand shear rates in the order of magnitude of those found in spray drying and therefore are not expected to be a source of instability (62). However, significant instability can be caused when shear stress is combined with the rapid formation of an air–water interface (63). It has been shown that proteins such as human growth hormone with a pronounced amphiphilic nature adsorb at the air/water interface where they tend to unfold and undergo aggregation by the interaction of the hydrophobic region. It has also been shown that addition of surfactant to the feedstock solution is effective in preventing the formation of insoluble aggregates. However, because commonly used surfactants are liquid at ambient conditions (i.e., nonionic surfactants such as polysorbates and pluronics) it leads to the formation of cohesive particles that easily fuse, limiting their applicability to parenteral formulations where the interparticle interactions are not critical (24,40,64,65). Recently, the use of trileucine, a surface active tripeptide which is a solid at ambient conditions, has been demonstrated to both displace protein and peptides from the air–liquid interface thus reducing protein aggregation and reduce interparticle forces as well as producing low-density particles (23).

Coating and Encapsulation

The surface activity of the protein is an important determinant for stability at the air–liquid interface. However, when the droplet size distribution, solution concentration and drying rates are kept constant, the main driving force determining the surface composition is the diffusivity and solubility of the formulation components (26). In the case of spray dried protein formulations the slow diffusivity due to the large molecular weight of the API enriches the surface when the other components are small molecule excipients with significant solubility in water (e.g., sucrose, trehalose, mannitol, etc.). However, small molecule excipients with lower aqueous solubilities (e.g., isoleucine, leucine, trileucine, etc.) or exicipients with larger molecular weight can be used to control the surface composition.

Using this concept, spray drying has been utilized to engineer the radial composition of particles to effectively "coat" individual protein particles and to reduce or prevent surface-induced conformational changes of the protein during spray-drying (23,42). Effective spray-drying coating agents which have been demonstrated to coat small molecule, peptide and protein APIs as well as non-viral gene vectors include: trileucine (23), leucine (66,67), and dipalmitoylphosphatidylcholine (68).

When the degree of segregation leads to a complete phase separation it can be considered encapsulation. Spray drying has been shown an effective technique to encapsulate active ingredients using biodegradable polymers to sustain or modify the release of the active ingredient for several applications (8,69).

Fast Dissolving/Disintegrating Tablets and Powders

Fast dissolving/disintegrating tablets (FDDT) have recently being developed as alternative oral dosage forms for patients who may have difficulties swallowing tablets or liquids. FDDTs disintegrate and/or dissolve rapidly in saliva without the need of water often within a few seconds and are true fast dissolving tablets. Others contain excipients to enhance rate of tablet disintegration in the oral cavity and are more appropriately termed fast disintegrating tablets (70). Several production methods have been utilized, such as low pressure direct compression, wet granulation, molding, freeze drying, sublimation, and more recently spray drying. In order to allow fast dissolving tablets to dissolve in the mouth, they are made of either very porous and soft-molded matrices or compressed into tablets with very low compression force, which makes the tablets friable and/or brittle, which are difficult to handle, often requiring specialized peel-off blister packaging. There are several examples of commercially available products using these technologies (71).

Spray-drying has been used to produce highly porous solids to provide fast disintegration along with an amorphous API solid state for rapid dissolution (17,18). In one instance, the formulations that were produced contained hydrolyzed and unhydrolyzed gelatin as a support agent for the matrix, mannitol as a bulking agent, and sodium starch glycolate or crosscarmellose as a disintegrant. Disintegration and dissolution was further enhanced by adding citric acid or sodium bicarbonate. Tablets manufactured from this powder disintegrated in less than 20 seconds in an aqueous medium. In another example spray dried formulations containing super disintegrants (such as Ac-Di-Sol, Kollidon CL, sodium starch glycolate), diluent (mannitol) along with sweetening agent (aspartame) were used to prepare orally dissolving tables of water soluble and water insoluble drugs (17).

Micro- and Nanoparticles

As the demand for particle based drug delivery systems increase (e.g., inhalation, needless injection, colloidal, nanosuspensions, etc.), spray drying has been introduced as an efficient one-step process to produce particles which are uniform in composition and have a well-controlled size distribution. Spray drying is a technologically superior process to the traditional methods used for the production of particles such as pulverization of large particles using ball or jet milling, crystallization or solidification of emulsions. Preparation of particles down to several hundreds of nanometers in size may be possible for water insoluble compounds using a wet grinding method which requires a large amount of cogrinding agents or surfactants, and where the final product is usually supplied as a suspension and contamination from the grinding media and residual cogrinding agent are common issues to this method. Spray drying offers an alternate process to isolate nanoparticle suspensions into micron sized matrices; avoiding the intrinsic cohesiveness of the nanoparticles. For example, the bioavailability of nanosized crystalline drug was improved when spray dried from a non-aqueous solution containing pluronic F127 (72). The reduction in the drug particle size, coupled with the surfactant wetting effect resulted in a fast onset formulation with bioavailablity comparable of that of a solution formulation. In addition, dispersion of the nanosized particles into a solid matrix improved its physical stability.

Spray drying has been proposed as a means of providing a carrier for efficient nanoparticle delivery (Fig. 26). A nanoparticle suspension was spray dried in the presence of lactose, used as a carrier, to demonstrate that nanoparticles remained in the nano-range size after spray drying and provide a means to improve their delivery by inhalation (73). Nanoparticles made out of polystyrene, colloidal silica (20) as well as gelatin and polycyanoacrylate (73) have been spray dried in the presence of lactose DPPC or DMP to improve their drug delivery efficiency.

Water insoluble nanoparticles embedded into water soluble carriers enable fast dispersion of the nanoparticles once in contact with the biological target. In the examples above nanoparticles suspended in a solution containing the soluble formulation components was spray dried. A one-step process to spray dry solution incompatible compounds based on a multinozzle system has been described (74). For example, chitosan dissolves in acid solutions forming a gel but it is insoluble in alkaline solutions, in contrast hydroxypropylmethylcellulose phthalate (HPMCP) is insoluble in acid solutions but soluble in alkaline solutions. Sustained release composite particles containing acetaminophen, chitosan and HPMCP as a carrier have been prepared using a 4-fluid nozzle spray-dryer (75). Acetominophen and chitosan were dissolved in the acidic solutions and HPMCP was dissolved in alkaline solutions and spray dried into three-component composite particles. Similarly polymeric submicron particles made out of PLGA or ethylcelluose, both water insoluble, alone or in combination with polyethylenimine and mannitol as a carrier have been prepared using the multinozzle spray drying approach (76).

Solid State Control

APIs are usually produced by extraction or chemical synthesis and isolated through a multiple step process comprised of controlled crystallization, solid–liquid separation, and drying. A post-drying step such as micronization is frequently needed to adjust particle properties such as size distribution and bulk density. Some pharmaceutical compounds are particularly difficult to micronize by conventional grinding or jet milling. For example, materials that have low-melting point or that are waxy can smear or form amorphous material. Spray drying is gaining popularity, replacing multi-step processes, to manufacture pharmaceutical materials where control of the particle size distribution, residual moisture content, bulk density and morphology is desired. Spray drying is notable for changing the solid state properties of drug compounds. To overcome these limitations, a multizonal spray drying process has been used to *purposefully control* the solid state of the drug compounds (15). This is achieved by controlling the residence time and the evaporation rate by adjusting the relative humidity or solvent vapor concentration during drying.

Solid Dispersions

Solid dispersions in water-soluble carriers have attracted considerable interest as a means of improving the dissolution rate, and oral bioavailability, of a range of hydrophobic drugs (77–80), however, commercialization has been limited because of

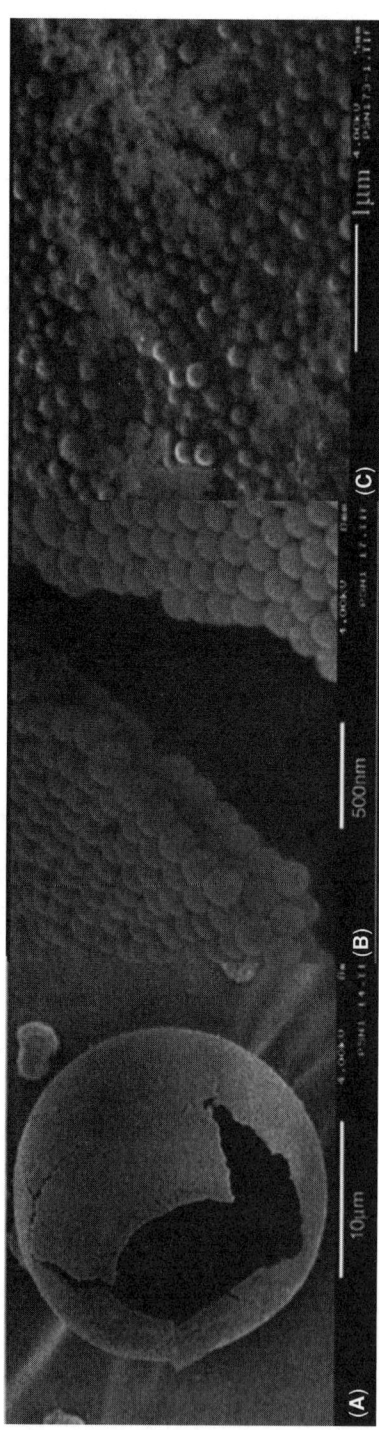

FIGURE 26 SEM images of (**A**) a typical carrier particle observed from spray drying a suspension of nanoparticles (170 nm), (**B**) a magnified view of particle surface, and (**C**) nanoparticles in solution after redissolving the carrier particles in a mixture of ethanol:water (70:30 v/v).
Source: From Ref. 20.

difficulties of conventional methods of preparation, mainly lack of feasibility for scaling up laboratory manufacturing process such as melt quenching or vacuum drying. The concept of using spray drying to produce solid dispersions for further processing into oral applications has been used since as early as 1980s (4,5,81,82), however, based on the increased number of academic and patent publications, there seems to be a renewed interest motivated by the increasing number of insoluble drugs which require a bioavailability improvement.

One perceived disadvantage of solid dispersions is the notion that they are unstable, because these are amorphous dispersions which tend to degrade faster and often crystallize upon storage. There are however published examples where the main purpose of enhancing dissolution rate of a poorly water soluble compound is achieved and long-term stability of tablets containing the solid dispersion has been shown (5). This was accomplished by spray drying oxazepman with Gelita collagel and lactose.

Other examples include spray drying amorphous simvastatin in the presence of PVP to improve the dissolution rate and oral bioavailability in rats (83) as well as the preparation of formulations for controlled delivery of a poorly soluble anticancer drug spray dried in the presence of TPGS and PEG (84).

Spray drying of a nonaqueous system has also been shown, a Gelucire 50/13 based solid dispersions have been prepared to stabilize and improve in vivo performance of hydrophobic drugs (79,80).

Other applications include the solid state stabilization of an inclusion complex by spray drying an aqueous solution of celecoxib and beta cyclodextrin which also results in an increase in dissolution rate.

Granulation

Use of spray drying to prepare granules for subsequent processing into a dosage form is not a new concept (85). Unlike the traditional granulation process where a granule is formed by agglomerating dry particles through compaction or addition of water and agglomerating excipients, spray drying has been utilized to form a granular product with adequate particle size control (50–150 µm) from a solution or a suspension. The solution or suspension may be of drug alone, a single excipient or a complete formulation. The resultant granules are free-flowing particles. Often the distribution of the binder in such granules favors the surface due to the solute migration during drying, which results in good compaction properties. This process can be used to make tablet granules, although it is probably economically justified for this purpose only when suitable granules cannot be produced by the other methods. Also, spray-drying can convert hard elastic materials into more ductile ones in the case of direct compression excipients as it is explained below. The primary advantages of the process are the short drying time and the minimal exposure of the product to heat owing to the short residence time in the drying chamber, as discussed above. Little deterioration of heat-sensitive materials takes place, and it may be the only process suitable for this type of product.

Spray drying has been integrated with fluidized bed systems. The integrated fluid bed can be either stationary with a back mix or plug flow design, depending on the cohesiveness of the product leaving the drying chamber. For example, products that can be directly fluidizable immediately after drying are appropriate for the stationary plug flow fluid bed whereas the back mix design is better for handling products that fluidize poorly due to their particle size distribution, morphology or moisture content or those that only flow after a short time in the fluidizing layer when the moisture content has been lowered.

Excipients

Spray drying has been used to produce excipients with improved performance. For example, spray dried lactose, obtained from spray drying a lactose aqueous suspension, has been available for many years and offers the advantage being directly compressible due to the more ductile amorphous lactose that is formed during drying by itself or in the presence of dicalcium phosphate (2,51). Microcrystalline cellulose is also another common pharmaceutical excipient that is available in a spray dried form. Spray dried mixtures of lactose and starch (85%/15%wt) as well as spray dried calcium carbonate and microcrystalline cellulose mixtures have been recently developed as direct compression excipient and are commercially available (86). Spray dried crystalline mannitol has been developed and show superiority in direct compression applications to other forms of crystalline mannitol (87). Other specialty excipients such as cyclodextrins that improve drug solubility forming an inclusion complex are also spray dried into a dry solid while maintaining solubility improvements (88,89).

CONCLUSIONS

The basic theory of spray drying is well understood and enables excellent control of the critical variables which affect product attributes. Judging by the number of recent publications described in the present chapter, which is not exhaustive by any means, one can conclude that spray drying is a process that meets the demand of sophisticated drug delivery systems through an efficient, one-step process capable or precise particle size and drug content control.

ACKNOWLEDGEMENTS

The authors would like to thank the following people at Nektar Therapeutics whose work contributed to this chapter: Andrew Boeckl, Dr. Christopher Varga, and Dr. Zhuoxiong Mao.

REFERENCES

1. Masters K. Applications of Spray Drying. Spray Drying Handbook. 3rd ed. New York: Halsted Press, 1979: 481–516.
2. Gunsel WC, Lachman L. Comparative evaluation of tablet formulations prepared from conventionally-processed and spray-dried lactose. J Pharm Sci 1963, 52:178–82.
3. Broadhead J, Rouan SKE, Rhodes CT. The spray drying of pharmaceuticals. Drug Dev Ind Pharm 1992; 18:1169–206.
4. Lo WY, Law SL. Dissolution behavior of griseofulvin solid dispersions using polyethylene glycol, talc, and their combination as dispersion carriers. Drug Dev Ind Pharm 1996; 22: 231–6.
5. Jachowicz R, Nurnberg E, Hoppe R. Solid dispersions of oxazepam. Int J Pharm 1993; 99: 321–5.
6. Vidgren P, Vidgren M, Paronen P. Physical stability and inhalation behavior of mechanically micronized and spray dried disodium cromoglcate in different humidities. Acta Pharmaceutica Fennica 1989; 98:71–8.
7. Maa Y-f, Nguyen P-A, Andya JD, et al. Effect of spray drying and subsequent processing conditions on residual moisture content and physical biochemical stability of protein inhalation powders. Pharm Res 1998; 15:768–75.

8. Vanbever R, Ben-Jebria A, Mintzes JD, Langer R, Edwards DA. Sustained-release of insulin from insoluble inhaled particles. Drug Dev Res 1999: 48:178–85.
9. Duddu SP, Sisk SA, Walter YH, et al. Improved lung delivery from a passive dry powder inhaler using an engineered PulmoSphere (R) powder. Pharm Res 2002; 19:689–95.
10. Ståhl K, Claesson M, Lilliehorn P, Linden H, Backstrom K. The effect of process variables on the degradation and physical properties of spray dried insulin inteded for inhalation. Int J Pharm 2002; 233:227–37.
11. Chan HK, Clark AR, Feeley J, et al. Physical stability of salmon calcitonin spray-dried powders for inhalation. J Pharm Sci 2004; 93:792–804.
12. White S, Bennett DB, Cheu S, et al. EXUBERA®: Pharmaceutical development of a novel product for pulmonary delivery of insulin. Diabetes Tech Ther 2005; 7:896–906.
13. Patton J. Breathing life into protein drugs. Nature Biotech 1998; 16:141–3.
14. Labrude P, Rasolomanana M, Vigneron C, Thirion C, Chillot B. Protective effect of sucrose on spray drying of oxyhemoglobin. J Pharm Sci 1989; 78:223–9.
15. Bennett DB, K. BT, Snyder HE, Platz RM, Inventors; Nektar Therapeutics, Inc., assignee. Spray drying process control of drying kinetics. US patent 20030044460, 2000.
16. Martino PD, Scoppa M, Joiris E, et al. The spray drying of acetozolamide as method to modify crystal properties and to improve compression behaviour. Int J Pharm 2001; 213:209–21.
17. Mishra DN, Bindal M, Singh S-K, Vijaya-Kumar S-G. Spray dried excipient base: A novel technique for the formulation of orally disintegrating tablets. Chem Pharm Bull 2006; 54:99–102.
18. Allen LV, Wang B, Davies JD. Inventors; The Board of Regents of the University of Oklahoma and Janssen assignee. Rapidly dissolving dosage form. US patent 6,066,337. July 6, 1998, 2000.
19. Hino T, Shimabayashi S, Nakai A. Silk microspheres prepared by spray-drying of an aqueous system. Pharm Pharmacol Commun 2000; 6:335–9.
20. Tsapis N, Bennett D, Jackson B, Weitz DA, Edwards DA. Trojan particles: Large porous carriers of nanoparticles for drug delivery. Proc Natl Acad Sci USA 2002; 99:1200–15.
21. Skalko-Basnet N, Pavelic Z, Becirevic-Lacan M. Liposomes containing drug and cyclodextrin prepared by the one-step spray-drying method. Drug Dev Ind Pharm 2000; 26:1279–84.
22. Lo Y-l, Tsai J-C, Kuo J-H. Liposomes and disaccharides as carriers in spray-dried powder-formulations of superoxide dismutase J Control Release 2004; 94:259–72.
23. Lechuga-Ballesteros D, Charan C, Stults CLM, et al. Trileucine improves aerosol performance and stability of spray-dried powders for inhalation. J Pharm Sci 2007; 96(5):1258–69.
24. Fäldt P, Bergenståhl B. The surface composition of spray-dried protein–lactose powders. Physiochem Eng Aspects 1993:183–90.
25. Millqvist-Fureby A, Malmsten M, Bergenstahl B. Surface characterization of freeze-dried protein/carbohydrate mixtures. Int J Pharm 1999; 191:103–14.
26. Vehring R, Lechuga-Ballesteros D, Foss WR. Particle formation in spray drying. J Aerosol Sci 2007, Submitted.
27. Raula J, Eerikäinen H, Kauppinen EI. Influence of the solvent composition on the aerosol synthesis of pharmaceutical polymer nanoparticles. Int J Pharm 2004; 284:13–21.
28. Elversson J, Millqvist-Fureby A. Particle size and density in spray drying-effects of carbohydrate properties. J Pharm Sci 2005; 94:2049–60.
29. Maa Y-F, Costantino HR, Nguyen P-A, Hsu CC. The effects of operating and formulation variables on the morphology of spray-dried protein particles. Pharm Dev Tech 1997; 2:213–23.
30. Vanbever R, Mintzes JD, Wang J, et al. Formulation and physical characterization of large porous particles for inhalation. Pharm Res 1999; 16:1735–42.
31. Varga CM, Snyder HE. High-magnification shadowgraphy characterization of rotary atomizer droplet production for pharmaceutical applications. Institute for liquid atomization and spraying systems conference. Toronto, Ontario, Canada; 2006.

32. Lefebvre AH. Atomization and Sprays. New York: Hemisphere Publishing Corporation, 1989.
33. Varga CM, Snyder HE. Impact of liquid viscosity on droplet sizes produced from air-assist atomizers. Institute for liquid atomization and spraying systems conference. Monterey, California, 2003.
34. Sonntag RE, Van Wylen GV. Introduction to Thermodynamics, Classical and Statistical. 2nd ed. New York: Wiley and Sons, 1982.
35. Fuchs NA. Evaporation and Droplet Growth in Gaseous Media. New York: Pergamon Press, 1959.
36. Crowe C, Sommerfeld M, Tsuji Y. Multiphase Flows with Droplets and Particles. Boca Raton, FL: CRC Press, 1998.
37. Straub JA, Chickering DE, Lovely JC, et al. Intravenous hydrophobic drug delivery: A porous particle formulation of paclitaxel (AI-850). Pharm Res 2005; 22:347–55.
38. Shekunov BY, Chow AHL, Feeley JC, Tong HHY, York P. Aerosolisation behaviour of micronised and supercritically-processed powders. Aerosol Sci 2003; 34:553–68.
39. Chew NY, Chan HK. Use of solid corrugated particles to enhance powder aerosol performance. Pharm Res 2001; 18:1570–7.
40. Adler M, Unger M, Lee G. Surface composition of spray-dried particles of bovine serum albumin/trehalose/surfactant. Pharm. Res. 2000; 17:863–70.
41. Abdul-Fattah A, Lechuga-Ballesteros D, Kalonia D, Pikal MJ. The impact of drying method and formulation on the physical properties and stability of methionyl human growth hormone in the amorphous solid state. J Pharm Sci 2007; Accepted.
42. Elversson J, Millqvist-Fureby A. In situ coating—An approach for particle modification and encapsulation of proteins during spray-drying. Int J Pharm 2006; 323:52–63.
43. Finlay WH ed. The Mechanics of Inhaled Pharmaceutical Aerosols. An Introduction. New York: Academic Press, 2001.
44. Heumann WL. Industrial Air Pollution Control Systems. New York: McGraw-Hill, 1997.
45. Clark AR, Egan M. Modelling the deposition of inhaled powdered drug aerosols. J Aerosol Sci 1994; 25:175–86.
46. Clark AR. Medical aerosol inhalers: past, present, and future. Aerosol Sci Tech 1995; 22: 374–91.
47. Hsu CC, Wu SS, Walsh AJ. The preparation of recombinant human deoxyribonuclease powder: comparative studies of spray drying versus lyophilization and application of microwave drying. In: Strumillo C, Pakowski Z, eds. Drying '96. Vol B. Krakow, Poland: Lodz Technical University, Dep. of Process and Environmental Engineering, 1996: 1229–36.
48. Labuza TP. The effect of water activity on reaction kinetics of food deterioration. Food Tech 1980; 34:36–41, 59.
49. Costantino HR. Excipients for use in lyophilized pharmaceutical peptide, protein, and other bioproducts. In: Pikal MJ, Costantino HR, eds. Lyophilization of Biomaterials. AAPS Press, 2004:139–228.
50. Franks F, Hatley RHM, Mathias SF. Material science and the production of shelf-stable biologicals. Pharm Technol Int 1991; 3:24–34.
51. Forbes RT, Davis KG, Hindle M, Clarke JG, Mass J. Water vapor sorption studies on the physical stability of a series of spray-dried protein/sugar powders for inhalation. J Pharm Sci 1998; 87:1316–21.
52. Naini V, Byron P, Phillips EM. Physicochemical stability of crystalline sugars and their spray-dried forms: dependence upon relative humidity and suitability for use in powder inhalers. Drug Dev Ind Pharm 1998; 24:895–909.
53. Abdul-Fattah A, Kalonia DS, Pikal MJ. The challenge of drying method selection for protein pharmaceuticals: Product quality implications. J Pharm Sci 2007, Online ahead of publication.
54. Maa Y-F, Prestrelski SJ. Biopharmaceutical powders: Particle formation and formulation considerations. Curr Pharm Biotech 2000; 1:283–302.

55. Lechuga-Ballesteros D, Miller DP, Zhang J. Residual water in amorphous solids, measurement and effects on stability. In: Levine H, ed. Progress in Amorphous Food and Pharmaceutical Systems. London: The Royal Society of Chemistry, 2002: 275–316.
56. Maa Y-F, Costantino HR, Nguyen P-A, Hsu CC. The Effect of operating and formulation variables on the morphology of spray-dried protein particles. Pharm Dev Tech 1997; 2:213–23.
57. Mumenthaler M, Hsu CC, Pearlman R. Feasibility study on spray-drying protein pharmaceuticals: Recombinant human growth hormone and tissue-type plasminogen activator. Pharm Res 1994; 11:12.
58. Broadhead J, Rouan SKE, Hau I, Rhodes CT. The effect of process and formulation variables on the properties of spray-dried galactosidas. J Pharm Pharmacol 1994; 64:458–67.
59. Hageman MJ. The role of moisture in protein stability. Drug Dev Ind Pharm 1988; 14: 2047–70.
60. Ståhl K, Claesson M, Lilliehorn P, Lindén H, Bäckström K. The effect of process variables on the degradation and physical properties of spray dried insulin intended for inhalation. Int J Pharm 2002; 233:227–37.
61. Maa Y-F, Nguyen P-A, Sweeney T, Shire SJ, Hsu CC. Protein inhalation powders: Spray drying vs. Spray freeze drying. Pharm Res 1999; 16(2):249–54.
62. Maa Y-F, Hsu CC. Effect of high shear on proteins. Biotech Bioeng 1996; 51:458–65.
63. Maa Y-F, Hsu CC. Protein denaturation by combined effect of shear and air-liquid Interface. Biotech Bioeng 1997; 54:503–12.
64. Maa Y-F, Nguyen P-A, Hsu SW. Spray drying of air-liquid interface sensitive recombinant human growth hormone. J Pharm Sci 1998; 87:152–9.
65. Adler M, Lee G. Stability and surface activity of lactate dehydrogenase in spray-dried trehalose. J Pharm Sci 1999; 88:199–208.
66. Chew NYK, Shekunov BY, Chow HHYTAHL, Savage C, Wu J, Chan H-K. Effect of amino acids on the dispersion of disodium cromoglycate powders. J Pharm Sci 2005; 94: 2289–300.
67. Li H-Y, Neill H, Innocent R, Seville P, Williamson I, Birchall JC. Enhanced dispersibility and deposition of spray-dried powders for pulmonary gene therapy. J Drug Target 2003; 11: 425–32.
68. Bosquillon C, Lombry C, Preat V, Vanbever R. Influence of formulation excipients and physical characteristics of inhalation dry powders on their aerosolization performance. J Control Release 2001; 70:329–39.
69. Fernandez-Carballido A, Herrero-Vanrell R, T. M-MI, Pastoriza P. Biodegradable Ibuprofen-loaded PLGA microspheres for intraarticular administration. Effect of Labrafil addition on release in vitro. Int J Pharm 2004; 279:33–41.
70. Bogner RH, Wilkosz MF. Fast-dissolving tablets. US Pharmacist. 2002, http://www.uspharmacist.com/oldformat.asp?url=newlook/files/feat/fastdissolving.htm
71. Patel PB, Chaudhary A, Gupta GD. Fast Dissolving Drug Delivery Systems: An Update. 2006, http://www.pharmainfo.net/exclusive/reviews/
72. Yin SX, Franchini M, Chen J, et al. Bioavailability enhancement of a COX-2 inhibitor, BMS-347070, from a nanocrystalline dispersion prepared by spray-drying. J Pharm Sci 2005; 94: 1598–607.
73. Shama JO-H, Zhang Y, Finlay WH, Roa WH, Löbenberg R. Formulation and characterization of spray-dried powders containing nanoparticles for aerosol delivery to the lung. Int J Pharm 2004; 269:457–67.
74. Snyder HE, Vosgber MJ, Varga CM, Inventors; Nektar Therapeutics, Inc., assignee. Spray drying methods and related compositions. US patent 20030124193, 2003.
75. Chen RC, Takahashi H, Okamoto H, Danjo K. Particle design of three-component system for sustained release using a 4-fluid nozzle spray-drying technique. Chem Pharm Bull 2006; 54: 1486–90.
76. Ozeki T, Beppu S, Mizoe T, Takashima Y, Yuasa H, Okada H. Preparation of polymeric submicron particle-containing microparticles using a 4-fluid nozzle spray drier. Pharm Res 2006; 23:177–83.

77. Serajuddin ATM. Solid dispersion of poorly water-soluble drugs: Early promises, subsequent problems, and recent breakthroughs. J Pharm Sci 1999; 88:1058–66.
78. Leuner C, Dressman J. Improving drug solubility for oral delivery using solid dispersions. Eur J Pharm Biopharm 2000; 50:47–60.
79. Chauhan B, Shimpi S, Paradkar A. Preparation and characterization of etoricoxib solid dispersions using lipid carriers by spray drying technique. AAPS Pharm Sci Tech 2005; 6: E405–E412.
80. Shimpi SL, Chauhan B, Mahadik KR, Paradkar A. Stabilization and improved in vivo performance of amorphous etoricoxib using Gelucire 50/13. Pharm Res 2005; 22:1727–34.
81. Bloch D. Spray-dried solid dispersions of hydrochlorothiazide and chlorthalidone in pentaerythritol. Pharm Acta Helvetica 1983; 58:14.
82. Corrigan O. Physicochemical properties of spray dried drugs: phenobarbitone and hydroflumethiazide. Drug Dev Ind Pharm 1983; 9:1.
83. Ambike AA, Mahadik KR, Paradkar A. Spray-dried amorphous solid dispersions of simvastatin, a low Tg drug: in vitro and in vivo evaluations. Pharm Res 2005; 22:990–8.
84. Mu L, Teo MM, Ning HZ, Tan CS, Feng SS. Novel powder formulations for controlled delivery of poorly soluble anticancer drug:application and investigation of TPGS and PEG in spray-dried particulate system. J Control Rel 2005; 103:565–75.
85. Kornblum SS. Sustained-action tablets prepared by employing a spray-drying technique for granulation. J Pharm Sci 1968; 58:125–7.
86. Gohel MC. A review of co-processed directly compressible excipients. J Pharm Pharm Sci 2005; 8:76–93.
87. Nuguru KS, Giambattisto D, Al-Ghazawi AK. Evaluation and characterization of spray-dried mannitol as an excipient for direct copression formulations of naproxen sodium. AAPS Pharm Sci 2001; 3:Abstract available from: http://www.aapspharmsci.org/
88. Hassan H, Kata M, Ers I, Aigner Z. Preparation and investigation of inclusion complexes containing gemfibrozil and DIMEB. J Incl Phenom Macrocyclic Chem 2004; 50:219–25.
89. Dollo G, Corre PL, Chollet M, et al. Improvement in solubility and dissolution rate of 1, 2-dithiole-3-thiones upon complexation with beta-cyclodextrin and its hydroxypropyl and sulfobutyl ether-7 derivatives. J Pharm Sci 1999; 88:889–95.
90. Lucas P, Anderson K, Staniforth JN. Protein deposition from dry powder inhaler: Fine particle mutiplets as performance modifiers. Pharm Res 1998; 15:562–9.

8
Pharmaceutical Granulation Processes, Mechanism, and the Use of Binders

Stuart L. Cantor, Larry L. Augsburger, and Stephen W. Hoag
School of Pharmacy, University of Maryland, Baltimore, Maryland, U.S.A.

Armin Gerhardt
Libertyville, Illinois, U.S.A.

INTRODUCTION

The wet granulation process has been impacted over the last 25 years by the development of improved equipment, innovative research, novel polymeric binders, and even Process Analytical Technologies (PAT) applications that accurately measure granule growth using a Lasentec® (Mettler Toledo, Inc. Columbus, Ohio, U.S.A.) focused beam reflectance measurement (FBRM) or through the use of near-infrared spectroscopy/ chemometrics and computer modeling. Changes such as the refinement of high shear granulators and fluid bed processors have enabled a faster throughput of batches and more accurate process monitoring. Furthermore, development of laboratory-scale models of these two pieces of equipment has made the production of many small batches of costly drugs possible for research purposes. Also, some binders for wet granulation are no longer widely used while other synthetic polymers with different functionalities have supplanted them largely due to regulatory concerns as well as their easier preparation and subsequent quality impact on both the granulation and final tablets.

Granulation has been defined as "any process whereby small particles are gathered into larger, permanent masses in which the original particles can still be identified (1)." It is an example of particle design intended to produce improved performance through the combination of formulation composition and manufacturing processes; and a modified particle morphology is achieved through the use of a liquid acting on the powder blend to form interparticulate bonds which then result in granules of varying sizes. For many centuries, medicinal powders have been combined with honey or sugar in a hand rolling process to produce pills. With the development of tablet presses in the 19th century and their ever-increasing production rates, the demands made on the powder feed materials increased commensurately, as did the understanding of the materials, the machinery and processes, and the subsequent evaluation techniques of the finished products. Granules are primarily used in the manufacture of tablets, though they may also be used to fill hard gelatin capsules, or they may become a sachet product when a large dose exceeds the capacity to swallow easily.

As practiced in the pharmaceutical industry, granulation is often the first processing step where multiple formulation components are combined. Performance during tablet compression is dependent on all prior unit operations; and as granulation is frequently the most complex and difficult process to control, it deserves special emphasis during formulation development. In addition, because suppliers of excipients prefer to have a relatively wide set of specifications for individual materials, this situation creates the necessity for the granulation operation to be sufficiently robust that it yields consistent product throughout the preparation of clinical supplies and through the entire commercial lifetime of the finished dosage form. This inherent variability of the neat components makes it imperative to evaluate multiple lots of the individual components (preferably at the limits of important specification parameters, e.g., particle size distribution and moisture content. This is typically done in the pilot plant with the aid of a statistically designed factorial experiment, and this may be required to be repeated intermittently as the manufacturing process/specifications evolve over time.

During formulation development of a new molecular entity, both the processing sequence and the composition of finished product are optimized. Typically, the final formulation composition is completed first, with subsequent optimization of the processing sequence continuing through Phase I and II clinical studies for a single formulation; the goal being delivery of Phase III clinical supplies that are representative of commercial product and can be validated prior to launch. As part of the processing sequence optimization, granulation may be incorporated to meet a number of objectives, as shown in Table 1. However, the main goals of granulation are to improve the flow and compression characteristics of the blend, and to prevent component segregation. Granules

TABLE 1 Selected Granulation Binders, Method of Incorporation, and Usage Levels

Binder	Method of addition	Formulation percentage
Natural polymers		
Starch	Wet mix	2–5
Pregelatinized starch	Wet mix	2–5
Pregelatinized starch	Dry mix	5–10
Gelatin	Wet mix	1–3
Alginic acid	Dry mix	3–5
Sodium alginate	Wet mix	1–3
Synthetic and semi-synthetic polymers		
PVP	Wet mix	0.5–5
PVP	Dry mix	5–10
Methyl cellulose	Wet mix	1–5
Methyl cellulose	Dry mix	5–10
HPMC	Wet mix	2–5
HPMC	Dry mix	5–10
Polymethacrylates	Wet mix	15–35 as solution (4.5–10.5% w/w solids)
Polymethacrylates	Dry mix	10–35
Sodium CMC	Wet mix	1–5
Sodium CMC	Dry mix	5–10
Sugars		
Glucose	Wet mix	2–25
Sucrose	Wet mix	2–25
Sorbitol	Wet mix	2–10

Abbreviations: CMC, Carboxymethylcellulose; HPMC, Hydroxypropylmethylcellulose; PVP, Polyvinylpyrrolidone.
Source: Modified from Ref. 62.

flow better and are usually more compactible than the original powders. Granulation also permits handling of powders without loss of blend quality, since after blending particles are locked in-place within granules in a form of ordered mix.

Wet granulation is a complex process with a combination of several critical formulation and process variables greatly affecting the outcome. For example, determination of the granulation endpoint is still considered by many to be an art, with knowledge only gained through years of hands-on experience. Moreover, the range of liquid that can be added during mixing is very narrow and overwetting a granulation can make the batch unusable.

Granulation is a process of size enlargement used primarily to prepare powders for tableting. It consists of homogeneously mixing the drug and filler powders together and then wetting them in the presence of a binder so that larger agglomerates or granules are formed. The moist granules are then dried to a low-moisture content, generally less than 3%, and either sieved to eliminate oversize and fines or passed through a mill to obtain the desired particle size and size distribution for tableting. The percentage of fines left behind after drying gives a good indication of the extent of granule growth. The wet mass can also be passed through a sieve while wet; especially, for quite cohesive powders this can help reduce the percentage of oversize particles.

Wet granulation can serve several important functions such as improving the release rate and bioavailability of poorly soluble drugs by forming a hydrophilic film of the binder over the surfaces of the drug granules; this improves their wettability and thus, dissolution rate (1). It also improves the flowability of powdered blends by reducing the cohesiveness of the powder particles, reduces the fines, thus improving the blend's electrostatic properties, and increases the average particle size; these factors can also improve the mechanical properties of the tablets. Wet granulation is an especially useful process for improving the content uniformity of tablets prepared using low-dose drugs (<20 mg).

The ability to deliver final product content uniformity of commercial batches and eliminate segregation during subsequent unit operations for a wide range of active pharmaceutical ingredient dosages are critical attributes, as is the delivery of consistent powder flow rates that yield minimal weight variability during the compression of tablets or plug formation for insertion within hard gelatin capsule shells. The capacity to control both raw material fluctuations and manufacturing parameters through numerous commercial batches throughout the product's life cycle is critical.

The decision on whether to include a granulation operation should also be based on knowledge of the potential disadvantages associated with it. Among these factors are higher production costs due to the increased time, labor, equipment, energy, and testing to control the process, additional processing steps to remove the added liquid and/or mill the resultant granules, variable granulation product quality, material loss, material transfer. In addition, the addition of a granulating fluid introduces disadvantages such as: controlling the time of solvent interaction with the powders, potential alteration of drug dissolution rate, drug stability, validation challenges, and the need for improved in-line, real-time endpoint detection that predicts total performance. When these disadvantages outweigh the advantages of granulation, it may be worthwhile to consider a direct compression sequence and eliminate not only the granulation/drying step, but also the milling/size reduction operation.

FORMULATION

At the initial stage of a tablet manufacturing project, the formulation team is required to produce product for both stability studies and human clinical studies. This is typically complicated by additional constraints of minimal drug quantity availability and aggressive timelines. It is important to recognize that formulators generally distinguish two phases in developing granulation formulations, i.e., the intra- and extragranular phases. Generally, the active, any filler(s), and perhaps certain other components as required are granulated. These components that form the granules are considered intragranular components. The disintegrant, lubricant, and glidant (if needed) are blended with the dried finished granulation to produce the running mix that will be compressed. These components make up the extragranular phase. Often, formulators will divide the disintegrant between the intra- and extragranular phases to optimize disintegration time (2). In theory, the extragranular disintegrant is expected to facilitate disintegration of the dosage form into granules, while the intragranular disintegrant is expected to facilitate granule disintegration into primary particles.

Microcrystalline cellulose can play a unique role in granulation. Usually regarded as a direct compression filler–binder because of its high compactibility, microcrystalline cellulose is sometimes also added extragranularly, often at a level of 10–25%, to enhance the compactibility of the running mix when the granulation itself lacks sufficient compactibility. Furthermore, even though it loses compactibility following wet granulation, microcrystalline cellulose may be added intragranularly as a granulation aid, often at a level between 5% and 20%, where its hydrophilicity and water holding capacity benefit the granulation and drying processes. Its presence intragranularly promotes rapid, even wetting and drying, which helps to avoid overrunning the granulation endpoint during high shear mixing and reducing the tendency toward uneven distribution of soluble colorants (and other soluble components) that can result from migration during granulation drying. Based on specific data from preformulation studies and other constraints, improved initial formulations may be utilized.

Currently the solvent of choice for wet granulation processes is water, namely, purified water, USP. As the formulation components typically contain large fractions of organic composition, it is necessary to minimize the potential for microbial contamination and growth by removing the water quickly once the granules have been formed. When a binder (e.g., povidone) is dissolved prior to the granulation step, adequate controls are required to limit the duration prior to use. Addition of the solvent is done via either spraying from a nozzle or pumping through an open tube. When a spray nozzle is employed, the solvent is distributed over a much larger surface area, whereas the open tube approach relies on the granulator to distribute the solvent, however, either approach may be successful.

Ethanol and hydroethanolic mixtures are alternative solvents, which may be utilized when a drug sensitive to hydrolysis is developed. However, there are certain drawbacks to using such solvents. Due to their increased lipophilicity, they impact powder wetting and granule properties. Furthermore, there is an increased safety hazard of potential detonation during drying, which requires associated venting and suppression equipment and facilities modification. In additional, environmental concerns and regulatory constraints that limit volatile organic compounds and requirements for residual solvent levels, documentation requirements, and costs, along with options to utilize dry granulation techniques, have limited their use; so that today, the wet granulation process is largely aqueous based, utilizing water or perhaps hydroalcoholic solutions containing a majority of water rather than solvents.

A binder may be included in the formulation to increase particle cohesion and acts to facilitate granule nucleation and growth; thus, the binder impacts flow properties and may also improve tablet crushing strength and reduce friability. The spreading of a hydrophilic binder over particle surfaces and subsequent drying during the granulation process may also improve the dissolution of hydrophobic or poorly soluble drugs from granulations by enhancing particle wettability. This process is sometimes referred to as hydrophilization (3–5). Excess binder must be avoided and care must be taken to control the quantity of binder employed to avoid any possible deleterious impact on tablet disintegration and dissolution rate.

Among the factors impacting binder performance in high shear equipment are the binder quantity, binder addition method (wet vs dry), solvent quantity, solvent addition rate and method (spray vs open tube), wet massing time, impeller speed, chopper speed, and equipment design; and these parameters need to be optimized during the development process, typically with the aid of a statistically designed set of experiments.

Improved understanding of the behavior of amorphous polymeric binders during the wet granulation process is critical to better formulation development. A model wet granulation system was recently developed containing lactose monohydrate granulated in a planetary mixer with an aqueous 12% w/v solution of polyvinylpyrrolidone (PVP) K30 and studied using high speed Differential Scanning Calorimetry (DSC) equipment which enabled very short run times. Buckton et al. (6) recently reported on the first measurement of in situ properties of a binder present in the granules. Furthermore, the authors also stated that this granulation process resulted in a solid dispersion of PVP and amorphous lactose and that changes in the binder properties over time such as crystallization could be expected and could impact tablet tensile strength.

A novel granulation technique was reported using steam instead of water as the binder in a high-shear mixer (7). The poorly soluble diclofenac (0.02 mg/mL) was used as the model drug at 10% w/w along with polyethylene glycol (PEG) 4000 as the excipient (90% w/w). Steam granules were compared with granules produced by other traditional techniques, namely, wet, and melt granulation. Steam granules had a more spherical shape and a larger surface area and DSC/powder X-ray diffraction confirmed that the drug was transformed from its original crystalline form into an amorphous form. Dissolution testing showed an increased dissolution rate of the drug from the granules as compared with either the pure drug or a physical mixture. This increased dissolution rate is likely due to the increased surface area of the steam granules.

On the other hand, the steam granulation process using acetaminophen at 15% was compared against two other wet granulation methods; using water, and using a PVP K30 binder solution at 5%. All three methods used a high shear mixer. The results indicated that the use of steam as a granulating liquid enabled a reduction in the drying time as a lower amount of water was used. The steam granules had the lowest dissolution rate over 10 hours as compared with the other two methods. Additionally, sensory evaluation results showed that the acetaminophen was successfully taste-masked in the steam granules (8). However, even with these latest technological innovations, "the lack of predictive behavior of the granulation process has complicated the development of suitable models, and consequently, the granulation process is often considered to require a trial-and-error approach (9)."

BINDER FUNCTIONALITY

Binders are just one of the critical excipients for a successful wet granulation formulation, as they are used to create an ordered mixture of all the ingredients by creating a cohesive network. While more than 30 different materials have been studied over the years, currently there are only about a dozen binders that are commonly used as granulating agents and these can be subdivided into three main categories, (i) sugars such as sucrose, glucose (10), or sorbitol (11), for use primarily in chewable tablets; (*ii*) natural polymers and gums such as pregelatinized starch (12–15), starch (16–18), acacia, gelatin, and sodium alginate, although the latter four are rarely used today; (3) synthetic polymers which include PVP (8,19–24), PEG (7,25–28), all the semi-synthetic cellulose derivatives (e.g., Hydroxypropylmethylcellulose (HPMC) (12,29–39), methylcellulose (40,41), hydroxypropylcellulose (HPC) (42–47), sodium carboxymethylcellulose (CMC) (48), and ethylcellulose (38,49–56); as well as the polymethacrylates (22,57–61), a class of materials sold as either aqueous dispersions, dry powders, or organic solutions under the trade names Eudragit® (Evonik Industries, Essen, Germany), Eastacryl® (Eastman, Kingsport, Tennessee, U.S.A.), Kollicoat® (BASF, Ludwigshafen, Germany), or Acryl-eze® (Colorcon, Inc., West Point Pennsylvania, U.S.A.). See Table 1 for a listing of common binders used in aqueous-based processes and their concentration ranges.

However, with the advent of newer synthetic polymers, several natural binders are no longer that popular. Gelatin usage has dramatically decreased due to health concerns over bovine spongiform encephalopathy or mad cow disease. Acacia or gum arabic, being a natural product, was found to be prone to batch-to-batch inconsistencies in its viscosity as well as having high-bacterial counts. Starch required an extra processing step of heating in order to form a paste. The high viscosity of the paste makes this ingredient more difficult to work with and incidentally, can lead to localized overwetting, which generates oversized granules. Consequently, it is difficult for the starch to become homogeneously distributed throughout the powder bed and many formulators have preferred to use pregelatinized starch instead for its easier use and improved impact on product quality. Much background information has been written over the years regarding the wet granulation process including some newer review articles (63–70).

Over the years, researchers have reported using polymeric binders along with other excipients in unique ways for targeted therapies or for controlled drug release; some of these techniques will be discussed further. The selection of the appropriate binder and levels for a certain application are usually empirical, involving some type of optimization; and based upon previous company results, functional characteristics, performance, cost, and availability. The ability of a binder to produce strong, non-friable granules is dependent on the binder itself and binder's distribution in the granulation. However, the use of too much binder or too strong and cohesive of a binder will produce harder tablets which will not disintegrate easily, hence, impairing drug release, and can even cause excessive wear on the punches and dies. On the other hand, using too low a quantity of binder will produce friable granules, can generate a large amount of fines, and produce tablets with lower crushing strengths as a result.

Binders can be added either as dry powders in the blend or prepared beforehand as solutions and added during mixing. Generally, a larger quantity of granulating liquid used will yield a narrower particle size range along with coarser, harder granules due to the formation of solid bridges as with excipients such as lactose. Using a low viscosity binder solution as opposed to a dry powder requires a much lower concentration of the binder in order to achieve a certain granule hardness. This is likely due to the fact that the polymer is already fully hydrated and dissolved in the solution; which enables it to be more easily homogeneously distributed within the blend. In general, it has been shown that the use of a dry binder added within to the powder blend results in smaller granule sizes and a high level of larger lumps (71). Holm (72) does not generally recommend adding a dry binder to the blend because the binder distribution throughout the powder bed cannot be assured. However, other researchers have recommended just the opposite (73,74).

When applying the binder solution during mixing, it is best to provide a uniform liquid spray with as small a droplet size as possible as this will have the largest surface area. This spray will have the greatest coverage throughout the powder bed and will prevent localized overwetting of the granules, which can result in oversized particles. The rate of binder addition is important as well since a consistent, steady rate is desired to obtain a narrower and consistent particle size distribution.

Typically, finer granules with lower bulk densities can be obtained when a smaller volume of liquid is added during mixing. Moreover, these granules of smaller particle size yield tablets with faster dissolution rates and lower hardness values (75). The mechanical properties of a binder film are important as well and a good tablet binder should be able to offer flexibility and plasticity and yield without rupturing in order to absorb the effects of elastic recovery (62).

The type of binder selected can also affect the mechanical properties of the granules and tablets (Fig. 1). While gelatin showed the highest granule crushing strength using the lowest binder levels during high shear granulation, PVP showed intermediate values for crushing strength. At the other end of the spectrum, PEG 4000, a waxy, plastic material exhibiting poor binding properties, showed not only the lowest granule crushing strength values but required the highest binder levels. Recently, it was similarly reported for lactose-based placebo granulations using aqueous binder solutions of 9% w/w in a fluid bed granulator, that the mechanical strength of PVP K30 granules was lower than that of granules prepared with either pregelatinized starch or gelatin; in fact, PVP granules were characteristically softer, more plastic, and readily deformable (24).

Gelatin, now widely phased out as a binder in the pharmaceutical industry, had some interesting properties. Gelatin is a protein-based polymer that undergoes gelation when cooled to ambient temperature. It is known to provide good adhesion properties in agglomerates, produce films with high tensile strength, and yield strong granules and tablets of intermediate hardness (62,67).

The binder selected also has implications for coating operations as it would be more advantageous to use a binder with a lower elastic recovery as this would diminish the likelihood that the common problems of tablet coating uniformity and cracking would occur. Figure 2 shows the positive correlation between the percentage of elastic recovery and the residual die wall pressure measured by compression of wet granulated

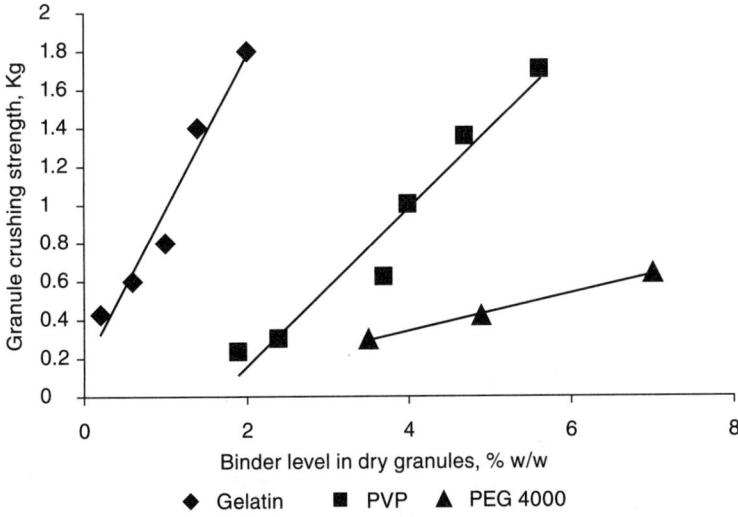

FIGURE 1 Crushing strength of wet granulated dicalcium phosphate granules using different binders (impeller speed, 400 rpm, chopper speed 3000 rpm). *Source*: Adapted from Ref. 76.

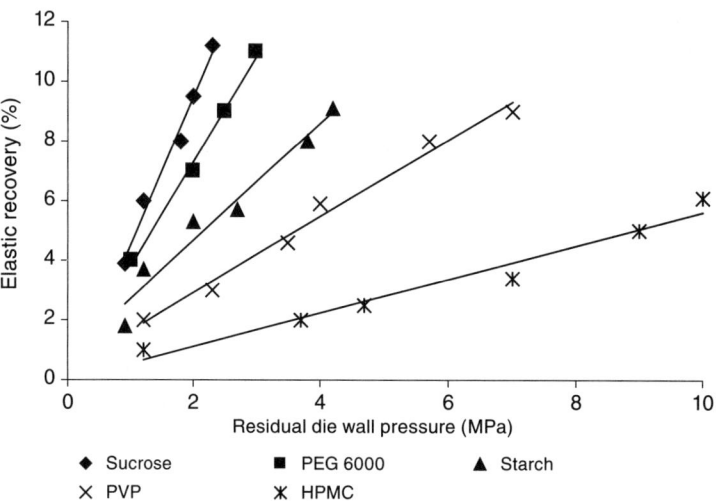

FIGURE 2 Tablet elastic recovery versus residual die wall pressure for acetaminophen tablets containing 4% w/w level of different binders. A high-shear mixer was used during wet granulation. *Source*: Adapted from Ref. 77.

acetaminophen. The binders studied exhibit a wide range of residual die wall pressures showing that binders can improve the plastic deformation properties of the tablet granulations. The graph shows that HPMC is a better binder for the brittle acetaminophen than is PVP; owing to the fact that HPMC tablets display the lowest elastic recovery values across the pressure range (62,77). In comparing PVP films with those of methylcellulose, Reading and Spring (78) found that PVP films had significantly lower values for tensile strength, toughness, and Young's modulus than methylcellulose, which showed significant elongation at fracture. This shows that methylcellulose is more elastic than PVP and such information can indicate the extent of a binder to improve the plasticity of the granules and thereby absorb the effects of elastic recovery. Furthermore, while adding a surfactant such as sodium laurel sulfate to acetaminophen granulated with PVP showed improvements in granule plasticity and gave lower elastic recovery values after tableting; the addition of glycerol to the granules gave even better results. Accordingly, the crushing strength of the corresponding tablets was also increased (77).

PARTICLE INTERACTIONS

Independent of the process employed, five distinct bonding mechanisms at the level of particle–particle interactions have been identified by Rumpf and co-workers (79) and they are:

1. Solid bridges—formation of bridges due to dissolution during granulation with subsequent solvent removal from drying. Solid bridges can also be formed by chemical reactions, and sintering/heat hardening.
2. Immobile liquids—addition of specialty binders that sorb the granulating solvent, soften, deform, and adhere to particles, then harden during drying.
3. Mobile liquids—liquid bridges at higher fluid levels that occupy void spaces.
4. Intermolecular and long-range forces—van der Waals forces, electrostatic forces.
5. Mechanical interlocking—fracture and deformation due to pressure that produces shape related bonding or intertwining of long fibrous particles.

Within the confines of the pharmaceutical industry, extensive use is made of immobile liquids. When a granulating liquid is utilized, it is distributed by mechanical action and can become concentrated in microscopic zones containing amorphous hydrophilic surfaces with strong sorptive capability and regions of increased molecular mobility. The presence of granulating liquid in these zones may lead to partial dissolution of soluble materials and regional softening of the particles. The physical movement of particles by mechanical action leads to random occurrences of such regions coming into close enough contact to produce bonding via a combination of these immobile liquid regions and/or capillary forces which may be capable of surviving further particle movement and agitation and may even strengthen as the solvent is removed. The granulation process is thus dependent upon the relative balance that exists between the construction and destruction of interparticulate bonds. This balance is largely influenced by the amount of granulating fluid utilized: as more fluid is added, the adhesion between like materials and cohesion between different materials swings toward more bonds being formed, thus moving the particle size distribution to larger size values.

Initially the particles are wetted by the granulating liquid, which leads to the formation of loose agglomerates. The relative liquid saturation of agglomerate pores, S, is the ratio of pore volume occupied by the liquid to the total agglomerate pore volume. It may be calculated by the following equation:

$$S = [H[(1-\varepsilon)/\varepsilon]\rho \tag{1}$$

where H is the ratio of liquid binder mass to the solid particle mass, ε the intragranular porosity, and is the true density of the solid material.

When $S < 25\%$, the agglomerates are said to be in a low-moisture or pendular state which is a stage of low-liquid saturation, S, with interparticulate voids still present and with particles held together by immobile liquid bridge bondings via surface tension at the liquid-air interface. Granulation proceeds through the intermediate funicular stage, where $25\% < S < 80\%$, and finally, the time interval when $S > 80\%$ where the granulation is in the capillary state. During this stage, all the air has been displaced from between particles and the particles are held together by capillary pressure. During drying, these liquid bridges become solid bridges as the solid material re-crystallizes and water is evaporated, first from the particle surface and subsequently from within the particle (67).

For a theoretical system of moist, spherical, monodisperse agglomerates, granule strength is given by the following equation:

$$\sigma_t = SC\,[(1-\varepsilon)/\varepsilon]\,(\gamma/d)\cos\theta \tag{2}$$

where σ_t is the moist agglomerate strength, S the liquid saturation level, C a material constant, ε the porosity, γ the surface tension, d the particle diameter, and θ is the contact angle between the liquid and solid.

The main value of this equation is the guidance it provides in controlling an actual granulation process when the components are neither monodisperse nor spherical. For example, when it is necessary to create a relatively larger granule size distribution, the moist agglomerate's strength is increased (to effect diminished granule attrition and greater consolidation/growth). Based on Equation (2), the formulation and processing options available to accomplish that end are increase the saturation level, decrease the porosity, decrease the surface tension, and decrease the particle diameter or increase the contact angle.

A high shear granulator will produce a relatively lower porosity granule than a low shear granulator, milling of the dry powders prior to granulation will produce smaller particle diameters, selecting formulation components that are relatively more hydrophilic when granulating with water will increase the contact angle, or it may be possible to add a surfactant that will increase the contact angle.

Whereas a relatively larger mean granule will possess better flow properties, the final granulation size in relation to the tablet diameter and die fill volume must be balanced to achieve the appropriate content uniformity, which from a theoretical standpoint is improved with a larger number of small granules. For a two-component system assuming that all granules have uniform drug content, the relative standard deviation is given by:

$$\text{RSD} = [X(1-X)/n]^{0.5} \qquad (3)$$

where RSD is the relative standard deviation, X the fraction of active ingredient, $1-X$ the fraction of the second component, and n is the number of particles. Thus, increasing the number of particles reduces the relative standard deviation, and therefore improves the tablet content uniformity. Approximate recommendations from Capes (80) for granule size intended for various tablet sizes are as follows:

Tablet size	Screen size
Up to 3/16 inch diameter	#20 U.S. mesh
7/32 to 9/32 inch diameter	#16 U.S. mesh
5/16 to 13/32 inch diameter	#14 U.S. mesh
7/16 inch and larger	#12 U.S. mesh

THE SOLID–LIQUID INTERFACE

Agglomeration of powders during the addition of liquid in wet granulation can be best described by several mechanisms and occurs in three phases; (*i*) nucleation of particles; (*ii*) consolidation and coalescence between agglomerates; and (*iii*) breakage and attrition. Nucleation occurs with fine particles that have been completely wetted by the granulating liquid; this leads to the formation of loose, porous nuclei composed of a small number of particles, then fine powders are coalesced between and around the wetted particles. During consolidation and coalescence, agitation force produces increasing granule size via bonding between multiple nuclei. However, this growth is eventually limited by the amount of solvent added and the abrasion from movement for both wet and dry states, which leads to some degree of breakage and attrition. A liquid droplet joins two or more particles together through mobile liquid bridges, which are held together by capillary pressure and surface tension; a schematic of a liquid bridge is presented in Figure 3. Our

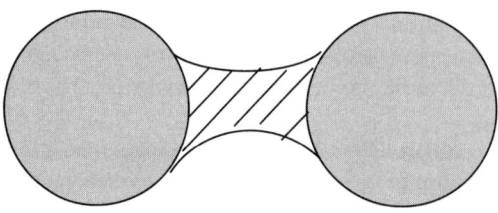

FIGURE 3 Schematic of a liquid bridge between two equal sized particles.

Pharmaceutical Granulation Processes, Mechanism, and the Use of Binders

understanding of the complexities of the granulation process has significantly improved over the last 15 years. This new understanding has lead to a change from the traditional view of that granulation process occurs in five stages (81), to the modern view which involves only three stages. These three sets of rate processes of granule growth are presented in Figure 4.

During nucleation, the particle growth rate increases with increased liquid content. Surface tension is a term used to describe the energy barrier between a liquid and air and is a measure of the attractive forces between molecules of a liquid. The higher the surface tension of a liquid, the more the liquid tries to reach the energetically most favored form, i.e., a droplet. The surface tension of the binder liquid tends to lower the total surface free energy by reducing the air–liquid interfacial area, which enhances the particle wettability. Decreasing the binder surface tension will decrease the capillary pressure holding the particles together. However, if the surface tension is too low, it can weaken the granules, allowing them to shear apart more easily. The magnitude of the surface tension of liquids used in granulation varies only between 20 and 80 mNm^{-1}, with the latter value close to the surface tension for purified water.

A low surface tension value correlates with a small contact angle. The binder with the smaller contact angle has improved spreadability and can wet powders more effectively (65,84). A surfactant can also be added to the binder solution to improve wettability, especially for hydrophobic powders, and functions to lower both the surface tension as well as the contact angle of the liquid. If the contact angle, θ, is less than 90°, then the powder wetting is spontaneous. However, if the contact angle is closer to 180° then the powder would be considered unwettable by the liquid. The pore space within a particle assembly can be simplistically considered as a model capillary. The capillary pressure, P_c, of a liquid is related to the surface tension by the following equation:

$$P_c = \frac{-2\gamma \cos \theta}{r} \tag{4}$$

(i) Wetting and nucleation

(ii) Consolidation and coalescence

(iii) Attrition and breakage

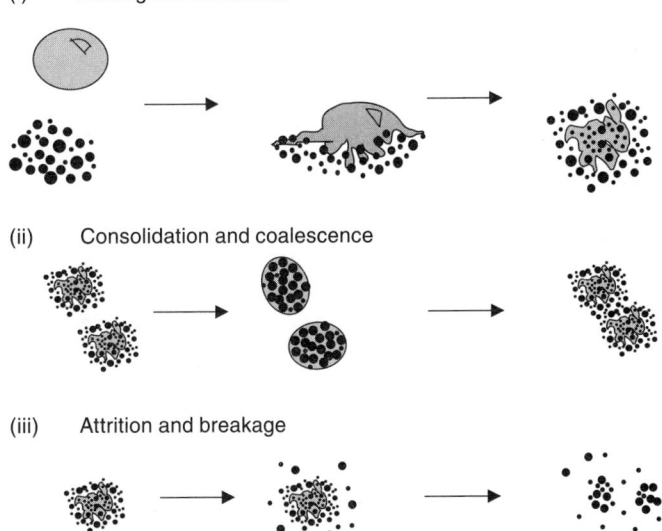

FIGURE 4 Modern approach schematic of the three rate processes for wet granulation. *Source*: From Refs. 65, 82, 83.

where γ is the surface tension of the liquid, θ the contact angle, and r is the radius of the capillary. The contact angle in this equation is an effective contact angle on the actual surface, which is likely to be rough, as distinct from that measured on a smooth surface. For a rough surface, and with a contact angle less than 90°, the effective contact angle is small and hence the approximation $\cos \theta \cong 1$ can be made (84).

Typical values for viscosity and surface tension of various binders in solution are presented in Table 2. It can be seen that although there are differences in viscosity between the two molecular weight grades of PVP, the values for surface tension are the same, and rather high, approaching that of water. The surface tension of the HPMC binder is significantly lower than for PVP, suggesting that the former polymer will offer enhanced spreadability and wettability of the particles, which can, in turn, improve granule strength. Data to support the surface tension lowering effect of a surfactant, polysorbate 80, is presented in Table 3. Granule growth proceeds further by consolidation and coalescence where collisions between agglomerates, granules and powder, or granules and equipment lead to granule compaction and growth and this mechanism is also favored by fine particles with a wide particle size distribution. Free liquid at the surface of an agglomerate aids in interparticulate bonding by contributing strength and this helps prevent particle separation while the mass is being mixed. However, in the third stage, breakage or attrition can occur as wet or dried granules break apart due to impact from the agitation occurring in the granulator (65,85).

GRANULATION PROCESSES

When classified on the basis of operating principle, eight types of granulation processes have been categorized, and they are:

1. Dry granulation—direct physical compaction densifies and/or agglomerates the dry powders.
2. Wet high-shear granulation—rotating high-shear forces via high-power-per-unit-mass with addition of a liquid.
3. Wet low-shear granulation—rotating low-shear forces via low-power-per-unit-mass with addition of a liquid.

TABLE 2 Binding Agents and Properties of Aqueous Solutions Used in Granulations

Material	Concentration % w/w	Viscosity[a] mPas (30°C)	Surface tension[b] mN/m (25°C)
Kollidon 90 PVP	3	9	68
	5	31	68
	8	109	68
Kollidon 25 PVP	3	1	68
	20	10	67
Methocel E5 HPMC	3	6	48
	6	43	48
	8	91	48

[a]Viscosity determined by Brookfield LVT Viscometer.
[b]Surface tension determined by drop weight method of Adamson.
Abbreviations: PVP, Polyvinylpyrrolidone; HPMC, Hydroxypropylmethylcellulose.
Source: Adapted from Refs. 86 and 87.

TABLE 3 Viscosities and Surface Tensions of an Aqueous 3% Kollidon 90 Solution with Various Concentrations of added Polysorbate 80

Polysorbate 80 level, w/w%	Viscosity mPas (30°C)	Surface tension mN/m(25°C)
0	9	68
0.02	9	57
0.4	9	46
0.8	10	44

Source: Adapted from Ref. 86.

4. Low shear tumble granulation—rotation of the vessel and/or intensifier bar via low-power-per-unit-mass with addition of a liquid.
5. Extrusion granulation—pressure gradient forcing a wetted or plasticized mass through a sized orifice with linear shear.
6. Rotary granulation—a central rotating disk, rotating walls, or both, cause centrifugal or rotational forces that spheronize, agglomerate and/or densify a wetted or non-wetted powder or extruded material, possibly incorporating a liquid and/or drying.
7. Fluid bed granulation—direct application of an atomized granulation liquid onto solids with little or no shear, while the powder is suspended by a continuous gas stream, with continuous drying.
8. Spray dry granulation—granulating liquid containing dissolved or suspended solids is atomized and rapidly dried by a controlled gas stream to produce a dry powder.

Many of these methods are important enough to have a chapter devoted to the topic, e.g., spray drying and dry granulation chapters.

High-Shear Granulation

The majority of high-shear granulators are composed of a cylindrical or conical mixing bowl, a three-blade impeller, an auxiliary chopper, a motor to drive blades and chopper and a discharge port. The bowl may be jacketed to control product temperature via circulating hot or cool liquids. The impeller's function is to mix the powder and spread the granulating liquid, it routinely rotates from 100 to 500 rpm. Functionally, the chopper is intended to reduce large agglomerates to granules, and it typically rotates from between 1000 and 3000 rpm. As a result of the success and popularity of this approach, a relatively large number of vendors offer this type of equipment. A picture of a laboratory-sized, Diosna® (Dierks Söhne GmbH, Osnabrück, Germany) high shear granulator with a 6-L mixing bowl is shown in Figure 5.

Major advantages of this technique include:

1. short processing time;
2. versatility in processing a wide range of formulations for both immediate and controlled/sustained release products;
3. reduced binder solution quantity (relative to low shear machines);
4. ability to process highly cohesive materials;
5. greater densification and reduced granule friability;
6. reproducibility of uniform granule size distribution;
7. dust reduction; and
8. predictable end-point determination.

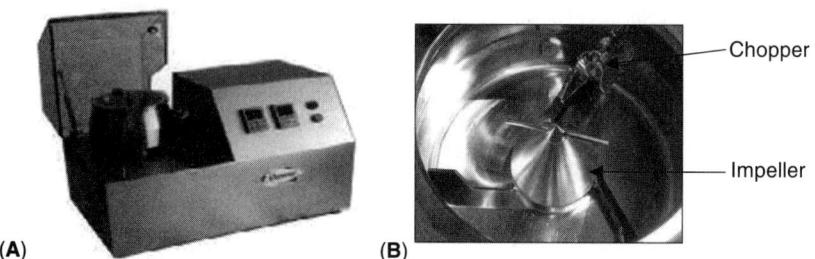

FIGURE 5 (A) Laboratory-scale Diosna® High shear granulator with 6-liter bowl, (B) chopper and impeller inside the mixing bowl.

Along with these advantages, there may be challenges due to:
1. reduced granule compressibility relative to low shear granulation;
2. narrow range of operating conditions.

Subsequent to the granulation step, it is necessary to employ a drying operation which is most frequently performed in a fluid bed dryer; and afterwards, a sizing/milling operation is needed to yield the final granulation. Equipment is available that allows for improved efficiency by employing a one-pot processing approach, where both the granulation and drying steps are performed in the same vessel through application of microwave radiation, vacuum drying, or gas-assisted drying to remove the granulating liquid.

One further option is called moisture-activated dry-granulation; in this approach, a reduced amount of binder liquid, approximately 1–4%, is added and mixed to cause agglomeration. Subsequently, additional moisture-absorbing powder such as microcrystalline cellulose, potato starch, and/or the highly porous silicon dioxide, is added and mixed to return the product to a free flowing powder, and following the blending of a lubricant, the granulation product may be compressed into tablets.

Primary process variables (and critical process parameters) include:
1. batch load in the granulator bowl,
2. impeller speed,
3. granulation liquid addition method,
4. granulating liquid addition rate,
5. chopper speed,
6. wet massing time.

In one example of a process optimization study, Badawy et al. (88) utilized a Plackett–Burmann experimental design to evaluate variables such as impeller speed, granulating solution addition rate, total amount of water added, wet massing time, etc., for a lactose-based formulation. Increasing the amount of water added, high-impeller speed, and short-massing time produced a relatively larger granule particle size distribution. By increasing the impeller speed or wet massing time, granule friability, and porosity were decreased; however, tablet hardness was also decreased.

An aqueous granulation of microcrystalline cellulose in a high-shear mixer produced increased granule hardness with increased granulation time and added water levels. This was attributed to disruption of long chain structures by the impeller's shear force, as determined by a combination of small-angle X-ray scattering and wide-angle powder diffraction techniques.

Low-Shear Granulation

By virtue of a machine's agitator speed, sweep volume or bed pressure, a granulator may produce relatively lower shear, which has implications for the operating conditions and resultant granule properties. Just as with high-shear machines, the unit operation of low-shear granulation may consist of a dry mixing phase, addition of granulating solvent which may contain a binder, kneading the mass to effect the required granules, followed by removal of the solvent to a target range. As a broad generalization, low-shear granulators tend to require longer run times, they yield lower density and higher porosity granules than those of high shear granulators, and the quantity of granulating solvent for a high shear machine may be reduced to 60–80% of that of a low shear machine (89). As a result of their design, the low shear machines are less capable of compressing the granules and reducing the void volume, and they require additional binder solution.

Granulators which operate by mechanical agitation include planetary mixers, ribbon or paddle blenders, orbiting screw mixers and sigma blade mixers. They cause particle movement through the rotational movement of a blade(s) or paddles, and have been adapted to perform wet granulation despite their original function as blenders. Planetary mixers may require a distinct dry blending step prior to wet granulation due to insufficient vertical mixing. The orbiting screw mixer may be fitted with a spray nozzle mounted on the agitator, it has a reputation of providing gentle action that may be advantageous when a formulation has diminished granule strength.

Rotating shape granulators are defined by a shell mounted on an axis, examples include double cone and V-shaped machines. Their peripheral rotation rate is typically 250–350 ft/min. To produce convective motion of the powder, a second rotating device is mounted on the shell rotation axis, this is known as an agitator or intensifier bar; and it may contain the granulating liquid addition system and normally spins at $10 \times$ greater peripheral speed than the shell. Among the parameters to optimize during product development are shell peripheral speed, agitator bar design, size and speed, batch load/range, liquid addition mode/spray droplet size, rate and quantity. It is possible for these vessels to be jacketed for heating or cooling, or they may be vacuum capable, thus permitting drying in a single pot processing sequence or flushing with nitrogen to provide an inert atmosphere when hydroethanolic solvents are necessary.

Applied to both low- and high-shear granulators, the term single-pot processor refers to granulators that have been fitted with various integral drying possibilities (90,91). Thus, single-pot processing make possible mixing, granulating, drying, and blending granulations in a single piece of equipment. The integration of these operations into a single unit provides a number of advantages (90–93); namely: (*i*) capital investment in equipment and space may be reduced, (*ii*) material handling steps may be reduced, (*iii*) reduced processing time, (*iv*) reduced personnel requirements, (*v*) as closed systems, environmental concerns such as relative humidity (RH), product contamination and environmental exposure to dangerous drug substances are minimized, and (*vi*) minimization of losses in product transfer. Moreover, many single-pot processors can be fitted with clean-in-place systems. Systems employing vacuum drying are of particular interest when flammable solvents or such compositions are involved.

Single-Pot Processes

Powders loaded into the single-pot processor are dry-mixed until appropriate uniformity is achieved; after mixing, the binder solution is sprayed in and wet massing ensues. Factors normally associated with the granulation process such as spray rate and volume, droplet size, nozzle distance and position, main impeller speed, chopper speed and time on, etc., should be controlled, as usual. Wet massing continues until an appropriate granulation endpoint is reached and the granulation is usually dried by vacuum drying or microwave-vacuum drying. Traditionally, single-pot processors are equipped with jacketed bowls that supply the energy for drying via circulated heated water. Vacuum drying allows for faster drying and lower temperatures, which may be suitable for many thermolabile materials (92). To facilitate solvent removal and promote uniform drying, the wet mass is generally agitated gently during drying by slowly rotating blades or by rotating the bowl itself. Overmixing should be avoided as partial mechanical damage to granules can result (91). In one study (94), 15% shorter drying times were found when a swinging bowl was used during vacuum drying. Stripping-gas systems have been developed for commercial single-pot processors that allow faster drying by introducing a gas flow through the powder bed (92,95). The gas improves wall-to-product heat flow and vapor removal.

The introduction of microwave/vacuum drying to single-pot processing was a significant development that makes possible rapid drying at lower temperatures (91,96–98). Microwave drying also allows linear scale-up in single-pot processes, something which is not possible in a traditional vacuum drying system (90,95,97,99). However, because of the highly energetic, deep penetration afforded by microwaves, component stability must be carefully considered (92). The appropriateness of each new formulation for microwave drying needs to be assessed (91).

The single-pot process concept has also been applied to melt granulation. In one example, in a solvent-free process that eliminated the drying step, Hamdeni et al. (100) described the manufacture of controlled release pellets containing a fatty-matrix and using a MiPro, Pro-C-ept processor. More recently, that laboratory (101) described the preparation of a melt granulation by a solvent-free, single-pot process as part of the development of floating, sustained release mini tablets. Table 4 describes the features of some commercially available single-pot processors.

Fluid Bed Granulators vs. High Shear Granulators

Starting with the quality of the raw materials and proceeding through to granulation, drying, and tableting, there are a number of different variables that affect both the tableting

TABLE 4 Some Commercially Available Single-Pot Processors

Processor	Features/options
Bohle VMA (10L–1200L) (L.B. Bohle, LLC)	Double jacket, vacuum, VAGAS© gas stripping system; optionally supported by microwave drying
Diosna VAC 20–2000 (20L–2000L) (Diosna Dierks and Söhne GmbH)	Double jacket, gas stripping, vacuum dryer
Collette Ultima (25L–1200L) (Niro Pharma Systems)	Double jacket, vacuum; gas-assisted vacuum (Transflo™); microwave/vacuum; swinging bowl.
Zanchetta (various models up to 1200L) (VimA Impianti S.r.l., subsidiary of IMA S.p.a.)	Double jacket, vacuum, tilting bowl, gas stripping (GA.ST. system)
Aeromatic-Fielder GP System (3L, 10L) (Niro Pharma Systems)	Double jacket, vacuum/gas assistance (AV model Aerovac™ Vacuum Dryer); microwave/vacuum dryer (SP model)

Source: Adapted from Ref. 93.

operation as well as the quality of the tablets obtained; these are listed under several categories from Faure (102) in Table 5. The two most important process variables with a high shear mixer are the impeller speed and the wet massing time. The chopper speed can also play a role but that depends on the size and shape of the chopper used, as chopper design can vary along with the type of high shear mixer employed. It is known that the higher mixing intensity of high shear mixers results in denser granules while those prepared in fluidized bed granulators (low shear conditions) are more porous and therefore more compressible (103). While the operation of a high shear mixer is fairly straightforward, fluid bed granulators have several important process parameters that need to be carefully monitored since these have a significant impact on the granules produced. Several figures will illustrate some important properties of granules prepared by either high-shear mixers or fluidized bed granulators.

The droplet size of the atomized binder solution is a very important process variable in fluidized bed granulation and depends on the viscosity of the binder solution. Furthermore, when the liquid evaporation is excessive due to a high inlet flow rate and/or high inlet air temperature or the liquid flow rate is low, the powder bed moisture content will be low. A spray dry process will occur where the granule size depends essentially on the droplet size of the binder (104). Granule agglomeration is controlled by the moisture content of the bed. If the moisture content is too high, the bed becomes overwetted and defluidizes rapidly; but if the moisture content is too low, no agglomeration will occur (67). However, with high-shear granulators the intense mixing agitation from impeller and chopper blades contributes to the spreading of the liquid and the droplet size has little effect upon the granule size.

There are other process parameters which are also important when dealing with fluid bed granulation such as the atomization air pressure and the binder addition rate; however, these have been studied with mixed results. While some authors have shown a decrease in granule size with increased atomization air pressure (105–107) Ormos et al., (108), found no effect. Similarly, while Davies and Gloor (105) found that an increase in binder addition rate resulted in a larger granule size, Schaefer and Worts (109) found no such effect.

Gao et al., (103) reported that granulations using an atomization air pressure of 1.5 bar, corresponding to a higher air-to-liquid mass ratio, had significantly more fines (20–34.5%) than those produced using 0.5 bar (<11% fines). This increase in the level of fines is attributed to the finer spray droplet formation of the binder solution as a result of increasing the air-to-liquid mass ratio during atomization. The result is the formation of weaker liquid binder-powder bridges on the surface of the particles, which limits granule growth.

A fairly good positive correlation ($R^2 > 0.87$) was observed between the droplet size of different binder solutions and their granule size as measured by the geometric mean diameter (Fig. 6). The use of gelatin showed the largest granule growth per droplet size likely due to the fact that this polymer has good adhesive properties and forms strong films. Methylcellulose showed the smallest granules while PVP was intermediate in its effect.

Although the lower molecular weight PVP K25 had the ability to be used across the widest concentrations, both gelatin and higher molecular weight PVP K90 possessed the best agglomeration properties of the binders studied as these showed the most granule growth with increased binder level (Fig. 7).

Particle agglomeration is mainly influenced by the degree of liquid saturation; which is, in turn, dependent on the intragranular porosity and volume of binder solution used. It was found that the primary factors affecting the density and porosity of lactose and calcium phosphate during high shear granulation were the amount of binder solution

TABLE 5 Main Variables Affecting the Quality of Tablets Obtained by Wet Granulation and Tableting

Material parameters	Granulation conditions	Drying conditions	Granule properties	Tablet properties
Powder particle size distribution	In high-shear mixing: Mixing/collision generation levels	In high-shear mixing: Extent of mixing	Particle size distribution	Tableting: Compaction force and speed
Wettability of the solid by the liquid	Process time	Mode of drying (microwave, infrared)	Bulk density and porosity	Extra-granular additions: e.g., lubricants, extra-granular disintegrants
Solid solubility and degree of swelling in binder liquid	Fill level	Energy input	Moisture content	
Binder concentration and viscosity	Liquid spray rate	Process time	Flow (usually good)	
	Quantity of solvent	In: fluid bed granulation: Inlet air temperature and RH	Drug content uniformity across the particle size distribution	
	Temperature (+/− controlled)	Air flow rate	Binder distribution	
	In fluid bed granulation: Spray droplet size Spraying surface and rate	Process time	Granule strength/friability	
	Quantity of solvent			
	Bed fluidity/airflow rate			
	Inlet air temperature and RH			
	Equilibrium temperature and RH in bed			
	Process time			

Abbreviation: RH, % relative humidity.
Source: From Ref. 102.

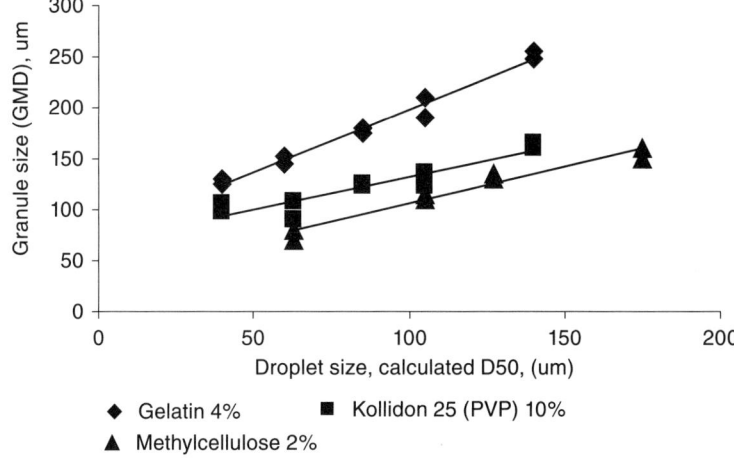

FIGURE 6 Correlation between droplet size calculated from an empirical droplet size equation (110) and granule size (GMD) after using three different binder solutions during fluidized bed granulator operation. *Abbreviation*: GMD, geometric mean diameter. *Source*: Adapted from Ref. 111.

added and the impeller speed. While lactose showed only a slight decrease in porosity during mixing, the porosity of calcium phosphate granules decreased significantly from 40% to 20% (112). Granule porosities begin to decrease very rapidly after the nucleation phase with binder solution volumes of about 28–30%, which is the same region where the granule growth by consolidation and coalescence starts (Fig. 8). It can also be seen that as the level of Methocel® E5 HPMC (Dow Chemical, Midland Michigan, U.S.A.) increases from 3% to 8% that the granule porosity also decreases. This effect is due to the fact that higher binder levels will produce solutions with higher viscosities and a thicker solution can more effectively adhere and fill the available pores; remaining on the particles following the mixing agitation.

The physicochemical properties of the binder solution also affect the power consumption during wet granulation, which is an indirect measurement of granule growth. The surface tension of the binder liquid affects the strength of the mobile liquid bridges

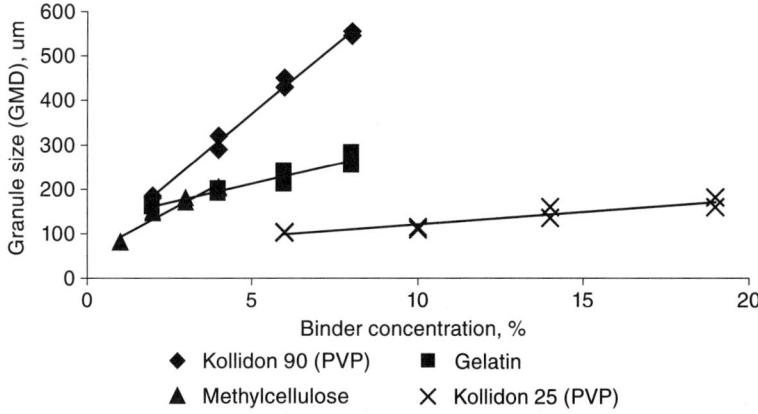

FIGURE 7 Effect of different binder solution concentrations on the granule size (GMD) in a fluidized bed granulator, Glatt WSG 15. Air-to-liquid mass ratio at the nozzle: 1.15. *Abbreviation*: GMD, geometric mean diameter. *Source*: Adapted from Ref. 111.

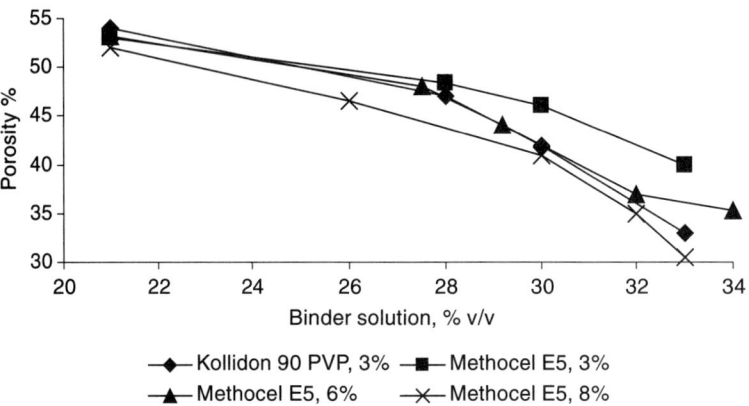

FIGURE 8 Correlation between intragranular porosity and the percentage of binder solution added in a high shear granulator (impeller speed 400 rpm, chopper speed 3000 rpm). *Source*: Adapted from Ref. 113.

holding the particles together. It has been shown that use of a lower surface tension liquid creates weaker liquid bridges between powder particles inside the wet agglomerate (114). This looser association of particles will lead to a greater amount of consolidation and coalescence which will expel more moisture from the granules. This explains the lower liquid requirements to attain overwetting when using lower surface tension binder solutions (115). An in-depth study of the properties of drying liquid bridges is presented by Farber et al. (116). They compared liquid bridges of only lactose or mannitol with pure HPC, HPMC, or PVP and found that bridges with only lactose or mannitol tend to expand upon solidification. In contrast, the polymeric bridges tended to compact. Bridges crystallized from solutions of the non-polymeric excipients were polycrystalline, brittle and had low strength, while bridges from the polymeric excipients were found to be amorphous, strong, and tough.

On the other hand, the use of high surface tension liquid binders will lead to a higher resistance of the wet granules against the mixer agitation with a resulting increase in the power consumption. For example, Figure 9 shows that when Methocel HPMC is used as a binder, both the power consumption and granule size are decreased compared to when PVP solutions are used. This is due to the fact that HPMC solutions have significantly lower surface tension values compared with PVP solutions. Although the two molecular weight grades of PVP have the same surface tension and similar power consumption, there is a significant increase in the geometric mean particle size with the higher molecular weight grade. The solution of the higher molecular weight PVP grade will be more viscous and adhere better to the particles, thus promoting increased granule growth.

The use of power consumption to monitor and attempt to identify the granulation endpoint continues to be very popular; however, newer techniques such as on-line probes using NIR spectroscopic techniques can also offer much assistance to the pharmaceutical formulator. The power consumption curve can be divided into five distinct regions or phases which also correspond to the amount of granulating liquid added (Fig. 10) (117,118).

In the initial Phase I, no increase in power consumption will be observed. The particles are moistened and liquid is absorbed without forming liquid bridges. Beginning with Phase II, there is a sharp increase in power consumption; the buildup of liquid

Pharmaceutical Granulation Processes, Mechanism, and the Use of Binders

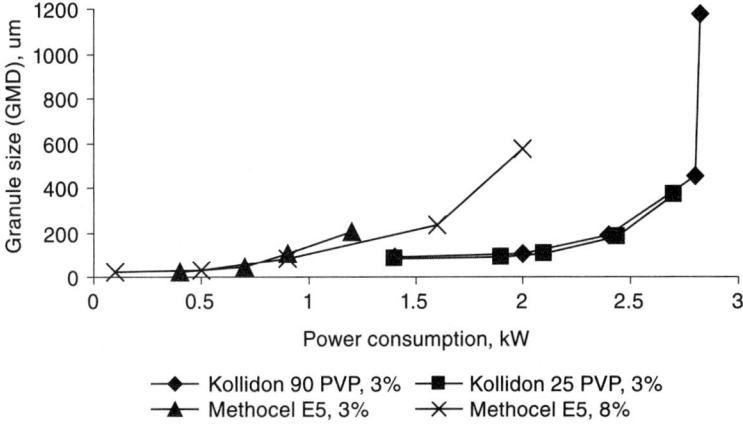

FIGURE 9 Correlation between power consumption and mean granule size during addition of different binder solutions using a high-shear granulator (impeller speed 400 rpm, chopper speed 3000 rpm). *Source*: Adapted from Ref. 86.

bridges begins and the first granules are formed. At Phase III, the power consumption levels off, the interparticle voids fill with granulating liquid and further agglomeration occurs with kneading and compaction. In Phase IV, overwetting leads to liquid saturation, with S > 80%. Finally, with Phase V, we see that the plot slope drops off precipitously and this indicates that a suspension is formed (droplet stage) (118,119).

A fluid bed processor uses the flow of air to keep the powder bed fluidized or in continuous motion while a binder solution is sprayed into the chamber. The gentle mixing action of fluidization aids in coating the particles uniformly and typically no milling step after granulation is required. The fluid bed processor is quite different from a high shear granulator and the critical process variables as well as the quality attributes of the final granulation are also different as would be expected. The granulation process is much faster with a high shear mixer compared to a fluid bed drier and the high shear mixer

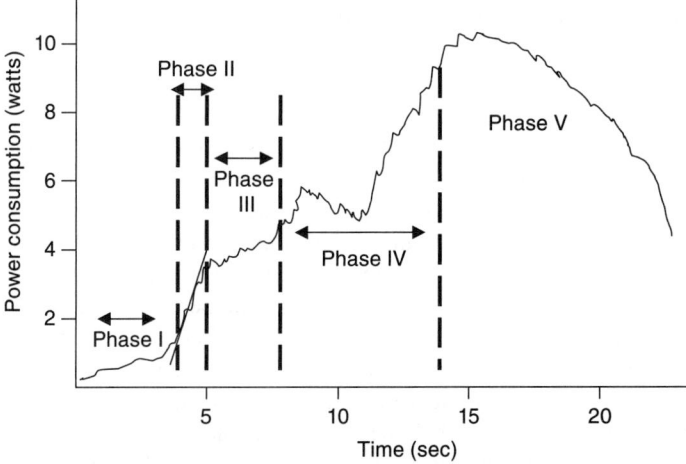

FIGURE 10 Regions of the power consumption curve during wet granulation. *Source*: Modified from Refs. 117, 118.

requires significantly less liquid, about two-thirds to three-quarters less, due to the greater densification of the granules brought about by the more intense agitation. Likewise, a mixer with less intensive agitation will produce granules with higher porosities and a narrower particle size distribution (120). In fact, Shaafsma et al., (121) stated that the porosity of granules from a fluid bed granulator is generally between 40% and 50% while those granules from a high shear mixer range from only 20% to 30%.

Another major difference between these two types of granulators besides the quantity of liquid used is the fact that with a fluid bed process the drying stage occurs simultaneously with the powder wetting. This greatly affects the binder distribution in the granules, and impacts the particle properties for each process; giving rise to differences in their morphology and structure. Innovative research has been conducted to examine the binder distribution in granules using population balance modeling and fluorescent markers with high-shear mixers (115,122,123) or with fluid bed granulators (121). For instance, with granules prepared by wet massing in a high-shear mixer the binder is distributed as a sponge-like matrix. While this same matrix is observed in granules from a fluidized bed granulator, the granule surfaces are now coated with a shell of binder from the spraying process. Tablets prepared from fluidized bed granulations were found to be stronger, and this finding was ascribed to the surface shell of binder surrounding the granules that contributed to enhanced interparticulate bondings (67,124).

Furthermore, due to the fact that the drying step occurs simultaneously with liquid addition in fluid bed granulators, the evaporation of liquid results in an increased concentration of binder in the liquid bridges holding the particles together; and consequently the liquid bridges become more viscous and immobile. As a direct result of this, the adhesive forces are markedly increased and the agglomerates are stabilized (125). Increasing the level of the binder added in a fluid bed granulator will cause the liquid bridges between particles to be more viscous and this will lead to increases in granule size (126,127). However, with high-shear mixers there is minimal solvent evaporation and the liquid bridges are typically mobile. Granules are instead stabilized by densification and deformation. Consequently, although Ritala et al. (113) found only a small effect of the concentration of five different binders on granule growth during liquid addition in a high shear mixer, it was noted that PVP and gelatin produced granules with the highest average particle size. However, it was also observed that a higher binder concentration resulted in lower power consumption, since the binder acts more effectively as a lubricant when its concentration is increased.

Melt Granulation

In this approach, the binder is added as a dry powder that melts with the application of heat. Generally 10–30% w/w of binder is utilized, within a typical melting range of 50–100°C. Binders with melting points below this range are seldom employed as they are prone to softening and/or sticking during handling and storage, whereas binders with higher melting points may accelerate drug decomposition. Powder addition and dry mixing are conducted at ambient temperature, then the system temperature is raised by the application of heat, often from a jacketed vessel, and/or by heat generated from interparticulate friction during high-speed movement; this induces a phase transition of the binder from a solid to a liquid or molten state and it then acts as the granulating liquid. Once the granulation process has been completed, the system is cooled, the binder reverts to a solid phase and it holds the granules together by means of solid bridges. (An alternative approach is to use a softened semisolid as the binder, this is frequently termed thermoplastic granulation).

Examples of hydrophilic binders in this category include PEGs and poloxomers, and they are preferred for immediate release dosage forms. Hydrophobic binders include fatty acids, fatty alcohols, waxes and glycerides, and they are preferred for prolonged-release formulations.

The two most prominent advantages of melt granulation are:

1. one step, one processor approach that does not require drying;
2. applicable to water sensitive products or processes (i.e., effervescent products).

This process is tempered with limitations from unsuitability for use with temperature sensitive materials and potential detrimental impact to rapid dissolution from high binder concentration. Considering the particle size distribution requirements, the optimal range is from 25 to 100 µm. Smaller particles may be problematic due to the need for high levels of liquid saturation required to overcome their cohesiveness, whereas larger particles have a proclivity to form weak agglomerates or fines.

BINDER SELECTION

Sugars

Poorly tasting and bitter over the counter drugs or nutraceuticals can be wet granulated with sweeter compounds such as sugars, sorbitol, mannitol, or maltodextrins to aid in their taste-masking when used in chewable tablet formulations. Binders such as PVP or various cellulose derivatives can also be added. In this case, the binder concentration should be somewhat higher than normal for optimal coating of the drug. A disintegrant may also be needed as part of the wet granulation formulation and can help break apart the tablet into primary particles in the stomach. It should be kept in mind that sorbitol is fairly hygroscopic and can have a laxative effect if levels are too high. Also, glucose (or dextrose) is a reducing sugar and high levels should not be used as the color of the tablets can become darker upon storage, especially at elevated temperatures. This darkening effect is due to the Maillard reaction, which occurs in the presence of primary amines (128,129). Intimately mixing the drug with a more palatable substance during granulation assists in lowering the surface area that the objectionable drug can react to on the tongue. The degree of taste masking obtained will depend upon the drug dosage as well as the inherent off-taste of the drug.

A physical mixture containing sodium diclofenac and lactose was mixed with a small amount of a concentrated saccharose solution (Emdex®, JRS GmbH, Rosenberg, Germany) in order to obtain a homogeneous paste similar to a solid dispersion. Cores of 0.5 cm diameter were then prepared. Tablets were prepared with the drug core at the center, surrounded by a matrix of Eudragit RS 100 and a channeling agent of 50% of different particle size fractions of either sodium chloride or Emdex. During dissolution testing in simulated gastric fluid (pH 1.2), the drug remains poorly soluble and unionized; however, in pH 7.4 buffer (to simulate conditions in the colon), the drug becomes soluble. The channeling agent had a significant effect on the drug release as the Emdex curve showed a typical sigmoidal profile, whereas the NaCl curve showed a longer lag time followed by a zero-order release profile (130).

Natural Polymers

Starch

While starch paste is rarely used in new products due to its high viscosity and therefore non-homogeneous distribution in granules during wet granulation, pregelatinized starch is an effective replacement with improved properties. Pregelatinized starch is starch that has been chemically or mechanically processed to rupture all or part of the starch grains and is available as fully or partly pregelatinized; however, fully pregelatinized starches tend to lose much of their disintegrant properties. Pregelatinized starch is thus easier to solubilize as it requires only cold water and can be used as a binder in dry form from 5% to 10% w/w with water added after dry blending, or prepared as a 10–15% solution and used at 2–5% w/w during wet granulation. Levels from 5% to 10% w/w offer optimal tablet disintegrant properties. As in other cases, however, adding the starch as a dry powder requires two to four times as much binder to achieve the same effect, compared with the use of a binder solution. The selection of the proper lubricant and levels is important for this excipient. If a lubricant is required in the formulation magnesium stearate may be used at levels below 0.25% w/w since concentrations greater than this may have adverse effects on tablet strength and dissolution following direct compression. Therefore, stearic acid is generally the preferred lubricant of choice for granulations containing pregelatinized starch that will be tableted using direct compression (131). However, other formulation parameters such as binder selection and levels can also impact tablet strength. Becker at al., (19) studied high shear granulation of 75% w/w acetaminophen using water and binders at levels of 0%, 2%, 6%, and 10%, and compared tablet crushing strength. The binders used were HPMC, PVP K30, HPC, maltodextrin, and pregelatinized starch. It was found that HPMC and PVP, especially at higher levels, functioned best to improve tablet strength; and significantly outperformed starch at the 10% level. They recommended that the minimum concentration of starch for their acetaminophen formulation should be no less than 10% w/w. However, while tablets containing HPMC or PVP granules took 1 hour to disintegrate, pregelatinized starch was able to show rapid tablet disintegration times.

Synthetic and Semi-Synthetic Polymers

Polyvinylpyrrolidone

Polyvinylpyrrolidone is an inert, synthetic polymer consisting of a linear chain of 1-vinyl-2-pyrrolidinone groups, and the varying degrees of polymerization of these groups gives rise to the wide range of molecular weights available from 2500 to 3M. PVP is generally used from 0.5% to 5% in a formulation on a dry weight basis and has the added advantage of being soluble in both water and alcohol.

Due to its low viscosity in solution with certain grades, higher binder levels can be used during granulation. However, caution should be exercised with higher levels as the residual aldehyde levels in PVP can cause pellicle formation in gelatin capsule shells (132). The aldehydes act to crosslink the gelatin causing a thin film to develop and this decreases the solubility of the capsule shells, thus, delaying drug release. The USP 25 sets a limit of ≤ 0.05% for aldehyde content (133). Moreover, PVP has been shown to be very hygroscopic, with significant amounts of moisture being absorbed at low relative humidities (134). When acetaminophen tablets granulated with either pregelatinized starch or PVP K30 were subjected to 8 weeks of storage at either 52% RH or 94% RH, it was found that the tablets containing PVP were more susceptible to humidity-related changes affecting tablet hardness, disintegration time, and drug dissolution (15).

Another unique physicochemical property of PVP solutions is their high-surface tension, which is close to purified water. Ritala et al. (86) reported that the use of PVP solutions to granulate dicalcium phosphate in a high shear mixer resulted in more dense granules with larger average particle sizes than compared with the use of HPMC solutions. Furthermore, low levels of PVP C15 ranging from 0.2% to 0.8% w/w were found to reduce the tackiness of 2.0% w/w HPMC solutions; without affecting the state of hydration of the HPMC. The lower molecular weight grade of PVP performed the best owing to its suitable hydrodynamic size to interdisperse among the HPMC polymer chains and reduce the extent of HPMC-HPMC bonding.

Polymethacrylates

The polymethacrylates are a diverse group of about twenty inert, sustained release polymers with unique properties that are available as either aqueous liquid dispersions, milled dry powders, or organic solutions; and are composed of synthetic cationic, anionic, or neutral polymers of dimethylaminoethyl methacrylates, methacrylic acid, and methacrylic acid esters in varying ratios. They are listed in the USP 29/NF24 and are defined under separate monographs. Their applications in pharmaceutical formulation have been primarily with solid oral dosage forms such as capsules, beads, and tablets as matrix film formers and film-coating agents, but they can also be used to form the matrix layers in transdermal delivery systems. However, polymethacrylates are also used as binders in both aqueous and solvent-based wet granulation processes. Wet granulation with these polymers is particularly suited for high-dose, water-soluble actives. Larger quantities (5–20%) of dry polymer solids corresponding to approximately 0.5 to 2 mg/cm^2 are used to control the release of an active substance from a tablet matrix. Dry powders can be used in direct compression formulations at levels ranging from 10% to 50%.

Eudragit RL 30D and Eudragit RS 30D copolymers are aqueous dispersions containing 30% w/w of dry polymer substance with a low content of quaternary ammonium groups (QAG) present as salts; it is the presence of these QAG in these polymers which impart hydrophilic properties. Despite their high solids content, these dispersions have low viscosities, permitting a sufficient quantity of polymer to be easily incorporated into a formulation. These two polymers differ in their level of QAG with Eudragit RS 30D containing a comparatively 50% lower amount of ammonium groups at 5% w/w, and consequently the films formed are less permeable to water. While film coatings prepared from either polymer give pH-independent drug release, these polymers are frequently blended together in order to adjust the film permeability and thereby the drug release profile. Plasticizers such as triethyl citrate (TEC) can also be added at levels of 10–20% w/w of dry polymer weight to improve film flexibility of the brittle acrylic polymers and to further delay drug release. The improved film flexibility from using plasticizers offers other benefits as well. Adding 20% w/w TEC to a high dose theophylline formulation that was wet granulated in a fluid bed drier using Eudragit RS powder as a matrix and 6% Eudragit® RS 30D as a binder, was found to improve the crushing strength of microtablets compared to formulations without TEC or using TEC at 10% w/w (60).

However, another type of polymethacrylate copolymer which is neutral and has good compressive properties is available commercially as either Eudragit NE 30D or Eudragit NE 40D, corresponding to 30% or 40% dry solids content, respectively. This polymer offers pH-independent drug release and forms very flexible films without the addition of a plasticizer. Moreover, enteric polymers which only dissolve readily and release drug above pH 5.5 are also available as an aqueous dispersion (Eudragit L 30D-55) or as a redispersible dry powder (Eudragit L 100-55). The overall effectiveness of these polymers in sustained release matrix applications is much more pronounced with the wet granulation process than with direct compression.

Enteric acrylic polymers were used as binders in high-shear wet granulation in order to target the colon and prevent drug from being released in the small intestine. Twenty percent ethanolic solutions of each of the following pH-dependent methacrylate polymers, Eudragit L, Eudragit S, and hydroxypropyl methylcellulose acetate succinate (HPMCAS) were added to either ibuprofen or furosemide during mixing. The matrix granules were further coated with additional HPMCAS and cellulose acetate phthalate in a fluid bed drier from 10 to 30% w/w. While the absorption of ibuprofen was adequate with a lag-time of approximately 2 hour and t_{max} values of 4–5 hours, the absorption of furosemide was negligible, due to the extra enteric coating on the granules (135).

The use of acrylic polymers in tablet formulations can also improve patient compliance by reducing the dose frequency through improved sustained drug release. Metformin HCl/Gliclazide was wet granulated using 1.25% PVP K30 and Eudragit® NE 30D as a binder; the level of acrylic polymer solids in tablets was 7.5% and 10.8% with respect to drug content. Drug release was found to follow a Higuchi square root of time kinetics profile showing a fairly rapid initial burst followed by a slower release as time progresses. The results indicated that with Gliclazide and Metformin HCl release at 6 and 8 h, respectively, that the formulation was successful to reduce the dosage frequency from two to three times a day to just once a day (57).

Likewise, other research used the wet granulation technique along with ethanolic solutions of ethylcellulose, Eudragit RS 100, Eudragit RL 100, and PVP as granulating agents in combination with hydrophilic matrix materials such as HPMC, sodium CMC, and sodium alginate; in order to develop a once-daily sustained-release matrix tablet of the highly water soluble drug, nicorandil. A hydrophilic matrix of HPMC alone could not control the nicorandil release effectively for 24 hours. However, the most effective formulation in the study utilized both HPMC and ethylcellulose with a drug:HPMC ratio of 1:4 and ethylcellulose at 4% w/v as a granulating agent. Drug release for this formulation was best fit using the Korsmeyer-Peppas ($R^2 = 0.999$) model with a n value of 0.718; indicating anomalous drug release of diffusion coupled with erosion (22).

Wet granulation was also performed in a fluidized bed granulator using only the highly water soluble drug, theophylline anhydrous, and Eudragit RS 30D mixed with triacetin as a plasticizer at 10% w/w. Theophylline was coated at levels of 11% and 22%, corresponding to 25% and 40% in the dried granules, respectively. It was found that increasing the polymer concentration resulted in an increase of the mean granule diameter, as the polymer behaved like a typical dissolved binder.

However, drug release was unable to be lowered simply by increasing polymer level. Curing of the granules in an oven for 2 hours at approximately 70° C was found to be necessary to form a coherent, non-porous film coating, but only showed an effect with granules containing a polymer load of 40%. The authors also found that the release rate of the cured granules is predetermined by the moisture content of the fluidized bed at the end of the granulation process; the higher the moisture content, the lower the release rate (59).

A fluidized bed system was also used to coat the water insoluble drug, sodium diclofenac. A wet granulation formulation was first used containing microcrystalline cellulose and PVP K-30 as a binder at 20% w/w. Granules were then enteric coated with a 12% solids level of Eudragit L 30D-55 using TEC as a plasticizer to a weight gain of either 5% or 8%. It was found that the process and formulation were very effective during dissolution testing at both preventing release under acidic conditions (0.1 N HCl) and with showing complete release in buffer at pH 6.8 (61).

Polyethylene Glycol

While PEG and its derivatives are typically used in hot melt granulation or solid dispersions, there have been recent articles written describing their use as binders in pharmaceutical wet granulation. PEG is available in either liquid or solid form in a wide range of grades with different average molecular weights. PEGs of relatively high molecular weight (6000 and above) are supplied as free-flowing, milled powders. They may be used as binders in direct compression tableting or by dry mixing and subsequent wet granulation with either water or ethanol.

Abdelbary et al. (25) used an oil-in-water emulsion of a PEG derivative, PEG-6-stearate, to granulate acetaminophen by two methods with the goal of producing rapidly disintegrating tablets. The results showed that while the tablets prepared from hot melt granulations gave improved hardness values, the disintegration time of tablets from wet granulated batches were relatively shorter at 40 ± 2 seconds. Other work has examined the use of different grades of PEG in both low shear and high shear wet granulation.

Solid PEG 1500 was used at levels between 12% and 19% to granulate different grades of calcium carbonate ranging in particle size from 4 to 23 µm using a high shear mixer. Three different methods of PEG incorporation were examined: (*i*) pouring molten PEG (60°C) onto the powder; (*ii*) spraying; and (*iii*) melting-in, where the PEG binder was added as a solid flake and is melted-in by the heat and torque generated through mixing. While all methods resulted in a bimodal distribution of granule sizes, the authors stated that this seems to be an intrinsic feature of all processes in which liquid is mixed into a finely powdered solid material. Moreover, the spray and melt-in methods gave a lower content of coarse granules than the pour method. The melt-in method also gave a significantly lower rate of granule growth as measured by their volume mean diameter (D[4,3]). The authors concluded by stating that the particle size of the solid starting material was critical during granule growth. As the particle size of the solid decreases, the bimodality becomes more pronounced and that the finer the solid material (ie., 4 µm), the slower the loss of pore volume. Fu et al. (26) also studied high shear wet granulation using similar particle size grades of calcium carbonate but used only the pour method with liquid PEG 400 at similar levels of 11.5–19%. Similarly, they found that the main factors affecting the size distribution of granules are the grade of powdered material used (initial particle size, shape, surface characteristics, etc.), and its porosity.

Cellulose-Based Polymers

This class of cellulose derivatives includes hydroxypropylmethylcellulose or HPMC, hydroxyethylcellulose (58), methylcellulose, HPC, and ethylcellulose. As mentioned earlier, most cellulose-based polymers except for PVP, have lower surface tension values in the range of 40–50 mN/m, thus similar adhesive and film-forming qualities will be seen.

Ethylcellulose

Not all cellulose derivatives are soluble in water. For example, ethylcellulose is an ethyl ether of cellulose and requires alcohol in order to dissolve; it can be used either dissolved in alcohol or as a dry binder, which is then wetted with alcohol. Ethylcellulose powder can be used as a binder in modified release formulations containing water-soluble drugs and also offers an advantage for use with materials that are moisture-sensitive. Ethylcellulose is available in a number of grades that differ in their degree of substitution and average molecular weight; and is also available as a micronized powder at three viscosity grades; namely 7, 10, and 100 cP. These low viscosity powdered grades can be used as binders in wet granulation and offer several advantages for the formulator.

Ethylcellulose produces hard tablets with low friability; tablets usually will disintegrate readily but drug dissolution will be impaired due to the fact that ethylcellulose acts as an inert, hydrophobic matrix; however, this can be advantageous for delaying release of water-soluble drugs. In fact, it has been shown that the lower viscosity grade of ethylcellulose (7 cP) allows for the production of harder tablets under similar compression forces (51, 52, 136). Lower viscosity ethylcellulose also displays the slowest drug release rate, as this grade is more compressible and therefore has a lower porosity (53, 56).

Furthermore, the lower viscosity grades also exhibited lower mean yield pressures than the higher viscosity grades following Heckel analysis, indicating the greater compressibility of the former. The higher viscosity grades were shown to be more elastic in their deformation behavior as a result of their higher molecular weight polymeric chains being more ordered and less prone to forming more permanent interparticulate bonds (136).

Research was undertaken to develop a controlled release tablet of naproxen using ethylcellulose and both methods of wet granulation and solid dispersion were compared for effectiveness. Naproxen level was kept constant at 16% while ethylcellulose content was varied from 6% to 28% in the formulations. While both methods were successful at producing formulations with drug release profiles of at least 12 hours, the amount of ethylcellulose required to prepare such formulations was 33% less using the solid dispersion method. While none of the formulations released 100% of the drug, a cumulative 88% of naproxen was released from the solid dispersion formulation, compared with 84% from the wet granulation formulation (50).

Ethylcellulose can also be added as a binder liquid during wet granulation in the form of an aqueous pseudolatex dispersion. Two products currently available are Aquacoat®, a 30% w/w ethylcellulose dispersion without plasticizers from FMC Corp., Philadelphia, Pennsylvania, U.S.A. and Surelease®, a 25% w/w ethylcellulose dispersion containing the hydrophobic plasticizers, dibutyl sebacate and oleic acid, available from Colorcon, West Point, Pennsylvania, U.S.A. Granule formulations of acetaminophen and lactose were wet granulated with and without using Surelease as a binder and tablets were prepared. As the level of total solids from the ethylcellulose formulations was increased, the compressibility was improved. Granulations with ethylcellulose also showed enhanced deformation and densification behaviors and gave tablets better mechanical strength compared to control tablets formulated without Surelease (49).

Hydroxypropyl Methylcellulose

The swelling properties of HPMC as a sustained release, hydrophilic matrix binder in tablets are well known. This polymer also has the ability to form a gel network to delay drug release (30,32,34,36,137). The use and efficiency of HPMC as a tablet and granule binder is comparable with methylcellulose. HPMC is available in a variety of grades with different solution viscosities and it is soluble in both water and hydroalcoholic solutions. However, HPMC is more soluble in cold water than hot but more dispersible in hot water than cold. Therefore, it is recommended to hydrate the HPMC powder in very hot water first, under agitation, and then to cool the solution down as quickly and as low as possible in order to avoid lumping problems.

The use of a fast hydrating "K" grade of HPMC (HPMC 2208) has been reported to have successfully provided 12-hour extended release to metoprolol tartrate tablets when used as a hydrophilic matrix. The three processes of direct compression, high-shear granulation, and fluid bed granulation were compared; and in the latter two processes another grade of HPMC, Methocel E5, was also selected as the binder of choice. It was found that while direct compression formulations exhibited poor flow, picking and sticking problems during tableting, high-shear granulation resulted in the formation of hard granules which were difficult to mill, however, the tablets were satisfactory. However, the best method of choice appeared to be fluid bed granulation as the granules showed the best flow and tablet properties, including a slower drug dissolution rate, when compared with the other two methods (138). This study was taken to the next level by using what was learned to identify the critical formulation and processing variables for these HPMC matrix tablets; and also to develop slow-, medium-, and fast-releasing tablets of metoprolol tartrate for further scale-up and in vivo studies (139). These landmark studies served an important role in providing model data in an experimental design space which then served as the scientific basis for regulatory policy development on scale-up and post-approval changes for modified-release dosage forms (SUPAC-MR) (140).

Dissolution results are known to be dependent on the solid state of the drug substance, formulation composition, and manufacturing conditions (141). Recently, it was discovered that HPMC at a level of 29% can affect the solid phase transformation of anhydrous ciprofloxacin in tablets following wet granulation. While the anhydrate showed a significantly higher dissolution rate than the hydrate form as expected, the anhydrate rapidly converted to the hydrate form when exposed to moisture. However, premixing the anhydrate with HPMC in the presence of either water or ethanol was found to inhibit the processing-induced phase transition (21). This phenomena has been reported previously with HPMC at a level of 50% inhibiting the transformation of carbamazepine to carbamazepine dihydrate in the gel layer of the hydrated tablets and also in aqueous solutions (142); and also has been observed with PVP at 5% w/w inhibiting indomethacin crystallization from molecular dispersions (143).

Another formulation variable that can have a significant outcome on tablet properties is the incorporation stage of the binder; whether it is added intra- or extragranularly (144). Wet granulation using water was performed in a high shear mixer with the drug level at 10%, HPMC K15M from 24% to 32% added intragranularly, and either 0%, 4%, or 8% HPMC added extragranularly. In addition, each formulation was prepared using two different amounts of water for granulation, normal versus overgranulated; and all tablets were compressed at two target hardness levels, namely 3.3 and 6.0 kP. These tablets were compared against a direct compression formulation which served as the control. The results showed that the best intragranular:extragranular HPMC ratio was a 24%:8% distribution which gave a robust product having good reproducibility; neither hardness nor overgranualtion seemed to have any major impact on the release profile of these tablets.

Methylcellulose

Methylcellulose is a methyl ether of cellulose and is available in a variety of different grades of substitution and average molecular weight. When used as a binder in wet granulation, low- or medium-viscosity grades are preferred. While methylcellulose powder is stable, although slightly hygroscopic; solutions are liable to microbial spoilage and antimicrobial preservatives should be used if storage delays are expected. Methylcellulose is a good tablet and granule binder and this ability improves with increasing molecular weight. Methylcellulose is practically insoluble in solvents and hot water. In cold water, methylcellulose swells and disperses slowly to form a viscous, colloidal dispersion. The use of a novel, chemically modified methylcellulose as a tablet matrix was recently reported to study release of theophylline, aspirin, and atenolol. This research involved the substitution of 50% of the hydroxyl groups of the methylcellulose with a hydrophobic acid derivative such as glutaric acid to produce methylcellulose glutarate (MC-GA). This was done in order to decrease the swelling rate of the polymer matrix in aqueous solution through reduced hydrogen bonding capacity. The drug to polymer ratio was kept at 4:1 (w/w). While all the drug tablets containing methylcellulose yielded an approximately 80% release between 2.5 and 3 hours, those tablets prepared with MC-GA gave a zero-order release profile over 12 hours. The reduced swelling of the MC-GA tablets was attributed to the reduced hydrophilicity of the MC-GA polymer (40).

Hydroxypropylcellulose

HPC is a partially substituted hydroxypropyl ether of cellulose and is used as an excipient in tableting and wet granulation due to its good affinity for water as well as for its binding abilities. There are a number of grades available that have different particle sizes and substitution levels. HPC is a stable material although it is hygroscopic after drying. It can be used as an extended-release matrix former at levels between 15 and 35% w/w or as a tablet binder from 2 to 6% w/w. The drug release rate can be decreased by decreasing the viscosity of HPC in the formulation, however, the addition of an anionic surfactant will increase the polymer viscosity and subsequently decrease the release rate of the drug. This excipient also has a low-substituted version (L-HPC containing 5–16% hydroxypropoxyl groups) which functions as a wet granulation binder in tablets but also has disintegrant properties. Higher levels of hydroxypropoxyl group substitution impart improved binding strength to this polymer.

While HPC is freely soluble in water, L-HPC is insoluble in aqueous media but swells when it comes into contact with water. It was discovered that another difference between HPC and L-HPC is the degree of side chain branching; which affects the cloud point, and serendipitously was also found to affect the dissolution rate of hydrochlorothiazide tablets containing 5% w/v of either HPC or HPC-L. HPC containing tablets had a higher dissolution rate due to the lower polymer cloud point at 39 °C. A phase separation occurs during dissolution and a less viscous layer surrounding the drug granules is responsible for the faster dissolution rate (44).

Other properties of these polymers have also been reported. For instance, it was noted that using acetaminophen along with HPC-L in high shear wet granulation led to a reduction in granule particle size even when used at a 10% level; and this was attributed to the small particle size of this binder (ca. 50 μm) as well as its poor binding properties. However, while granule strength was quite low, and in many cases even lower than that achieved when no binder was present; crushing strength of acetaminophen tablets containing HPC-L was comparable with the use of pregelatinized starch or maltodextrin as binders (19).

In contrast, the liquid bridges formed from pure HPC were found to be very strong and tough due to the fact that it is non-crystalline. Furthermore, it was found that a liquid bridge of ideal qualities and strength was formed from the combination of 18% anhydrous lactose and 5% HPC (Klucel® EXF) (116). Previously it was thought from traditional granulation theory that only the binder level was key in assuring appropriate granule strength. However, recent research has shown that excipients, which are strongly soluble in the liquid binder, play a major role in the formation and strength of solid bridges inside a granule (145).

This data is further supported by research on granule growth of mannitol and anhydrous dibasic calcium phosphate conducted in a fluid bed drier using HPC as the binder solution at levels from 5 to 15% w/w. Mannitol with the lowest binder level of 5% showed a prolonged lag time followed by slow but steady growth; however, using 15% HPC showed an immediate and prolonged rapid increase in granule size. This is in sharp contrast to the results for anhydrous dicalcium phosphate, which showed no growth at all at a 10% HPC level. At a binder level of 15%, however, a rapid granule growth was observed but only after a longer protracted lag time. The insolubility of the calcium phosphate in water and the weaker liquid bridges thus formed likely contribute to the generally slower granule growth for this excipient (47).

The effect of different levels of binder solution (PVP K-30 at 3%, and Methocel E5 from 3% to 8%) added during high-shear mixing on dicalcium phosphate porosity was reported earlier by Ritala et al. (113). They found that as the wet massing time increases and as the mean granule size increases with the addition of increased levels of binder, that the intragranular porosity decreases (86).

The effect of increased level of binder solution on the total porosity (summation of the mannitol internal porosity plus the granule porosity) of mannitol granules was studied. Unlike dicalcium phosphate, mannitol is water-soluble and is expected to show differences in porosity during granule growth. It was found that as the level of binder applied to the granules increased, that the total porosity also steadily increased; in fact a clear correlation between the total granule porosity and the binder concentration was observed for the mannitol granules (47) This work provides an important addition to our knowledge base of wet granulation technology and granule growth mechanisms of materials with differing physical and chemical properties.

The selection of the proper excipients in a wet granulation formulation is important to prevent deleterious phase transformations of drug, which can lead to problems of physical stability and bioavailability. It was recently reported that neither silicified microcrystalline cellulose, which is partially crystalline, or lactose monohydrate, which is crystalline, were able to control and prevent hydrate formation of nitrofurantoin anhydrate in the presence of high water levels involved during the wet granulation process. However, the amorphous binder L-HPC was able to hinder the conversion of this drug to its hydrate form by absorbing the water and preventing it from entering into chemical reactions (42).

PAT AND ENDPOINT DETERMINATION

Based on the higher success rate of manufacturing processes outside of the pharmaceutical industry, PAT are being applied to provide an objective, sensitive and improved definition of the optimal wet granulation endpoint at the pilot scale, and also improved control of other critical process parameters as well. This then forms the basis for planning ever-increasing scales of production, which is then verified with data from increasingly larger machines, thus forming the basis for regulatory filings and future manufacturing.

As the final product of the granulation process is a compressed tablet, the definition of an appropriate endpoint may include a combination of tablet manufacturing properties (e.g., compression force, tablet weight variation, dissolution time, content uniformity) and granulation properties (e.g., mean particle size, particle size distribution, flow rate), and this represents a compromise of the many factors yielding the final tablet. Frequently, the most important parameters demanded of a granulation are improved flow properties and homogeneous distribution of drug without future segregation; yet these are assessed after the completion of the granulation and drying steps. Currently, real time measurements are made of parameters that have a correlation to flow properties of the dried granulation and drug distribution, however, the strength of this correlation needs a more critical assessment. While this approach has resulted in significant improvements from the era of empirical operator-defined endpoints, there remains the opportunity for further improvements in the determination of the granulation endpoint.

Various techniques are available for the assessment of a granulation operation, of these the "on-line" measurements are significantly more valuable than either "at-line" or "off-line" characterization, this due to the possibility for controlling the granulation operation and applying logical adjustments that have been defined *a priori* to deliver optimal, consistent results. Parameters that can be measured "on-line" include current, voltage, capacitance, conductivity, probe vibration, granule momentum, chopper speed, impeller or motor shaft speed, impeller tip speed, main impeller relative swept volume, motor slip, temperature, binder addition rate, power consumption on the main motor, impeller torque, and reaction torque on the motor base (146).

Of these, power consumption has emerged as a popular method (118,147–150), due to its low cost, economical operation, non-obtrusive installation, and most importantly, its correlation with the extent of densification (86) and granule growth (149). Though up to 30% of motor power consumption may be due to machine function (e.g., cooling fan, air drag, bearing friction) and there may be long-term drift as the machinery wears, this has become routinely available. Tershita et al. (151) used a bottom drive granulator to produce a power profile during granulation. Based on this work, four distinct phases were identified; in Phase I, power consumption grows rapidly, during Phase II there is fluctuation with the maximum power draw, in Phase III, the power consumption declines, and finally in Phase IV there is constant power. Temperature was also recorded; and it increased steadily by approximately 25°C in 8 minutes.

A second popular approach is measurement of the main impeller torque, which reflects the increasing cohesive force of the powders via addition of liquid and agglomerate tensile strength. This requires strain gauge installation on the impeller shaft, retrofit installation is more involved than power instrumentation, yet it has the distinct advantage of a direct link to the impeller load and thus the status of the granulating powders, and it is not impacted by mixer conditions.

Recent research attempting to improve on these techniques includes efforts with measurement of acoustic emissions (152–154). This approach utilizes placement of piezoelectric sensors at multiple locations, and has the advantages of being non-invasive, does not contact the product, and is relatively inexpensive. The authors showed that the optimum endpoints occurred near the start of a plateau region, however they also noted that data from trials in a PMA-10 model did not give profiles that corresponded to changes in the granulation process.

Additionally, near-infrared spectroscopy has been utilized to monitor moisture for endpoint determination (155,156), though this technique is limited to detecting only moisture at the bed surface. The FBRM is a technique for particle size determination; in a study by Dilworth et al. (157), comparing power consumption, FBRM, and acoustic signals, these measurements were found to be complimentary. Thermal effusivity is a material property that combines thermal conductivity, density and heat capacity. Fariss et al. (158) used "at-line" samples and found colinearity between power consumption and thermal effusivity.

SCALING

The challenge of scaling a granulation process from laboratory to commercial production has been completed successfully innumerable times, yet it remains a daunting challenge in that no single, broadly applicable model or theory accurately predicts the process parameters; thus it remains for each product's development team to create the body of knowledge through extensive laboratory or pilot plant trials. Due to cost limitations of conducting experiments at the production scale, a limited number of confirmatory trials often yields a paucity of data, this may be marginally adequate and lead to frequent difficulties during the commercial life cycle, which may drive a re-formulation or secondary process optimization/re-validation effort.

On the assumed basis of a fixed formulation with the ratios of each powder component defined explicitly and a clearly defined goal for the commercial manufacturing phase, the scaling effort may be launched. Included in the commercial manufacturing goal are the expected manufacturing equipment and batch size(s) at specific manufacturing sites. Following from this, a thorough understanding of the full scale facility and equipment necessary is required, including batch ranges and fill level, impeller design and rotation speed(s), bowl geometry, liquid addition system capability, PAT equipment, and material transfer techniques and time requirements for both loading and discharging. Intermediate scale equipment and pilot scale equipment and sites also need to be selected, preferably retaining a single design/mode of granulation from one machinery manufacturer, this allows the development team access to the substantial experience and expertise of that manufacturer's technical support team, who may provide significant guidance.

For a series of PMA high shear granulators, work by Rekhi et al. (75,159) recommended the following three factors be considered in scaling:

1. maintain constant impeller tip speed (radial velocity);
2. linearly scale the granulating fluid to the batch size;
3. adjust granulation massing time based on the ratio of impeller speed from one scale to the next.

Though maintenance of constant impeller tip speed is rarely feasible, this approach may lead to long processing times.

An alternative approach from Kristensen et al. (68,160) suggests addition of relatively larger amounts of granulating liquid, due to reduced mixing efficiency and less densification at larger scale. Saturation level was found to be the link between median granule diameter and machine scale.

A third option is based on the relative sweep volume, which is the space through which an impeller pass per second is divided by the mixer volume. While this has been correlated to the specific energy consumed by the granulation (161), the d_{50} was unable to be correlated.

Dimensionless power relationships have been investigated by Faure et al. (102,162,163). Power number (impeller drag force to inertial stress ratio), Reynolds number (inertial forces relative to viscous forces), and Froude number (ratio of centrifugal acceleration to gravitational constant) were utilized, and under certain conditions it was possible to prepare a master curve from data at various bowl capacities. With the master curve, determination of the power consumption could be performed to define the granulation endpoint. For scaling low shear rotating shell granulators, maintenance of constant peripheral speed is an option. Pilot scale vessels may turn at 25–30 rpm, and production vessels 4–8 rpm. An alternative technique from work by Chirkot (164) with a V-type granulator is to maintain a constant cumulative torque to mass ratio.

Frequently the scaling process becomes a customized effort for each individual product/formulation, standards are seldom available due to the unique physical characteristics of the formulation components and of the granulation process and equipment. As the resources required for full scale lot manufacture are significantly larger than for pilot scale work, a minimum number of statistically optimized confirmatory trials may be performed prior to initiation of validation and commercial manufacturing to give an idea of the variability in the design space.

REFERENCES

1. Lerk C, Lagas M, Fell JT, Nauta P. Effect of hydrophilization of hydrophobic drugs on release rate from capsules. J Pharm Sci 1978; 67:935–9.
2. Augsburger L, Brzeczko AW, Shah U, Hahm H. Characterization and functionality of superdisintegrants. In: Swarbrick J, Boylan JC, eds. Encyclopedia of Pharmaceutical Technology, New York: Marcel Dekker, 2002; 285–6.
3. Lagas M, deWit HJC, Woldring MG, Piers DA, Lerk CF. Technetium labelled disintegration of capsules in the human stomach. Pharm Acta Helv 1980; 55: 114–9.
4. Lerk C, Lagas M, Huen L, Broersma P, Zuurman K. In vitro and in vivo release of hydrophilized phenytoin from capsules. J Pharm Sci 1979; 68:634–7.
5. Lerk C, Lagas M, Fell JT, Nauta P. Effect of hydrophilization of hydrophobic drugs on release rate from capsules. J Pharm Sci 1987; 67:935–9.
6. Buckton G, Adeniyi AA, Saunders M, Ambarkhane A, HyperDSC studies of amorphous polyvinylpyrrolidone in a model wet granulation system. Int J Pharm 2006; 312(1–2): 61–5.
7. Rodriguez L, Cavallari C, Passerini N, Albertini B, Fini A. Preparation and characterization by morphological analysis of diclofenac/PEG 4000 granules obtained using three different techniques. Int J Pharm 2002; 242(1–2): 285–9.
8. Albertini B, Cavallari C, Passerini N, Voinovich D, Rodriguez L. Characterization and taste-masking evaluation of acetaminophen granules: comparison between different preparation methods in a high-shear mixer. Eur J Pharm Sci 2004; 21(2–3):295–303.
9. Keary CM, Sheskey PJ. Preliminary report of the discovery of a new pharmaceutical granulation process using foamed aqueous binders. Drug Dev Ind Pharm 2004; 30(8):831–45.
10. Juslin L, Yliruusi J, Effect of fluidized bed granulation on the crystal properties of lactose, glucose and mannitol. S.T.P. Pharm Sci 1996; 6(3):173–8.
11. Johnson J, Wang LH, Gordon MS, Chowhan ZT. Effect of formulation solubility and hygroscopicity on disintegrant efficiency in tablets prepared by wet granulation, in terms of dissolution. J Pharm Sci 1991; 80: 469–71.
12. Cao Q, Choi YW, Cui JH, Lee BJ. Formulation, release characteristics and bioavailability of novel monolithic hydroxypropylmethylcellulose matrix tablets containing acetaminophen. J Control Rel 2005; 108(2–3):351–61.
13. Di Martino P, Censi R, Malaj L, Martelli S, Barthelemy C. Influence of metronidazole particle properties on granules prepared in a high-shear mixer-granulator. Drug Dev Ind Pharm 2007; 33(2):121–31.
14. Joachim J, Kalantzis G, Joachim G, Reynier JP, Ruiz JM. Pregelatinized starches in wet granulation: experimental design and data analysis. Part 2. Case of tablets. S.T.P. Pharma Sci 1994; 4(6):482–6.
15. Sarisuta N, Parrott EL. Effects of temperature, humidity, and aging on the disintegration and dissolution of acetaminophen tablets. Drug Dev Ind Pharm 1988; 14(13):1877–81.
16. Chowhan Z, Yang IC. Effect of intergranular versus intragranular cornstarch on tablet friability and in vitro dissolution. J Pharm Sci 1983; 72:983–8.
17. de Castro A, Vicente JA, Mourao SC, Bueno JH, Gremiao MP. Effect of maize starch concentration on in vitro acetaminophen release from tablets. Brazil J Pharm Sci 2003; 39(3): 289–97.
18. Vojnovic D, Moneghini M, Chicco D. Nonclassical experimental design applied in the optimization of a placebo granulate formulation in high-shear mixer. Drug Dev Ind Pharm 1996; 22(9–10):997–1004.

19. Becker D, Rigassi T, Bauer-Brandl A. Effectiveness of binders in wet granulation: Comparison using model formulations of different tabletability. Drug Dev Ind Pharm 1997; 23(8):791–808.
20. Dias V, Pinto JF. Identification of the most relevant factors that affect and reflect the quality of granules by application of canonical and cluster analysis. J Pharm Sci 2002; 91(1):273–81.
21. Li X, Zhi F, Hu YQ. Investigation of excipient and processing on solid phase transformation and dissolution of ciprofloxacin. Int J Pharm 2007; 328(2):177–82.
22. Reddy K, Mutalik S, Reddy S. Once-Daily Sustained-Release Matrix Tablets of Nicorandil: Formulation and In Vitro Evaluation. AAPS Pharm Sci Tech 2003; 4(4):Article 61.
23. Wong T, Heng PWS, Yeo TN, Chan, LW. Influence of polyvinylpyrrolidone on aggregation propensity of coated spheroids. Int J Pharm 2002; 242;357–60.
24. Yueksel N, Karatas A, Baykara T. Comparative evaluation of granules made with different binders by a fluidized bed method. Drug Dev Ind Pharm 2003; 29(4):387–95.
25. Abdelbary G, Prinderre P, Eouani C, Joachim J, Piccerelle P. The preparation of orally disintegrating tablets using a hydrophilic waxy binder. Int J Pharm 2004; 278(2): 423–33.
26. Fu J, Cheong YS, Reynolds GK, Adams MJ, Salman AD, Hounslow MJ. An experimental study of the variability in the properties and quality of wet granules. Powder Technol 2004; 140(3):209–16.
27. Knight P, Instone T, Pearson JMK, Hounslow MJ. An investigation into the kinetics of liquid distribution and growth in high shear mixer agglomeration. Powder Technol 1998; 97:246–57.
28. Rezaei H, Sakr A. Effect of molecular weight of polyethylene glycol binders on acetaminophen tablets: low shear wet granulation. Pharm Ind 2001; 63(9):974–84.
29. Bravo S, Lamas MC, Salomon CJ. Swellable matrices for the controlled-release of diclofenac sodium: Formulation and in vitro studies. Pharm Dev Tech 2004; 9(1):75–83.
30. Hogan J. Hydroxypropylmethylcellulose sustained release technology. Drug Dev Ind Pharm 1989; 15:975–99.
31. Kiortsis S, Kachrimanis K, Broussali T, Malamataris S. Drug release from tableted wet granulations comprising cellulosic (HPMC or HPC) and hydrophobic component. Eur J Pharm Biopharm 2005; 59(1):73–83.
32. Li C, Martini LG, Ford JL, Roberts M. The use of hypromellose in oral drug delivery. J Pharm Pharmacol 2005; 57:533–46.
33. Qiu Y, Hui HW. Cheskin H. Formulation development of sustained-release hydrophilic matrix tablets of zileuton. Pharm Dev Tech 1997; 2(3):197–204.
34. Sako K, Sawada T, Nakashima H. Influence of water soluble fillers in hydroxypropylmethylcellulose matrices on in vitro and in vivo drug release. J Control Rel 2002; 81:165–72.
35. Saravanan M, Nataraj KS, Ganesh KS. Hydroxypropyl methylcellulose based cephalexin extended release tablets: Influence of tablet formulation, hardness and storage on in vitro release kinetics. Chem Pharm Bull 2003; 51(8):978–83.
36. Shah A, Britten NJ, Olanoff LS, Badalamenti JN. Gel-matrix systems exhibiting bimodal controlled release for oral delivery. J Control Rel 1989; 9:169–75.
37. Shah N, Railkar AS, Phuapradit W, Zeng FW, Malick AW. Effect of processing techniques in controlling the release rate and mechanical strength of hydroxypropyl methylcellulose based hydrogel matrices. Eur J Pharm Biopharm 1996; 42(3):183–7.
38. Tiwari S, Murthy TK, Pai MR, Mehta PR, Chowdary PB. Controlled release formulation of tramadol hydrochloride using hydrophilic and hydrophobic matrix system. AAPS Pharm Sci Tech 1993; 4(3) Article 31.
39. Xu G, Fang F, Zhang R. Sunada H. Granulation of aspirin sustained release formulation with hydroxypropyl methylcellulose as rate controlling agent. Drug Dev Ind Pharm 1997; 23(11):1105–10.
40. Khairuzzaman A, Ahmed SU, Savva M, Patel NK. Zero-order release of aspirin, theophylline and atenolol in water from novel methylcellulose glutarate matrix tablets. Int J Pharm 2006; 318(1–2):15–21.

41. Wan L, Prasad KP, Influence of quantity of granulating liquid on water uptake and disintegration of tablets with methylcellulose. Pharma Ind 1989; 51(1):105–9.
42. Airaksinen S, Karjalainen M, Kivikero N, Westermarck S, Yliruusi J. Excipient selection can significantly affect solid-state phase transformation in formulation during wet granulation. AAPS Pharm Sci Tech 2005; 6(2):Article 41.
43. Badawy S, Gray DB, Hussain MA. A study on the effect of wet granulation on microcrystalline cellulose particle structure and performance. Pharm Res 2006; 23(3):634–40.
44. Desai D, Rinaldi F, Kothari S, Paruchuri S, Both D. Effect of hydroxypropyl cellulose (HPC) on dissolution rate of hydrochlorothiazide tablets. Int J Pharm 2006; 308(1–2):40–5.
45. Kato H, Ono Y, Yonezawa Y, Sunada H. The effect of binder particle size on granule and tablet properties in high shear and extrusion granulation. J Drug Deliv Sci Tech 2006; 16(6):461–6.
46. Kawashima Y, Takeuchi H, Hino T, Niwa T, Ohya M. Preparation of prolonged-release matrix tablet of acetaminophen with pulverized low-substituted hydroxypropylcellulose via wet granulation. Int J Pharm 1993; 99:229–38.
47. Rajniak P, Mancinelli C, Chern RT, Stepanek F, Hill BT. Experimental study of wet granulation in fluidized bed: Impact of the binder properties on the granule morphology. Int J Pharm 2007; 334(1–2):92–102.
48. Emeje M, Kunle OO, Ofoefule SI. Effect of the molecular size of carboxymethylcellulose and some polymers on the sustained release of theophylline from a hydrophilic matrix. Acta Pharm 2006; 56(3):325–35.
49. Ghaly E, Ruiz NR. Compressibility characteristics of matrices prepared with ethylcellulose aqueous dispersion. Drug Dev Ind Pharm 1996; 22(2):91–5.
50. Iqbal Z, Babar A, Ashraf M. Controlled-release naproxen using micronized ethyl cellulose by wet-granulation and solid-dispersion method. Drug Dev Ind Pharm 2002; 28(2):129–34.
51. Katikaneni P, Upadrashta SM, Neau SH, Mitra AK. Ethylcellulose matrix controlled release tablets of a water soluble drug. Int J Pharm 1995; 123(Aug. 29):119–25.
52. Katikaneni P, Upadrashta SM, Rowlings CE, Neau SH, Hileman GA. Consolidation of ethylcellulose: effect of particle size, press speed, and lubricants. Int J Pharm 1995; 117(Apr. 4):13–21.
53. Khan G, Meidan VM. Drug release kinetics from tablet matrices based upon ethylcellulose ether-derivatives: A comparison between different formulations. Drug Dev Ind Pharm 2007; 33(6):627–39.
54. Kulvanich P, Leesawat P, Patomchaiviwat V. Release characteristics of the matrices prepared from co-spray-dried powders of theophylline and ethylcellulose. Drug Dev Ind Pharm 2002; 28(6):727–39.
55. Ruiz N, Ghaly ES. Mechanisms of drug release from matrices prepared with aqueous dispersion of ethylcellulose. Drug Dev Ind Pharm 1997; 23(1):113–7.
56. Shileout G, Zessin G. Investigation of ethylcellulose as a matrix former and a new method to regard and evaluate the compaction data. Drug Dev Ind Pharm 1996; 22(4):313–9.
57. Arno E, Anand P, Bhaskar K, Saravanan M, Vinod R. Eudragit NE30D based Metformin/Gliclazide extended release tablets: Formulation, characterisation and in vitro release studies. Chem Pharm Bull 2002; 50(11):1495–8.
58. Khidr S. Preparation and evaluation of controlled-release sodium valproate/valproic acid (valdisoval) tablets. Bull Pharm Sci 2003; 26(Part 2):179–86.
59. Radtke G, Knop K, Lippold BC. Manufacture of slow-release matrix granules by wet granulation with an aqueous dispersion of quaternary poly(meth)acrylates in the fluidized bed. Drug Dev Ind Pharm 2002; 28(10):1295–302.
60. Rey H, Wagner KG, Wehrle P, Schmidt PC. Development of matrix-based theophylline sustained-release microtablets. Drug Dev Ind Pharm 2000; 26(1):21–6.
61. Silva O, Souza CR, Oliveira WP, Rocha SC. In vitro dissolution studies of sodium diclofenac granules coated with Eudragit L-30D-55(R) by fluidized-bed system. Drug Dev Ind Pharm 2006; 32(6):661–7.

62. Kristensen H. Binders. In: Swarbrick J, Boylan JC, eds. Encyclopedia of Pharmaceutical Technology. New York: Marcel Dekker, 1988.
63. Boerefijn R, Hounslow MJ. Studies of fluid bed granulation in an industrial R&D context. Chem Eng Sci 2005; 60:3879–90.
64. Cameron I, Wang FY, Immanuel CD, Stepanek F. Process systems modeling and applications in granulation: a review. Chem Eng Sci 2005; 60:3723–50.
65. Iveson S, Litster JD, Hapgood KB, Ennis J. Nucleation, growth and breakage phenomena in agitated granulation processes: a review. Powder Technol 2001; 117:3–39.
66. Knight P. Challenges in granulation technology. Powder Technol 2004; 140:156–62.
67. Kristensen H, Schaefer T. Granulation: review on pharmaceutical wet granulation. Drug Dev Ind Pharm 1987; 13(4–5):803–72.
68. Kristensen H, Schaefer T. Granulations. In: Swarbrick J, Boylan JC, eds. Encyclopedia of Pharmaceutical Technology. New York: Marcel Dekker, 2002:121.
69. Litster J, Ennis BJ, Liu L, ed. The Science and Engineering of Granulation Processes. Dordrecht: Kluwer Academic Publishers; 2004.
70. Reynolds G, Fu JS, Cheong YS, Hounslow MJ, Salman AD. Breakage in granulation: a review. Chem Eng Sci 2005; 60:3969–92.
71. Tapper G, Lindberg NO. The granulation of some lactose qualities with different particle size distributions in a domestic-type mixer. Acta Pharm Suec 1986; 23:47–56.
72. Holm P. High shear mixer granulators. In: Parikh D, ed. Handbook of Pharmaceutical Granulation Technology. New York: Marcel Dekker, 1997.
73. Laicher A, Profitlich T, Schwitzer K, Ahlert D. Modified signal analysis system for end-point control during granulation. Eur J Pharm Sci 1997; 5(1):7–14.
74. Lindberg N, Jonsson C. The granulation of lactose and starch in a recording high speed mixer, Diosna P25. Drug Dev Ind Pharm 1985; 11:917–30.
75. Rekhi G, Caricofe RB, Parikh DM, Augsburger LL. A new approach to scale-up of a high shear granulation process. Pharm Technol Yearbook 1996; 58:67.
76. Armstrong N, March GA. Quantitative assessment of factors contributing to mottling of colored tablets. 1. Manufacturing variables. J Pharm Sci 1976; 65(Feb):198–200.
77. Krycer I, Pope DG, Hersey JA. An evaluation of tablet binding agents part II. Pressure binders. Powder Technol 1983; 34(1):39–51.
78. Reading S, Spring MS. Effects of binder film characteristics on granule and tablet properties. J Pharm Pharmacol 1984; 36(July):421–6.
79. Rumpf H. The strength of granules and agglomerates, Knepper W, Editor. Interscience: New York. 1962: 379–414.
80. Capes C. Particle size enlargement. Elsevier Scientific: Amsterdam. 1980: 91.
81. Sastry K, Fuerstenau DW. Mechanisms of agglomerate growth in green pelletization. Powder Technol 1973; 7:97–105.
82. Ennis B, Litster JD. Particle size enlargement. 7th ed. Perry's Chemical Engineer's Handbook R. Perry Green D. ed. New York: McGraw-Hill, 1997.
83. Tardos G, Irfan-Khan M, Mort PR. Critical parameters and limiting conditions in binder granulation of fine powders. Powder Technol 1997; 94:245–58.
84. Knight P. Structuring agglomerated products for improved performance. Powder Technol 2001; 119:14–25.
85. Simons S, Fairbrother RJ. Direct observations of liquid binder–particle interactions: the role of wetting behaviour in agglomerate growth. Powder Technol 2000; 110(1–2):44–58.
86. Ritala M, Holm P, Schaefer T, Kristensen HG. Influence of liquid bonding strength on power consumption during granulation in a high shear mixer. Drug Dev Ind Pharm 1988; 14(8):1041–1060.
87. Adamson AM. Physical Chemistry of Surfaces. 3rd ed. New York: Wiley; 1976.
88. Badawy S, Menning MM, Gorko MA, GIlbert DL. Effect of process parameters on compressibility of granulation manufactured in a high-shear mixer. Int J Pharm 2000; 198:51–61.

89. Chirkot T, Propost C. Low-shear granulation. In: Parikh D, Handbook of Pharmaceutical Granulation Technology. Boca Raton, FL: Taylor & Francis, 2006: 230.
90. Robin P, Lucisano LJ, Pearswig DM. Rationale for selection of a single-pot manufacturing process using microwave/vacuum drying. Pharm Tech 1994; 18(5):28–36.
91. Stahl H. Single-pot systems for drying pharmaceutical granules. Pharm Tech 2000; 24:32–40.
92. Bauer K, Vadagnini M. New developments in wet granulation. Pharm Tech Eur 1997; 9(3):27–34.
93. Giry K, Gentry M, Viana M, Withrich P, Chulia D. Multiphase versus single pot granulation process: influence of process and granulation parameters on granule properties. Drug Dev Ind Pharm 2006; 32:509–30.
94. Vaerenbergh V. The influence of a swinging bowl on granulate properties. Pharm Tech Eur 2001; 13(3):36–43.
95. Stahl H. Comparing different granulation techniques. Pharm Tech Eur 2004; 11:23–33.
96. Lucisano L, Poska RP. Microwave technology- fad or future. Pharm Tech 1990; 14(4):38–42.
97. Poska R. Integrated mixing granulating and microwave drying: a development experience. Pharm Eng 1991; 11(1):8–13.
98. Waldren M. Microwave drying of pharmaceuticals–the development of a process. Pharm Eng 1988; 8(1):9–13.
99. Pearswig D, Robin P, Lucisano LJ. Situation modeling applied to the development of a single-pot process using microwave/vacuum drying. Pharm Tech 1994; 18(6):44–60.
100. Hamdani J, Moes AJ, Amighi K. Development and evaluation of prolonged release pellets obtained by the melt pelletization process. Int J Pharm 2002; 245(1):167–77.
101. Goole J, Vanderbist F, Amighi K. Development of new multiple-unit sustained-release floating dosage forms. Int J Pharm 2007; 334(1–2):35–41.
102. Faure A, York P, Rowe RC. Process control and scale-up of pharmaceutical wet granulation processes: a review. Eur J Pharm Biopharm 2001; 52(3):269–77.
103. Gao J, Jain A, Motheram R, Gray DB, Hussain MA. Fluid bed granulation of a poorly water soluble, low density, micronized drug: comparison with high shear granulation. International Journal of Pharmaceutics 2002; 237:1–14.
104. Schaefer T, Worts O. Control of fluidized bed granulation. V. Factors affecting granule growth. Arch Pharm Chemi Sci Ed 1978b; 6:69–82.
105. Davies W, Gloor WT. Batch production of pharmaceutical granulation in a fluid bed I: effects of process variables on physical properties of final granulation. J Pharm Sci 1971; 60:1869–74.
106. Rambali B, Baert L, Thone D, Massart DL. Using experimental design to optimize the granulation process in fluid bed. Drug Dev Ind Pharm 2001b; 27:53–61.
107. Schaefer T, Worts O. Control of fluidized bed granulation I. Effects of spray angle, nozzle height and starting materials on granule size and size distribution. Arch Pharm Chemi Sci Ed 1977b; 5:51–60.
108. Ormos Z, Pataki K, Csukas B. Studies on granulation in fluidized bed. II. The effects of amount of the binder on the physical properties of granules formed in a fluidized bed. Hung J Ind Chem 1973; 1:307–28.
109. Schaefer T, Worts O. Control of fluidized bed granulation III. Effects of inlet air temperature and liquid flow rate on granule size and size distribution. Arch Pharm Chemi Sci Ed 1978a; 6:1–13.
110. Schaefer T, Worts O, Control of fluidized bed granulation. 2. Estimation of droplet size of atomized binder solutions. Arch Pharm Chemi Sci Ed 1977a; 5:178.
111. Schaefer T, Worts O. Control of fluidized bed granulation. 4. Effects of binder solution and atomization on granule size and size distribution. Arch Pharm Chemi Sci Ed 1978c; 6(1):14–25.
112. Jaegerskou A, Holm P, Schaefer T, Kristensen HG. Granulation in high speed mixers. Part 3. Effects of process variables on the intragranular porosity. Pharm Ind 1984; 46(3):310–4.

113. Ritala M, Jungersen O, Holm P, Schaefer T, Kristensen HG. Comparison between binders in the wet phase of granulation in a high shear mixer. Drug Dev Ind Pharm 1986; 12(11–13): 1685–700.
114. Lian G, Thornton C, Adams MJ. A theoretical study of the liquid bridge forces between two rigid spherical bodies. J Coll Interface Sci 1993; 161:138–47.
115. Pepin X, Blanchon S, Couarraze G. Power consumption profiles in high shear wet granulation. Part 1. Liquid distribution in relation to powder and binder properties. J Pharm Sci 2001; 90(Mar):322–31.
116. Farber L, Tardos GI, Michaels JN. Micro-mechanical properties of drying material bridges of pharmaceutical excipients. Intl J Pharm 2005; 306(1–2):41–55.
117. Bier H, Leuenberger H, Sucker H. Determination of the uncritical quantity of granulating liquid by power measurements on planetary mixers. Pharm Ind 1979; 41:375–80.
118. Leuenberger H, Bier HP, Sucker HB. Theory of the granulating-liquid requirement in the conventional granulation process. Pharm Tech 1979; 6:61–8.
119. Corvari V, Fry WC, Seibert WL, Augsburger LL. Instrumentation of a high-shear mixer: evaluation and comparison of a new capacitive sensor, a watt meter, and a strain-gage torque sensor for wet granulation monitoring. Pharm Res 1992;9(12):1525–33.
120. Pont V, Saleh K, Stinmetz D, Hemati M. Influence of the physicochemical properties on the growth of solid particles by granulation in fluidized bed. Powder Technol 2001; 120:97–104.
121. Schaafsma S, Vonk P, Kossen NW. Fluid bed agglomeration with a narrow droplet size distribution. Int J Pharm 2000; 193(5).
122. Pepin X, Blanchon S, Couarraze G. Power consumption profiles in high shear wet granulation. Part 2. Predicting the overwetting point from a spreading energy. J Pharm Sci 2001; 90(Mar):332–9.
123. Reynolds G, Biggs CA, Salman AD, Hounslow MJ. Non-uniformity of binder distribution in high-shear granulation. Powder Tech 2004; 140(3):203–8.
124. Ragnarsson G, Sjogren J. Influence of the granulating method on bulk properties and tabletability of a high dosage drug. International J Pharmaceut 1982, 12(Oct): 163–71.
125. Jager K, Bauer KH. Polymer blends from PVP as a means to optimize properties of fluidized bed granulates and tablets. Acta Pharm Technol 1984; 30(1):85–92.
126. Alkan M, Yuksel A. Granulation in a fluidized bed. Part 2. Effect of binder amount on the final granules. Drug Dev Ind Pharm 1986 12(10):1529–43.
127. Nouh A. Effect of variations in concentration and type of binder on the physical characteristics of sulfadiazine tablets and granulations prepared by wet and fluidized bed granulation method. Pharma Ind 1986; 48(6):670–3.
128. Daruwala J. Chewable tablets. In: Lieberman H, Lachman L, eds. Pharmaceutical Dosage Forms: Tablets. New YorK: Marcel Dekker, Inc, 1980: 289–337.
129. Peters D, Medicated Lozenges, in Pharmaceutical Dosage Forms: Tablets, Lieberman H, Lachman L, Editor. Marcel Dekker, Inc.: New York.1980 339–466.
130. Gonzalez-Rodriguez M, Maestrelli F, Mura P, Rabasco AM. In vitro release of sodium diclofenac from a central core matrix tablet aimed for colonic drug delivery. Eur J Pharm Sci 2003; 20:125–31.
131. Rowe R, Sheskey PJ, Weller PJ, eds. Handbook of Pharmaceutical Excipients. 4th ed. Grayslake, IL: Pharmaceut Press, 2003.
132. Singh S. Alteration in dissolution characteristic of gelatin containing formulations: A review of the problem, test methods and solutions. Pharm Technol 2002; 26(4):36–58.
133. United States Pharmacopeia 29/NF 24. 2005, Rockville, MD: United States Pharmacopeial Convention.
134. Stubberud L, Forbes RT. Use of gravimetry for the study of the effect of additives on the moisture-induced recrystallization of amorphous lactose. Int J Pharm 1998; 163(Mar 18): 145–56.
135. Marvola M, Nykanen P, Rautio S, Isonen N. Autere A-M, Enteric polymers as binders and coating materials in multiple-unit site-specific drug delivery systems. Eur J Pharm Sci 1999; 7:259–67.

136. Upadrashta S, Katikeneni PR, Hileman GA, Neau SH, Rowlings CE. Compressibility and compactability properties of ethylcellulose. Int J Pharm 1994; 112:173–79.
137. Dahl T, Calderwood T, Bormeth A, Trimble K, Piepmeier E. Influence of physicochemical properties of hydroxypropylmethylcellulose on naproxen release from sustained release matrix tablets. J Control Release 1990; 14:1–10.
138. Nellore R, Rekhi GS, Hussain AS, Tillman LG, Augsburger LL. Development of metoprolol tartrate extended-release matrix tablet formulations for regulatory policy consideration. J Control Release 1998; 50:247–56.
139. Rekhi G, Nellore RV, Hussain AS, Tillman LG, Malinowski HJ, Augsburger LL. Identification of critical formulation and processing variables for metoprolol tartrate extended release (ER) matrix tablets. J Control Release 1999; 59:327–42.
140. FDA, Guidance for industry-modified release solid oral dosage forms/Scale-up and post approval changes: chemistry, manufacturing, and controls. In Vitro Dissolution Testing and In vivo Bioequivalence Documentation, Guidance effective October 6, 1997.
141. Zhang G, Law D, Schmitt EA, Qiu YH. Phase transformation considerations during process development and manufacture of solid oral dosage forms. Adv Drug Del Rev 2004; 56(3):371–90.
142. Katzhendler I, Azoury R, Friedman M. Crystalline properties of carbamazepine in sustained release hydrophilic matrix tablets based on hydroxypropylmethylcellulose. J Control Release 1998; 54:69–85.
143. Matsumoto T, Zografi G. Physical properties of solid molecular dispersions of indomethacin with poly(vinylpyrrolidone) and poly(vinylpyrrolidone-co-vinyl-acetate) in relation to indomethacin crystallization. Pharm Res 1999; 16:1722–8.
144. Huang Y, Khanvilkar KH, Moore AD, Hilliard-Lott M. Effects of manufacturing process variables on in vitro dissolution characteristics of extended-release tablets formulated with hydroxypropyl methylcellulose. Drug Dev Ind Pharm 2003; 29(1):79–88.
145. Farber L, Tardos GI, Michaels JN. Evolution and structure of drying material bridges of pharmaceutical excipients: studies on a microscopic slide. Chem Eng Sci 2003; 58:(4515–25).
146. Levin M. Wet granulation: End-point determination and scale-up. Encyclopedia of Pharmaceutical Technology, Third Edition 2006, J. Swarbrick, Ed. Boca Raton, FL: Taylor & Francis.
147. Betz G, Buergin PJ, Leuenberger H. Power consumption profile analysis and tensile strength measurements during moistu agglomeration. Int J Pharm 2003; 252(1–2):11–25.
148. Betz G, Buergin PJ, Leuenberger H. Power consumption measurement and temperature recording during granulation. Int J Pharm 2004; 272(1–2):137–49.
149. Holm P, Schaefer T, Kristensen HG. Granulation in high-speed mixers. Part IV. Effects of process conditions on power consumption and granule growth. Powder Technol 1985; 43:225.
150. Landin M, Rowe RC, York P. Characterization of wet powder masses with a mixer torque rheometer. Nonlinear effects of shaft speed and sample weight. J Pharm Sci 1995; 84(5):557–80.
151. Tershita K, Kato M, Ohike A, Miyanami K. Analysis of end-point with power consumption in a high speed mixer. Chem Pharm Bull 1990; 38(7):1977–82.
152. Belchamber R. Acoustics- a process analytical tool. Spec Eur 2003; 15(6):26–27.
153. Briens L, Daniher D, Tallevi A. Monitoring high-shear granulation using sound and vibration measurements. Int J Pharm 2007; 331:54–60.
154. Rudd D. The use of acoustic monitoring for the control and scale-up of a tablet granulation process. J Proc Anal Tech 2004; 1(2):8–11.
155. Miwa A, Toshio Y, Itai S. Prediction of suitable amount of water addition for wet granulation. Int J Pharm 2000; 195(1–2):81–92.
156. Otsuka M, Mouri Y, Matsuda Y. Chemometric evaluation of pharmaceutical properties of antipyrine granules by near-infrared spectroscopy. AAPS PharmSciTech 2003; 4(3):Article 47.

157. Dilworth S, Mackin LA, Weir S, Claybourn M, Stott PW. In-line techniques for end-point determination in large scale high shear granulation. In 142nd British Pharmaceutical Conference. 2005.
158. Fariss G, Keintz R, Okoye P. Thermal effusivity and power consumption as PAT tools for monitoring granulation endpoint. Pharm Tech; June 2006. http://pharmtech.findpharma.com
159. Rekhi G, Caricofe RB, Parikh DM, Augsburger LL. A New Approach to Scale-up of a High-Shear Granulation Process. Pharm Tech 1986; 20(Suppl):2–10.
160. Kristensen H. Particle agglomeration in high shear mixers. Powder Technol 1996; 88: 197–202.
161. Horsthuis G, van Laarhoven JAH, van Rooji RBM, Vromans H. Studies on upscaling parameters of the Gral high shear granulation process. Int J Pharm 1993; 92:143–50.
162. Faure A, Grimsey IM, Rowe RC, York P, Cliff MJ. Applicability of a scale-up methodology for wet granulation processes in Colette Gral high shear mixer-granulators. Eur J Pharm Sci 1999a; 8(2):85–93.
163. Faure A, Grimsey IM, Rowe RC, York P, Cliff MJ. Process control in a high shear mixer-granulator using wet mass consistency. The effect of formulation variables. J Pharm Sci 1999b; 88(2):191–5.
164. Chirkot T. Scale-up and endpoint issues of pharmaceutical wet granulation in a V-type low shear granulator. Drug Dev Ind Pharm 2002; 28:871.

9
Dry Granulation

Garnet E. Peck, Josephine L. P. Soh, and Kenneth R. Morris
Department of Industrial and Physical Pharmacy, College of Pharmacy, Nursing and Health Sciences, Purdue University, West Lafayette, Indiana, U.S.A.

INTRODUCTION

In the production of pharmaceutical dosage forms, granulation is one of the most common unit operation employed to improve the flow and compressibility of particulate material by size enlargement and densification. Granulation can be divided into wet and dry methods. Wet granulation methods are more often chosen over dry granulation because of dust elimination, single-pot processing and obtaining predictable granulation end-point determination. Examples of wet granulation methods include fluid bed, high shear, pelletization techniques such as extrusion-spheronization, spray drying, rotary processing and so forth. In wet granulation, a liquid is used to agglomerate powder particles with constant agitation into a coherent mass which is subsequently dried and sized for subsequent processing. Despite their advantages, wet granulation methods are not suitable for thermo-labile and moisture sensitive materials or materials that are highly cohesive. In such instances, dry granulation or granulation by compression become the method of choice as it eliminates the need for an extra drying step which is detrimental to actives that degrade or convert to a less stable form under elevated temperatures.

Most drug actives do not possess adequate flow properties and compressibility to produce a final dosage form (often a tablet) of desired physical and mechanical properties. These properties include content uniformity, low friability, strong enough for subsequent handling and processing such as coating and packaging and good dissolution profiles to achieve the requisite bioavailability. Hence, other materials or excipients are often added to the powdered active to improve the tabletability of the overall blend. Depending on the nature of the active, excipients such as microcrystalline cellulose (MCC), dicalcium phosphate, lactose monohydrate can be added to provide a balance of plasticity and brittle fracture needed to bring about successful bonding within a tablet.

MATERIAL SCIENCE
Deformation of Pharmaceutical Powders

To achieve the goals of dry granulation as discussed above, it is necessary to induce plastic deformation of the powders of interest to facilitate bonding into a compact for subsequent milling into granules. While the theory of deformation is well understood for many materials (1), it is less well described for powders and even less for powders of molecular organic particles.

Stress–Strain Relationships

Even with the gaps in the theory, the fundamental concepts developed for continuum systems are substantially the same for systems of pharmaceutical powders. Powders confined and subjected to a compressive stress will rearrange until there is insufficient free volume to allow translation of particles. As the stress increases, particles make contacts which increase in area with stress, they will deform elastically (i.e., reversibly) with Young's modulus (E) as the linear proportionality constant. The normal strain (e_1) in the loading direction for a material undergoing elastic deformation under uniaxial tension (σ) may be expressed as (2):

$$e_1 = \frac{\sigma_1}{E} \tag{1}$$

where E is the proportionality constant for the elastic deformation range and is commonly referred to as the modulus of elasticity or Young's modulus.

At very high applied loads or when the material shows poor elastic deformation, the elastic limit or the yield point, Y, is reached (Fig. 1). Beyond Y, the subsequent deformation becomes permanent in nature and is not recoverable upon removal of the applied load. This is known as plastic deformation and is predominantly observed in materials where the shear strength is less than the tensile or breaking strength. Further volume reduction occurs during this stage as the interparticulate voids are filled by the particles undergoing plastic deformation.

Apart from a permanent change in particle shape, plastic deformation also leads to an increase in the strength and hardness of the material. This change in the shape under stress is the strain and may be defined as the change in dimension relative to the initial dimension (i.e., engineering strain). As the stresses of interest to most dry granulation are compressive and/or shear stresses, the resulting strain will typically have some shear and some compressive contribution. The stress–strain relationship in this region deviates from the linearity defined by Hooke's law but shows a power law dependence:

$$\sigma = K\varepsilon^n \tag{2}$$

where $\varepsilon = \ln(1+e)$ is the true strain, e is the nominal strain and K and n are material constants termed as *strength* coefficient and *strain-hardening exponent*, respectively.

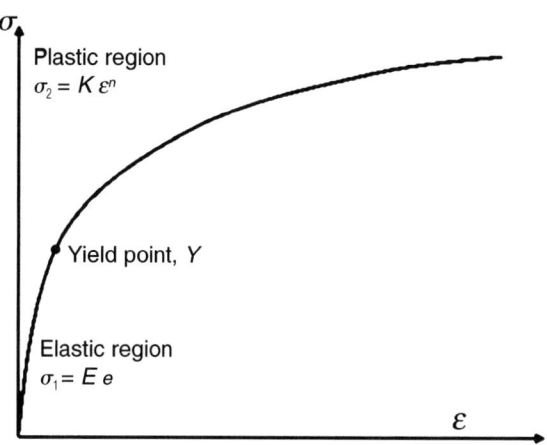

FIGURE 1 Stress–strain profile of a material undergoing uniaxial compression.

Dry Granulation

From a plot of true stress–true strain behavior on logarithmic coordinates, K and n can be found where K is determined by extrapolating the curve to unit strain value while the n is defined by the slope of the plastic region.

The relationship between the mechanical response of an individual particle to a directly applied stress and that of a powder of the particles is complex because the force transmission to an individual particle is mediated by other particles. As an example consider an amorphous excipient and assume the particles are spherical and have a monodisperse size. The response to an applied stress of an individual particle should be independent of the direction of application as we're assuming the particle structure is isotropic (unlike a crystal which may exhibit a different response to stress in different directions due to the anisotropic structure dictated by periodic packing constraints).

For a confined powder which is composed of the particles, the response to the application of stress follows the steps discussed above. That is, before the transmission of stress to an individual particle in the body of the powder is the same as if it were directly stressed, the particles have to rearrange to allow multiple points of inter-particulate contact and approach the "fully dense" state (relative to the individual particles). This results in a lag in the stress–strain profile however; the yield point and energy of deformation should remain close to that of the individual particle property once corrected for the number of particles in the powder. A schematic stress–strain profile for a particle and for a powder made up of the particles is illustrated in Figure 2A. Figure 2B shows the same plots normalized.

When compressing a heterogeneous system of powders the situation is yet more complex as the force distribution experienced by, for example, a crystal (probably a crystalline API) in the presence of an excipient (e.g., MCC) will differ from that experienced by the same crystal in a powder consisting only of crystallites.

Yield Behavior

The behavior of real component powders may be estimated using a yield criterion (1), which requires a knowledge of the magnitudes of the directional response to stress of the particle and knowledge of the particle size distribution and particle orientation. Much of this information is not readily available for molecular organic solids and is the subject increasing attention of academic materials scientists. Even knowing the crystal structure, the dynamic response to mechanical stresses is not currently predictable without exhaustive effort (3). However, yield behavior may be measured and correlated to the

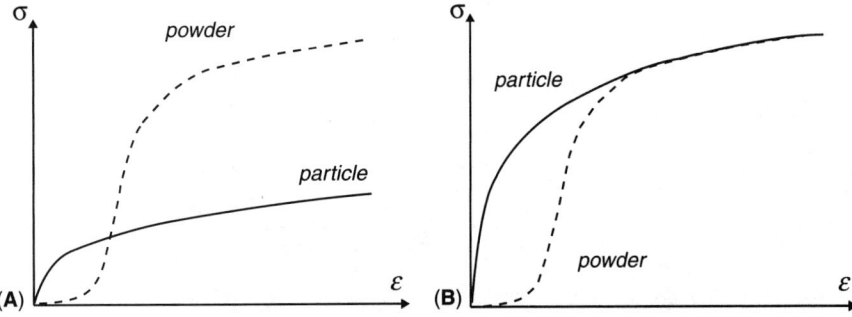

FIGURE 2 (**A**) Stress–strain profiles for a particle and a powder bed, (**B**) corresponding normalized stress–strain profiles.

micromeritic properties to anticipate/estimate the behavior of powders with variable properties (4). Of these, particle size is typically the most important micromeritic property impacting yield and ultimately bonding.

Fragmentation

When the applied stress exceeds the tensile strength of the material, particles begin to fracture under load, into smaller, discrete particles. Particle fragmentation creates new surfaces, additional contact points and multiple potential sites for bonding. Owing to the change in particle size and shape, a certain degree of particle rearrangement may occur and results in further volume reduction. Fragmentation commonly occurs in hard, brittle particles such as sucrose and acetaminophen. Thus, it can also be referred to as brittle fracture. Subsequently, fragmented particles may undergo several cycles of elastic and/or plastic deformation. The increase in the surface area and the rearrangement of particles into closer proximity greater facilitates interparticulate bond formation (5).

Bonding

After the yield stress is applied and the powder is deforming plastically, the particles can bond or fuse to form a strong compact. Bonding is usually ascribed to particle interaction through van der Waals forces (6). Looking at a packing diagram of a crystal structure such as acetaminophen (APAP) shown in Figure 3, it is clear that there is very little room to bring the molecules in the lattice closer together than they already are. However, if we consider that the *aoc* (020 crystallographic) plane shown in Figure 3 can be displaced along the *o–c* direction, the potential for portions of different crystals to interact through the new surfaces created by the slip. Many such planes may be "activated" upon the application of mechanical stress through compaction or milling. Alternately, crystals with

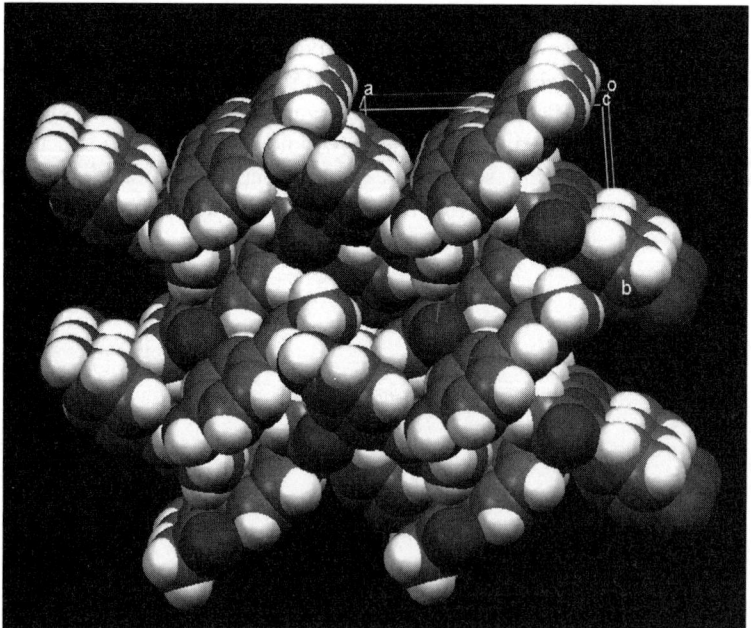

FIGURE 3 APAP Packing diagram down the c crystallographic axis. *Source*: CSD REFCODE HXACANø1 displayed in Mercury Version 1.5.2.

Dry Granulation

a dominant *aoc* face may exhibit an increase in the plane perpendicular to it, that is, the *boc* plane (001 crystallographic)

In fact, looking at the powder X-ray diffraction patterns of APAP as received and after uniaxial compression, it is clear that many of the peaks have changed in *relative* intensity (Fig. 4). The 001/020 (*boc/aoc*) ratio has increased dramatically and while some of this is due to alignment under pressure, in a properly prepared sample, much of the change is attributable to the fracturing of the crystals. The relative intensities of key reflections are labeled illustrating the point.

The shear stress during grinding in mortar and pestle produces more dramatic effects as shown in Figure 5. The relatively larger energy is capable of disrupting even strong interactions in the crystal's structure giving rise to largely unpredictable intensity changes.

A similar but milder trend is observed for granules from roller compaction. Figure 6 shows the PXRD pattern for the dry blend and the granules make from the blend. The APAP particle size is much smaller than that used in the above examples (approximately 35 μm as opposed to approximately 250 μm). Again the 001/020 (*boc/aoc*) ratio has increased significantly in the granules.

Analysis of other planes, i.e., the increase in the 21-1/020 and decrease in the 011/020 peak ratios leads to the observation that the 020 plane has been sheared during the process resulting in the final material. This can understood qualitatively using the reference planes in Figure 7 showing that the 020 coplanar or near coplanar planes decrease while those more perpendicularly related increase in their peak intensities.

These results show that even with possible differences in stress transmission due to the excipient, the basic response must (as expected) be dictated by the underlying crystal structure of the API. Also, all of the crystal structure related analysis gives the formulator the tools needed to estimate or at least anticipate which crystal structures should deform most easily and for a given structure, which shape is the most likely to behave well

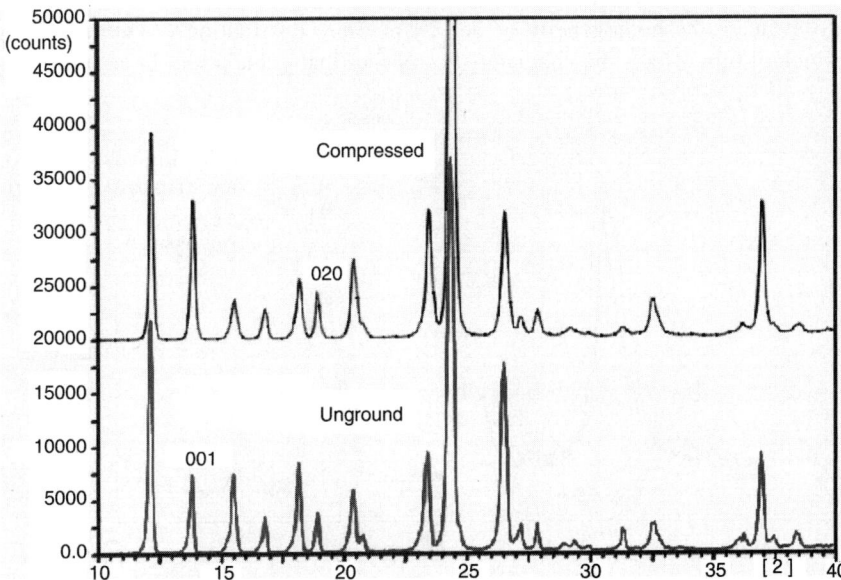

FIGURE 4 X-ray diffraction patterns of APAP powder and compact. *Source*: Courtesy of Morris.

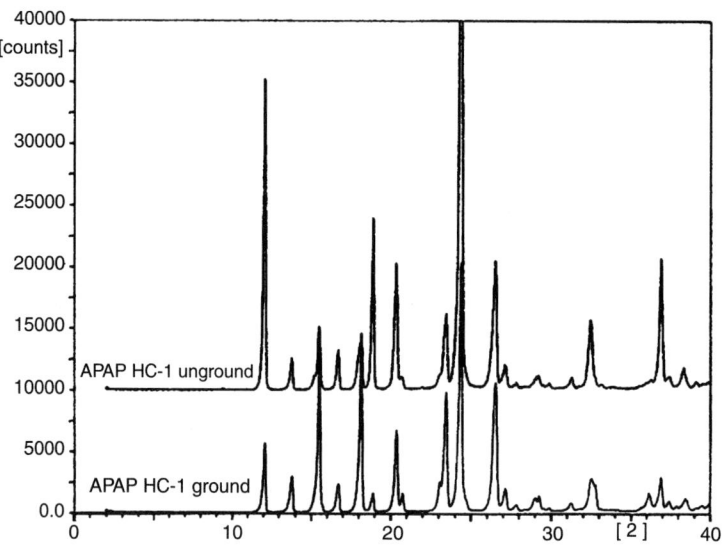

FIGURE 5 X-ray powder diffraction patterns of ground and unground APAP. *Source*: Courtesy of Morris.

(i.e., deform and bond) under mechanical stress. For a given sample of material, the particle size distribution and shape may impact on performance and this dependency is sometimes difficult to anticipate unless the analysis here is applied.

Micromeritics

The density of granules used in tablet production is influenced by the densification of the slugs or compacted ribbon (7–9). To determine the porosity and pore size distribution of a ribbon or granules, mercury intrusion porosimetry may be used. This technique can also be used to evaluate the homogeneity of density/pressure distribution on a compact or granule which in turn affects the characteristics of the final granulation. In addition, gas

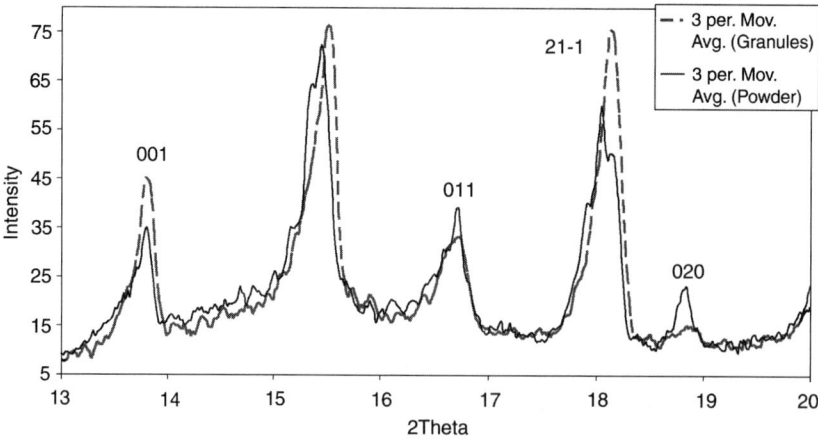

FIGURE 6 X-ray powder diffraction patterns of powder and granules of 50% APAP/MCC before and after roller compaction/milling. *Source*: Courtesy of Soh and Morris.

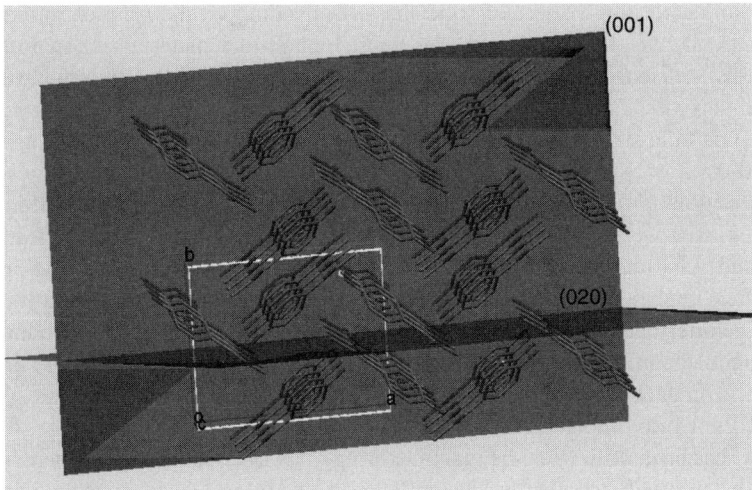

FIGURE 7 A packing diagram showing perpendicular planes through the APAP lattice (Mercury, Version 1.5.2).

adsorption measurements may also be used to estimate surface area which may be coupled with particle size determinations (usually sieve, diffraction based) to assess the impact of compaction and milling conditions on granule properties.

The ultimate goal of a granulation process is to improve the tableting properties of the active drug substance. Granule characteristics such as flow, friability, and density have an important influence on the characteristics of the tablets produced. The bulk density of the granulation will have an effect on the flow properties of the granulation. The granule friability can give an indication of the compression behavior of the granules. Measurements of granule friability may also be used to determine granule strength. The flow of a granulation will influence the die fill and uniformity of the tablets produces. Examining the granule characteristics will not only provide information on the granulation properties but will also provide information on the use of roller compaction as a granulation method.

METHODS OF DRY GRANULATION

Slugging—Batch

Slugging is the process of compressing a powder blend into large tablets (1 in. diameter, ¼ in. thickness) using large-diameter flat-faced punches at hydraulic pressures of 4–6 tons. The resultant compact is known as a slug and is typically milled into smaller particles known as granules. Slugging results in considerable dust production which poses a problem for good containment and reduction of cross contamination. Other main shortcomings of slugging include: batch processing, low throughput (30–50 kg/hr), poor process control, frequent maintenance changeovers and poor economy of scale. Otherwise, considerations for slugging are the same as for roller compaction discussed below.

Roller Compaction—Batch or Continuous

A more efficient form of dry granulation is roller compaction. It is a process where a flowing powder bed is continuously fed between two counter-rotating rolls where it is densified and consolidated into a sheet of solid mass. Depending on the type of rollers used, the feed material may be compacted into dense ribbon-like materials known as flakes (smooth rolls) or dense briquettes (almond or stick-shaped) if the rollers have grooved or etched surfaces. For pharmaceuticals, the ribbons are further milled to give granules of desired particle size, size distribution, flow and bulk density for tableting and capsule filling (10–12).

Roller compaction is a relatively simple and inexpensive process which offers distinct advantages over wet granulation, particularly for moisture-, solvent-, or heat-sensitive compounds. In the pharmaceutical industry, it is an attractive granulation alternative as it offers considerable cost savings due of its high production throughput (up to 100,000 kg/hr), shorter cycle times and fewer processing steps. Moreover, elimination of a drying step reduces production and development time as well as ease of scale-up (13). While roller compaction is simpler than wet granulation methods in terms of operation, it is still not fully understood or explored (14).

Although RC has been utilized in the manufacturing of a variety of products, there is currently no well-established, "quality-by-design" type methodology to account for raw material variation in the efficient and controlled operation the roller compactor. Thus, RC formulation and process development still relies largely on experience, trial-and-error and empirical design of experiment (DoE), though some researchers have begun to model the process (14–16), including newer attempts using finite element modeling (17). The model developed by Johanson (15) was used to predict material behavior undergoing continuous shear deformation between the rollers. In his model, the material was assumed to be cohesive, compressible, and isotropic. The latter method using finite element modeling was found to be more versatile because it incorporates information pertaining to powder behavior, geometry and frictional interactions (17). Nevertheless, practical applications of these models in the actual production settings are rare.

Pharmaceutical Applications

The earliest reported pharmaceutical applications of roller compaction were published in 1966 (12). A typical formulation for roller compaction will contain a fragmenting material (e.g., lactose), a plastically deforming material such as MCC or corn starch, binder (e.g., hydroxylpropylmethylcellulose, HPMC), actives, and lubricants (magnesium stearate).

In a study conducted by Li and Peck (18), granulation of maltodextrin using roller compaction and fluid bed granulation was compared. Roller compacted granules were less porous, more dense and flowed better. They were more resistant to deformation (indicated by the higher yield pressure value in Heckel plot). The corresponding tablets produced from these granules were also weaker and this was attributed to work hardening effect. This also gave rise to tablets with lower tensile strength caused by work hardening.

In the presence of several low-viscosity grades of HPMC, dissolution rates of poorly soluble actives such as carbamazepine, naproxen and nifedipine were markedly improved when the physical blend was roller compacted (19). The compaction process was believed to have facilitated the drug dissolution rate because the drug particles kept in close contact with the HPMC particles. Creation of high local surfactant concentrations of HPMC in the boundary layers surrounding drug particles during dissolution provided a lower-energy pathway to enhance drug dissolution and release.

A bio-adhesive material used in the preparation of buccal tablets was prepared using roller compaction (20). A fractional factorial design was employed to investigate the effects of the roller compactor operating parameters and the tablet compression pressure on the dissolution profiles and bio-adhesive properties of the tablets. Drug release rate was significantly influenced by the roll pressure, roll type and tablet compression force. A high compression pressure and a ribbed roller tended to produce more linear dissolution profiles. The buccal tablet properties were dependent on the roller compaction processing parameters. The gap between the rollers and compaction force affected the bio-adhesive force significantly.

Milled crude plant materials do not compress well into tablets because of their poor compressibility and adverse flow properties hence, the milled plant material needs to be formulated with additives into granules for tableting. Herbal materials are often hygroscopic due to the presence of resins and gums which tend to be sticky on contact with water. Moreover, the presence of thermo-labile actives make them unsuitable for processing using wet or high shear granulation methods. However, dried herbal materials often exhibit poor flow during to their fibrous shape and the tendency to interlock which further impedes flow during compression.

In the study by Heng et al. (21), the anti-viral herb, *baphicacanthus cusia* was roller compacted in the presence of polyvinylpyrrolidone (PVP). The effects of roller compactor operating parameters, PVP concentration and the effect of co-milling were also investigated in that study. The authors reported that a higher roll speed was beneficial to the overall strength of the ribbon due to longer dwell times available for particle rearrangement and bonding. Addition of PVP decreased the flowability of the herbal powder blend which subsequently affected the size and friability of the granules. Granules properties were affected by two opposing factors, the flowability and binding capacity of herbal powder blend.

A PVP (low-molecular weight) concentration of less than 10% (w/w) was insufficient for any marked improvement in binding properties of the herbal powder. Co-milling of primary-milled herbal powder and PVP improved the flowability of the powder blend. The enhanced flow properties, coupled with the increased binding capacity due to increasing PVP concentration, contributed favorably to the mechanical strength and handling properties of the granules.

Other herbal materials prepared by roller compaction included St. John's wort (22) and *Eschscholtzia californica* Cham (23). Tableting of the granulated extract markedly reduced the problems associated with dust and material feed as well as the incidence of capping. Tablets produced from granulated extracts disintegrated three times faster than those tabletted from the powder blend. Hygroscopicity of *E. californica* Cham. extracts decreased after roller compaction due to decreased material surface area.

Equipment

Machine design varies between manufacturers with claimed advantages for each (Fig. 8). Mainly, the machines differ in the configuration and relative positioning of the rollers as illustrated in Figure 9. Typically, only one roll is fixed in relation to the frame while the other is movable by controlling the adjustable hydraulic force. This feature enables slight adjustments in the roll gap and also extends the range of the compression pressures that can be delivered to the roll surface, in turn, to the feed material present between the rolls (24). When both rollers are axially fixed, the compression pressures tend to fluctuate with the varying material feed.

Clearly, the design and configuration of the rollers can impact the final ribbon quality and yield although a certain degree of powder leakage (up to 30%) is observed

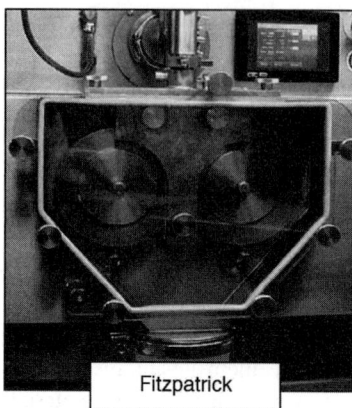 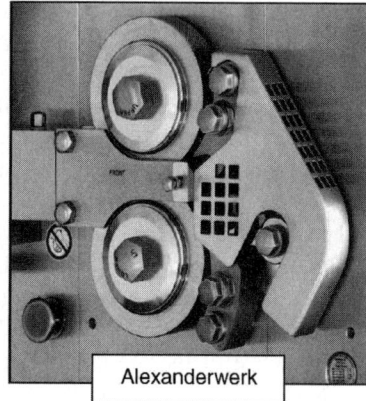

FIGURE 8 Examples of roller compactors from different manufacturers. *Source*: Courtesy of Alexanderwerk.

with most compactors (5). To circumvent this problem, vacuum deaeration and roll gap control have been incorporated into newer compactors.

Application of a vacuum to the feed material just prior to the rollers eliminates air pockets within the powder bed. This result in better venting and a more homogenous material feed into the compression zone. Regardless of roller orientation, vacuum deaeration was shown to reduce the leakage rate significantly (5). The location of the deaeration relative to the rolls/feed screws may impact its effectiveness.

DESIGNING THE PROCESS

Designing a roller compaction process requires the same approach as designing a process for any dosage form. That is, knowing the characteristics of the API, the desired dose, and the ultimate use of the granules, a determination must be made as to whether or not the process is viable and if so, what conditions are necessary/optimal for production. So the approach requires identifying critical variables, designing and executing experiments, and the selection of optimal conditions.

Identifying the Critical Equipment Variables

Critical variables may be characteristic of the materials and/or the process. Materials properties have already been discussed briefly and of course the equipment variables for the unit operations will depend upon differences in the raw materials. However, there are general relationships between the roller compaction process variables and the properties of the resulting ribbons and granules that can aid in process design.

Roll Design

In older roller compactors, the feed screw did not always adequately deliver the powder to the gripping and compaction zone due to stationary side seals which resist the flow. Factors affecting uniform distribution of compaction pressures were investigated by Funakoshi et al. (25). The distribution of compaction pressures across the entire ribbon was estimated by determining the force needed to drill the ribbon at various locations.

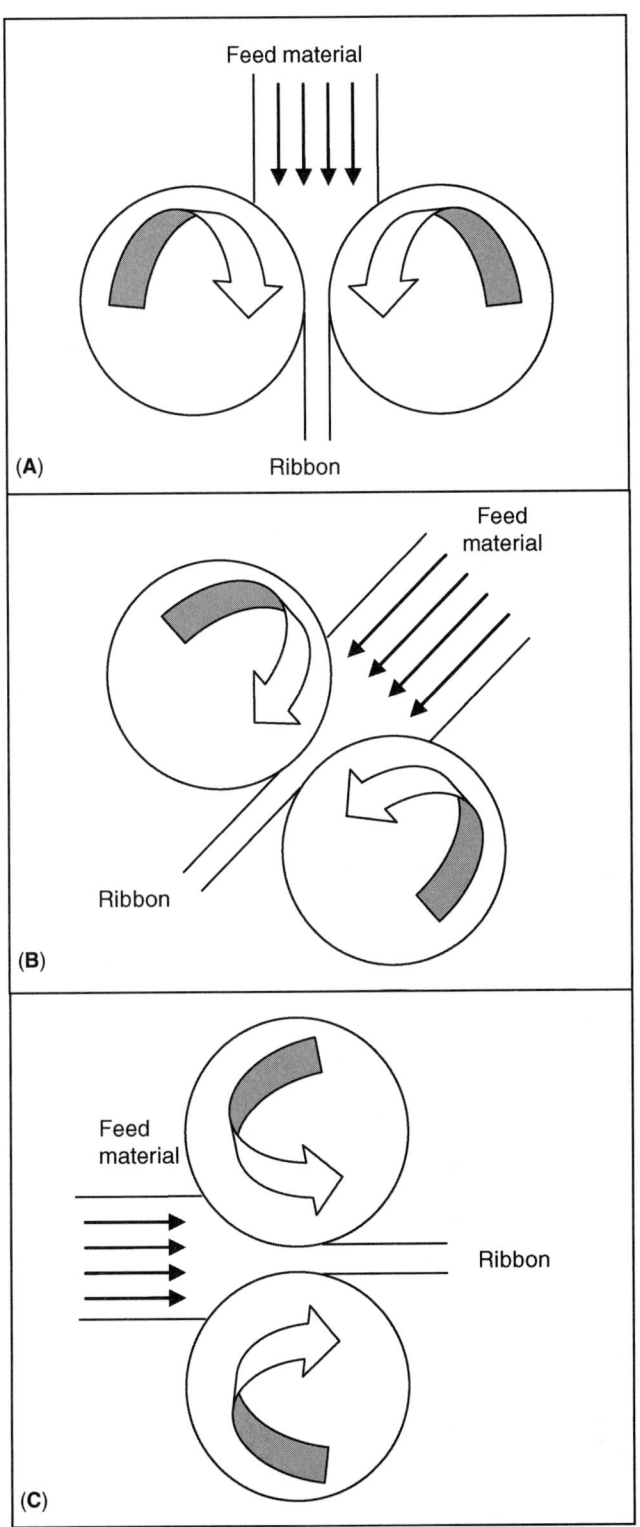

FIGURE 9 Common roller configurations: (**A**) horizontal, (**B**) inclined, and (**C**) vertical.

Lactose was the model substance used while a small amount of riboflavin was added to act as a secondary pressure indicator.

A concave-convex roller pair was used which maintained their mutual fit when rotating. The rims of the concave roller were varied with different wall slopes (ω) from 45° to 90°. The study found the compaction pressures to be uniform over the whole width of the rollers and the amount of uncompacted material (leakage) was reduced when the wall slope of 65° was used. These findings were later supported by another study by Parrott (26).

The type of roll surfaces has a marked effect on the overall production throughput of a roller compaction process (Fig. 10). A variety of roll surfaces and configurations are available depending on the compaction behavior of the material. For instance, powders that tend to stick or cling to the roll surface requires the use of smooth or circumferential grooved surfaces, while materials that release cleanly from the roll after compaction may be pressed with one of the pocketed design or rolls with grooves in the axial direction.

However, differences between smooth and axially grooved roller surfaces were compared in study by Sheskey and Hendren (27). No observable differences were found in the particle size distribution of granules milled from these ribbons. Friability, crushing strength and drug release profiles of the tablets prepared from the respective granules were also comparable.

Feed System

Roller compaction of pharmaceutical powder involves force-feeding with one or more feed screws due to their poor flowabilities. Force feeding also ensures a constant and uniform delivery of powder material to the roll surfaces, increasing the efficiency of the process. The powder may be force-fed through the rolls using only one feed screw, but multiple feed screws are also commonly used.

When the feed screws are positioned perpendicularly to each other, they are generally designated as the horizontal feed screw (HFS) and the vertical feed screw (VFS)

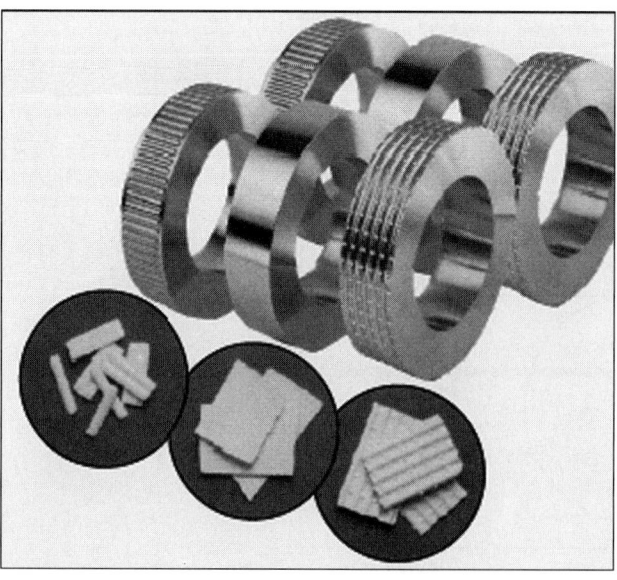

FIGURE 10 Different roll types and surfaces. *Source*: Courtesy of www.fitzmill.com.

Dry Granulation

based on the direction of their motion. Depending on the scale of the roller compactor, the HFS and the VFS assemblies may be composed of multiple feed screws to transfer the powder from the storage hopper over longer distances to the compaction zone. A single feed screw has been reported to result in uneven delivery of powder onto the roll surfaces, giving regions of heterogeneous density on the ribbon that and can affect the product quality. In fact, researchers (14,28) have found sinusoidal variations on sodium chloride ribbons produced using a single HFS set up. The periodicity of this density variation in the compact density was found to be the same as the periodicity of the HFS speed (Fig. 11).

The final feed screw will determine the force with which the powder is delivered to the nip region of the compactor. This again can result in "starving" the rolls or pre-compacting the powder. The rate should be high enough to provide sufficient friction with the roll so it can pull the material in yet not so high as to bog down the rolls.

The vacuum deaeration system was introduced by Miller (29) and involves modifying the feed screw assembly just before the nip region to include a vacuum deaeration port. Vacuum is applied through sintered plates with openings of a few microns. Air entrapment in interparticulate voids of the powder material undergoing compaction is a major problem that leads to poor feed homogeneity. During compaction, these pockets of air will attempt to escape through the powder bed causing it to fluidize and resulting in uneven and reduced material delivered to the roll gap.

The escaping air also causes excessive fines during milling due to the formation of thin and weakly formed edges which break perpendicularly to the compaction direction. The resultant compact edges appear "saw toothed" and varies in length depending on the inherent material properties, the amount of entrained air as well as the roll speed. In extreme case, the compact may even rupture and fall back into powders much like the feed material. Such problems occur when the compacted ribbon is not sufficiently strong to withstand the pressures caused by the entrapped air (30).

Based on the equilibrium of forces acting on the materials, a number of theories have been proposed to describe the behavior of materials undergoing deformation and compaction between the rolls. The first complex model to account for the behavior of materials between roll presses was proposed by Johanson (15). In his model, the flow of powder material through the roller compactor was divided into three regions characterized by their position relative to the rolls, the forces acting on the compacting mass, and the timing of material passing through each zone (Fig. 12).

Slip Region: The slip region, as the name implies, is characterized by material slipping onto the roll surface with a corresponding elastic deformation of the particles. Frictional forces on the roll surface impart a forward motion to the bulk material and cause it to flow further into the region between the rollers.

Nip Region: Powder begins to pre-densify as it is fed into the roll gap; region where powder particles are rearranged and densified, and plastic deformation occurs.

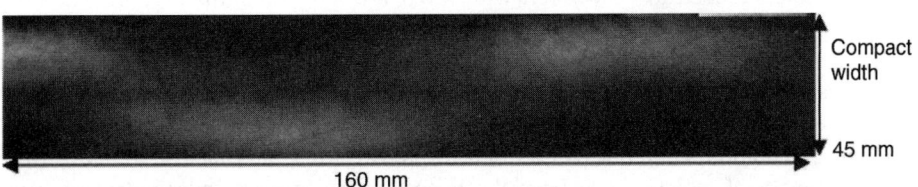

FIGURE 11 Sinusoidal variation in the density of sodium chloride compacts (14). *Source*: Courtesy of Elsevier.

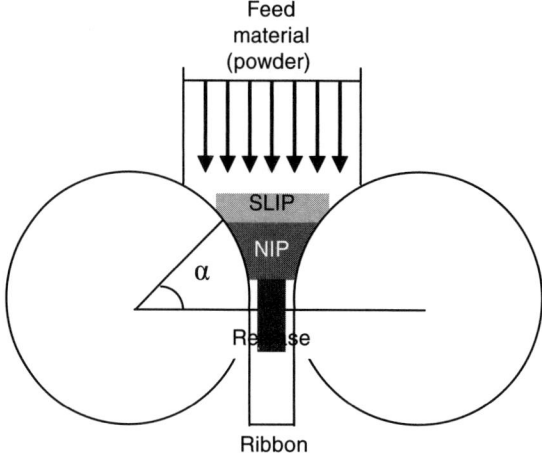

FIGURE 12 Different regions in a roller compactor.

This region is described using the nip angle, α. This angle is directly affected by the roll diameter and is established in a line through the rolls' center to a point on either roll where the powder is starting to move at the same speed as the roll surface (Fig. 12). Since the nip angle is independent of roll diameter, a bigger roller will lead to greater material densification given a constant roll gap.

The roll diameter, roll speed, roll surface, and feeding method can be selected to maximize the nip angle for obtaining the desired ribbon or granule characteristics. The nip angle varies with physical properties of the powder which include: compressibility, gas permeability, and flow. Very compressible powders are often associated with large nip angles (approx. 30°) while the poorly compressible powders give small nip angles of between 7° and 10°. The nip angle also depends on the nature of the feeing mechanism and the physical characteristics of the rollers and their surfaces.

The density of the material, at the point of the nip angle approaches its tapped density value and the material begins to undergo compression between the rolls. The material is then forced through the region of maximum pressure where it undergoes a rapid increase in the density resulting in the formation of the compacted mass.

Release Region: Once the ribbon is formed, the release region which starts at the point of maximum pressure on the roll surface occurs. This region depends on the elastic properties of the feed material.

Roll Pressure and Roll Speed

When different powder blends of HPMC were compacted at different roll pressures, higher compaction pressures were found to produce larger granules and the corresponding tablets tended to be weaker, with lower crushing strengths (31,32). The drug release profiles were, however, not affected by the processing variables. Jerome et al. (33) demonstrated the significance of the ratio between roll speed to feed screw speed on mechanical strength and friability of ribbons. In a later study, Simon and Guigon (34) also showed the importance of feed screw speed on the compaction throughput of lactose. Different granulation techniques were used to prepare MCC and lactose granules (35). Tensile strength of tablets made from the lactose granules were independent of granulation technique used although this could not be said for MCC granules. In general MCC granules prepared by extrusion or dry granulation gave stronger tablets. Slugging was

Dry Granulation

reported to have a negative influence on compressibility of MCC (36). Inghelbrecht and Remon (13) rank-ordered the influence of roll pressure, roll speed, and horizontal screw speed in the compaction of lactose. The same researchers also reported good granule properties when a ratio of roll speed: HFS speed of 0.5 was used for drum-dried waxy starch.

Roll pressure and combined speed variable (fixed ratio of roller speed and feeding screw speed) were studied at three levels in the roller compaction of ibuprofen (37). The operating variables were not found to have a significant effect on tablet crushing strength or disintegration time. As this was a high dose formulation, the authors concluded that the effect of varying roller compactor parameters was largely influenced by the compactability of ibuprofen. The interaction between roller pressure and combined speed variable was reportedly significant in the drug release profiles.

Dwell Time

Dwell time can be defined as the period during which a dynamic process remains constant in order that another process may occur. In the case of roller compaction, the dwell time under pressure results in the consolidation of the powder mass to give rise to a solid compacted ribbon. The dwell time is mainly determined by the roll speed and it is generally accepted that a certain time under pressure is necessary to allow particle rearrangement and bonding which in turn, eliminates the occurrence of lamination and capping (in tablets). On the contrary, when the dwell time is too long, over compression or over granulation can occur and the compacts instead start to flatten out and laminate.

Roll Gap

Roll gap is defined the narrowest distance between the two rolls. At any given compaction pressure, a specific roller gap will yield a corresponding fixed flake thickness (allowing for some product expansion). A fixed feed rate for a fixed roller speed and compaction pressure maintains the flake thickness. Rollers get too close if the material feed is too low and vice versa. Therefore, in principle, acceleration or deceleration of product delivery system can cause variations in the ribbon thickness and density. By monitoring the roll gap in a feedback loop, a constant material feed can be achieved.

Mill

Milling is the mechanical process of breaking particles into smaller pieces via one or more particle size reduction mechanisms. In roller compaction, the ribbons produced are milled into free flowing granules which can then be filled into capsules or compressed into tablets. Particle size reduction or comminution can occur via four main mechanisms: attrition, compression, cutting and impact, and differ by the direction and magnitude of the force applied. In attrition, a force is applied in the direction parallel to the particle surface while compression is directed towards the center of the particle. Cutting is simply the application of a shear force to a material. Lastly, particle size reduction by impact requires the application of an instantaneous force perpendicular to the particle/agglomerate surface. The force can result from particle-to-particle or particle-to-mill surface collision (40).

Location: In a roller compactor, the mill or granulator is often located after the rolls (as the formed ribbons exit) and before a screen. The mill reduces the ribbons into granules which pass through the screen which separates the over-sized granules from those that are of the desired size. It can also be a separate piece of equipment instead where the formed ribbons are transferred to and milled separately.

Type: Mills can be classified into many different types based on their operating principles. In general, they can be divided into fluid energy, impact, cutter, compression, screening, and tumbling mills (Fig. 13). Impact (hammer), cutter, and screening mills are most commonly found in roller compactors manufactured by Hosokawa Bepex, Fitzpatrick and Alexanderwerk AG. Screening mills can be further sub-classified into rotating impeller and oscillating bar for roller compactors.

A hammer mill is typically composed of a delivery device to introduce the material into the path of the hammers. This is achieved through a rotor that is made up of a series of machined disks mounted on the horizontal shaft. Materials are introduced into the paths of the hammers by a variable speed vein feeder. The speed of the feeder is controlled to maintain optimum amperage loading of the main motor. Freely rotating hammers suspended from rods running parallel to the shaft and through the rotor disks

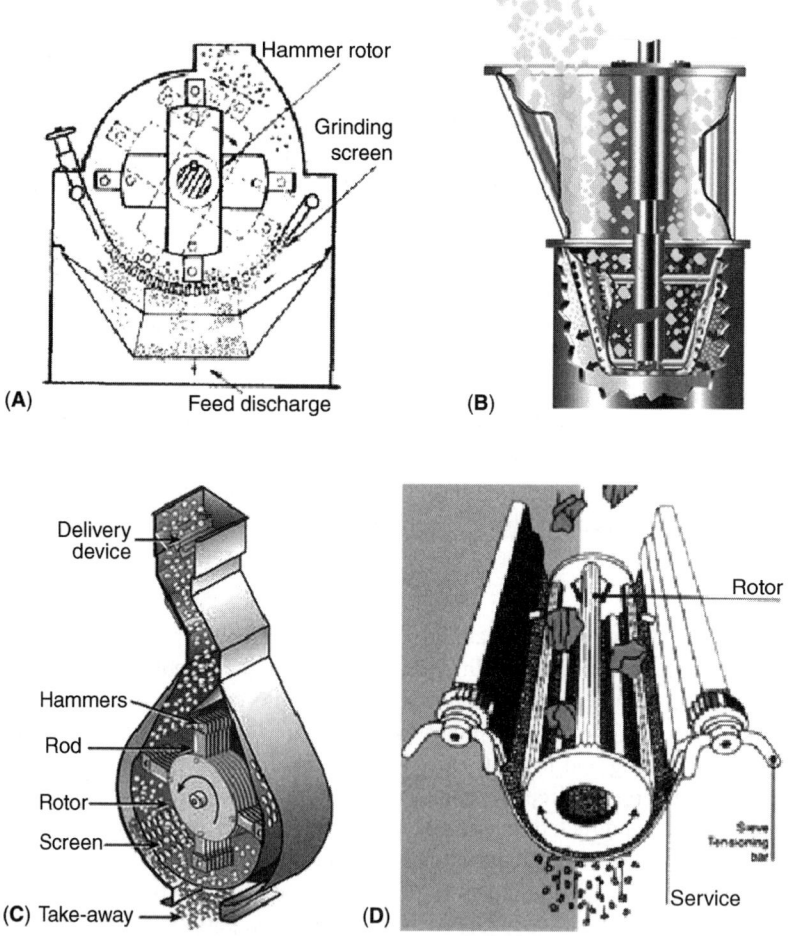

FIGURE 13 Types of mills commonly encountered in roller compaction. (**A**) Hammer, (**B**) cone, (**C**) hammer-cutter, (**D**) oscillating granulator (oscillating impeller). *Sources*: (**A**) www.feedmachinery.com; (**B**) courtesy Keith McIntosh of Quadro; (**C**) courtesy Dr. Kim Koch, Northern Crops Institute; (**D**) www.granualtorsindia.com/products.htm.

Dry Granulation

perform the function of smashing the feed material into smaller particles. A perforated mesh helps to perform coarse sieving and helps to sieve out particles of the desired size range. Cutter mills are very similar in operation except that that sharp blades are used in place of blunt surfaces. Hammer and cutter mills are especially suited for brittle or fibrous materials and can be considered the most commonly encountered mills for roller compaction.

Other mills that are used in roller compaction include cone milling and oscillating granulators. Design-wise, cone milling is distinctly different from hammer or cutter mills in that the impeller is shaped to rotate around a cone-shaped sieve. The main advantages of cone-milling over hammer or cutter mills are the: higher milling throughput due to wider in feed diameter, minimum contact surface area to ensure maximum product flow and lower cleaning costs, compact design and ease of scalability.

Oscillating granulator mills the material through a screen using a rasp or hole screen. The particle size range and crushing intensity are governed by rotor speed, while upper particle size limit is dictated by the screen size. It is mainly advantageous in that it imparts a gentle milling action.

Recent work by Smith, Bowman, and Morris (unpublished) show that hammer milled granules may produce stronger tablets while tablets from comilled granules are less sensitive to changes in milling variables.

Variables: *Hammer Design and Placement.* The choice, design and positioning of hammers within the mill is dictated by the rotor speed, motor power, and screen size. The design and placement is optimized to yield maximum contact with the feed material so as to achieve maximum milling efficiency. Depending on rotor speed, the size of hammers varies. Generally, lower rotor speeds require bigger hammers and the number of hammers is also lower per unit horsepower. For instance, a rotor speed of approximately 1,800 rpm is best used with hammers that are around 10 in. long, 2.5 in. wide and 0.25 in thick and there should be one hammer for every 2.5–3.5 horsepower. They should be arranged on rods and balanced so that the distance between hammers is optimized. The distance between hammers and screen must also be adjusted to give adequate contact and impact.

Screen. The final product particle size is governed by the extent of open area in screen. Screens are designed to be strong and maintain their integrity (no change in aperture size) with maximal open area. The optimal orientation and alignment of screen apertures is one where they are positioned in a 60° staggered pattern which provide an open area of 40% for 1/8 in holes aligned on 3/16 in. centers (feed machinery.com). The ratio of open screen area to horsepower is another important consideration where a low ratio results in poor ventilation and excessive heat generation which is detrimental to thermolabile actives and reduces milling throughput.

Milling Speed. Tip speed of the hammers dictates the overall particle size reduction and ranges between 80 and 120 m/s. It is calculated by multiplying the rotational speed of the drive source (shaft rpm) by the circumference of the hammer tip arc.

$$\text{Tip speed (m/s)} = \frac{\pi D \times \text{rpm}}{60} \tag{3}$$

where D is the diameter (m) and rpm and milling speed in revolutions per minute.

Collection. Once the material is milled, it is important to ensure that the milled particles are properly exited from the milling zone in a timely and effective manner. Usually, this is not a problem when the appropriate screen and hammer-to-screen distance is selected. Particles that are retained on the screen after milling begin to fluidize due to the high rotational speed of the hammers and are swept across the screen surface. As the particles grind across the screen surface, they are continually attrited into very fine particles. Excessive fines production leads to energy waste, heat and dust generation.

In the newer designs, an air-assist system that draws air into the milling zone is introduced. These systems are designed such that lower pressures are present on the exit of the screen to prevent fluidization and ensure that the particles do not remain on the screen. It is possible to use two screens in succession with the screen with larger apertures on top. This helps to reduce the amount of material retained on the face of the screen.

Gauge R&R: Having identified some critical equipment variables it should be pointed out that the state of reliability and accuracy of modern compactors is very high. For example, during a gauge R&R, Pinal et al. in our labs showed the reproducibility and accuracy of roll speed on the Fitzpatrick IR220 (Fig. 14). This means that the majority of unanticipated variation in product must be a function of the materials and formulation.

Identifying the Critical Formulation Variables

With respect to process design, these formulation variables will largely be determined by the required dose (concentration) of the active ingredients and its mechanical and micromeritic properties. This is summarized in Figure 15.

For low-dose formulations, the mechanical properties are largely determined by the mechanical properties of the excipients (39). Therefore, selection of chemically inert excipients that flow, deform, and bond well such as MCC are the most commonly used and content uniformity is the most common concern. This can occur through segregation of the API from the excipients in pre-blending or agglomeration of the API during handling with the same result. The use of flow aids or glidents such as fumed silica or talc aid in achieving homogeneity and dissipating electrostatic charging that may cause agglomeration.

Most often, as discussed in the introduction, roller compaction is used for higher dose compounds that when formulated either will not flow well enough to achieve homogeneous blends and/or do not form acceptable tablets in direct compression. In this

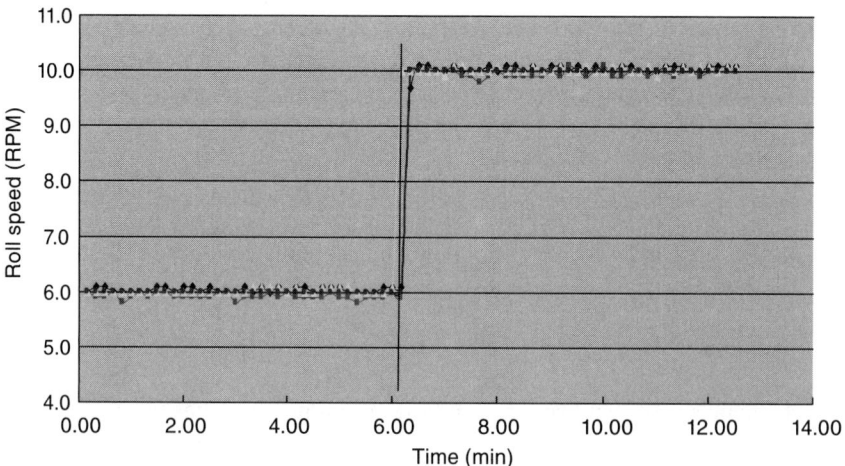

FIGURE 14 Reproducibility and accuracy of roll speed for three replicate roller compactor tests. *Source*: Courtesy of Pinal et al.

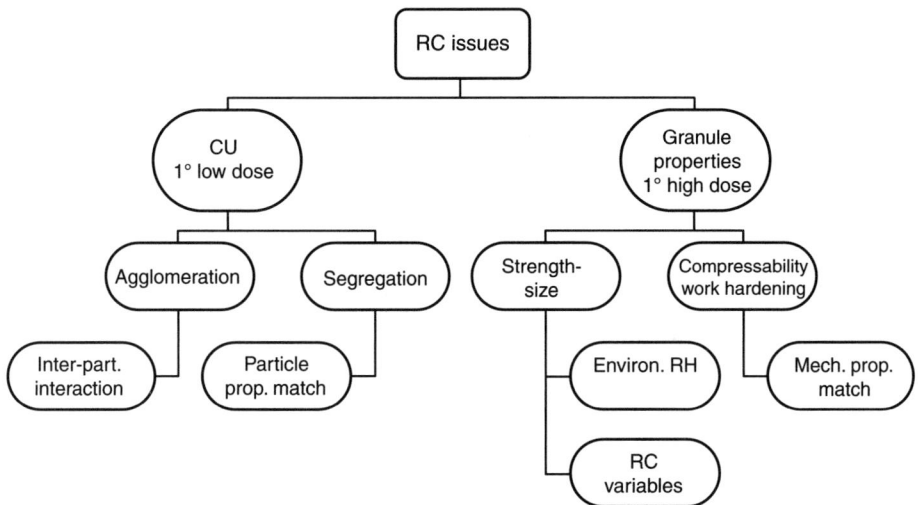

FIGURE 15 Formulation-based issues for process design.

situation, the mechanical properties of the formulation depend in a larger measure on the mechanical properties of the API. Whether or not an acceptable ribbon and granules can be produced then depends on the material properties interacting with the equipment variables discussed in the earlier section (40).

Impact of Micromeritic Properties

A smaller particle size grade of a plastic deforming material, Sta-Rx 1500 and a fragmenting material-lactose was found to give stronger tablets (41) though this result was not observed when MCC of different particle size was used. When binary mixtures of different particle size fractions of α-lactose monohydrate were used (42), the crushing strength and specific surface area of tablets prepared using the binary mixtures were lower than those values determined from linear interpolation of tablets compacted using single sieve fractions.

The degree of fragmentation was found to diminish with smaller sieve fractions at the same compression load when several sieve fractions of unmilled crystalline α-lactose monohydrate was used. The authors concluded that particle fragmentation would reduce as porosity approached zero and elastic behavior would start to dominate the consolidation process (43). With a decrease in particle size, yield pressure decreased and the strain rate sensitivity index increased (44) which suggested a reduction in the extent of fragmentation. The transition from brittle to ductile material was thought to occur for a median particle size of around 20 μm (45).

Several authors reported increase in tablet crushing strength when the particle size of α-lactose monohydrate was smaller (43,46,47). Fell and Newton (48) prepared tablets from three particle size fractions of crystalline lactose at 2 compaction speeds. The fraction with the smallest particle size was found to undergo the largest degree of particle rearrangement when calculated using both the Heckel and Cooper and Eaton plots. Vromans et al. (47) also showed that tablets prepared from smaller particles tended to be thicker than those produced using large particles. This observation was attributed to the higher porosity of tablets prepared using smaller particles.

The effect of lactose particle shape was also investigated in the study by Fell (48) where the addition of increasing amounts of spherical, spray-dried lactose fines to a tablet can be assumed to be made up of spherical isometric particles whose strength is mainly influenced by van der Waals forces acting at the coordination points of the particles. The proportionality between tensile strength of brittle lactose tablets and the internal specific surface area was established in a theoretical model proposed by Leuenberger et al. (49). Over a size range of 32–400 μm, A linear increase in tablet pore surface area with compaction force was found for all types of crystalline lactoses (α-lactose monohydrate, anhydrous β-lactose, anhydrous α-lactose) (50). This was based on the assumption that the change in pore surface area and actual binding surface varied proportionately (43).

Depending on the type of excipient used and their deformation behavior, the optimal operating parameters for roller compaction differed. For instance, Inghelbrecht et al. (11,13) found that lactose 200M needed a high roller speed: horizontal screw speed ratio whereas maize starch which is a plastic material, performed better at a lower roll speed: HFS ratio. A comparative study using seven different grades of MCC with the ibuprofen was conducted by Inghelbrecht and Remon (11). At an ibuprofen content of 25%, poorer granule quality was observed with all MCC types except Avicel CE-15 (co-processed with guar gum). When the ibuprofen concentration was increased, the granule quality was regained. Hence, it was suggested that the presence of low amount of ibuprofen (fragmenting) disrupted the bonding between plastically deforming MCC particles. However, this weakening of bonding ability between MCC particles was compensated by the fracture and sintering ability of ibuprofen at higher concentrations.

Lactose Grade

Crystalline lactose monohydrate is the most widely used diluent for tablet formulation. In direct compression, sieved crystalline fractions of α-lactose monohydrate, particularly the 100-mesh grade, is used because of its better flowability. The crystalline nature of lactose has been shown to strongly influence the compaction process and affect the mechanical properties of the compacts produced (51). Fragmentation is generally accepted as the predominant mechanism during consolidation for all types of crystalline lactose. Furthermore, water of crystallization, α:β ratio or degree of crystallinity were not found to affect the bonding mechanism significantly (50).

Vromans et al. (52) established a direct relationship between the compactibility and extent of fragmentation of crystalline lactose with the initial powder surface areas. It was suggested that the compactibility of crystalline lactose was dependent on the particle surface properties which was dictated in part by the crystallization process. Single crystals with low specific surface area and poor compaction properties are often associated with slow crystallization (e.g., α-lactose monohydrate). On the contrary, aggregates of microcrystals (anhydrous lactose) obtained from rapid crystallization followed by dehydration or roller drying showed better bonding due to their higher specific surface areas.

Conventionally processed lactose (104–150 μm, wedge-shaped) resulted in harder tablets than those prepared by conventionally processed lactose fines (<75 μm) alone. In another study by Roberts and Rowe (53), it was concluded that α-lactose monohydrate was more brittle than the directly compressible lactose grades (granulated grade and spray-dried grade) because of its higher yield pressure. They attributed this to the less spherical shape of α-lactose monohydrate as compared to the processed lactose grades. From scanning electron micrographs and surface area measurements of raw materials and tablets, isotropic ratio and Heckel analysis, α-lactose monohydrate particles was concluded to consolidate by plastic deformation and fragmentation (54).

Dry Granulation

Effects of Binder Properties

Binders are added for the purpose of improving the binding properties of granules and their compactability, in turn, giving rise to granules of desired mechanical strength (55). In the study conducted by Sheskey and Dasbach (32), nine different binders were evaluated for immediate-release tablets prepared by roller compaction. Higher binder concentrations resulted in stronger tablets that were less friable. Interestingly, it was the binder concentration rather than the applied roll pressures that governed affected the drug release rates from tablets prepared with many of these binders.

When a coarser grade of binder was used, the mechanical strength of tablets containing various crystalline materials such as lactose, acetaminophen and sodium chloride were weakened (56). With the exception of sodium chloride which undergoes plastic deformation, the other materials were extensively fragmented. This extent of particle fragmentation in turn, altered the effect of binder particle size. Larger surface areas associated with finer lactose granules gave rise to more contact points for bonding which in turn, produced harder tablets that had finer pore structures (46,57,58).

CHARACTERIZATION OF RIBBONS

It has been shown that the tensile strength of roller compacted ribbons is reflected in the density of the compacts (59). A three point beam bending approach (69) was used to determine both tensile strengths and Young's moduli for both ribbons and uniaxial compacted "surrogates" for ribbons (Fig. 16) (4) which have been used to determine compaction properties when material is limiting.

$$\text{Tensile Strength} = \frac{3Fl}{2bh^2} \tag{4}$$

$$\text{Young's Modulus} = \frac{Fl^3}{4\xi h^3 b} \tag{5}$$

where F is the applied force, l is the distance between the supports, b is the depth, h is the height of the sample, and ξ is the deflection (bending) of the beam.

Gupta also showed that for a given set of milling conditions in a Comil™ the post milled particle size distribution is related to the tensile strength of the ribbon (Fig. 17). This is a key in designing and controlling a roller compaction process as will be discussed later in the monitoring section.

Of course granules must not be so dense that they no longer perform as desired. They must dissolve as required for the dosage form and more pertinent to this discussion,

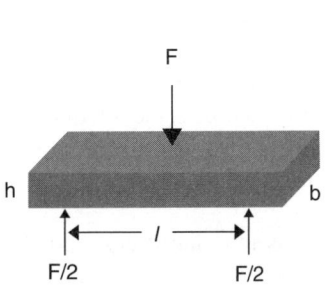
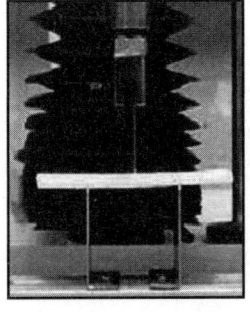

FIGURE 16 Three point beam bending set-up.

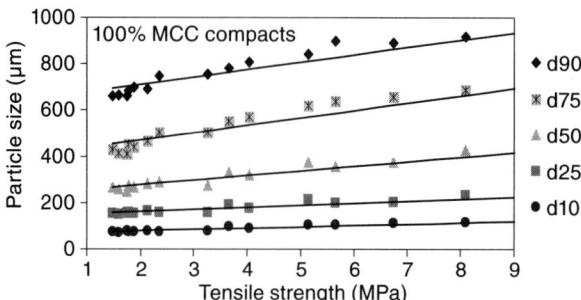

FIGURE 17 Ribbon tensile strength and particle size distribution. *Source*: Based on Ref. 60.

they must retain sufficient plasticity to deform and bond to yield an acceptable tablet. Referring to Figure 1, this means that the desired ribbon should be past the yield stress so it will bond but not at the extreme of the stress-strain behavior. At the extreme, the material may be strain or work "hardened". In the materials science literature, work hardening is typically associated with cyclic strain and recovery cycles with progressively less recovery. However, the same effect can be observed if the ribbon is over compressed resulting in granules that will no longer plastically deform under the uniaxial compression in the tablet press. This will be discussed further in the process design section.

DESIGN OF EXPERIMENTS AND DESIGN SPACE

Armed with a first principles or phenomenological model, one can identify potentially critical variables of a process. These may then be used in the designing of experiments to probe the sensitivity of the process to changes in these variables and to identify operating ranges which produce product with the desired attributes. This was illustrated for drying by Wildfong et al. (61) who used heat and mass transfer relationships for fluid bed trying to develop a method of assessing the implementation of accelerated drying.

Once identified all possible combination of the variables could of course be tested, however, this is typically prohibitively resource intensive to be practical. DoE is a class of statistically based methods to select combinations of variables that may be tested to yield the same information using a reduced number of experiments. DoE is often used in a totally empirical manner; however, the knowledge of potentially critical variables can greatly simplify the process. DoEs may take the form of simple experiments which bracket the extremes of variable combinations, the so called extreme vertices method, or may be more intricate. Commonly, a partial matrix type screening DoE will be executed to zero in on the ranges in variables that show the maximum impact and/or that most closely bracket the desired responses from the process. This is followed by a more focused matrix DoE to determine optimum ranges of operations.

An example of a "Latin Squares" DoE is shown below in the results table probing reasonable ranges of some of the variables for roller compaction (62). As the relationship between density and tensile strength, and subsequent post-milled particle size was established (as discussed above), density was identified as the primary response variable of interest.

The acceptable or desired density ranges are defined as introduced conceptually earlier and are based upon:

Dry Granulation

1. whether the ribbon is too dense leading to strain or work hardened granules on the upper end,
2. on the lower end where the density is too low to form a ribbon or granules.

Once we are this far in our understanding and demonstration of the impact of the variables on the chosen response, creation of a design space is possible (ala, ICH Q8). Figure 18 shows the schematic for design space from Table 1. The level curves in between the filled areas represent the range of densities that is acceptable and the combinations of the roll speed and moisture (i.e., the %RH of exposure) that will work to produce the product (or intermediate at this stage).

This looks (and really is) straight forward and only slightly more effort than those skilled in development do presently. However, there are some differences between the way process design is currently performed and associated issues with the design space approach that should always be addressed in this formalism. In short they are: controlling, monitoring, and modeling.

Process Control

Process control is critical as the use of the design space means maintaining the process within the bounds of acceptable response. This is a departure from the industry's usual time only based control, however, recent advances in regulatory opinion, science and technology now makes this a real possibility. The idea is not to document failure but to avoid failure by near real-time corrective action when the process tends toward deviation.

Process Monitoring

Monitoring goes hand-in-hand with control as one must know when the process is trending out of control to be able to affect an adjustment to remain in the design space. This means real-time or near real-time data. The key point so often missed is that the interval of data collection of the critical variables must be short relative to the total time of the operation to allow for adjustment. Real-time may mean anything from using traditional laboratory testing in a timely manner to in-line monitoring. A thermometer and a manual temperature adjustment may be fine depending upon the process.

It is important to know which variables are the meaningful variables to your process for control as well as the proper monitoring interval. For roller compaction we will discuss three types of monitoring for control:

1. Off-line monitoring using traditional tests for physical and chemical properties as well as less or non-traditional testing such as NIR. To repeat an earlier comment,

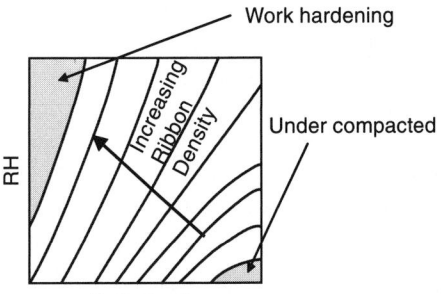

FIGURE 18 Schematic for design space created from Table 1. *Source*: Courtesy of Gupta, Clark and Morris.

TABLE 1 Results of DoE for roller compaction study

Attribute	RH(%)	Roll speed (rpm)		
		5.0	6.0	7.0
Moisture Content (% w/w)	25	3.3	3.3	3.3
	45	5.0	5.0	5.0
	65	6.3	6.3	6.3
Relative Density	25	0.76	0.70	0.68
	45	0.79	0.76	0.72
	65	0.81	0.77	0.73
Tensile Strength (MPa)	25	4.9	3.2	2.6
	45	5.5	3.9	2.9
	65	6.9	5.3	3.3

Source: From Ref. 62.

there is nothing wrong with doing off-line measurement during development or even manufacturing if the data are collected at proper time interval for control. This can be quite challenging with roller compaction however, given the rate of material flow.
2. Equipment readout feedback control is often used in the form of monitoring the roll gap as a function of the feed screw and roll speeds.
3. On-line monitoring the ribbon and/or granules with NIR or other techniques (e.g., Raman) to follow critical material properties is only recently being implemented outside of research labs (60). The principles of diffuse reflectance NIR show how the monitoring of a variable proportional to density is possible. First looking at the schematic of diffuse reflectance in Figure 19 makes it obvious that if the sample density varies so must the path of the radiation through it. Second, the Kubelka–Munk function used to describe the reflectance phenomenon contains material factors that enter into the denominator as shown.

The principle has been demonstrated by Drennen (69) for determining tablet hardness and the principle is the same in that the slope of the NIR spectra change as the density (or particle size) change. This is illustrated in Figure 20 for roller compacted ribbons of MCC.

Going from the top to the bottom of the figure the spectra represent decreasing ribbon densities (increasing roll speed therefore an effectively lower dwell time). The slopes are decreasing with decreasing density which is consistent with the predictions of

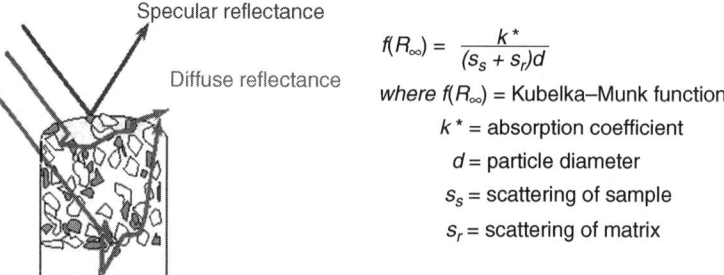

$$f(R_\infty) = \frac{k^*}{(s_s + s_r)d}$$

where $f(R_\infty)$ = Kubelka–Munk function
k^* = absorption coefficient
d = particle diameter
s_s = scattering of sample
s_r = scattering of matrix

FIGURE 19 Schematic of diffuse reflectance.

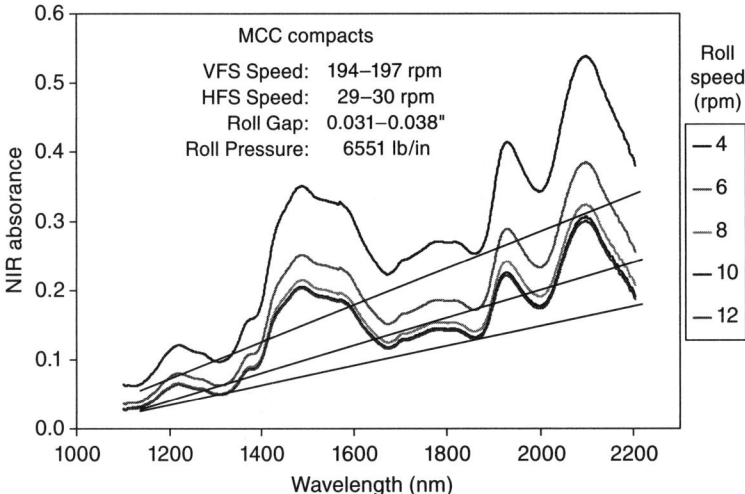

FIGURE 20 Dependence of NIR spectral slope on roll speed (i.e., density).

the Kubelka–Munk relationship. There is additional dependence in the wavelength relationship but a simple regression of the spectra yield a good correlation with the density which shown in Figure 21 and as discussed earlier this was found to correlate with the post-milled particle size distribution.

The contribution of equipment drift is very small as discussed in the chemometrics section. To illustrate this, consider the variability of a real-time NIR signal from a ribbon as it is compacted on the Fitzpatrick IR520 as shown in Figure 22. The variation in slope is on the order of 0.5 units introducing only a small error in the measurement. Of course once quantified this contribution can be corrected for in the data.

The price of being able to observe the process in near real-time with NIR or other monitors is dealing with the large amount of data and the interpretation. This requires the use of multivariate methods to reduce the dimensions of the data into something that can be handled. This is accomplished through the use of chemometrics.

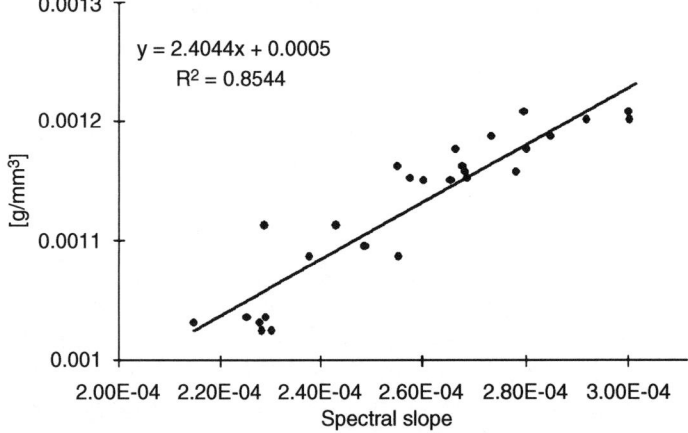

FIGURE 21 Correlation of density with the spectral slope for roller compacted ribbons.

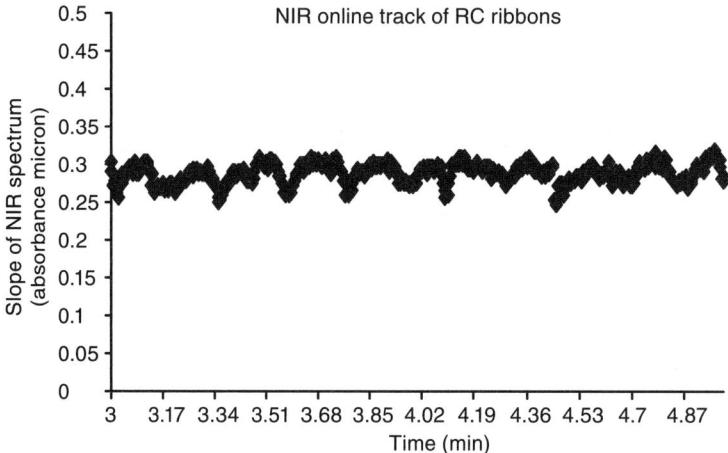

FIGURE 22 Variation in NIR slope due to roll RPM. *Source*: Courtesy of Pinal et al.

Process Modeling

Modeling is also a requirement for the design space. However, what constitutes a model can vary from an almost totally empirical model to a first principles model. All may be valid if the assumptions upon which the model was created are clear and adhered to. For example, the model presented above is an empirical model based upon selection of variables that seem logical based upon the science and statistical analysis of the data collected. If we had a physics equation (constitutive relationship) and the ability to predict all of the variables, it would be a first principles model. In between empirical and first principles are so called "hybrid" models that may have known relationships between variables but require calibration or determination of coefficients. The differences are that:

1. first principles models are:
   a. scaleable,
   b. useable beyond the range over which they were tested (within the assumptions of the model); while
2. empirical models are:
   a. valid only for the system on which they were developed (including material and equipment),
   b. only over the ranges tested (should include dimensional analysis);
3. Hybrid models are:
   a. more scalable as there is a predictive relationship with which to change some variables, and/or
   b. more able to vary materials ranges.

As an example of a hybrid model, consider that we know that granule drying is a describable by heat and mass transport equations, yet the impact of the porosity and tortuosity of granules being dried while known critical variables to the mass transfer stage drying are usually not predictable. We may still scale-up (or down) the first heat transfer stage of drying and with fairly little effort, estimate the starting point for the mass transfer stage. However, if the granulation and/or formulation is changed there will be work needed to verify the variations in the physical properties of the new granulation.

CHEMOMETRICS

Overview

Chemometrics refer to any mathematical or statistical method applied to chemical measurements to improve data interpretation. Often, the term chemometrics is used when referring to multivariate data analysis techniques such as principal component analysis (PCA) and partial least squares projection (PLS). Advantages of multivariate analysis methods are: (*i*) pattern recognition, (*ii*) unraveling hidden relationships establishing the correlation between multiple variables, (*iii*) reduce data dimensionality, and (*iv*) allow identification and correction of systematic noise (pre-treatment). The following paragraphs will give a brief overview of PCA and PLS followed by a specific example of how PLS is applied to deconvolute the NIR signals obtained during monitoring for calibrating ribbon density.

PCA is a pattern recognition technique that searches for systematic variation in a given data matrix. As background noise is random in nature, it will not be captured by the principal components (PC). PCA is performed by decomposing a complex data matrix (**X**) into a summation of different factors or components (**tp**) and an error matrix (**E**) as illustrated in Figure 23. A factor or component is the outer product of a column and row vector; the column vector refers to the scores (**t**) and explain the relationship among samples during process; the row vector is known as the factor loadings (**p**) and explains the relationship among variables during the process. The loadings will identify the variables that are affected by the process and how they are affected (63).

Loadings (**p**) is determined from cosine of the angles, θ, between the variable and the vector and it represents the Influence of variable on **p**. Scores (**t**), on the other hand, represents the sample projections onto the loading vector by the relationship:

$$\mathbf{t} = \frac{Xp}{p'p} \tag{5}$$

A detailed explanation on the derivation of PCA is available in a review paper by Svante (63). In many ways, PLS is similar to PCA except that it looks for correlations between matrices or a matrix and a vector. Robust calibrations can be created using PLS because the correlation is multivariate in nature, making it less susceptible to random noise. PLS captures the highest variance in the data set and correlates both data blocks simultaneously. Unlike PCA where independent score sets for each data block is calculated, a common link or weight loading vector (**w**) is calculated. A regression coefficient, **c**, is used to predict independent variables.

$$\mathbf{t} = \frac{Xw}{w'w} \tag{6}$$

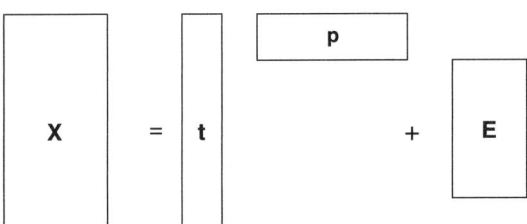

Where **X** = data matrix, **t** = scores, **p** = loadings and **E** = error matrix.
A factor or component (**tp**) is defined as the product of **t** and **p**.

FIGURE 23 Overview of PCA. *Abbreviation*: PCA, principal component analysis.

$$\mathbf{c} = \frac{t'y}{t't} \tag{7}$$

For further information on PLS and PCA, the reader is encouraged to see Refs. 64, 65, and 66.

Application to Roller Compaction

Density Monitoring

In the study conducted at Purdue University, the feasibility of using PLS for density calibration and monitoring in roller compaction was investigated using surrogate ribbons containing 50:50 blend of MCC and APAP. Surrogates were prepared at different compaction pressures (4500–12500 lb) in a Carver press to yield compacts of different densities. NIR spectra of the surrogates were taken on both faces, at an integration time of 0.035 seconds. PLS calibration was performed using the compaction pressures used in the preparation of the surrogates.

Absorbance of the NIR spectra increased expectedly with as the surrogates became denser (Fig. 24B). In the first PC, the loadings plot closely resembled the averaged spectra of the blends (Fig. 25A). This indicated that the main variability could be attributed to intensity (absorbance) of the spectra which was in turn caused by the density variation. As shown in Figure 25B, both the 1st and 2nd PCs captured changes in the spectral slopes.

The root mean square error of calibration was 534.9 lb, with an R^2 of 0.982 while the root mean square error of prediction by cross validation was 617.7 lb with an R^2 of 0.976. These results demonstrate the feasibility and usefulness of PLS calibration in density monitoring and prediction in surrogate ribbons. The next step will be to implement this algorithm on real time, online NIR measurements taken from actual ribbons prepared in roller compaction.

Identifying Critical Raw Material Properties

A recent study conducted by Soh et al. (67) clearly established the importance of raw material properties in modeling the ribbon, granule, and tablet properties prepared in roller compaction using multivariate analysis. The material properties evaluated included particle size, size distribution, flow and compressibility as well as density. In the absence of raw material properties, roller compactor operating parameters (roll speed, HFS, and roll pressure) alone were unable to predict the ribbon density, granule particle size, and tablet tensile strength satisfactorily. The overall effect of every material property on the respective ribbon and granule quality was illustrated using the coefficient overview plot in the multivariate analysis software. Raw material tabletability, MCC fraction, tapped density, Kawakita constant ($1/b$), angle of fall, and span were found to exert dominant effects on the various RC responses (Fig. 26).

Scale-Up

In theory, scale-up can be performed by applying the similarity principle from data collected on the smaller unit (68). Based on the similarity principle, two processes can be considered similar when they occur in similar geometric space and all dimensionless groups required to describe the process have the same numerical values.

Dry Granulation

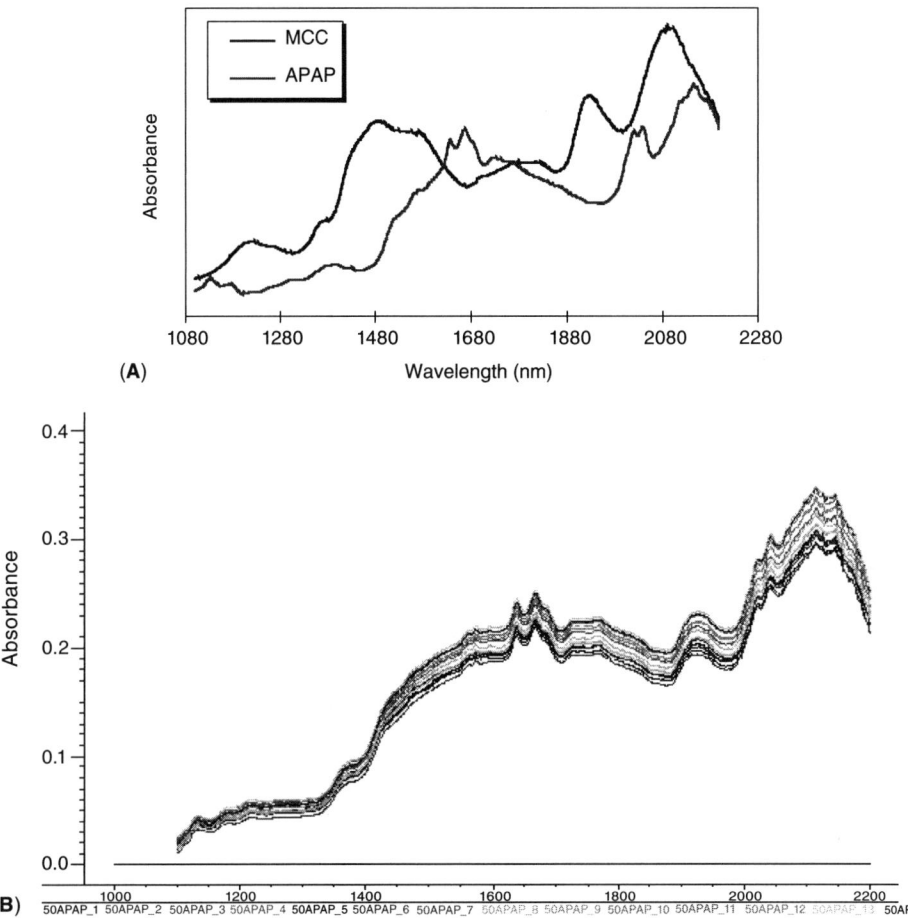

FIGURE 24 NIR spectra of (**A**) pure MCC and pure APAP; (**B**) surrogate ribbons containing 50:50 blend of MCC and APAP prepared at different densities. *Abbreviation*: MCC, microcrystalline cellulose. *Source*: Courtesy of Morris et al.

The Buckingham-Pi theorem is a systematic way of reducing the number of dimensionless groups and is central to the concept of dimensional analysis. In this theorem, if an equation containing K variables is dimensionally homogenous, it can be reduced to a relationship containing $K - r$ independent products referred to as π terms where r is the minimum number of reference variables required to describe the variables. To determine the dimensionless variables, the method of repeating variables is used (68).

Raw material properties (such as density, particle size, yield strength, Young's modulus, and Poisson ratio) and roller compactor operating parameters (feed screw speed, roll pressure, roll speed, and roll gap) can be expressed in the form of reference variables. In this chapter, roll gap is expressed as a function of roll pressure, roll speed, feed screw speed, diameter of rolls, true density, young modulus, Poisson ratio, yield strength, and particle size as shown in the following equation:

$$\frac{RG}{D} fcn \left(\frac{RP}{TrueDens * RS^2 * D^{2'}} \frac{HFS}{RS'} \frac{D}{d'} \frac{E}{TrueDens * RS^2 * D^{2'}} \frac{Y}{E'} PoissonRatio \right)$$

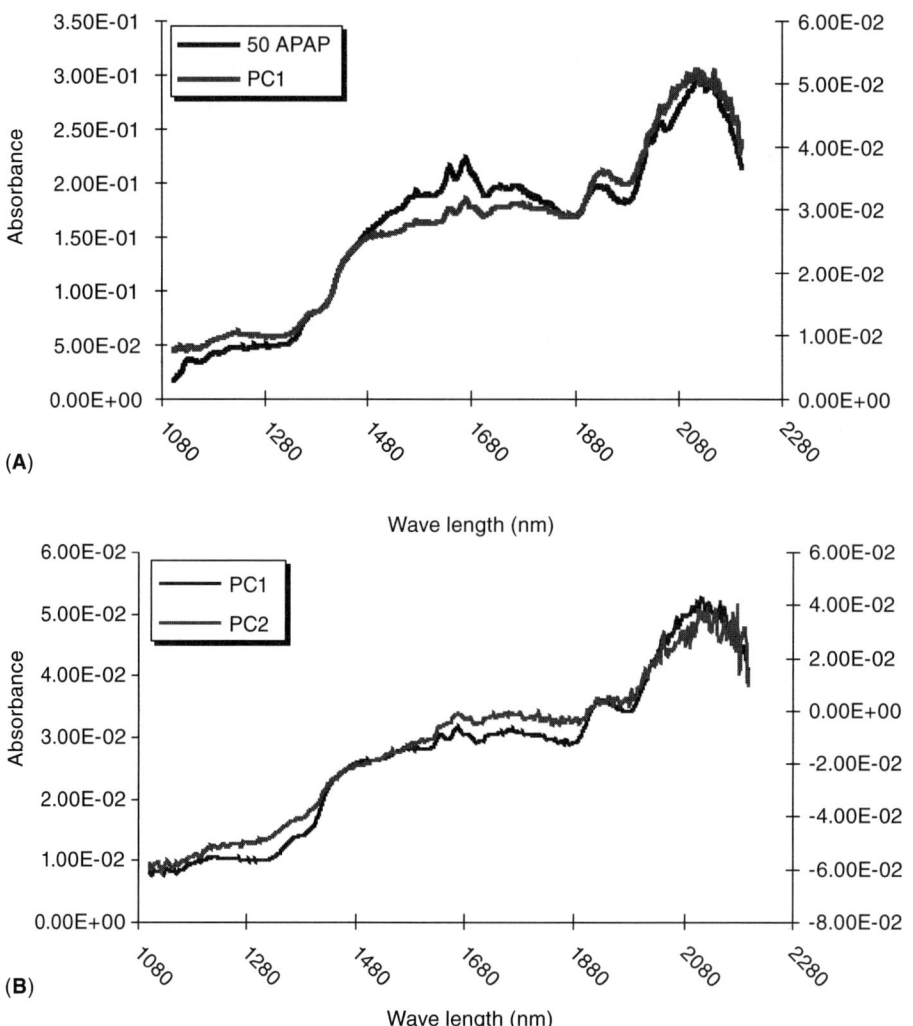

FIGURE 25 (**A**) Loadings plot of 1st PC compared to the averaged NIR spectra of a 50:50 blend of MCC:APAP on the 1st PC, (**B**) Loadings plot of 1st and 2nd PC. *Abbreviations*: MCC, microcrystalline cellulose; PC, principle component.

where RG is the roll gap, RP is the roll pressure, RS is the roll speed, HFS is the horizontal feed screw speed, D is the roll diameter, d is the particle size, TrueDens is the true density of feed material, E is the Young's modulus, and Y is the yield strength.

Since the true density, Young's modulus, Poisson ratio, and particle size of the feed material are inherent material properties and cannot be readily altered, the remaining terms and relationships left to be kept constant are: $D_2/D_1 = d_1/d_2$, $HFS_2/HFS_1 = RS_1/RS_2$ and $RG_2/RG_1 = D_1/D_2$ where the subscripts "1" and "2" denote two different roller compactors. In other words, at a given roll pressure and the same material/formulation, the roller compaction process can be scalable when these dimensional terms have the same numerical values.

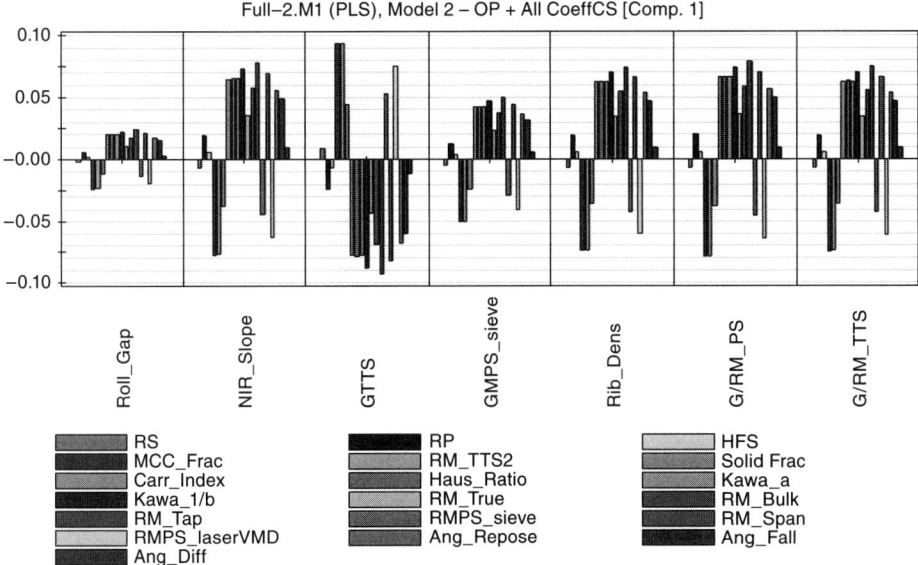

FIGURE 26 Coefficient overview plot showing the effects of raw material properties on measured roller compaction responses. *Source*: From Ref. 67.

ACKNOWLEDGEMENTS

The authors gratefully acknowledge the Consortium for the Advancement of Manufacturing of Pharmaceuticals (CAMP) and the National Science Foundation-Engineering Research Center for Solid Organic Particulate Systems (ERC-SOPS) for the financial support. The works of Drs. Ronald Miller (Bristol-Myers Squibb Company), Abhay Gupta (FDA-CDER), Saly Romero-Torres (Schering-Plough Corporation) have been referred to in the preparation of this manuscript.

REFERENCES

1. Bowman KJ. Mechanical Behavior of Materials. New Jersey: John Wiley, 2004.
2. Hosford WF, Robert MC. Metal Forming: Mechanics and Metallurgy, Englewood Cliffs, NJ: PTR Prentice Hall, 1993.
3. Beyer T, Day GM, Price SL. The prediction, morphology, and mechanical properties of the polymorphs of paracetamol. J Am Chem Soc 2001; 123:5086–94.
4. Hancock BC, Zografi G. Characteristics and significance of the amorphous state in pharmaceutical systems. J Pharm Sci 1997; 86(1):1–12.
5. Miller RW. Roller compaction technology. In: Parikh DM, Ed. Handbook of Pharmaceutical Granulation Technology. New York: Marcel Dekker, 2005: 159–90.
6. Podczeck F. Particle–Particle Adhesion in Pharmaceutical Powder Handling. London: Imperial College Press, 1998: 13.
7. Khan KA, Musikabhumma P. Effect of slugging pressure on the properties of granules and tablets prepared from potassium phenethicillin. J Pharm Pharmacol 1981; 33:627.
8. Levy G, Antkowiak JM, Procknal JA, White DC. Effect of certain tablet formulation factors on dissolution rate of active ingredient II. J Pharm Sci 1963; 52(11):1047.

9. Malkowska S, Khan KA, Lentle R, Marchant J, Elger G. Effect of recompression on the properties of tablets prepared by moist granulation. Drug Dev Ind Pharm 1983; 9(3):349.
10. Hariharan M, Wowchuk C, Nkansah P, Gupta VK. Effect of formulation composition on the properties of controlled release tablets prepared by roller compaction. Drug Dev Ind Pharm 2004; 130:565–72.
11. Inghelbrecht S, Remon, JP. Roller compaction and tableting of microcrystalline cellulose/drug mixtures. Int J Pharm 1998; 161:215–24.
12. Cohn R, Heilig H, Delorimier A. Critical evaluation of the compactor. J Pharm Sci 1966; 55:328–31.
13. Inghelbrecht S, Remon J P. The roller compaction of different types of lactose. Int.J Pharm 1998; 166:135–44.
14. Guigon P, Simon O. Roll press design-influence of force feed systems on compaction. Powder Technol 2003; 130:41–8.
15. Johanson JR. A rolling theory for granular solids. Trans ASME J Appl Mech 1965; 32:842–8.
16. Turkoglu M, Aydin I, Murray M, Sakr A. Modeling of a roller-compaction process using neural networks and genetic algorithms. Eur J Pharm Biopharm 1999; 48(3):239–45.
17. Dec RT, Zavaliangos A, Cunningham JC. Comparison of various modeling methods for analysis of powder compaction in roller press. Powder Technol 2003; 130:265–71.
18. Li LC, Peck GE. The effect of agglomeration methods on the micromeritic properties of a maltodextrin product, Maltrin 150^{TM}. Drug Dev Ind Pharm 1990; 16:1491–503.
19. Mitchell SA, Reynolds TD, Dasbach TP. A compaction process to enhance dissolution of poorly water-soluble drugs using hydroxypropyl methylcellulose. Int J Pharm 2003; 250:3–11.
20. Rambali B, Baert L, Jans E, Masseart DL. Influence of the roll compactor parameter settings and the compression pressure on the buccal bio-adhesive properties. Int J Pharm 2001; 220:129–40.
21. Heng PWS, Chan LW, Liew CV, Chee SN, Soh JLP, Ooi SM. Roller compaction of crude plant material: Influence of process variables, polyvinylpyrrolidone and co-milling. Pharm Dev Tech 2004; 9(2):135–44.
22. von Eggelkraut-Gottanka SG, Abed SA, Muller W, Schmidt PC. Roller compaction and tabletting of St. John's Wort plant dry extract using a gap width and force controlled roller compactor. I. Granulation and tabletting of eight different extract batches. Pharm Dev Technol 2002; 7:433–45.
23. Schiller M, von der Heydt H, März F, Schmidt PC. Enhanced processing properties and stability of film-coated tablets prepared from roller-compacted and ion-exchanged Eschscholtzia californica Cham. Dry extracts. STP Pharm Sci 2003; 13:111–7.
24. Wennerstrum S. Ten things you need to consider when choosing and installing a roller press system. Powder Bulk Eng 2000; 14(2).
25. Funakoshi Y, Asogawa T, Satake E. The use of a novel roller compactor with a concavo-convex roller pair to obtain uniform compacting pressure. Drug Dev Ind Pharm 1977; 3:555–73.
26. Parrott EL. Densification of powders by concavo-convex roller compactor. J Pharm Sci 1981; 70:288–91.
27. Sheskey PJ, Hendren J. The effects of roll compaction equipment variables, granulation technique, and HPMC polymer level on a controlled-release matrix model drug formulation. Pharm Technol 1999; 23:90–106.
28. Adeyeye MC. Roller compaction and milling pharmaceutical unit processes: Part I. Am Pharm Rev 2000; 3:37–42.
29. Miller RW. Advances in pharmaceutical roller compactor feed system designs. Pharm Technol 1994; 18:154–62.
30. Johanson JR, Cox BD. Fluid Entrainment Effects in Roll Press Compaction. Proc Inst Briq Agglom 1987; 20:251–63.
31. Sheskey PJ, Cabelka TD, Robb RT, Boyce BM. Use of roller compaction in the preparation of controlled-release hydrophilic matrix tablets containing Methylcellulose and Hydroxypropyl Methylcellulose polymers. Pharm Technol 1994; 18:132–50.

32. Sheskey PJ, Dasbach TP. Evaluation of various polymers as dry binders in the preparation of an immediate-release tablet formulation by roller compaction. Pharm Technol 1995; 19:98–112.
33. Jerome E, Delacourte A, Guyot JC, Hervieu P, Dehont F. Granulation of pharmaceutical powders by compaction an experimental study. Drug Dev Ind Pharm 1994; 20:65–74.
34. Simon O, Guigon PrP. Interaction between feeding and compaction during lactose compaction in a laboratory roll press. KONA 2000; 18:131–8.
35. Horisawa E, Danjo K, Sunada H. Influence of granulating method on physical and mechanical properties, compression behaviour and compactibility of lactose and microcrystalline cellulose granules. Drug Dev Ind Pharm 2000; 26:583–93.
36. Beten DB, Yüksel N, Baykara T. The changes in the mechanic properties of a direct tableting agent microcrystalline cellulose by recompression. Drug Dev Ind Pharm 1994; 20:2323–31.
37. Murray M, Laohavichien A, Habib W, Sakr A. Effect of process variables on roller-compacted ibuprofen tablets. Pharm Ind 1998; 60:257–62.
38. FDA-CDER. Guidance for industry. SUPAC-IR/MR: Immediate release and modified release solid oral dosage forms. Manufacturing equipment addendum, 1999.
39. Rogers TL. Content considerations for low dosage drug formulations processed by roller compaction. Ph.D Thesis, Purdue University, West Lafayette, Indiana, USA, 1999.
40. Falzone AM, Peck GE, McCabe GP. Effects of changes in roller compaction parameters on granulations produced by compaction. Drug Dev Ind Pharm 1992; 18:469–89.
41. McKenna A, McCafferty DF. Effect of particle size on the compaction mechanism and tensile strength of tablets. J Pharm Pharmacol 1981; 34:347–51.
42. Riepma KA, Veenstra J, de Boer AH, et al. Consolidation and compaction of powder mixture: II. Binary mixtures of different particle size fractions of α-lactose monohydrate. Int J Pharm 1991; 76:9–15.
43. de Boer AH, Vromans H, Lerk CF, Bolhuis GK, Kussendrager KD, Bosch H. Studies on tabletting properties of lactose. III. The consolidation behaviour of sieve fractions of crystalline α-lactose. Pharm Week. Sci Ed 1986; 8:145–50.
44. York P. Particle slippage and rearrangement during compression of pharmaceutical powders. J Pharm Pharmacol 1978; 30:6–10.
45. Roberts RJ, Rowe RC. The effect of the relationship between punch velocity and particle size on the compaction behaviour of materials with varying deformation mechanisms. J Pharm Pharmacol 1986; 38:567–71.
46. Fell JT, Newton JM. The tensile strength of latose tablets. J Pharm Pharmacol 1968; 20:657–9.
47. Vromans H, De Boer AH, Bolhuis GK, Lerk CF, Kussendrager KD. Studies on tabletting properties of lactose. Part I. The effect of initial particle size on binding properties and dehydration characteristics of lactose. Acta Pharm Sucica 1985; 22:163–72.
48. Fell JT. The Influence of fines on the flow and compaction properties of lactose. J Pharm Pharmacol 1973; 25(Suppl.):109P.
49. Leuenberger H, Bonny JD, Lerk CF, Vromans H. Relation between crushing strength and internal specific surface area of lactose compacts. Int J Pharm 1989; 52:91–100.
50. Vromans H, De Boer AH, Bolhuis GK, Lerk CF, Kussendrager KD, Bosch H. Studies on tabletting properties of lactose. Part II. Consolidation and compaction of different types of crystalline lactose. Pharm Week Sci Ed 1985; 7:186–93.
51. Busignies V, Tchoreloff P, Leclerc B, Hersen C, Keller G, Couarraze G. Compaction of crystallographic forms of pharmaceutical granular lactoses. II.Compacts mechanical properties. Eur J Pharm Biopharm 2004; 58:577–86.
52. Vromans H, Bolhuis GK, Lerk CF, Kussendrager KD. Studies of tableting properties of lactose. IX. The relationship between particle structure and compactibility of crystalline lactose. Int J Pharm 1987; 39:207–12.
53. Roberts RJ, Rowe RC. The effect of punch velocity on the compaction of a variety of materials. J Pharm Pharmacol 1985; 37:377–84.

54. Duberg M, Nyström C. Studies on direct compression of tablets VI. Evaluation of methods for the estimation of particle fragmentation during compaction. Acta Pharm Suec 1982; 19:421–36.
55. Symecko CW, Rhodes CT. Binder functionality in tabletted systems. Drug Dev Ind Pharm 1995; 21:1091–114.
56. Nyström C, Mazur J, Sjögren J. Studies on direct compression of tablets II. The influence of the particle size of a dry binder on the mechanical strength of tablets. Int J Pharm 1982; 10:209–18.
57. Selkirk AB, Ganderton D. Influence of wet and dry granulation methods on the pore structure of lactose tablets. J Pharm Pharmacol 1970; 22:86S–94S.
58. Riepma KA, Vromans H, Zuurman K, Lerk CF. The effect of dry granulation on the consolidation and compaction of crystalline lactose. Int J Pharm 1993; 97:29–38.
59. Gupta APG, Miller RW, Morris KR. Real-time near-infrared monitoring of content uniformity, moisture content, compact density, tensile strength, and young's modulus of roller compacted powder blends. J Pharm Sci 2005; 94(7):1589–97.
60. Gupta APG, Miller RW, Morris KR. Nondestructive measurements of the compact strength and the particle-size distribution after milling of roller compacted powders by near-infrared spectroscopy. J Pharm Sci 2004; 93(4):1047–53.
61. Wildfong PLD, Samy AS, Corfa J, Peck GE, Morris KR. Accelerated fluid bed drying using nir monitoring and phenomenological modeling: method assessment and formulation suitability. J Pharm Sci 2002; 91(3):631–9.
62. Gupta APG, Miller RW, Morris KR. Effect of the variation in the ambient moisture on the compaction behavior of powder undergoing roller-compaction and on the characteristics of tablets produced from the post-milled granules. J Pharm Sci 2005; 94(10):2314–26.
63. Wold S. Principal component analysis. Chemomet Intell Lab Syst 1987; 2:37–52.
64. Beebe KR, Kowalski BR. An introduction to multivariate calibration and analysis. Anal Chem 1987; 59(17):1007–17.
65. Gabrielsson J, Lindberg N-O, Lundstedt T. Multivariate methods in pharmaceutical applications. J Chemometrics 2002; 16:141–60.
66. Haaland DM, Thomas EV. Partial least-squares methods for spectral analyses. 1. Relation to other quantitative calibration methods and the extraction of qualitative information. Am Chem Soc 1988; 60:1193–202.
67. Soh JLP, Wang F, Boersen N, et al. Modeling the effects of raw material properties and operating parameters on ribbon and granule properties prepared in roller compaction using multivariate data analysis. Drug Dev Ind Pharm. Submitted.
68. He Y, Liu X, Litster JD. Scale up considerations in granulation. In: Parikh DM, ed. Handbook of Pharmaceutical Granulation Technology. Boca Raton, Florida: Taylor and Francis Group, 2005:459–90.
69. Kirsch JD, Drennan JK. Nondestructive tablet hardness testing by near-infrared spectroscopy: a new and robust spectral best-fit algorithm. J Pharm Biomed Anal 1999; 19(3–4):351–62.

10

The Preparation of Pellets by Extrusion/Spheronization

J. M. Newton
The School of Pharmacy, University of London, and Department of Mechanical Engineering, University College London, London, U.K.

HISTORICAL INTRODUCTION

The process of extrusion/spheronization originated in Japan and was introduced into Europe and the United States in the early 1960s as the process of "Maurumerization," which was the trademark of the Fuji Denki Koyo Co Ltd. Eli Lilly & Co sold them under license and the first description in the literature by Reynolds (1) in Europe and Conine and Hadley (2) in the United States were from this company. The advantages for the process listed by Reynolds (1) were "regularity in shape, consistency of size, definite surface characteristics, low friability, flexible in respect of sphere size which can be produced, capable of high throughput and easy operation." These claims can still be justified in most instances and the ability to produce pellets with relatively high drug load, up to +80% and the ability to carry out formulation studies on relatively small samples of material, can be added. The claim to the flexibility of possible sizes does not mention the possible range and in practice, it is quite limited. For example, Clarke et al. (3) found that while pellets in the range of 0.5–5.0 mm could be prepared on a small scale, the preparation of such a range on a large scale would be very difficult. At the lower end, it is difficult to provide uniform holes of less than 0.5 mm in diameter, which are rigid enough to withstand the extrusion forces. It is also difficult to provide satisfactory formulations that would extrude through such dies. At the upper end, there is very limited information as to how larger diameter extrudate functions. There is work by Rough and Wilson (4) with 3-mm dies, but some of the products are hardly of suitable quality. A range of about 0.7–2.5 mm is a more realistic range. While several major pharmaceutical products are made by this process, even their scale is dwarfed by the requirements of other industries. I was once asked to advise a chemical company who wished to produce in 1 day what would have represented the annual production of a major pharmaceutical product. Also, the fact that the process involves several stages requiring different pieces of equipment and is difficult to convert to a fully continuous process, has lead to some limitation of the application of the process. There is a recent publication titled "Evaluation of the performance of a new continuous spheronizer" would indicate that this had been solved (5). The paper, however, only describes its use as a batch process and the information as to how it would be used in a continuous mode is scanty. On a manufacturing scale, the process, therefore, must be considered as a batch process.

Nevertheless, it is an extremely useful addition to the armory of pharmaceutical processes for the preparation of pellets. While formulation is still strongly experience dependent, as more successful preparations are reported, the formulation possibilities are continuing to expand. To be able to apply the information from the literature to aid formulation, it is important to remember however that, while the generic term "extrusion/spheronization" is used in many publications, there are considerable differences in the principles by which the equipment functions and differences in the operating conditions of a given piece of equipment (especially the extruders). Thus, findings can be very specific to a given set of equipment, operating conditions, and formulation. There is as yet no all-embracing solution to converting any given drug into a high drug loaded pellet. For example, for one drug I was able to produce good pellets from the racemate but could not produce pellets from either the R or the S isomer.

PROCESS OUTLINE AND PREPARATION OF PELLETS

The process consists of the following stages: mixing, extrusion, spheronization, and drying. Mixing and drying are standard unit operations used in pharmaceutical technology and the standard type of equipment is available and generally used in the process. The equipment involved in the extrusion and spheronization stages were not standard processes when the process was introduced and therefore these require detailed consideration. The extrusion process is extensively used in several industries and extruders vary considerably in the way material is processed. Several types have been used in pharmaceutical industry and it is very important to identify what type has been used and how it has been operated as the extrudate, which is produced can be very different in quality. The spheronization equipment is very similar, comprising of a plate rotating within a cylinder. The plate designs do vary but there is little fundamental work on their design and limited experimental work. The difference in the pellets produced when a radial and cross hatch plates were used to process the same extrudate, was found to be dependent on the length of die used to produce the extrudate (6). For the shorter die length (length to radius 1:6.1) there was an effect, but for extrudate produced with a longer die (length to radius ratio 1:11), there was no difference in the pellets produced. In another study, the actual surface design was found to be less important than the other stages of the process and the formulation (7). The speed of operation is related to the dimensions of the spheronizer and has been related to the velocity at the periphery of the plate (8). In most cases for a given diameter of spheronizer, the rotational speed is not critical but for the preparation of pellets, which included a high percentage of croscarmellose sodium (Ac–Di–Sol®, FMC Corporation, Philadelphia, Pennsylvania, U.S.A.), it was found necessary to reduce the rotational speed by a factor of 10 (9).

Most systems function with "paste" but Young et al. (10) described the use of a process whereby the extrusion was with a hot-melt system, the extrudate cut in a pelletizer (Randcastle RCP-2.0, Randcastle Inc. Cedar Grove, New Jersey, U.S.A.) into cylindrical pellets, which were then spheronized on a conventional spheronizer (Caleva Model 120, AC Compacting LLc, North Brunswick, New Jersey, U.S.A.) heated with a heat gun to 65–70°C while dusting with microcrystalline cellulose (MCC) to prevent agglomeration. The picture of the pellets shown to illustrate the product appears round but the process times of 45 and 80 minutes are considerably longer than those involved with the paste systems.

MIXING

The preparation of the wet mass used to produce the extrudate can be carried out by established techniques. It has been known for some years that, when studying the properties of pastes, good mixing was required. It is common for ceramic paste systems to be subjected to "pugging," i.e., passing the mixed wet mass through a wide bore extruder as well as standard planetary mixing (11). As the consistency of the mass involved in extrusion is rather wetter than that used in the preparation of granules used for tablets or capsules and must be uniformly consistent, it might be expected that high shear mixer/granulators would be required. Although there is certainly something to be said for this kind of approach, and is certainly essential for some formulations, a simple planetary mixer can be quite adequate, especially if the extruder used has a long die (i.e., length to radius ratio of 1:8). In a study of the influence of the mixing stage prior to extrusion Schmidt and Kleinebudde (12) compared the influence of four mixing regimes: planetary, high shear, and a twin screw extruder with two different screw assembles. The extruder for the second stage extrusion was a ring-die extruder with a die diameter 1.0 mm and a length of 2.5 mm, i.e., "short" dies, which had been described in earlier papers (7,12). The optimum water content required for what they defined as "good" pellets (aspect ratios not less than 1:10) was found to vary with the amount of energy put into the initial system. Thus, the water content as well as the mixing process differs for the different systems for which results are available, which makes identification of the influence of the premixing process difficult.

There are systems, which provide a dedicated mixing system. The use of mixing within a co-rotating twin-screw extruder system is described by Kleinebudde et al. (13). This system also claims the ability to be able to adjust the water content to the appropriate level and because it acts as both mixer and extruder, reduces the number of items of equipment required. This system is not widely employed in screen extruder systems, which without careful formulation can generate considerable heat that could be detrimental to heat sensitive formulations. Hellen et al. (14) describe the use of a granulator (Nica M6L, Nica systems AB, Molndal, Sweden) that functions with a high speed turbine to mix the powder with the water prior to extrusion.

EXTRUSION

The greatest variation in the process is in the extruders used. As the name of the process implies, it would be thought that it is essential to extrude a formulation to produce spherical pellets. This, however, is not the case. Chopra et al. (15) found that for a given formulation, it was possible to produce good quality pellets from a particular formulation if the wet mass was subjected to simple oscillating granulator or even direct spheronization after mixing in a high shear/mixer granulator. Just as it is not always necessary to extrude, it cannot be concluded that if a good extrudate can be formed that this can be processed to provide spherical granules (16,17).

The types of extruders and their characteristics are described by Newton (18). In assessing any paper claiming to study the process of extrusion/spheronization, it is important to identify just which type of extruder was used and what were the operation conditions. It may not be possible to generalize on the validity of the findings to processing by other extruders.

Most extruders are adapted for use from other areas of technology, and it is essential to ensure that if they are to be used for a pharmaceutical product, they are suitable for GMP use. Extruders are not interchangeable and some formulations can be better suited to one than another, while in some cases it is only necessary to make a small adjustment in the liquid level to achieve successful interchange of extruders (19). The basis of the process of extrusion is to force a material from a large cross section through a small cross section (the die). The first stage is to compress the wet mass, which consists of liquid, solid and air such that the air is removed. Effort is then required to force the material from the large diameter to a small diameter the amount of effort depending on the extent of this reduction, the "reduction ratio." Having achieved this, effort is also required to force the material along the length of the die. The most important difference between the different types of extruders is the system that provides reduction ratio, the length of the die and the speed at which the system operates. Most wet masses are non-Newtonian in their rheological properties; hence, their extrusion is rate dependent. Therefore, the quantitative descriptions of the forces involved are complex and rate dependent (20–29). In long dies (length to radius ratios at least 1:6), paste formulations are also often subjected to phase separation, i.e., the liquid is displaced to different regions of the mass and can be even expelled from the mass when subjected to the forces involved with measuring its rheological properties or being processed (30,31). Modeling the process involved with water/microcrystalline cellulose (MCC) systems, considering the initial compaction, followed by paste convection after the onset of flow has been described (32). Tomer et al. (33) detected by magnetic resonance imaging, that in a capillary rheometer (a ram extruder) there was evidence for both radial and axial migration of the fluid during extrusion which was extrusion rate and formulation dependent. The same technique indicated that there was a uniform distribution of water within the extrudates of the model formulations collected in the steady state stage of the extrusion in a ram extruder (34). It was found possible to calculate a percolation threshold, which decreased as the extrusion speed increased and that there was a relationship between percolation threshold and the extrusion force.

In screen extruders (i.e., short dies; length radius ratios less than 1:5) the major forces involved are in bringing the mass to the screen and therefore the "squeeze flow" properties of the wet mass may be more relevant. These can be measured as described by Mascia et al. (35).

There has been for some time, clear evidence that in long dies, there is considerable consolidation of the wet mass (21). This has a major contribution to the consistency of the extrudate, which is very different to the extrudates produced by short dies (i.e., screen extruders). This could well account for the differences in the performance of formulations processed by different types of dies. There is evidence, that for paste systems, the type of flow is "plug flow" (20). Here there is migration of the fluid to the wall of the die to form a layer of liquid, and it is the properties of this liquid layer that are very important. Thus, some migration of the fluid during extrusion may not be a bad thing.

Working with a ram extruder as a capillary rheometer, Raines et al. (23) were able to show that the quality of the extrudate, in terms of surface roughness could be related to the yield pressure at zero velocity, of the wet mass, determined as described by Benbow et al. (11). The wet masses with a high value for this parameter were smooth and regular in appearance. Unfortunately, several of these smooth surface extrudates did not spheronise. As yet, it is not possible to quantify exactly the rheological parameters and their values, which control whether a formulation can be processed into spheres yet they clearly can be very different and still form pellets. Yet a small change in either composition or process can sometimes have a dramatic effect on the performance, changing a successful process into a disaster. A recent publication (36) suggesting that "the torque rheometer provides a simple reliable and competent preformulation tool to predict the quality of MCC pellets prepared by extrusion/spheronization" may be somewhat premature. The properties of the pellets that are reported provide no information of the properties of the pellets that really matter, i.e., size, size distribution and shape; also the extrusion system was not what one would usually associate with the process of extrusion/spheronization. In our experience (37), the mixer torque rheometer is not simple to operate and while it provides "numbers," these cannot be related to classical rheological theory. As with other papers, which claim to use this technique to evaluate the ability to predict the performance of formulations in a quantitative manner, it has not been established. It certainly seems possible to apply this system to measuring what is considered to be the liquid saturation of the wet mass (37). Just how this fits into ensuring that a formulation will both extrude and spheronise has yet to be established. The lack of fundamental rheological measures also restricts the use of the "powder rheometer" as applied to wet powder masses by Luukkonen et al. (38). The application of oscillatory rheometry on wet powder mass formulations did provide an indication that the elastic properties of the mass could be an important characteristics, and that there appeared to be an optimum region (27). This is despite the very much lower shear rates involved with oscillation than those involved in the extrusion process. Again this is not an easy technique to use and simple experimentation remains the most common approach to formulation.

The selection of the extruder is an important issue as once set as part of the product registration process, a change in type could be costly. There are several issues involved. Scalability will be discussed latter. The screen extruders provide low resistance to processing and are easy to clean. They can be manufactured by punching the holes or laser drilling. The latter are preferable, as the holes produced are more likely to have uniform diameter along the length. Punching can produce holes that have a non-uniform bore dimension. The extrudate they produce is not highly compressed and is much more likely to suffer from surface impairment, a phenomenon reported some time ago (39,40) with short dies. There is some debate as to whether these irregularities in the surface actually aid the process by allowing the extrudate to fragment readily. This may be the case with some formulations, but the irregularities can cause the breaking of the extrudate into a wide range of lengths, which results in pellets with a wide range of sizes. In my experience extrudate produced by screen extruders are often more sensitive to the variations in spheronization conditions. They are also subject to wear and distortion, which could result in varying extrudate quality with time. They can also generate considerable quantities of heat and screen temperatures in the range of 40°–70°C have been reported (41). This could have serious implications for drug stability. This type of extruder is, however, extensively used in the pharmaceutical industry.

In choosing which extruder to use, it is important to consider the availability of the material for trials. Working with materials that are inexpensive or limited in their availability makes the use of larger scale manufacturing equipment difficult. The use of experimental extruders could present problems of scaling up the process. The ram extruder can be used with as little as 20 g of wet mass (42). This type of extruder is expensive to use for conventional pellet products, although for products, which require a precision extrudate, e.g., the implant Zolodex® (AstraZeneca PLC, London, U.K.) they are the system of choice. The ease of transferring such a formulation from the ram extruder to a manufacturing scale should not present problems if a long die extruder is to be used in manufacturing. It is possible to transfer the formulation almost directly to a screen extruder system (19), and comparisons with long die gravity feed extruders have been published (30,43). These, however, may be formulation dependent.

Even within a single type of extruder, variations in the operating procedures can result in extrudates, which can be very different in consistency. At a low speed, it is possible for liquid migration to occur, resulting in extrudates of different liquid content and hence consistency, at differing stages as the ram progresses down the barrel (29,30). This could result in an extrudate, which differs in terms of its spheronization properties. To avoid this, the speed should be increased. It must be remembered, however, that as the speed increases, so does the force required to maintain the ram speed and the possibility of producing extrudate with an irregular, rough or even "sharked skinned" surface (39,40). There could be, therefore, optimum operating conditions, which could differ from one formulation to another.

Baert et al. (44) related the extrusion forces measured with a specially instrumented "gear" extruder, which had been previously described (45), to the ability to make satisfactory spherical pellets from ternary mixtures of MCC with α or β lactose or calcium phosphate and water. Their definition of pellet quality in terms of shape was a little optimistic. There was no indication of the presence or absence of surface impairment of the extrudate and they failed to provide details of the diameter and length of the dies fitted to the extruder. Nevertheless, the work does illustrate that for this type of extruder, it would be possible to provide a quantification of the functioning of the extruder system to control product quality. A power-consumption-controlled extruder to identify the correct water content required for mixtures of MCC/lactose monohydrate extruded with a co-rotating screw extruder, fitted with an end plate containing 48 holes 2.5 mm long and 1.0 mm in diameter (i.e., at the upper end of a "short" die), has been described by Kleinebudde et al. (13). There is no description of the quality of the extrudate in terms of surface quality. The higher the MCC content the higher the power consumption. The higher the power consumption, the less spherical the pellets as judged by the aspect ratio. In fact most of the pellets had aspect ratio values greater than 1.1, which are not really spherical. Again, however, it does provide a method of quantifying aspects of the extrusion process.

SPHERONIZATION

Operating Conditions

The design of the spheronizer is quite simple. It consists of a plate, which rotates within the confines of cylindrical walls. The process is illustrated in Figure 1. As the plate rotates, it carries the wet mass towards the wall of the cylinder where it then rises up the wall, then falls back over the mass in the form of a "torus." These interactions between the wall, plate, and other parts of the extrudate mass combine to produce the rounding of the pellets. Intuitively one would expect the time on the plate, the load of extrudate, speed of rotation and the plate texture to influence the performance of the system.

The extrudate is "cut" at the edge of the plate, hence the design of the plate with reference to its influence on the edge should be important, yet there is no work to show how design can influence this aspect of the process. Again one would expect the surface texture of the plate to be important. There does not appear to be any fundamental work on the design of the surface of the plate. The surface of the plate takes different forms, but these appear to be more related to ease of manufacture and product identity than fundamental understanding of what is required. The mass occupies little more than a quarter of the diameter of the plate, once it is functioning yet the plate surface is usually of the same design across the whole diameter. It is certainly very helpful to have the same surface irrespective of plate diameter to remove a variable associated with scaling up. In addition to the papers previously mentioned (6,7), there is a study, which describes the

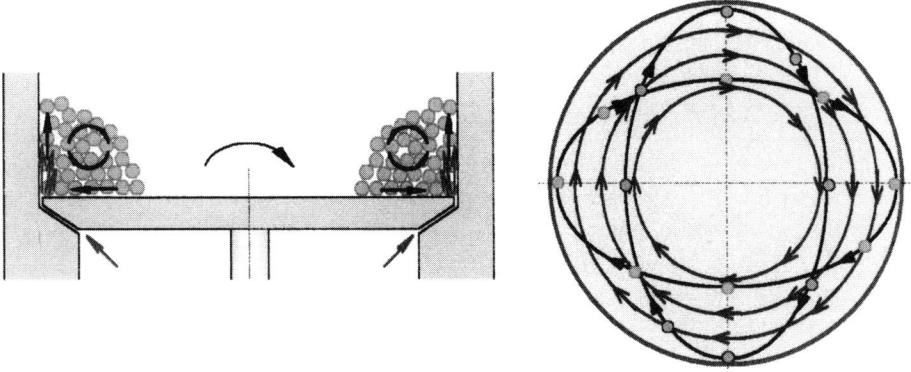

FIGURE 1 Design of a spheronizer and spheronization process. *Source*: Courtesy of Hosakawa.

use of plates with differing surfaces (46). The work was associated with a rotary processor system and it is not possible to know whether these findings on plate design can be transferred to other extrusion/spheronization systems. I would tend to think it would be the formulation that is the major factor in determining the performance and it would be difficult to generalize from this limited study.

The speed at which the plate rotates is such that it forces the mass towards the wall of the spheronizer by centrifugal force. Too low a speed fails to produce rounding, while too high a speed results in considerable size reduction, even though the extrudate used was prepared in long dies (6). As this is related to the speed of rotation and the radius of the plate, the rotation speed will vary with the diameter of the plate. Newton et al. (8) found that it was the performance of a formulation in terms of rounding that could be related to the linear velocity of the plate at the tip, hence as the diameter of the plate increased, the speed of rotation of the plate should be decreased. Based on the basic plate used in their studies, 22.5 cm diameter, which was used at 1000 rpm, the rotational speed of larger and smaller systems could be calculated. Most systems follow this rule, because the bulk densities of a wet mass are reasonably consistent. Papers, which consider the speed as a variable, are not very useful. There are only a few papers that show significant effects. Speed is important when the bulk density of the wet mass is very low, as in the case where the formulation contained a high proportion of Ac–Di–Sol in the wet mass (9). With such a system, at the normal speeds, the low density of the wet mass causes it to be thrown too readily to the wall such that it rises up the wall and hits the lid of the spheronizer, resulting in a very irregular motion. Reducing the rotational speed to provide the usual pattern, a factor of 10 was required, resulted in good quality pellets.

For a standard extrudate, it was found that there is an optimum load of extrudate (7). Too low a load produces too many interactions with the plate and the wall, while too high a load produces too little interaction between the pellets and the plate/wall. For a 22.5-cm diameter plate, the optimum load was 300 g, but with longer processing times, loads of up to 1000 g could be processed satisfactorily if the formulation was suitable.

There are papers, which report different responses to these process variables (47–50) but these all use short die screen extruders, rather than a long dies to produce the extrudate, which would provide very different quality extrudate. Here it appears that speed can have an influence. For example, some early work with a given formulation did report a speed effect but while the diameter of the die was specified, the length was not so it is not possible to say if the effect is due to the properties of the extrudate or not (50). The authors commented that the formulation was probably the most important variable in their study.

Baert et al. (51) reported an investigation of parameters important in the spheronization process with extrudates produced by a gravity feed extruder, Avicel PH101 and various water levels. They used five sets of the conditions; varying time and speed of rotation to provide the optimum yield of pellets of satisfactory roundness values for a given water content, by the application of mathematical modeling.

For health and safety reasons, the usual spheronizer operates with a lid. In some instances, if the formulation contains an excess of water, condensation will appear on the lid. This is usually an indication that "free" water is present. This is to be avoided if possible by reducing the level of water or by the provision of a means of removing the excess water vapor from the spheronizer. Equally important for efficient functioning of the system, there should be no sticking of the wet mass to the plate or the walls of the spheronizer. This is usually a formulation issue but needs to be addressed if efficient production is to be achieved.

Mechanism of Spheronization

By taking samples and characterizing the width, length, density, and sphericity of the pellets as a function of time, Chapman (52) found that, under the correct conditions, the extrudate was chopped into cylinders, whose ends were then rounded and pushed together to form a "dumbbell" shape, which were further compressed along their length, to form round pellets. This was confirmed by photographing the pellets on the rotating plate with a camera fitted with a high-speed shutter, and observing the changes with time (43,53). The time over which the changes occur varies with the formulation. With some systems, it could take as little as 1 minute, while in other cases; it could take up to 30 minutes. Once rounded, a good formulation can stay on the plate for a prolonged time without any change in size or shape. In some cases, the pellets never become round retaining their dumbbell or ovoid shape, usually an indication that the formulation is too "dry." If a formulation will not form round pellets within 30 minutes, it is very unlikely to round no matter how long it remains on the spheronizer plate. Very "dry" formulations never even achieve elongated cylinders. They disintegrate back into powder and fall down the gap between the plate and the wall. At the other end of the fluid content, if the formulation is too wet, the pellets will grow in size with time, due to migration of fluid to the surface of the pellets, which allows their agglomeration. Depending on the formulation they can round into larger spherical pellets but usually there is a lack of control and the product is very irregular in size, size distribution, and shape. The sensitivity of a formulation to moisture content is formulation dependent. Some can tolerate quite a wide range of fluid contents, while others only function over a very narrow range, as little as 0.5% change in fluid content.

Vervaet et al. (54) reported that they had observed a formulation in which the extrudate coiled on itself to form a pellet. I have never observed such an occurrence and their report may be representative of a particular formulation. What I have seen is a formulation where the extrudate broke into powder when added to the plate: this mass re-agglomerated to form excellent pellets. This was presumably due to a particular combination of circumstances. Vervaet et al. (54) also suggested that the dumbbells break into two parts, which then round separately. I have never seen this with any formulations.

DRYING

It is usually by standard tray or fluid bed systems. For specific use, freeze-drying has been used. The pellets prepared from MCC (Avicel PH101) mixed with a water/ethanol system, were found to have different porosity and mechanical strength depending upon how they were dried (55).

The pellets generally produced by the process are usually quite robust and therefore handling by fluid bed dryers is possible for most formulations without causing any damage or loss due to friability. For oven or fluid-bed drying, it was found that, for pellets containing 25% Avicel CL-611 and 75% theophylline, higher drying temperatures provided a faster drying rate, smaller the mean pellet size and higher the crushing strength (56). The opposite was true for microwave drying. The authors attributed this to the shrinkage of pellets, which had been reported previously by Kleinebudde (57) with systems of 30% of three model drugs and either 69.5% Avicel PH101 or 49.5% Avicel and 20% low substituted hydroxyproplyl cellulose. The author found that it was necessary to use image analysis to identify these changes. Based on the determination of the width of the pellets, there was clear evidence that freeze drying produced larger size pellets than those dried by oven or fluidized dryer, where considerable reduction in the median values of the width can be seen. The authors claim that good quality round pellets could be produced appears optimistic when reference to the graphs shows that for most systems, more than 50% of the pellets had an aspect ratio of greater than 1.2, which is far from round. Nevertheless it is clear that for some formulations, especially those containing high levels of MCC, drying will result in shrinkage of the pellets. By careful monitoring pellet dimensions, Berggren and Alderborn (58) confirmed the shrinkage of pellets during slow drying in the atmosphere, for pellets prepared by a screen extruder, Avicel PH101 and mixtures with either water or 25/75% ethanol/water mixture. Those produced with water, showed a higher degree of shrinkage and a greater degree of densification. The rate of drying was found to influence the properties of the pellet (59). Using a specially constructed convective drier to dry pellets prepared with a screen extruder from mixtures of MCC (Avicel PH101) with either water or ethanol/water mixtures, Berggren and Alderborn (59) concluded that, "increasing the rate of drying did not affect the shape and surface texture of the dried pellets and did not cause fracturing of the pellets: an increase in drying rate gave more porous pellets due to decreased pellet densification: an increased drying rate gave pellets that were more deformable, as assessed from Kawakita 1/b values, and which formed tablets of a higher tensile strength."

The rate of drying has also been shown to influence the mechanical properties of pellets in the same size fraction, prepared from a MCC (Avicel PH101) (55). Slow drying was found to produce the strongest pellets, while the weakest were those that had been subjected to rapid drying by freeze-drying. These effects were due to the different structure produced by the different rates of drying, rapid drying producing a porous structure. These results apply to pellets formulated with MCC. For other materials, this may not be true.

PROPERTIES OF PELLETS

Pellet Size and Size Distribution

As discussed earlier, the usual pellet size produced ranges from approximately 0.5 to 2.5 mm. From the early reports (1,2), one of the important advantages claimed for the process was that the pellets produced were very uniform in size illustrating this with size distributions showing the majority of pellets in one sieve fraction. Most workers usually report the size and size distributions produced as an indication of the quality of the product. It is not always possible to make exact comparisons of the results as the method of describing the size and its distribution varies from researcher to researcher. While sieving is a very common method and relates well to the needs of the production process for the further use of pellets, the way results are presented is not always appropriate. The sieving process provides a measure of the "width" of the pellet as it measures the minimum dimension that will pass through the square aperture formed by the mesh. The distribution represents a "weight" distribution. Some papers that express the results in mesh size rather than the aperture dimension fail to provide the standard used to define the sieves, fail to use appropriate combination of sieves, fail to provide an appropriate description of the distribution of the central tendency (mean, mode, or median), and the spread. When a central value and spread are given it is sometimes in the form of a geometric distribution, without demonstrating that the size distribution is in fact that associated with this function, i.e., left skewed (60–63).

As an alternative to sieving, size distributions are sometimes presented from image analysis. It must be remembered that, unless special mounting is used, the pellets will be positioned in their plane of maximum stability, which will allow their longest dimension to be measured. These systems should allow a good description of the distribution functions, especially if associated with statistical packages, but they will of course be number distributions as opposed to the weight/volume distributions provided by sieving which have been clearly shown to differ (6,43). They are also not very helpful if the samples analyzed have been pre-sieved before determination of their size characteristics by image analysis (64,65).

Neither sieving nor image analysis can measure the third dimension of the pellets, i.e., the "thickness" of the pellets. For a set of pellets of different shape, there was clear evidence that measuring the thickness by a ring gap sizer indicated that the pellets were slightly thinner in this dimension (15).

The size and distribution of size produced by the process is a complex function of the process, the processing conditions and the formulation. The influence of the drying conditions has been mentioned previously. Exact predictions are not possible but there are clearly factors, which can be used to try and control these properties. There are several stages at which the final pellet size can be influenced.

From the early work, Reynolds (1) clearly illustrated the influence of the size of screen used when the extrudate was produced with a screen extruder, the smaller the screen the smaller the pellets. One would expect this to be a general rule, and for a given formulation it is probably correct. For different formulations the sizes for a given screen could differ from one formulation to another. Also for the same formulation, the pellet size produced by a screen extruder could differ from that for extrudate produced by a long die extruder. Even with long dies of equal diameter, it was found possible to produce pellets of different size characteristics if the long die was associated with a ram extruder rather than a rotary cylinder extruder (43) and this effect was further modified by the particle size of the model drug (lactose), used in combination with MCC (53). The rate of extrusion of the same formulation was shown to influence the median pellets diameter (66). This could be associated with the liquid migration, which can occur with some formulations when extruded at slow rates with long dies. This can result in extrudates of variable water content (66). It can also be recognized by observing forced flow in the extrusion process with a ram extruder. The variable water content results in sections of the extrudate being too wet, providing opportunities for agglomeration to take place. Some of the extrudate is too dry, which can result in small spheres. It does not happen for all formulations. Chatchawalsaisin et al. (67) found that, although several formulations displayed forced flow and hence fluid migration, they gave acceptable pellets.

For a given die and a constant set of extrusion conditions, one would expect the pellet size to be constant. This is however not the case. Even the extrudate is not of constant diameter, being formulation dependent, varying with the excipient, drug (even only at a 10% level) and water content (67). The dry extrudate was found to range in diameter from 97% to 113% of 1.13 mm diameter of the extruder die. The smaller diameter could be due to shrinkage of the extrudate on drying, while the larger diameter could be due to 'die swell', where the extrudate has been subjected to mechanical contraction as it passes through the die and releases this contraction on exiting the die. A linear increase in pellet diameter with extrudate diameter, which had different values for the slope and the intercept, was observed for each of the four drugs used in the study (67). This increase in diameter could be associated with the extrudate breaking into different lengths during the spheronization stage, or differences in the degree of compression during the spheronization phase.

The quantity of liquid used in the formulations for extrusion/spheronization, usually water, is greater than that used in conventional granulation and reaches levels of between 30% and 40% of the solids content. The solubility of the drug might therefore be expected to be involved in the size of the final pellet as the drug will dissolve during the extrusion/spheronization stages and re-crystallizes in the drying stage. In a study with different model drugs mixed with an equal quantity of MCC, the median pellet size produced, using the optimum water content and a standard set of extrusion conditions with a long die (ram extruder), followed by standard spheronization conditions, was not related to drug solubility, which ranged from 14.3 to 1000 g/L(68). Even when the pellets contained 80% of the model drug, the pellets formed from the less soluble model (lactose) where larger than those formed form the more soluble model (ascorbic acid) (29). Therefore, the solubility of the drug is not the controlling factor. For four formulations, which contained the same ratio of a water insoluble component of approximately the same particle size, the same proportion of MCC and water extruded under the same conditions, the pellets had the same modal sieve fraction value but differed between 1.1 and 1.3 mm in their median diameter (69).

PELLET SHAPE

The object of the process is to provide pellets, which are of a spherical form and when the process functions correctly, this is what is obtained. There is however, no uniformity in the literature as to what is an acceptable definition of what is considered as "spherical" and even a recent paper relies solely on descriptive terms for the shape of the pellets they produce without any attempt at the quantification of the shape (70). Such an approach is not very helpful. In practical terms, Chopra et al. (71) found that for both uncoated and coated pellets of sieve size fraction 1–1.4 mm, as long as the "aspect ratio" (here defined as the ratio between the longest caliper distance and the caliper distance perpendicular to the longest one) was less than 1.2, then pellets could be filled into size 0 capsules to meet official weight uniformity standards. For a QC procedure the aspect ratio could be considered to be a satisfactory measure. Clearly however, any pellet with an aspect ratio of 1.2 can be visually seen as non-spherical, and it is not appropriate to work to this standard in formulation studies as has been suggested by Abdulla and Mader (63).

Simple indirect methods such as the variations in bulk density and several standard measures of circularity were shown by Chapman et al. (72) to be insensitive to changes in pellet shape. These workers developed a system based on producing and digitizing an image of the pellets, which could be processed to identify the angle to which a plane would have to be tilted to induce instability in a particle placed in a plane of maximum stability. This was termed "the one plane critical stability" (OPCS). At the time it represented a solution to the problem, but required considerable effort and skill of operation. The work however did show the lack of sensitivity of measures of circularity such as the often-used measures 4π area/Perimeter^2. The advent of improved image analysis systems has brought new approaches to the problem but not a consistent solution to the problem. Podczeck et al. (73) have discussed the issues involved in ensuring that a correct image is obtained. Again this work demonstrated the lack of sensitivity of the shape factors usually available in image analyzers, yet these continue to be used by workers in the field, which makes some of the claims to producing spherical pellets rather suspect. The shape factor e_R proposed by Podczeck and Newton (74) was further modified by simply analyzing an image of the pellet at right angles to the first image, to allow a three-dimensional shape factor (75) to be determined, giving a more detailed characterization of pellet shape. While the work of Podczeck et al. (73) identified an aspect ratio of 1.10 as representing an acceptable value for the pellets shape, Ericksson et al. (76) clearly demonstrated that this measure of roundness is far less discriminating than the shape factor e_R in identifying variations in pellet roundness (Fig. 2). The range of normalized values for the aspect ratio of the same 100 pellets was far less than that for e_R. This is sometimes interpreted as a lack of precision, when in fact it is a demonstration of being more discriminatory. Almeida-Prieto et al. (77) criticized the use of this shape factor saying that it could not distinguish between a square and a circle, which is just not true (74) and that it could not resolve differences between more complex shapes. As it was not intended to do this but assess differences from the spherical form, it is perhaps not surprising. They also question the various values quoted. It is very important to compare like with like. The values obtained with pellets themselves are very different to those obtained with model figures created in only two dimensions (74).

DENSITY/POROSITY

An important property of the pellets is the structure that they posses as this influences their performance as a dosage form in terms of the way that they can be further processed and can influence their drug release properties. Most systems produced will be as oral controlled release dosage forms, achieved by application of coatings. Thus, the pellets must be capable of being processed by the various techniques available for the application of coatings.

As described previously, the process, especially if long dies are used in the extrusion process will result in compaction of the system. If the spheronization of the extrudate follows that described earlier, there will be further consolidation of the mass. In fact, Chapman (52) used evidence of an increase in density of the pellets as part of his proof of the mechanism of spheronization. The liquid content of formulations is quite high, often 35–40%, hence the rate of removal of this and the potential influence of shrinkage can all influence the final structure. In some formulations, not all the liquid is removed from the pellets, which again can influence the final density. The density of the materials incorporated into the formulation will also influence the density of the pellets. Hence, it is not always possible to predict the final density of the pellets. Because of the influence of the material density, it is preferable to express the property as "porosity."

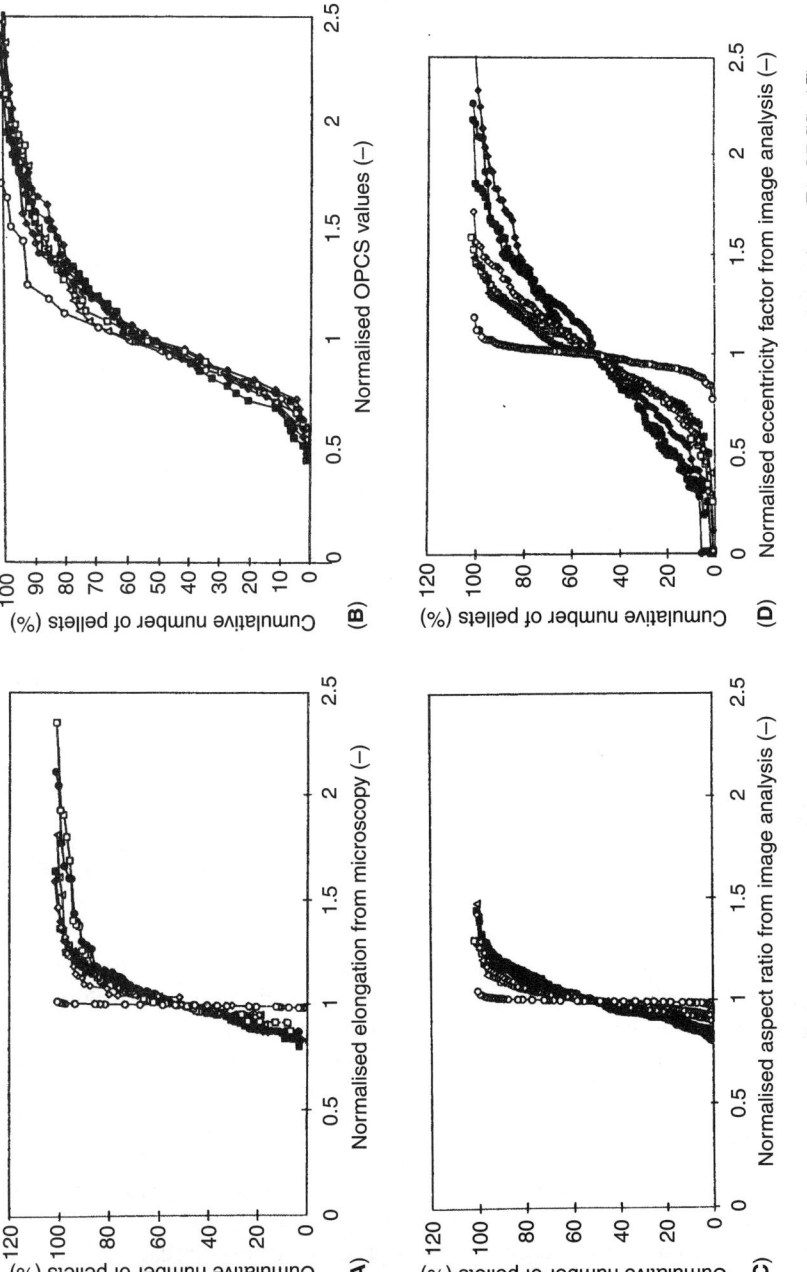

FIGURE 2 Cumulative distribution functions of pellet shapes using different shape factors: (**A**) elongation, (**B**) OPCS, (**C**) aspect ratio, and (**D**) e_R. *Abbreviation*: OPCS, one plane critical stability. *Source*: From Ref. 76.

Chapman (52) found that the estimation of the pellet density by air/helium comparison pycnometer was equivalent to those measured by a mercury pycnometer method (78). As the former method is far more convenient, this has been used in our laboratories to determine the pellet density and the porosity calculated as:

Porosity = 1–relative density,

where the relative density is the ratio of the pellet density to the apparent particle density of the powder components.

Considering the data available on the use of long dies, the porosity of pellets varies over a considerable range, 3–35% (66). The constituents of the pellets have a very important influence (67). In general, the higher the level of MCC or glyceryl monostearate (GMS) the lower will be the porosity (67) while the presence of high levels of water insoluble materials, tends to increase the porosity (15,66). The greater the quantity of water used in the process, the higher the porosity of pellets based on different formulations (66). If an aqueous solution of alcohol is used as the fluid, then the pellets based on MCC formulations will be more porous when produced with either a short (79,80) or long (81) die extruder. As mentioned previously, the use of different drying methods can result in pellets of different porosity (56), freeze-drying producing pellets that were more porous than tray drying.

MECHANICAL PROPERTIES

Pellets will need further handling before they can be administered to patients. In their wet state, there is usually no difficulty with handling to transfer to the drying processes. In their dry state, there is the possibility that the pellets may be liable to attrition during fluid bed drying or fluid bed coating. If the pellets are to be filled into capsules or formed into tablets, then fracture becomes the more important issue. In the former case, this is due to trapping of the pellets in the moving parts of the equipment. In the latter case, it could be a matter of design in order to produce tablets containing coated pellets, which are not damaged on compaction, to allow the intact pellets to be released on administration.

Friability

Some of the early papers on the process were concerned with the use of the pellets in the preparation of tablets (82,83). The extrusion aid was Avicel RC581, not the best of materials for forming spherical pellets; the extruder was a thin screen system and the time on the spheronizer plate was very short, 60 seconds. There was no indication of the size or shape of the pellets. It is perhaps therefore, not surprising that the friability reported was quite high, especially as a vigorous method of adding glass beads to the system was adopted. Even with the presence of glass beads and pellets that were produced with a screen extruder, Hellen et al. (14) found that friability ranged from 0.3% to 2.7%. There is also the possibility of a formulation effect. When Chopra et al. (84) subjected a 500 g batch of pellets, which had been produced from the same basic formulation but with different processing methods (15), to the process of fluidization equivalent to that used in their coating, the loss in weight was less than 1% for all samples. In general, it appears that for good formulations, especially pellets produced from extrudate of long dies, there is no problem with the friability of the pellets.

Mechanical Strength

Fracture by Diametral Compression

The standard method to test the mechanical properties of pellets is to crush them in some form of tablet strength tester or physical testing instrument and record the force at which the pellets fracture. To ensure reproducible values, it is important to ensure that the rate of force application is not too rapid, that the method of detecting the force is sensitive enough, that the surfaces of the platens are free from debris, otherwise spreading of the load can occur, which can influence the load at which the pellet breaks. Even with all these conditions satisfied, there could be variation in the value of the fracture load as it is a property of brittle materials to be variable in their breaking load. Whether or not the pellets are brittle can be identified by a sharp peak in a load/time or displacement graph taken from the testing device, or checking that the pellets are breaking into two distinct portions across the diameter. If these conditions hold, then it is possible to convert the breaking load into a surface tensile strength (85).

The mechanical properties of pellets will be a complex function of the composition and method of manufacture. Formulations consisting of MCC and using water as the fluid form strong pellets, which is associated with the relatively low porosity of the pellets (80,81). Preparing the pellets with water/ethanol systems reduced their porosity and their mechanical strength (58,59,80,81). The influence of the addition of materials to MCC will depend on the quantity added and the nature of the material. For example, adding lactose equivalent to the amount of MCC with 10% of a model drug (paracetamol) reduced the surface tensile strength slightly, whereas addition of the same quantity of glyceryl monostearate (GMS) produced a considerable reduction in the value of the surface tensile strength (86). Addition of a liquid, glycerol, which was retained in the pellets after drying, reduced the value of the surface tensile strength even further (86).

Shear Strength

The value of the shear strength of a bed of pellets can be determined by the method described by Adams et al. (87), which involves compressing a bed of pellets and relating the deformation of the bed of pellets to force applied. For the systems studied by Bashaiwoldu et al. (86) the shear strength of the pellets with low values of surface tensile strength had even lower values of shear strengths.

Elastic Modulus

The recoverable deformation of the pellets was quantified from the linear portion of the load/deformation profile obtained when measuring the strength of pellets by Aulton et al. (88). Alternatively, the elastic properties as a "storage modulus" can be measured by the application of dynamic mechanical analysis (DMA) (89). The values obtained by this method for a series of pellet formulations were found to be considerably greater than those obtained by application of the former method (81), which must therefore be considered as an estimate of the real value. It did rank the pellet formulations in the same order as the DMA.

Viscoelasticity

The further advantage of the use of DMA to measure the mechanical properties of pellets is that it can also measure the "loss modulus" of the system, which when related to the storage modulus allows the derivation of the "Phase Angle" (89). A value of 0 will be obtained for fully elastic materials while a value of 90° will indicate a fully viscous material. There were only small changes in the value of the phase angle for the same formulation processed differently (89). For a series of pellets of different formulations, processed by the same method, those formulations, which contained the softer GMS or glycerol, had the higher values for the phase angle (81). Thus, a quantitative measure of the deformability of the pellets can be made with improved accuracy over that of measuring the slope of the diametric compression/displacement curve used by Aulton et al. (88).

Yield Value

By compressing pellets in a punch and die system, the changes in density as function of the pressure applied can be used to derive their yield pressure as described by Heckel (90,91). For pellets of the same diameter, produced from the same formulation processed by the same method, but dried by different processes, there were only slight differences in the value of the yield pressure (55). For pellets of the same diameter produced from different formulations however, there were considerable differences in the yield pressure (81).

CAPSULE FILLING

Pellets produced by extrusion/spheronization are predominantly used as controlled release preparations; therefore, the ability to be filled into hard shell capsules is an important feature of their performance. This can be achieved as described by Podczeck (92). The filling into hard shell gelatin capsules by the slide filling mechanism (92) of uncoated and film coated pellets prepared from the same formulation was found to be significantly influenced by their shape (71). The failure in performance was always under filling, and if a value of 1% was considered as the limiting value, then it was found that the pellets need not be ideally spherical to provide satisfactory results. Therefore, a simple shape factor such as the aspect ratio is acceptable, and the limiting value appears to be just above 1.2 (71). It was observed that the development of static electricity on the coated pellets had a far greater influence on the filling performance of the pellets than their shape (71). This could be overcome by mixing the pellets with 1% of powdered talc, as had been suggested previously (93). Surface roughness of the pellets, as measured by a laser profilometer, was found to influence the filling performance presumably by increased friction and increased sensitivity to electrostatic charging. A value of rugosity (Ra) greater than 2 µm was found to influence the fill weight and the proportion of under-filled capsules (71).

TABLETING

The early work on the tableting properties of pellets was associated with comparing their performance with conventional granulations (82,83). The authors found that there was some advantage to be gained with the pellets produced containing 80% model drugs and 20% MCC (Avicel RC581) by the extrusion/spheronization process involving a screen extruder and short spheronization times (60 seconds). There is no quantification as to the roundness of the pellets produced, but they had a narrower size distribution and better flow properties than granules made from the same ingredients by a conventional process.

The tablets produced from the granules were satisfactory in terms of mechanical strength, reported with the usual misnomer of "hardness," and disintegration (less than 10 seconds). Variables of the process did influence the properties of the tablets, but the increased complexity of the process was unlikely to replace the conventional granulation procedures. Studies on the compaction properties of pellets show that the materials, which constitute the pellets, have a very important influence on the properties of the tablets produced. Evidence that pellets containing high levels of MCC produced tablets which had lower tensile strength values than tablets produced at the same compaction pressure with the same level of powdered MCC was provided by Maganti and Celik (94). These pellets were however produced by a rotary processor, not by extrusion/spheronization. This loss of strength appears to be associated with the loss of compactability caused by wetting of the MCC. Thus, it might be expected that this loss of strength would also occur for pellets produced by extrusion/spheronization. Several workers (58,59,79,95) have described work into the compaction of pellets, which used them as models for studies into the compaction of granular materials. This work linked the properties of the tablets to those of the well-characterized pellets prepared from Avicel PH101. They clearly demonstrated that the porosity of the pellets and their associated loss of structure was necessary to form strong tablets. They also demonstrated that pellets containing only Avicel PH101 do not make good tablets, which was confirmed by later studies with differing types of pellet (96).

With the development of the extrusion/spheronization process to provide pellets for controlled release products, an interest in making these coated pellets into tablets as opposed to filling them into capsules developed, and products have reached the market. Just to tablet coated pellets can result in products which do not disintegrate into their original pellets or have lost their controlled release function (96). Whether the coat or the core will fracture when the stress of compaction is applied will probably depend on the relative elastic properties of the coating and the core, if the same principles shown to exist for coated tablets (97) are assumed. As mentioned previously, it is now possible to measure the elastic properties of pellets and the coat when applied to pellets (89), hence the measurements on cast free films and the associated problems have been eliminated. It should, therefore, now be possible to design systems from first principles from measured properties of the core and the coat, rather than the current system of trial and error which is currently used. Bodmeier (98) has reviewed the compaction of coated pellets. This review did not consider the influence of the method which was used to prepare the pellets, and while some of the issues discussed will be relevant, the influence of the properties of the core cannot be forgotten. Equally, the properties of the film coat, as predicted by Stanley et al. (97), would be important, as demonstrated by Beckert et al. (99). The basic concept used is to mix the coated pellets with a "cushioning" material to prevent the fracture of the film coat. The in vivo performance of a commercial product containing metoprolol is described by Ragnarsson et al. (100) and Sandberg et al. (101). The pellets were not, however, prepared by extrusion/spheronization and how it was possible to achieve the absence of pellets at the surface of the tablet is not clearly described. The cushioning material can take the form of powder, granules (88) or other pellets (69,102–105). The addition of powder has the problem of potential segregation in the tableting process because of the large difference in size between the pellets and the powder. In this respect, granules offer a better option. Similarly, the use of pellets of equal size should also be a better option than powder; except that free flowing equidimensional pellets are known to be a segregating system (106). In examining the claims made for the ability to produce tablet systems from coated pellets, it is important to examine if the ability to form uniform content has been evaluated. Whether the material added is granules or powder, they usually take the form of "soft," highly deformable systems. The relative degree of deformability is not always assessed and sometimes the softening material, such as GMS, can produce a system which inhibits disintegration of the pellets. This was overcome by added disintegrating pellets to the system, rather than powder disintegrant, to provide a three-component system of drug, disintegrant and soft pellets, the proportions of each being optimized to ensure good content uniformity, tablet disintegration and limiting the damaging of the coat (104). It could also be worth testing if the addition of powdered disintegrant will influence the maintenance of weight uniformity.

DRUG RELEASE

An immediate release product would require some special feature to warrant the increased cost of production when compared to a conventional capsule or tablet. Therefore, the major commercial use of pellets prepared by extrusion/spheronization is in the preparation of controlled release products and there are several highly successful products available. In particular the ability to produce pellets with a high drug loading offers advantages over alternative methods of forming pellets.

Controlled Release Pellets

The type of controlled release products reported are those which provide targeted release to the gastrointestinal tract such as enteric coated and colon targeted, and those which provide prolonged release. There are several ways of controlling the release of drug from pellet formulations, such as the formation of a hydrophobic matrix, the formation of a hydrophilic matrix or the application of a coating, either polymer or hydrophobic melt. The product Surgam SA® (SanoFi-Aventis, Paris, France) consists of a drug mixed with GMS and MCC to form pellets with a slow release profile. Tests with other drugs have demonstrated that this is not a solution to all problems as none of the drugs tested with even up to 80% of GMS, provided a delayed drug release profile (67,107). The involvement of a hydrophilic matrix which would swell to form a hydrophilic gel presents the problem of being able to handle this material in the process, as most of these materials form gels at the stage of water addition. There are therefore two issues: can pellets be formed and if so, will the release of drug be delayed sufficiently? The first issue has been solved with a range of materials such as, chitosan (108,109) alone and mixed with sodium alginate (110), CarbopolR 974P (Lubrizol Co., Wickliffe, Ohio, U.S.A.) (111), and croscarmellose sodium (9) sodium carboxymethyl cellulose (112) and xanthan gum (113). In some instances, water (107) can be used, but in others, it is necessary to use ethanol/water mixtures (109), and in the case of Carbopol (111), a solution in an electrolyte was necessary to avoid high viscosity due to swelling or stickiness. The degree of control of release is variable, but the system containing croscarmellose sodium is being used in a colon targeted product (9).

The spherical nature of the pellets provides the minimum surface/volume ratio for the application of a coating, which is usually a polymer. The shape of the pellets was not found to be critical for pellets coated with a solution of a polymer in non-aqueous solvent (114). There was, however, a relationship between the specific surface area of the pellets and the mean dissolution time (MDT) for a series of pellets which had been prepared by different techniques (15): the higher the value of the specific surface area, the lower the value of the MDT. For pellets coated with polymer dispersion, there was a complex relationship between drug, the level of drug and the excipients used as filler (115). For a specific colon delivery system, the water solubility of the drug was important in ensuring that the coat met the correct control performance. In this case the thickness had to be considerably thicker and the inclusion of GMS was required for the highly water soluble model drug glucose (116) compared to the less water soluble 5-aminosalicylic acid (117). A thicker coat alone was sufficient for an alternative colon delivery system (118). Clearly the properties of the film will be particularly relevant to the type of release profile and can be modified by the usual techniques of changing the pore forming material added (119). Thus, the formulation of the core and the coat have to be matched if a successful performance is to be achieved.

Enhanced Dissolution Pellets

The possibility of enhancing the drug release of highly water insoluble drugs, i.e., those in Classes 2 and 4 of the biopharmaceutical classification system and providing a solid dosage form is an attractive proposition. If solubilizing liquids could be incorporated into the system, then this goal could be achieved. Vervaet et al. (120) found that both PEG 400 and a non-ionic surfactant (Cremophor) could be incorporated into pellets and enhanced the release of a model water insoluble drug. They went on to show that when hydrochlorthiazide was dissolved in PEG 400 and incorporated into pellets, they had a significantly higher in vivo bioavailability in human volunteers than a marketed tablet (121). Pellets without the PEG 400 had a lower bioavailability than the marketed tablet. It has been found possible to form pellets containing a range of PEGs with molecular weights up to 35,000 (107). It would therefore presumably be possible to incorporate insoluble drugs into these materials as a solid solution, where appropriate, and to form pellets from the resultant mixture. Other liquid systems, which can be used to enhance the bioavailability of water insoluble drugs, are the self-emulsifying systems (SES) (122). It has been shown that these can in fact be incorporated into pellets at quite high levels (123–125). To use the formulations effectively, there has to be a compromise between SES content and pellet consistency as a high level of SES (35%) produces rather soft pellets, which would be difficult to handle by processing equipment. These systems are very unusual in that it does not matter how the liquid components are added to the MCC, either as the SES water mixture or as SES and water separately. It has been established that, such pellets prepared to include progesterone (water solubility 0.1 g/l) had the same in vivo bioavailability as the drug in the SES itself and a far better bioavailability than a fine suspension of the drug when administered to dogs (126). It has recently been shown that the individual components of the self-emulsifying system can be incorporated into the pellets (127). The ability to apply a coating to pellets containing a water insoluble drug and SES has established that it is possible to enhance the drug release and then control the drug release rate (128).

An alternative approach to this problem is to incorporate β-cylcodextrins into pellets. Debunne et al. (129) found that such an approach was limited when the drug was piroxicam (solubility 43.8 µg/ml in phosphate buffer pH 6.8). Even when incorporated either in the form of powder or as an inclusion compound, the drug release from the pellets was no better than a formulation based on Avicel PH 101 and Avicel CL611.

Mechanism of Drug Release from Pellets

There are several approaches to identifying the mechanism of drug release from pellets. For example, O'Connor and Schwartz (130) applied the approach of Higuchi (131) to show that for a series of pellet formulations, they behaved as an inert matrix with a linear relationship between the percentage released as a function of time. The application of statistical moments has been used to identify the release mechanism of several types of pellet formulations (132) and utilized by other workers (67,69,104,107,110,114). This approach utilizes the whole of the dissolution curve as opposed to the limited percentage release data considered by Higuchi (131) analysis. It does however consider the whole data for the system, which assumes that the individual pellets have the same mechanism of release, which may not always be true (133). This concept has been developed by Bergqvist et al. (134) to develop a single-pellet model, which can give predictions of the release from multiple-pellet systems and describe the release from single pellets. The authors claim that "The model for predicting dose-release profiles could be of great value in optimizing the performance of an existing formulation, as well as in the development of new controlled release pharmaceuticals." The analysis was based on the data from the release profile of 200 individual pellets and therefore an accurate evaluation of the drug release from the pellets could require the analysis of very low levels of drug. There is no published information of the distribution of drugs within pellets produced by extrusion/spheronization. Although the uniformity of the content clearly meets the official standards for the products on the market, from preliminary experiment, I have observed that the content uniformity of individual pellets can vary quite appreciably.

FORMULATION ASPECTS

Compared with other pharmaceutical dosage forms, the preparation of pellets by extrusion/spheronization is relatively new. Information on the formulation of the systems is therefore, less widely known and the level of what the lawyers would describe as "common general knowledge" is not very high. In my experience, the only single material that I have found capable of forming good pellets without any additive, other than the liquid used to form the paste for processing, is MCC and even here, the addition of some materials can in fact enhance its performance. A question which remains unanswered is: are we looking for an excipient that functions and retains this function in the presence of appreciable quantities of other additives, or are we looking for a material, which may not function by itself but is capable of ensuring that added materials, especially high levels of drugs, will function? As yet there is no clear answer, therefore the way that the experiments are conducted to investigate the performance of a "spheronization" aid involves various approaches to the problem, making comparisons difficult. There is also the need to ensure that the formulation can be made on a manufacturing scale and that the drugs which are incorporated are chemically and physically stable and have the required clinical performance. From the literature, it is clear that the formulation process generally takes the usual route, that if the formulation does not function, then you add something else, and if that does not work, add further material until success or failure is reached.

The formulation exercise is complicated by the fact that the detailed aspects of the process can have a very strong influence on the outcome. This makes statistically designed experiments difficult, as it is quite easy to provide a combination of variables that do not function at all, which restricts the analysis. I have seen formulations which will function well with one set of conditions on a given set of equipment, but be unsuccessful if the process conditions, e.g., extrusion rate, are changed. I have also seen several examples where a change in the type of extruder can result in effects ranging from loss of yield to total loss of product. This certainly makes the formulation exercise difficult, especially if there is only a small quantity of the active material to work with, as many of the practical systems require appreciable quantities of material. This is why I favor the ram extruder system for initial formulation work. We have found formulations developed from such a system with long dies that can be scaled up to full production equipment (8). We have also found it possible to ensure a successful transfer of a formulation developed with this approach to a screen extruder by modifying the water content (19).

An important first step is to know the level of drug the pellets are required to contain. If this is low (less than 10%) then the drug should present little if any problem. Above this level, problems can start to occur, and by 50% these could be appreciable. The upper limit is less clear and levels as high of 80% (27,29,67,119) and 90% (67) have been achieved, but these tend to be the exception rather than the rule.

To ensure that the formulation will function, it is necessary to provide a wet mass which has the correct consistency and retains this consistency during the various stages of the process. Just what this consistency is, as has been discussed earlier, is not as yet known. There are certainly wide ranges of consistencies, as measured by the classical rheological approach, which will function as clearly shown by the references listed in the earlier section. Maintenance of this consistency throughout the various stages of the process is associated with ensuring that the fluid and solid component do not separate. Separation during extrusion is well known (20). As well as the previously reported method of collecting extrudate fractions while at the same time monitoring the extrusion force with a ram extruder (29–31), a pressure membrane (66,135) and a centrifugal method (136) have been reported to measure this tendency. Migration of the liquid during the spheronization stage results in the coalescence of the pellets, the degree of which can vary from slight enlargement to complete agglomeration to from one large mass. The range of water content over which formulations will function is an important issue. When it becomes sensitive to less than 0.5% of water, it is quite difficult to identify and control a formulation; therefore, a lack of water sensitivity could be considered as an important property to evaluate, either for a formulation or in judging a new spheronization aid. There is also the issue of: what is an acceptable preparation? For capsule filling, the size range usually required is in the range of about 700–1400 µm, which is usually achievable with appropriate choice of extruder hole dimensions. The issue of the degree of "roundness" is less clear. In the literature there is the tendency to accept the aspect ratio as a measure, and since Chopra et al. reported that pellets with values for the aspect ratio below 1.2 could be satisfactorily filled into a capsule, this seems to be becoming what is acceptable (63). I find this unsatisfactory as pellets with this value for the aspect ratio are clearly not round. In my experience, formulations which do not provide good round pellets are variable in shape from batch to batch. Only those formulations that have a satisfactory "roundness" are reproducible. The other quality criteria, such as drug content, stability and drug release are as for other pharmaceutical preparations.

SPHERONIZATION AIDS/BINDERS

The major spheronization aid used since the early work (1,2) has been MCC. Just why this material functions so well is not clear. It is certainly been known for some time to be able to hold water (137), but so can other natural polymers, such as starch, but this does not produce good pellets. The interaction between water and cellulose materials is known to be complex (138). Thermal evidence appears to indicate that the water is present as "free" water which can be readily removed, but approximately 0.865 mol of water per 100 g of MCC appears to be absorbed as structured water (139). This gave rise to the concept that MCC acts as a "molecular sponge" (139). *The New Shorter Oxford English Dictionary* defines a sponge as "a soft light porous absorbent substance," and this description fits MCC very well. The individual particles of MCC can absorb and hold water even when pressure is applied (29,31,66,135,136), providing a deformable structure which functions effectively within the constraints of the whole process. That extrusion may influence the interaction that occurs is possible. We have found that allowing the water and the MCC to stay in contact for a longer time period, results in a different extrusion pressure (23), and in making capillary rheology measurements, we always leave the MCC and water in contact for at least 12 hours to reach equilibrium. Repeated measurement on a sample that has been extruded does not change the extrusion force recorded. We have found that the difference in the rheological properties of the fresh and stored samples did not influence the ability to form pellets by the process.

Kleinebudde (140) suggested that with MCC the process of extrusion induced a "microcrystallite-gel" state in the MCC/water system, which aided the process. Chopra et al. (15) found that for certain formulations, good quality pellets could be prepared without extrusion of the wet mass. Kleinebudde (140) offered no direct experimental evidence that the extrusion in any way changed the crystallinity of the MCC, nor that the system had different rheological properties, nor, for that matter, it was a gel. Thus the whole concept is seriously flawed and, even in a later paper, it was concluded that the use of Fourier transform Raman spectroscopy did not confirm the existence of a microcrystallite-gel (141). The water holding capacity is not the sole property involved, the consistency of the wet mass must also be important, as discussed previously.

Having noted that MCC is an important material for the process, there are several sources and several grades available, the details of which are available in the *Handbook of Pharmaceutical Excipients* (142). The different grades are associated with different particle size and moisture contents, and the presence of carboxymethyl cellulose sodium and/or colloidal silicon dioxide. It is important to identify which grade and brand of MCC has been used in any publication reporting formulations, as they have been shown to be different in their ability to produce pellets when mixed with an equal quantity of lactose (16,143). In some cases, it may be just an issue of modifying the amount of water required in the formulation, but with others, especially those with added colloids, the total behavior may be very different. That the colloidal grades failed to produce good quality pellets contrasts with their ability to produce good quality extrudate (23). El Saleh et al., using just MCC and water with a long die extruder, confirmed the difficulty of making pellets with the colloidal grades and that some other grades of MCC required different water levels to Avicel PH101 to ensure satisfactory pellets (144). To judge by the illustrations of the pellets produced however, the quality of the pellets in terms of shape is questionable (144). With the use of a screen extruder and a 3:7 MCC/lactose mixture confirmed that different MCC grades responded differently to the quantity of water required to produce satisfactory pellets, although again the illustrations of the pellet produced show that many are far from being round (145). Another study from the same laboratory of further MCC types is not helpful as the wet mass was not extruded but pushed through a 1-mm aperture sieve by hand, hardly controlled extrusion (146). The solution to the choice of MCC would appear to be to use a standard grade and stick to a given source.

An alternative approach is to modify the MCC in some way. One such approach is to reduce the particle size of the MCC. This was undertaken by ultra-sonic homogenization of a suspension of Avicel PH101 in the presence and absence of sodium lauryl sulfate, followed by spray drying (147). The evaluation of the performance of three such materials, which had a mean particle size of approximately 15 µm, at a 30% content in terms of preparing pellets from indomethacin (30%) and lactose (40%), with long die extrusion has been undertaken (148). In terms of the yield of pellets, (there appears to be no measure of shape), the reduced particle size material performed better than the original Avicel PH101 (148). Another way to change the properties of the MCC is via the degree of polymerization (PD). Testing samples with values ranging in PD from 166 to 365 (most conventional products have a value of about 230), the water content required to produce pellets, increased with the value of PD (149) but the paper presented very limited data on the quality of the pellets. This approach therefore does not appear to have a potential. Much more promising is the modification of the MCC by inclusion of additional polymers to yield a special grade (Avicel 955). Working with long dies and 80% of 20 model drugs with ranges of values of solubility, pK_a and freezing point depression, mixed with 20% of the modified MCC, pellets of satisfactory shape, as judged by the shape factor e_R, and with a limited size range could be produced (150). The size varied from material to material and it was clear that variations in the steady state extrusion force occurred with some drugs, indicating liquid migration during the extrusion process. It was not possible to identify how the drug properties influenced the performance by analysis of variance, as there were interactions between the factors. Principal component analysis identified that the drug properties influenced the spread of the pellet size and shape of the pellets. There were drugs forming a common cluster and those drugs which did not have a steady state extrusion force lay outside these values. Canonical analysis of the results allowed the quantity of water required to produce the best pellets to be identified with a non-linear model having a root mean square of 17.7%, which is very reasonable for such complex formulations. When comparing the addition of hydrophilic polymers as physical mixtures or as a co-spray dried product with MCC (polymer:MCC ratio 1:19), Law and Deasy (151) found that the latter performed better when processing a 20%:80% MCC:lactose system with long dies. They recommended hydroxypropyl methylcellulose and poyvinylpyrrolidone as hydrophilic polymers as these were less 'sticky' than sodium carboxymethyl cellulose. They used as a shape factor the reciprocal of the perimeter squared divided by $4\pi \times$ area, which is not very discriminating. My experience is that sodium carboxymethyl cellulose is the most useful polymer, but have no detailed evidence for this, but I can agree with comments of Law and Deasy (151) that the hydrophilic polymers can induce sticking of the wet mass to the spheronizer plate. As an alternative to polymers, I have sometimes found it useful to add bentonite at about the 5% level to improve the performance. It was used to aid the preparation of pellets of 5-aminosalicylic acid (117).

The early work with powdered cellulose, as a spheronization aid was not too promising as many of the pellets were not particularly spherical (152). A recent paper (153), however, suggests that powdered cellulose in the form of Elcema P100 (Degussa AG, Frankfurt Germany) can provide satisfactory pellets with 25% and 50% of a model water insoluble drug (frusimide) in terms of shape, although this was assessed by a rather insensitive shape factor. The pellets had a more rapid drug release profile than those produced with conventional MCC. There is the possibility that this difference in performance may be related to the fact different types of extruders were used in the two studies. The improved performance was achieved with a screen extruder. The powdered cellulose systems had considerably lower torque levels than the MCC systems when measured with a mixer-torque rheometer (153).

GMS added to MCC to provide a delay in drug release has proved to be valuable in assisting the preparation of pellets (19,67,107,116,154,155). It appears to function by assisting the material to form pellets rather than being a pellet former in its own right. It aids extrusion, although the forces are often quite high with these systems. I have often observed that during the spheronization stage of the process, the extrudate brakes down into powder, which then reassembles into granules, which then proceed to round into pellets.

The claim that various grades of pectin can replace MCC appears to be rather optimistic as very few of the formulations described produce pellets which could be described as spherical (156–159). The pellets produced with carrageenan appear to have a somewhat better potential although the aspect ratio was used as criteria of acceptable shape, and there are as yet only a restricted number of materials and levels tested (63,64,160). Also looking at the images of the pellets containing 20% of either MCC or κ-carrageenan and 80% acetaminophen, it is clear just how poor the pellets actually are, yet those containing MCC have aspect ratios below 1.1, which is claimed to be acceptable (Fig. 3). I am not convinced that this material offers a credible alternative to MCC. Steckel and Mindermann-Nogly (161) have reported formulations of chitosan mixed with MCC and chitosan alone. With water, the maximum level of chitosan which allowed reasonable pellets to be produced was 50%. This could be increased to 100% chitosan if solutions of acetic acid were used as the binder liquid. As this material, along with MCC forms pellets by itself, the ability to retain this property when drugs are added is an important issue. There were no details of the carrying capacity for drugs or the influence of the acetic acid on the stability of drugs in such formulations.

Prieto et al. (162) investigated the possible use of Starch-dextrin mixtures as an alternative to MCC. Only 2 of the 18 formulations they investigated had satisfactory roundness, as judged by their own shape factor, hardly a system with a high potential. The performance of formulations based on a high amylose starch (UNI-PRE EX starch) with 25% theophylline appears to offer some possibilities in terms of yield in a usable size fraction and shape (163). The actual values for the aspect ratio appear rather high and the shape factor e_R rather low for good quality spheres. Again to claim that the shape factors are acceptable from the work on the ability to fill pellets into capsules is not a good standard by which to judge the performance of formulations. Nevertheless, this system does appear to have potential.

A system, which does offer a considerable potential is that described by Podczeck (164). Here the excipient is colloidal silicon dioxide plus a surfactant, which appears to be able to provide formulations with high drug loading and pellets that are round and have a narrow size distribution (compare the pellets in Figure 4 with those in Figure 3).

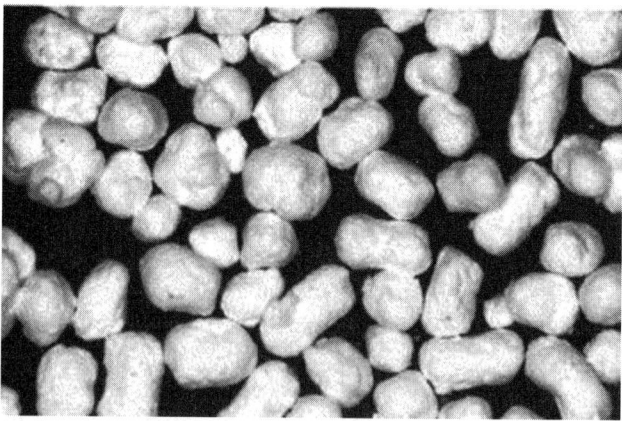

FIGURE 3 Pellets obtained from a mixture of Acetaminophen and microcrystalline cellulose, having an aspect ratio below 1.1. *Source*: From Ref. 64.

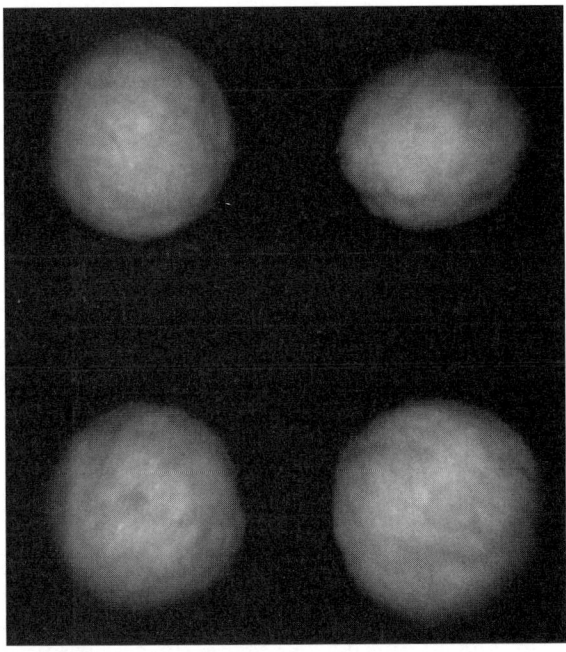

FIGURE 4 Pellets produced from colloidal silicon dioxide as spheronizing aid, drug, and surfactant. *Source*: Courtesy of F. Podczeck.

Non-aqueous Spheronization

The requirement for considerable water content to form a paste with a suitable consistency has lead to search for the ability to find an alternative solvent to water. This in turn has lead to the testing of materials other than MCC as the spheronization aid. The use of ethanol systems with MCC has already been mentioned (e.g., 55,71,79,80,86,95), but these all require the presence of some water. This was also the case with isopropyl alcohol (19). High levels of self-emulsifying systems could restrict the water content to as little as 5%, but the pellets then contain quite a high level of liquid and can be quite soft (123). Pellets can be prepared with up to 80% glycerol (81), but again the product is a soft pellet and one that is quite hydrophilic. A completely non-aqueous, hydrophobic pellet system was reported to provide a stable pellet formulation of a very water sensitive bleach activator (165). The liquid binder was white spirit and the spheronization aid was a hydrophobic clay, which was not registered for use in humans, but with suitable effort, this problem could be overcome. A system also based on mixtures of lactose, kaolin, Aerosil® (Aerosil, Parsippany, New Jersey, U.S.A.), bentonite, magnesium stearate, and light liquid paraffin was reported to be able to produce pellets of enteric coprecipitate of nifedipine with hydroxypropylmethylcellulose phthalate (166). The shape of the pellets appears to be "rounded," rather than spherical.

INFLUENCE OF DRUG

The large variations in the process conditions make the concept of being able to identify the critical properties of drugs extremely difficult. This is illustrated by the study of closely related model drugs (17,167). In terms of the force required to extrude the wet mass through a ram extruder, the behavior could be divided into two groups. Methyl, propyl, and butyl parabens formed a system, which provided a linear relationship between the steady state extrusion force (generally higher than the other group) and the percentage of drug and water present. Propyl gallate and 4-hydroxybenzoic acid formed a non-linear relationship between the extrusion force and the water and drug content (167). When it came to the spheronization stage of the process, two combinations of drug, MCC and water could be identified: (*i*) a combination, which produced pellets from all the model drugs and (*ii*) a combination which was too wet to produce pellets with any of the model drugs. Between these two extremes, it was found that "whether pellets could be made and their quality varied with the model drug" (17). It was not possible to relate the performance of these model drugs to any of their physico-chemical parameters such as molecular free energy. Cluster analysis again was the only way to provide any insight into the complex system, and indicated that water level and the type of model drug were the most important factors involved in the pellet size produced. Thus, the best that appears possible in terms of determining how to deal with a drug is to provide an indication of the quantity of water required as described for MCC (68) or a modified MCC (Avicel 955) (150).

One might expect there to be little difference between drugs that are highly water insoluble. The use of different water insoluble inorganic fillers in preparing pellets provided systems that did not perform equally (69). For highly water soluble drugs, an approach I have some times found useful is to dissolve the drug in water and use this with an equal quantity of MCC as the starting point. What is important is the use of a fine particle size as larger sizes encourage liquid migration during the extrusion process and allow water to come to the surface of the pellets, resulting in agglomeration, in the spheronization stage (53).

FILLERS

Many formulations can consist simply of drug and MCC, processed with an appropriate quantity of water. To decrease the cost, especially when the quantity of drug is relatively low, MCC can be replaced in some instances with filler. Those used are standard materials used in conventional oral formulations, such as lactose, mannitol, and calcium carbonate. The different fillers can influence the performance of the pellet formulation (115) but may not (168). In one study, we found it actually beneficial to include a quantity of lactose in a formulation, which contained a high level (80%) of drug, when one might expect the remainder of the formulation should be MCC (119). Thus, it appears necessary to take each formulation as an individual case.

DISINTEGRANTS

It is usual to characterize solid dosage forms in terms of their ability to disintegrate into the original drug particles, as the objective is to ensure that the patient receives the required dose of drug as efficiently as possible. For pellet formulations, this may not actually be an issue as they are used in the form of coated systems, either to protect from the environment, gastric acid intestinal enzymes or control the rate of drug release. Thus, the performance of the pellets will be controlled by mechanisms other than disintegration and their performance judged on different criteria than the usual immediate release preparation. Nevertheless reports (57) that formulations with MCC do not readily disintegrate are generally correct. There are two approaches to overcome this problem, add something to induce disintegration or to replace the MCC as a spheronizing agent. Traditional disintegrants such as starch and even "superdisintegrants" (169–171), do not seem to function very well, while one study claimed that the addition of superdisintegrants did not cause disintegration but did provide some enhancement of drug release (171). This is somewhat surprising as the addition of Ac–Di–Sol (croscarmellose sodium), due to its high swelling capacity, has been found to provide a controlled release pellet formulation (9). The inclusion of inorganic fillers can be used (103,104) but this requires an appreciable content, 20–30% to be effective, which may be too restrictive for some products.

To date, the approach of replacing the MCC with pectin has had limited success (64,65,157,158). The pellets do disintegrate, but the limited ability to form pellets appears to be rather restrictive. The use of colloidal silicon dioxide appears to be more encouraging as the pellets formed by this system do disintegrate readily (164).

STABILITY

Much of the work discussed above concentrates on the ability of the formulations to form satisfactory pellets, and in fact many studies do not include a drug at all. One of the most important features of formulation studies is to ensure that the product is stable. I am sure there is a considerable amount of data on file in industrial laboratories, but this is often not in a suitable format for publication in scientific journals and the information could be of a confidential nature. Conventional stability studies do not lend themselves readily to publication and the limited number of publications may be associated with the problem of providing results that illustrate that the drug is not stable to the process. As mentioned previously, the relatively high water content makes the process difficult to use for drugs that undergo hydrolysis. This can be overcome by moving to a non-aqueous liquid, but as explained this is as yet not fully resolved. One way to overcome this is to employ a system, which reduces the quantity of water required to form the paste and this was the approach described by Fitzpatrick et al. (19). This was also probably involved in the work of Basit et al. (154), who found that a conventional formulation of the drug ranitidine, lactose, and MCC resulted in pellets, which contained an impurity that did not occur when the same ingredients were used in a tablet formulation. These workers overcame the problem by replacing the lactose with barium sulfate and either reducing the level of MCC or removing it altogether and adding GMS instead.

Another source of instability could be the involvement of pressure during the extrusion part of the process, especially if long dies are used. This is also a potential problem if materials such as bacteria or enzymes are involved. There are varying degrees of success reported. When this was assessed for a series of different bacteria by Kouimtzi et al. (172) it was found that: "spores (*Bacillus subtilis*) were able to survive all stages of the process. The level of survival of gram-positive organisms after extrusion, spheronization and drying (60°C overnight) were significantly higher than the Gram-negative *E. coli*, with *B. angulatum* remaining viable in the final dried pellets." For *E. coli*, the level of killing was not affected by extrusion speed or die length, but the survival was inversely proportional to the extrusion pressure in the range 1–800 kPa. Huyghebaert et al. (173) reported that with *Lactococus lactis*, viability fell to 1% when processed by extrusion/spheronization. This loss was related to the drying stage of the pellets and occurred irrespective of whether the pellets were fluid–bed or freeze dried. Thus, it appears that the type of bacteria present during processing is a critical feature of whether or not it is possible to use the process.

FINAL REMARKS

The above survey shows that the process of extrusion/spheronization has developed since its introduction in the 1960s to a viable system for making pellets for controlled release dosage forms. It has some disadvantages compared to other methods of pellet preparation such as layering in coating systems, rotary processing, or use of direct pelletization in high speed granulators, in that it requires multiple items of equipment and is difficult to operate as a continuous process. The product, however, is usually of a high quality, reproducible and with the correct robust formulation there is little need for complex in process control. A robust, stable formulation can be identified with small quantities of material (19,42), which could be quite difficult for some drugs with the alternative pellet production processes.

Much of the literature is still descriptive and qualitative in nature and the area would benefit from fundamental studies. Standardization of the equipment, its description plus improvements in the methods of assessment of the pellets would make it easier to compare the findings from different workers.

REFERENCES

1. Reynolds AD. A new technique for the production of spherical particles. Manuf Chem Aer News 1970; 41(6):40–4.
2. Conine JW, Hadley HR. Preparation of small solid pharmaceutical spheres. Drug Cosmet Ind 1970; 106(4):38–41.
3. Clarke GM, Newton JM, Short MD. Gastrointestinal transit of pellets of differing size and density. Int J Pharm 1993; 100:81–92.
4. Rough SL, Wilson DI. Extrudate fracture and spheronization of microcrystalline cellulose pastes. J Mat Sci 2005; 40:4199–219.
5. Pinto JF, Abreu CN. Evaluation of the performance of a new continuous spheronizer. Drug Dev Ind Pharm 2006; 32:1067–78.
6. Newton JM, Chapman SR, Rowe RC. The influence of process variables on the preparation and properties of spherical granules by the process of extrusion and spheronization. Int J Pharm 1995; 120:101–9.
7. Schmidt C, Kleinebudde P. Comparison between a twin-screw and a rotary ring die press. Part II: influence of process variables. Eur J Pharm Biopharm 1998; 45:173–9.
8. Newton JM, Chapman SR, Rowe RC. Assessment of the scale up performance of the extrusion/spheronization process. Int J Pharm 1995; 120:95–9.
9. Speirs, C. Prednisolone metasulphobenzoate preparation for the treatment of inflammatory bowel disease. US Patent 5834021, 1998.
10. Young CR, Koleng JJ, McGinity JW. Production of spherical pellets by hot-melt extrusion and spheronization process. Int J Pharm 2002; 242:87–92.
11. Benbow JJ, Oxley EW, Bridgwater J. The extrusion mechanics of pastes- the influence of paste formulation on extrusion parameters. Chem Eng Sci 1987; 42:2151–62.
12. Schmidt C, Kleinebudde P. Comparison between a twin-screw extruder and a ring die press. I. Influence of formulation variables. Eur J Pharm Biopharm 1997; 44:169–76.
13. Kleinebudde P, Solvberg AJ, Linnder H. The power-consumption controlled extruder: A tool for pellet production. J Pharm Pharmacol 1994; 46:532–46.

14. Hellen L, Yliruusi J, Merkku P, et al. Process variables of instant granulator and spheroniser: I. Physical properties of granules, extrudate and pellets. Int J Pharm 1993; 96:197–204.
15. Chopra R, Newton JM, Alderborn G, et al. Preparation of pellets of different shape and their characterization. Pharm Dev Tech 2001; 6:495–503.
16. Newton JM, Chow AK, Jeewa KB. The effect of excipient source on spherical granules made by extrusion/spheronization. Pharm Tech Int 1992; 4(10):52–9.
17. Tomer G, Podczeck F, Newton JM. The influence of model drugs on the preparation of pellets by extrusion/spheronization: II spheronization parameters. Int J Pharm 2002; 231:107–19.
18. Newton JM. Extruders and extrusion. In: Swarbrick J, Boylan JC, eds. Encyclopaedia of Pharmaceutical Technology. Vol. 2, 2nd ed. New York: Marcel Dekker, 2002; 1220–36.
19. Fitzpatrick S, Taylor S, Booth SW, et al. The development of a stable, coated pellet formulation of a water sensitive drug, a case study: Development of a stable core formulation. Pharm Dev Tech 2006; 11:521–8.
20. Benbow JJ, Bridgwater J. Paste Flow and Extrusion. Oxford: Clarendon, 1993.
21. Harrison PJ, Newton JM, Rowe RC. The characterization of wet powder masses suitable for extrusion/spheronization. J Pharm Pharmacol 1985; 37:686–91.
22. Harrison PJ, Newton JM, Rowe RC. The application of capillary rheometry to the extrusion of wet powder masses. Int J Pharm 1987; 35:235–42.
23. Raines CL, Newton JM, Rowe RC. Extrusion of microcrystalline cellulose formulations. In: Carter R, ed. Rheology of Food, Pharmaceuticals and Biological Materials with General Rheology London: Elsevier Applied Science, 1990: 248–57.
24. Anderson AH, Newton JM. Influence of moisture content and particle size of barium sulfate on the extrusion properties of mixtures with microcrystalline cellulose. In: Carter, R, ed. Rheology of Food, Pharmaceutical and Biological Materials with General Rheology. London: Elsevier Applied Science, 1990: 258–67.
25. Chohan RK, Newton JM. Analysis of extrusion of some wet powder masses used in extrusion/spheronization. Int J Pharm 1996; 131:138–41.
26. Luukkonen P, Newton JM, Podczeck F, et al. Use of capillary rheometry to evaluate the rheological properties of microcrystalline and silicified microcrystalline cellulose. Int J Pharm 2001; 216:147–57.
27. MacRitchie KA, Newton JM, Rowe RC. The evaluation of the rheological properties of lactose/microcrystalline cellulose and water mixtures by controlled stress rheometry and the relationship to the production of spherical pellets by extrusion/spheronization. Eur J Pharm Sci 2002; 17:43–50.
28. Newton JM, Bazzigialuppi M, Podczeck F, et al. The rheological properties of self-emulsifying systems, water and microcrystalline cellulose. Eur J Pharm Sci 2005; 26:176–83.
29. Podczeck F, Knight P. The evaluation of formulations for the preparation of pellets with high drug loading by extrusion/spheronization. Pharm Dev Tech 2006; 11:263–74.
30. Baert L, Remon JP, Knight P, et al. A comparison between the extrusion forces and sphere quality of a gravity feed extruder and a ram extruder. Int J Pharm 1992; 86:187–92.
31. Tomer G, Newton JM. Water movement evaluation during extrusion of wet powder masses by collecting extrudate fractions. Int J Pharm 1999; 182:71–7.
32. Rough SL, Wilson DI, Bridgwater J. A model describing liquid phase migration within an extruding microcrystalline cellulose paste. Trans IChemE 2002; 80:701–14.
33. Tomer G, Newton JM, Kinchesh P. Magnetic resonance imaging (MRI) as a method of investigating movement of water during the extrusion of pastes. Pharm Res 1999; 16:666–71.
34. Tomer G, Mantle MD, Gladden LF, et al. Measuring water distribution in extrudates using magnetic resonance imaging (MRI). Int J Pharm 1999; 189:19–28.
35. Mascia S, Patel MJ, Rough SL, et al. Liquid phase migration in the extrusion and squeezing of microcrystalline cellulose pastes. Eur J Pharm Sci 2006; 29:22–34.
36. Soh JLP, Liew CV, Heng PWS. Torque rheological parameters to predict pellet quality on extrusion/spheronization. Int J Pharm 2006; 315:99–109.

37. Luukkonen P, Schaefer T, Hellen L, et al. Rheological characterization of microcrystalline cellulose and silicified microcrystalline cellulose wet masses using a mixer torque rheometer. Int J Pharm 1999; 188:181–92.
38. Luukkonen P, Schaefer T, Podczeck F, et al. Characterization of microcrystalline cellulose and silicified microcrystalline cellulose wet masses using a powder rheometer. Eur J Pharm Sci 2001; 13:143–9.
39. Harrison PJ, Newton JM, Rowe RC. Flow defects in wet powder mass extrusion. J Pharm Pharmacol 1985; 37:81–3.
40. Fielden KE, Newton JM. Extrusion and extruders. In: Swarbrick J. Boylan, JC, eds. Encyclopaedia of Pharmaceutical Technology. Vol. 5. New York: Marcel Dekker Inc., 1992: 395–442.
41. Malinowski HJ, Smith WE. Use of factorial design to evaluate granulations prepared by spheronization. J Pharm Sci 1975; 64:1688–93.
42. Cummings JH, Milojevic S, Harding M. et al. In vivo studies of amylose and ethylcellulose coated [^{13}C] glucose microspheres as a model for drug delivery to the colon. J Control Release 1996; 40:123–31
43. Fielden KE, Newton JM, Rowe RC. A comparison of the extrusion and spheronization behavior of wet powder masses processed by a ram extruder and a cylinder extruder. Int J Pharm 1992; 81:225–33.
44. Baert L, Fanara D, Remon JP, et al. Correlation of extrusion force, raw materials and sphere characteristics. J Pharm Pharmacol 1992; 44:676–8.
45. Baert L, Fanara D, Baets, De, et al. Instrumentation of a gravity feed extruder and the influence of the composition of binary and ternary mixtures on the extrusion forces. J Pharm Pharmacol 1991; 43:745–9.
46. Heng PWS, Liew CV, Gu L. Influence of teardrop studs on rotating base plate on spheroid quality in rotary spheronization. Int J Pharm 2002; 241:183–4.
47. Wan LSC, Heng PWS, Liew CV. Spheronization conditions on spheroid shape and size. Int J Pharm 1993; 96:50–65.
48. Hellen L, Yliruusi, J, Kristoffersson E. Process variables of instant granulator and spheronizer: II size and size distribution of pellets. Int J Pharm 1993; 6:205–16.
49. Elbers JAC, Bakkenes HW, Fokkens JG. Effect of amount and composition of granulation liquid on mixing, extrusion and spheronization. Drug Ind Pharm 1992; 18:501–17.
50. Woodruff CW, Nuessle NO. Effect of processing variables on the particles obtained by extrusion-spheronization processing. J Pharm Sci 1972; 61:787–90.
51. Baert L, Vermeersch H, Remon JP, et al. Study of parameters important in the spheronization process. Int J Pharm 1993; 96:225–9.
52. Chapman SR. Influence of process variables on the production of spherical granules. PhD thesis, University of London, 1985.
53. Fielden KE, Newton JM, Rowe RC. The influence of lactose particle size on the spheronization of extrudate processed by a ram extruder. Int J Pharm 1992; 18:205–24.
54. Vervaet C, Baert L, Remon JP. Extrusion-spheronization. A literature review. Int J Pharm 1995; 116:131–46.
55. Bashaiwouldu AB, Podczeck F, Newton JM. A study of the effect of drying techniques on the mechanical properties of pellets and compacted pellets. Eur J Pharm Sci 2004; 21:119–29.
56. Perez JP, Rabiskova M. Influence of the drying technique on theophylline pellets prepared by extrusion-spheronization. Int J Pharm 2002; 242:349–51.
57. Kleinebudde P. Shrinkage and swelling properties of pellets containing microcrystalline cellulose and low substituted hydroxypropyl cellulose: I. Shrinking properties. Int J Pharm 1994; 109:209–19.
58. Berggren J, Alderborn G. Drying behavior of two sets of microcrystalline cellulose pellets. Int J Pharm 2001; 219:113–26.
59. Berggren J, Alderborn G. Effect of drying rate on the porosity and tabletting behavior of cellulose pellets. Int J Pharm 2001; 227:81–96.

60. Heng PWS, Wan LSC, Chia CGH. Effect of off-bottom clearance on properties of pellets produced by melt pelletization. Pharm Dev Tech 1999; 4:27–33.
61. Heng PWS, Choo OMY. A study of the effects of characteristics of microcrystalline cellulose on performance in extrusion/spheronization. Pharm Res 2001; 7:39–49.
62. Koo OMY, Heng PWS. The influence of microcrystalline cellulose grade on shape and size distributions of pellets produced by extrusion-spheronization. Chem Pharm Bull 2001; 49:1383–7.
63. Abdulla A, Mader K. Preparation and characterization of a self-emulsifying pellet formulation. Eur J Pharm Biopharm 2007; 66:220–6.
64. Thommes M, Kleinebudde P. Use of K-Carrageenan as an alternative pelletization aid to microcrystalline cellulose in extrusion/spheronization. I. Influence of type and fraction of filler. Eur J Pharm Biopharm 2006; 63:59–67.
65. Thommes M, Kleinebudde P. Use of K-Carrageenan as an alternative pelletization aid to microcrystalline cellulose in extrusion/spheronization. II. Influence of drug and filler type. Eur J Pharm Biopharm 2006; 63:68–75.
66. Boutell S, Newton JM, Bloor J et al. The influence of liquid mobility and preparation of spherical granules by the process of extrusion/spheronization. Int J Pharm 2002; 238:61–76.
67. Chatchawalsaisin J, Podczeck F, Newton JM. The preparation by extrusion/spheronization and the properties of pellets containing drugs, microcrystalline cellulose and glyceryl monostearate. Eur J Pharm Sci 2005; 24:35–48.
68. Lustig-Gustafsson C, Johal HK, Podczeck F, et al. The influence of water content and drug solubility on the formation of pellets by extrusion and spheronization. Eur J Pharm Sci 1999; 8:147–52.
69. Lundqvist AEK, Podczeck F, Newton JM. Influence of disintegrant type and proportion on the properties of tablets produced from mixtures of pellets, Int J Pharm 1997; 147:95–107.
70. Sriamornsak P, Nunthanid J, Luangtana-anan M, et al. Alginate-based pellets prepared by extrusion/spheronization: A preliminary study on the effect of additive in granulating liquid. Eur J Pharm Biopharm 2007; 67:227–35.
71. Chopra R, Podczeck F, Newton JM, et al. The influence of pellet shape and film coating on the filling of pellets into hard shell capsules. Eur J Pharm Biopharm 2002; 53:327–33.
72. Chapman SR, Rowe RC, Newton JM. Characterization of the sphericity of particles by the one plane critical stability. J Pharm Pharmacol 1988; 40:503–5.
73. Podczeck F, Rahman SR, Newton JM. Evaluation of a standardized procedure to assess the shape of pellets using image analysis. Int J Pharm 1999; 192:123–38.
74. Podczeck F, Newton JM. A shape factor to characterize the quality of spheroids. J Pharm Pharmacol 1994; 46:82–5.
75. Podczeck F, Newton JM. The evaluation of a three-dimensional shape factor for the quantitative assessment of the sphericity and surface roughness of pellets. Int J Pharm 1995; 124:253–59.
76. Eriksson M, Alderborn G, Nystrom C, et al. Comparison between and evaluation of some methods for the assessment of the sphericity of pellets. Int J Pharm 1997; 148:149–54.
77. Almeida-Prieto S, Blanco-Mendez J, Otero-Espinar FJ. Image analysis of the shape of granulated powder grains. J Pharm Sci 2004; 93:621–34.
78. Strickland CW, Nussle NO. The physics of tablet compression: XI determination of porosity of tablet granulations. J Am Pharm Assoc Sci Ed 1956; 45:482–6.
79. Millili GP, Schwarz JB. The strength of microcrystalline cellulose pellets- the effect of granulating with water ethanol mixtures. Drug Dev Ind Pharm 1990; 16:1411–26.
80. Johansson B, Wikberg M, Ek R, et al. Compression behavior and compactability of microcrystalline cellulose pellets in relationship to their pore structure and mechanical properties. Int J Pharm 1995; 117:57–73.
81. Bashaiwoldu AB, Podczeck F, Newton JM. Application of dynamic mechanical analysis (DMA) to determine the mechanical properties of pellets. Int J Pharm 2004; 269:329–42.
82. Jalal IM, Malinowski HJ, Smith WE. Tablet granulations composed of spherical shaped particles. J Pharm Sci 1972; 61:1466–8.

83. Malinowski HJ, Smith WE. Effects of spheronizer process variables on selected tablet properties. J Pharm Sci 1974; 63:285–8.
84. Chopra R, Podczeck F, Newton JM, et al. The influence of film coating on the surface roughness and specific surface area of pellets. Part Part Syst Charact 2002; 19:277–83.
85. Shipway PH, Hutchings IM. Fracture of brittle spheres under compression and impact loading: I Elastic stress distributions. Phil Mag 1993; A67:1389–404.
86. Bashaiwoldu AB, Podczeck F, Newton JM. Factorial designed experiment to study the effects of excipients on the mechanical properties of pellets. J Pharm Pharmacol 2006; 58:1305–9.
87. Adams MJ, Mullier MA, Seville JPK. Agglomerate strength measurement using a uniaxial confined compression test. Powder Technol 1994; 78:5–13.
88. Aulton ME, Dyer AM, Khan, KA. The strength and compaction of millispheres: the design of a controlled-release drug delivery system for ibuprofen in the form of a tablet comprising compacted coated polymer coated millispheres. Drug Dev Ind Pharm 1993; 20:3069–104.
89. Podczeck F, Almeida SM. Determination of the mechanical properties of pellets and film coated pellets using dynamic mechanical analysis. Eur J Pharm Sci 2002; 16:209–14.
90. Heckel W. An analysis of powder compaction phenomena. Trans Metal Soc AIME 1961; 221:671–5.
91. Heckel W. Density-pressure relationships on powder compaction. Trans Metal Soc 1961; 221:1001–8.
92. Podczeck F. Dry filling of hard capsules. Chapter 5. In: Podczeck F, Jones BE, eds. Pharmaceutical capsules. 2nd.ed. London: Pharmaceutical Press, 2004: 119–38.
93. Pfeifer W, Marquardt HG. Investigations of the frequency and causes of dosage errors during the filling of hard gelatin capsules. Drugs made in Germany, 1986; 29:217–220.
94. Maganti L, Celik M. Compaction studies on pellets. I Uncoated pellets. Int J Pharm 1993; 95:29–42.
95. Johansson B, Alderborn G. Degree of pellet deformation during compaction and its relationship to the tensile strength of tablets formed of microcrystalline pellets. Int J Pharm 1996; 132:207–20.
96. Bashaiwoldu AB. Studies on the influence of composition and processing on the mechanical properties of pellets and compacted pellets. PhD Thesis, University of London, 2002.
97. Stanley P, Rowe RC, Newton JM. Theoretical considerations of the influence of polymer coatings on the mechanical strength of tablets. J Pharm Pharmacol 1981; 33:557–60
98. Bodmeier R. Tableting of coated pellets. Eur J Pharm Biopharm 1997; 43:1–8.
99. Beckert TE, Lehmann K, Schmidt PC. Compression of enteric-coated pellets to disintegrating tablets. Int J Pharm 1996; 143:13–23.
100. Ragnarsson G, Sandberg A, Jonsson UE, et al. Development of a new controlled release metoprolol product. Drug Dev Ind Pharm 1987; 13:1495–509.
101. Sandberg A, Ragnarsson G, Jonsson UE, et al. Design of a new multiple-unit controlled–release formulation of metoprolol CR. Eur J Clin Pharmacol 1988; 33(Suppl):S3–S7.
102. Pinto JF, Podczeck F, Newton JM. Investigation of tablets prepared from pellets by extrusion/spheronization Part I: the application of canonical analysis to correlate the properties of the tablets to the factors studied in combination with principal component analysis to select the most relevant factors. Int J Pharm 1997; 147:79–93.
103. Pinto JF, Podczeck F, Newton JM. Investigation of tablets prepared from pellets produced by extrusion/spheronization. Part II Modeling the properties of the tablets produced using regression analysis. Int J Pharm 1997; 152:7–16.
104. Lundqvist AEK, Podczeck F, Newton JM. Compaction of and drug release from coated pellets mixed with other pellets. Eur J Pharm Biopharm 1998; 147:369–79.
105. Vergote GJ, Kiekens C, Vervaet C, et al. Wax beads as cushioning agents during the compression of coated diltiazem pellets. Eur J Pharm Sci 2002; 17:145–51.
106. Twitchell A. Mixing Chapter 13. In: Aulton ME, 2nd ed. The Science of Dosage Form Design. Edinburgh: Churchill Livingstone, 2002: p. 181–96.

107. Blanque D, Sternagel H, Podczeck F et al. Some factors influencing the formation and in vitro drug release from matrix pellets prepared by extrusion/spheronization. Int J Pharm 1995; 119:203–11.
108. Tapia C, Buckton G, Newton JM. Factors influencing the mechanism of release from sustained release matrix pellets produced by extrusion/spheronization. Int J Pharm 1993; 92:211–8.
109. Santos H, Veiga F, Pina M, et al. Physical properties of chitosan pellets produced by extrusion-spheronization: influence of formulation variables. Int J Pharm 2002; 246:153–69.
110. Chatchawalsaisin J, Podczeck F, Newton JM. The influence of chitosan and sodium alginate and formulation variables on the formation and drug release from pellets prepared by extrusion/spheronization, Int J Pharm 2004; 275:41–60.
111. Neau SH, Chow MY, Durrani MJ. Fabrication and characterization of extruded and spheronised beads containing Carbapol^R 974, NF resin. Int J Pharm 1996; 131:47–55.
112. Goskonda SR, Hillman GA, Upadrashta SM. Development of matrix controlled release beads by extrusion-spheronization technology using statistical design. Drug Dev Ind Pharm 1994: 20:279–92.
113. Santos H, Veiga, Pina, ME, et al. Compaction, compression and drug release characteristics of xanthan gum pellets of different compositions. Eur J Pharm Sci 2004; 21:271–81.
114. Chopra R, Alderborn G, Podczeck F, et al. The influence of pellet shape and the surface properties on the drug release form uncoated and coated pellets. Int J Pharm 2002: 239:171–8.
115. Sousa JJ, Sousa A, Podczeck F, et al. The influence of core material and film coating on the drug release from coated pellets. Int J Pharm 2002; 232:111–22.
116. Milojevic S, Newton JM, Cummings JH, et al. Amylose as a coating for drug delivery to the colon; preparation and evaluation of glucose pellets. J Control. Release 1996; 38:85–94.
117. Milojevic S, Newton JM, Cummings JH, et al. Amylose as a coating for drug delivery to the colon: preparation and in vitro evaluation using 5-aminosalicylic acid pellets. J Control. Release 1996; 38:75–84.
118. Vier-Lopez ME, Nieto-Reyes L, Anguiano-Igea S, et al. Formulation of triamcinolone acetonide pellets suitable for coating and colon targeting. Int J Pharm 1999; 179:229–35.
119. Yuen KH, Deshmukh AA, Newton JM. Development and in vitro evaluation of a multiparticulate sustained release theophylline formulation. Drug Dev Ind Pharm 1993; 19:855–74.
120. Vervaet C, Baert L, Remon JP. Enhancement of in vitro release by using polyethylene glycol 400 and PEG-40 hydrogenated castor oil in pellets made by extrusion/spheronization. Int J Pharm 1994; 108:207–12.
121. Vervaet C, Remon JP. Bioavailability of hydrochlorothiazide from pellets, made by extrusion/spheronization, containing polyethylene glycol 400 as a dissolution enhancer. Pharm Res 1997; 14:1644–6.
122. Pouton C. Liquid formulations for oral administration of drugs: Non-emulsifying, self-emulsifying, and "self-microemulsifying" drug delivery systems. Eur J Pharm Sci 2000; 11:S93–S98.
123. Newton M, Pettersson J, Podczeck F, et al. The influence of formulation variables on the properties of pellets containing a self-emulsifying mixture. J Pharm Sci 2001; 90:987–95.
124. Newton JM, Godinho. A, Clarke AH, et al. Formulation variables on pellets containing self-emulsifying systems. Pharm Tech Eur 2005; 17(6):29–32.
125. Newton JM, Genis E, Clarke A, et al. Improving pellet extrusion. Pharma 2006; 1(2):56–60.
126. Tuleu C, Newton M, Rose J, et al. Comparative bioavailability study in dogs of a self-emulsifying formulation of progesterone presented in a pellet and liquid form compared with an aqueous suspension of progesterone. J Pharm Sci 2004; 93:1495–502.
127. Newton JM, Pinto MR, Podczeck F. The preparation of pellets containing a surfactant or a mixture of mono and diglycerides by extrusion/spheronization. Eur J Pharm Sci 2007; 66: 83–94.

128. Serratoni M, Newton M, Booth S, et al. Controlled drug release form pellets containing water-insoluble drugs dissolved in a self-emulsifying system. Eur J Pharm Biopharm 2007; 65:94–8.
129. Debunne A, Vervaet C, Remon JP. Development and in vitro evaluation of an enteric-coated multiparticulate drug delivery system for the administration of piroxicam to dogs. Eur J Pharm Biopharm 2002; 54:343–8.
130. O'Connor RE, Schwartz JB. Drug release mechanisms form a microcrystalline cellulose pellet system. Pharm Res 1993; 10:356–61.
131. Higuchi T. Mechanism of sustained-action medication. J Pharm Sci 1963; 52:1145–49.
132. Pinto JF, Podczeck F, Newton JM. The use of statistical moment analysis to elucidate the mechanism of release of a model drug from pellets produced by extrusion/spheronization. Chem Pharm Bull 1997; 45:171–80.
133. Hoffman A, Donbrow M, Gross ST, et al. Fundamentals of release mechanism interpretation in multiparticulate system: Determination of substrate release form single microcapsules and relation between individual and ensemble release kinetics. Int J Pharm 1986; 29:195–211.
134. Bergqvist P, Nevsten P, Nilsson B, et al. Simulation of the release from multiparticulate systems validated by single pellet and dose release experiments. J Control Release 2004; 97:453–65.
135. Fielden KE, Newton JM, Rowe RC. Movement of liquids through powder beds. Int J Pharm 1992; 79:47–60.
136. Tomer G, Newton JM. A centrifuge technique for the evaluation of the extent of water movement in wet powder masses. Int J Pharm 1999; 188:31–8.
137. Battista OA. Microcrystalline Polymer Science. London: McGraw Hill. 1975.
138. Li T-Q, Henricksson O, Klasen T, et al. Water diffusion in wood pulp cellulose fibers studied by means of pulsed gradient spin-echo method. J Colloid Interface Sci 1992; 154:305–15.
139. Fielden KE Newton JM, O'Brien P, et al. Thermal studies of the interaction of water and microcrystalline cellulose. J Pharm Pharmacol 1988; 40:674–8.
140. Kleinebudde P. The crystallite-gel model for microcrystalline cellulose in wet granulation, extrusion and spheronization. Pharm Res 1997; 14:804–9.
141. Fenchner PM, Wartewig S, Futing M, et al. Properties of microcrystalline cellulose and powder cellulose after extrusion/spheronization as studied by Fourier transform Raman spectroscopy and environmental scanning electron microscopy. AAPS PharmSci 2003; 5(4):article 31.
142. Rowe RC, Sheskey, PJ, Owen SC. Handbook of Pharmaceutical Excipients, 5th ed. London, Chicago: Pharmaceutical Press/APhA 2006:p132–5; 139–41.
143. Raines C. Rheological properties of different grades of microcrystalline cellulose. PhD. Thesis, University of London, UK, 1990.
144. El Saleh F, Jumaa M, Hassan I, et al. Influence of cellulose type on the properties of extruded pellets II Production and pellet properties. STP Pharm Sci 2000; 10:379–85.
145. Koo OMY, Heng PWS. The influence of microcrystalline cellulose grades on shape and shape distribution of pellets produced by extrusion/spheronization. Chem Pharm Bull 2001; 49:1383–7.
146. Heng PWS, Koo OMY. A study of the effects of the physical characteristics of microcrystalline cellulose on performance in extrusion/spheronization. Pharm Res 2001; 18:480–7.
147. Levis SR, Deasy PB. Production and evaluation of size reduced grades of microcrystalline cellulose. Int J Pharm 2001; 213:13–24.
148. Levis SR, Deasy PB. Pharmaceutical applications of size reduced grades of surfactant co-processed microcrystalline cellulose. Int J Pharm 2001; 230:25–33.
149. Kleinebudde P, Jumma M, El Saleh F. Influences of degree of polymerization on the behavior of cellulose during homogenization and extrusion/spheronization. AAPS PharmSci 2000; 2:article 22.

150. Jover I, Podczeck F, Newton M. Evaluation, by statistically designed experiment, of an experimental grade of microcrystalline cellulose, Avicel 955, as a technology to aid the production of pellets with high drug load. J Pharm Sci 1996; 85:700–805.
151. Law MFL, Deasy PB. Use of hydrophilic polymers with microcrystalline cellulose to improve extrusion/spheronization. Eur J Pharm Biopharm 1998; 45:57–65.
152. Lindner H, Kleinebudde P. Use of powdered cellulose for the production of pellets by extrusion/spheronization J Pharm Pharmacol 1994; 46:1–7.
153. Alverez L, Concheiro, A, Gomez-Amoza JL, et al. Powdered cellulose as excipient for extrusion-spheronization pellets of cohesive hydrophobic drug. Eur J Pharm Biopharm 2003; 55:291–5.
154. Basit AW, Newton JM, Lacy LF. Formation of ranitidine pellets by extrusion/spheronization with little or no microcrystalline cellulose. Pharm Dev Tech 1999; 4:499–505.
155. Newton JM, Chatchawalsaisin J, Podczeck F. The influence of monoglycerides, mixtures and derivatives on the formation of pellets by extrusion/spheronization. Pharm Tech Eur 2005; 17(12):38–43.
156. Tho I, Kleinebudde P, Sande SA. Extrusion/spheronization of pectin formulations. I. Screening of important factors. AAPS PharmSciTech 2001; 2(4):article 26.
157. Tho I, Kleinebudde P, Sande SA. Extrusion/spheronization of pectin-based formulations. II. Effect of additive concentration in the granulating liquid. AAPS PharmSciTech 2001; 2(4):article 27.
158. Tho I, Sande SA, Kleinebudde P. Pectinic acid, a novel excipient for the production of pellets by extrusion/spheronization; preliminary studies. Eur J Pharm Biopharm 2002; 54:95–9.
159. Tho I, Anderssen E, Drystad K, et al. Quantum chemical descriptors in the formulation of pectin pellets produced by extrusion/spheronization. Eur J Pharm Sci 2002; 16:143–9.
160. Bornhoft M, Thommes M, Kleinebudde P. Preliminary assessment of carrageenan as excipient for extrusion/spheronization. Eur J Pharm Biopharm 2005; 59:127–31.
161. Steckel H, Mindermann-Nogly F. Production of chitosan pellets by extrusion/spheronization Eur J Pharm Biopharm 2004; 57:107–14.
162. Prieto SA, Mendez JB, Espinar FJO. Starch-dextrin mixtures as base excipients for extrusion/spheronization. Eur J Pharm Biopharm 2005; 59:511–21.
163. Dukie A, Mens R, Adriansens P, et al. Development of starch-based pellets via extrusion/spheronization. Eur J Pharm Sci 2007; 66:83–94.
164. Podczeck F. Formulations. International Patent Application PTC/GB2007/050567; Publication number WO/2008/001140.
165. Barton DJ, Macduff MPJ, Newton JM. Bleach activator formulations. European Patent 0 482 806 A1, 1992.
166. Deasy PD, Gouldson MP. In vitro evaluation of pellets containing enteric coprecipitates of nifedipine formed by non-aqueous spheronization. Int J Pharm 1996; 132:131–41.
167. Tomer G, Podczeck F, Newton JM. The influence of type and quantity of model drug on the extrusion/spheronization of mixtures with microcrystalline cellulose. I. Extrusion parameters. Int J Pharm 2001; 217:237–48.
168. Palmer RMJ, Newton M, Basit, B, et al. Colonic release composition. US Patent 2005; US 2005/0220861.
169. Lovgren K. Disintegrants and fillers in the manufacture of spheres. The influence on the dissolution rates and binding properties. Lab-Pharm-Prob Tech 1984; 32:110–4.
170. Schroder M, Kleinebudde P. Influence of formulation parameters on dissolution of propylphenazone pellets. Eur J Pharm Biopharm 1995; 41:382–7.
171. Souto C, Rodriguez A, Parajes S, et al. A comparative study of the utility of two superdisintegrants in microcrystalline cellulose pellets prepared by extrusion/spheronization. Eur J Pharm Biopharm 2005; 61:94–9.
172. Kouimtzi M, Pinney RJ, Newton JM. Survival of bacteria during extrusion/spheronization. Pharm Sci 1997; 3:347–51.
173. Huyghebaert N, Vermeire A, Neirynck S, et al. Evaluation of extrusion/spheronization, layering and compaction for the preparation of an oral, multi-particulate formulation of viable, hIL-10 producing *Lactococus lactis*. Eur J Pharm Biopharm 2005; 59:9–15.

11
Coating Processes and Equipment

David M. Jones
Ramsey, New Jersey, U.S.A.

INTRODUCTION—FLUIDIZED BED AND PERFORATED PAN COATING

In solids manufacturing, many products require coating to provide the desired properties (1). Contemporary fluidized bed equipment is widely used to coat substrates in a broad range of particle sizes, from below 100 µm up to and including tablets. The fluidized bed is available in various configurations, depending on the vendor, but principally, they are based either on a conventional top spray, bottom spray (usually a variation of the Wurster though other types of bottom spray are available), or tangential spray, referred to as a rotor or centrifugal processor. A few iterations of the fluidized bed have been configured for tablet coating, particularly for modified release products or the application of a potent outer layer. This is primarily due to the very random and rapid mixing capability of air suspension systems and the absence for consideration of the spatial orientation of the tablets as they enter and exit the so-called "coating zone." The mechanical stress to which tablets are exposed is comparatively high and tablets and their coatings should be formulated specifically for their intended use in the fluidized bed. Although air suspension systems have enjoyed renewed interest for coating or layering of tablets, the perforated pan remains the preferred method for most tablet coating applications.

Films may be applied for identification, to improve core strength, aesthetics, taste masking, enteric release, stability (protection from environment), or to provide sustained or controlled release. For many products, development of latex coating materials has eliminated the safety hazards and emissions problems related to the use of organic solvents. A further characteristic is that these materials have higher solids concentrations and low viscosity and may be easier and faster to apply than films from solution. However, the use of organic solvents proliferates, and there are additional considerations unique to their use.

Successful film coating depends on a number of product and process considerations. Core or substrate material may be prepared using a variety of techniques including extrusion/spheronization; solution or suspension layering, granulation, etc. These processes are covered in other chapters of this text and will not be described herein. Factors such as substrate size, size distribution, shape, porosity, friability, and solubility may influence the release properties of the coated dosage form. The goal in coating is to apply the film in such a way that its release is governed by the intrinsic properties of the film, and not imperfection (core penetration, surface pores and defects, fines imbedded in the film, non-uniformity of distribution, etc.). In addition to the properties of the substrate and the coating material, the type of process selected may have a significant impact on the behavior of the finished product.

The basic differences between the various fluidized bed techniques and the perforated pan coating process will be elucidated. The coating methods described have common process variables. All require application of liquid, evaporation of the coating media and mixing of the core material to assure uniform distribution of the material being applied. These variables and their influence on product quality and the process will be discussed in detail.

DESCRIPTION OF THE TOP SPRAY PROCESS

The top spray fluidized bed is well known for its drying efficiency, as it has been used for drying and spray granulating for many years. It also has abilities in core material manufacture (via solution or suspension layering) and for coating. The counter-current spray technique typically discourages the use of volatile organic solvents (due to very rapid evaporation of the application media). However, it is effective at applying films from an aqueous solution or latex, and it is a premier method for application of a coating via hot melt. Solution and suspension layering, as well as film coating require the use of an application vehicle such as water or organic solvent. Hot melt coating involves melting of the coating material, spraying it in its molten state, and congealing it in a controlled manner onto the surface of the substrate (2,3). For small particles, top spray is the method of choice. The reason is that the coating is the least permeable when it is applied at a core product temperature that is as close to the congealing temperature of the coating material as possible. Under this condition, the bed is viscose and resistant to flow. In top spray, the product container is an open vessel with no impediment to flow. Therefore, the product temperature can be higher than that achievable using other types of fluidized beds, such as the Wurster or rotor tangential spray processor.

Substrate particle size and density may play a significant role in the ability to succeed in scale-up from lab to pilot and commercial size machines, principally due to the change in fluidization behavior. This is related to the increase in bed depth and loss of "wall effects" (the condition by which the process air is no longer constrained by the narrow walls of the small lab machine).

The gas fluidization and bubble characteristics have been defined in the literature (4–10). They are affected by the properties of the materials being fluidized and the design characteristics of the equipment being used, which vary with equipment vendors. Only the fundamentals of these phenomena will be described because of this dependence. Figure 1 illustrates typical fluidization characteristics for substrates of various particle sizes and densities encountered in air suspension processing.

Ignoring product attributes (particle size and density), the air distribution plate design influences the size and number of air bubbles entering the product bed, which in turn affects its mixing characteristics. Machines are typically designed to maximize the number of bubbles to result in effective mixing.

The conventional top spray method shown in Figure 2 has been used for layering and coating for decades. It evolved from the fluidized bed dryers commercialized more than 40 years ago. The substrate is placed in the product container, which is typically an unbaffled, inverted, truncated cone with a fine retention screen and an air or gas distribution plate at its base. Perforated plates such as a Conidur or Gill plate may also achieve air distribution and product retention. These types of plates may have directed holes for guiding the airflow horizontally in the product container (for side discharge as an example). Process air is drawn through the distribution plate and into the product.

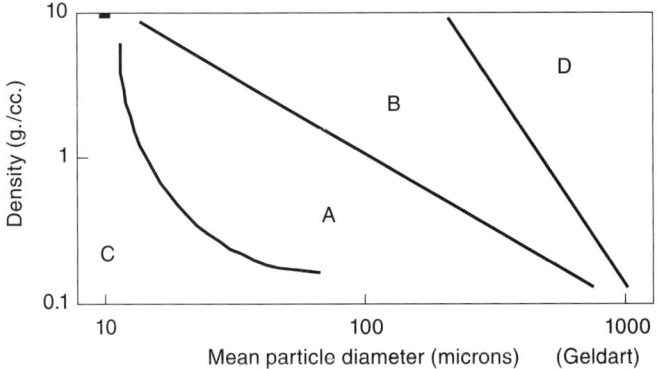

FIGURE 1 Typical fluidization characteristics for substrates of various particle sizes and densities. *Source*: From Ref. 4.

As the volume of air is increased, the bed no longer remains static but begins to expand, ultimately becoming fluidized in the air stream. The point at which the bed becomes just fluidized is known as incipient fluidization. In this condition, mixing and heat transfer are effective, assuming that the particles flow freely in response to the air stream. However, in practical terms, the velocity of particles in the bed under this condition is unnecessarily low for nearly all types of spraying processes. Increasing the air volume (and hence particle velocity) results in a wider fluidization range known as bubbling fluidization, in which the bed can be defined as containing two phases: a particulate phase, containing

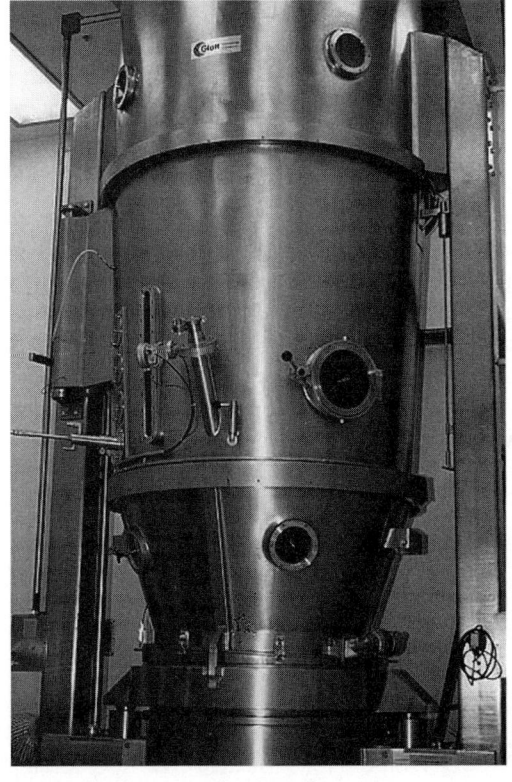

FIGURE 2 A representative example of a conventional top spray fluidized bed processor. *Source*: Courtesy of Glatt Air Techniques, Inc.

particles and air, and a bubble phase, which contains the excess air. The wide range of air velocities between the minimum fluidization velocity and pneumatic transport (for the majority of the particles to avoid retention in the product filters) is where processing typically occurs. The higher air velocities and volumes assure fluidization of the entire batch and permit faster spray application rates, and hence, a more economical process.

The particles are accelerated from the product container past the nozzle, which sprays liquid counter-currently onto the randomly fluidized particles. The wetted particles travel through this spraying "zone" into the expansion chamber, which is wider in diameter than the base of the product container. This results in a decreasing air velocity that allows deceleration of the particles to below entrainment velocity. The particles fall toward the wall and back into the product container and continue cycling throughout the duration of the process.

BOTTOM SPRAY PROCESSING

In 1959, Wurster, then at the University of Wisconsin, introduced an air suspension technique now known as the Wurster system (11,12). The Wurster process enjoys widespread use in the pharmaceutical industry for pellet core manufacturing (solution or suspension layering) and film coating of particles and pellets. Recently, it has seen a revived interest in tablet coating for modified release or the application of a potent API outer layer (where distribution uniformity is critical). Inserts typically range in size from 3.5 in. (100–500 g batch sizes) to 46 in. (up to approximately 800 kg). This process is used commercially for coating particles from less than 100 µm to tablets and for solution or suspension layering to produce core materials.

Basic Design Considerations

The basic design components of a Wurster system are shown in Figures 3 and 4. The product container is typically cylindrical or slightly conical, and houses a cylindrical partition (open on both ends) that is about half the diameter of the bottom of the container (up to 24 in. Wursters). At the base of the product container is an orifice plate that is divided into two regions. The open area of the portion of the plate beneath the partition is very permeable. This permits a high volume and velocity of air to pneumatically transport the substrate vertically. Particles accelerate upwards, past a spray nozzle that is mounted in the center of this up-bed orifice plate. The nozzle is usually pneumatic—liquid is delivered to the nozzle port at low pressure and is atomized by compressed air. The spray pattern is generally a solid cone of droplets, with a spray angle ranging from approximately 30° to 50°. The so-called "coating zone" formed is a narrow ellipse, and varies in volume depending on the nozzle type, the size of the substrate being sprayed and the pattern density in the partition.

The view inside of the Wurster insert in Figure 3 illustrates the regions of flow in the process. The region outside of the partition is referred to as the down-bed. The configuration of the orifice plate in this area depends on the size and density of the material to be processed. The purpose of the airflow in the down-bed region is to keep the substrate in near-weightless suspension, irrespective of its distance to either the wall of the product container or the partition. The goal is to have it travel rapidly downward (to minimize cycling time), and then be drawn horizontally toward and ultimately into the gap at the base of the partition. In general, tablets require significantly more air to

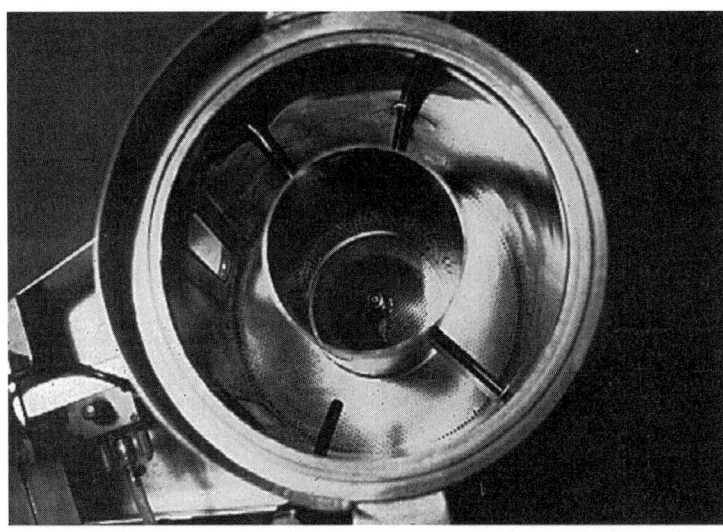

FIGURE 3 Interior view of components for a conventional 18 in. Wurster processor. *Source*: Courtesy of Glatt Air Techniques, Inc.

produce this condition than pellets or fine particles - the orifice plate must be selected accordingly (no single down-bed plate can achieve good fluidization properties for all substrates). As mentioned previously, the up-bed or partition plate controls the material flow inside of the partition. In general, this plate is considerably more permeable than the

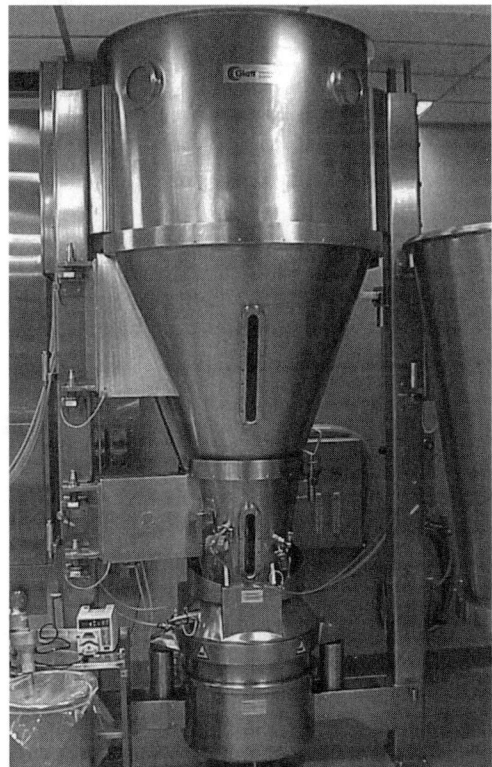

FIGURE 4 A representative example of a Wurster bottom spray fluidized bed processor. *Source*: Courtesy of Glatt Air Techniques, Inc.

down-bed plate. In pilot and production scale Wursters the up-bed plates may be removable such that one or the other may be changed to "fine-tune" the relationship of the substrate flow in these individual regions.

A second key process variable in Wurster coating is the height that the partition sits above the orifice plate, which controls the rate of substrate flow horizontally into the coating zone. Typically, the smaller the particles to be coated, the smaller the gap will be. When the Wurster coating chamber is assembled properly, the resulting flow pattern should be relatively smooth and rapid in the down-bed. Mass flow in the up-bed or partition region should be very dense and rapid to facilitate a maximum spray rate and coating efficiency.

The substrate exits the partition at a high rate of speed, requiring a region to decelerate. Above the product container is the expansion area, which is typically conical to allow for decreasing air and particle velocity. Wurster machines designed for pellets and small particles employ elongated expansion chambers to essentially enhance deceleration in the air space rather than by high velocity impact against machine components in the filter housing. By contrast, tablets do not need much expansion height, and in fact, attrition may be a severe problem. The orifice plate and partition height should be optimized so that the tablets travel upward only a very short distance out of the partition before beginning their descent. As a result, a mesh bonnet can be used in the expansion chamber, just above the product container, to keep the tablets from colliding with the steel walls of the expansion chamber. The coarse mesh is intended to allow the fines from the cores and any spray dried coating to exit the process area, avoiding incorporation in the layers of film. A conventional Wurster is not used extensively for tablet coating due to the comparatively high stress to which the tablets may be exposed (collisions with perpendicular surfaces and the expansion chamber). However, it is recommended when the film quality (minimal defects), and good film or active component distribution uniformity is very important, especially for modified release tablets. The films applied by Wurster are high in quality due to the concurrent spray and high drying efficiency of this air suspension process. There have been modifications to the Wurster process specifically for tablet coating. In addition to the collision bonnets in the expansion chamber (described previously), these include ramped spray nozzle surrounds, a change in partition geometry and air flow adjustability at the interface between the wall of the product container and the down-bed orifice plate.

Pellets and small particles are layered or coated extensively with the Wurster process using water, organic solvents, or to a limited extent by spraying molten materials. All fluidized bed techniques are known for high rates of heat and mass transfer, and the Wurster is also very effective in this regard. Highly water-soluble substrate materials can be coated using water-based applications without concern for core penetration. Droplets applied to the surface spread to form a continuous film or layer, and then quickly give up their moisture to the warm, dry air. After a thin layer or film has been applied, spray rates can be increased since the soluble core has been isolated. Films applied with volatile organic solvents are also high in quality because the formed droplets impinge on the substrate very quickly, minimizing the potential for spray drying of the film. Finally, there are limited applications involving the use of molten coatings. In this case, the coating or layer is applied by spraying a molten substance that subsequently congeals on the substrate surface. For a variety of reasons, the Wurster is not the process of choice for molten coating. If the substrate particle size is such that the Wurster is favored for its fluidization properties (generally coarser core materials) a molten coating may be applied reproducibly. Otherwise, top spray fluidized bed processing is a better choice for hot melt coating.

Coating Processes and Equipment

HS Wurster Considerations

HS Wurster technology, shown in Figure 5, is a product of Glatt Air Techniques, Inc. in Ramsey, NJ, and involves the use of a proprietary device to influence the behavior of the substrate in proximity to the coating zone (13). Unfortunately, the liquid spray application rate is not controlled merely by the drying capacity of the fluidization air, but by other factors. The nature of the coating material, particularly as it transitions from liquid droplets to a dried film (tackiness) will strongly impact the application rate. A second consideration involves the region immediately surrounding the top of the spray nozzle. In all Wurster inserts, the high volume of air rushing through the gap at the base of the partition creates suction through this gap. As a consequence, particles entering have a horizontal component to their flow—some travel towards the spray nozzle instead of simply making the transition from horizontal to vertical flow. A compounding factor is that the atomizing air has a very high velocity (it is likely supersonic) that creates streamlines drawing the substrate to the base of the developing spray pattern. In a standard Wurster, the nozzle is elevated above the orifice plate, at a position just below the confluence of fluidizing substrate particles. A portion of the developing up bed stream of product can pass the nozzle tip either closely or at a further distance. Particles that are very close to the nozzle tip encounter a heavy liquid stream and tend to be over-wetted. If they contact other particles, agglomerates are formed. Initially held together by liquid bridges of the coating liquid, the bridges are solidified as the application media is quickly evaporated, and the agglomerate becomes more rigid. The mechanical stresses of

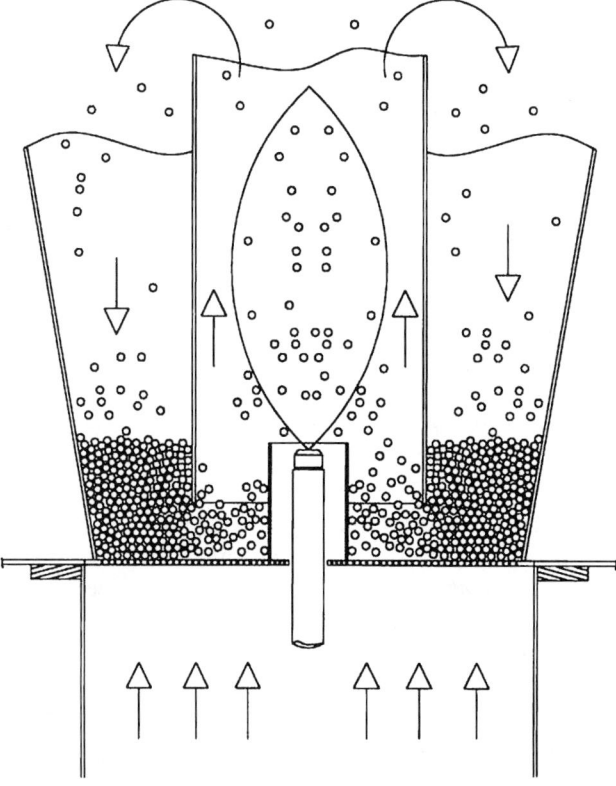

FIGURE 5 Diagram of components showing the HS Wurster. *Source*: Courtesy of Glatt Air Techniques, Inc.

fluidization may not be sufficient to break the formed agglomerate back into individual particles. To control what could otherwise be severe agglomeration, a typical response is to reduce the spray rate. This leaves a large amount of the process air's drying capacity unused. Other commonly used agglomeration control techniques include raising the inlet (and product) temperature to increase the drying rate, or raising the atomizing air pressure to shrink droplet size—options which are in conflict with producing high quality films. In fact, elevating the atomizing air pressure will increase the kinetic energy exerted by the spray nozzle. While this may decrease the amount of agglomeration, it accomplishes this task by shear. Unfortunately, the increased shear force may cause damage to a fraction of the batch. Some impact on the release properties of the coated material is inevitable. Even using these corrective measures, a quantity of agglomeration in traditional Wursters is almost unavoidable.

The HS Wurster was developed to keep particles away from the spray nozzle until the spray pattern is more fully developed. This is achieved by the use of a physical barrier that also forms a column of air around the nozzle. The elliptical void formed prior to the convergence of substrate at a distance from the nozzle results in a significant increase in the area of contact between the droplets and accelerating substrate. As a result, more of the process air's available drying capacity can be used, and the application rate increased substantially (more than doubled in many pilot scale lab trials). Because the particles are kept away from the wettest portion of the pattern agglomeration is also substantially diminished or eliminated. An additional benefit is that the high atomizing air velocities necessary to produce very small droplets for coating of particles smaller than 100 μm may be useable without pulverizing the substrate. The velocity of this air diminishes dramatically with distance from the nozzle, and even a few centimeters are significant. Keeping the product away from the nozzle tip allows the atomization air velocity to decrease significantly before contacting the substrate, reducing the likelihood of attrition, especially during the early stages of coating when the core material is in its most friable state.

Coating of substrates smaller than 100 μm has been achieved more effectively by using the HS Wurster. Success depends on many factors, both process and product related. Product considerations such as flow properties of the substrate (generally poor in this size range, which must be improved), as well as the liquid, which must be amenable to atomizing to droplets well below 10 μm, must be addressed. The tremendous surface area of such fine particles also requires very high coating quantities and, consequently, a low potency of the final coated product (often less than 50%).

Coating and Process Characteristics

The coating liquid is sprayed in the direction of motion of the fluidizing particles (concurrently). In general, the fluidization is orderly: very rapid, dilute phase pneumatic transport in the up bed, and relatively smooth and rapid descent in the down bed region (outside of the partition). Because the liquid is sprayed into a well-organized pattern of substrate moving relatively close to the nozzle, droplet travel distance is minimized. In this manner, droplets reach the substrate prior to any appreciable evaporation. By retaining their low viscosity, they are able to spread on contact and the resultant films are excellent, even when using organic solvents as an application medium. The drying efficiency of the fluidized bed also minimizes the potential for core penetration, and the sample shown in Figure 6 clearly shows a well-defined boundary layer between the substrate and the coating material.

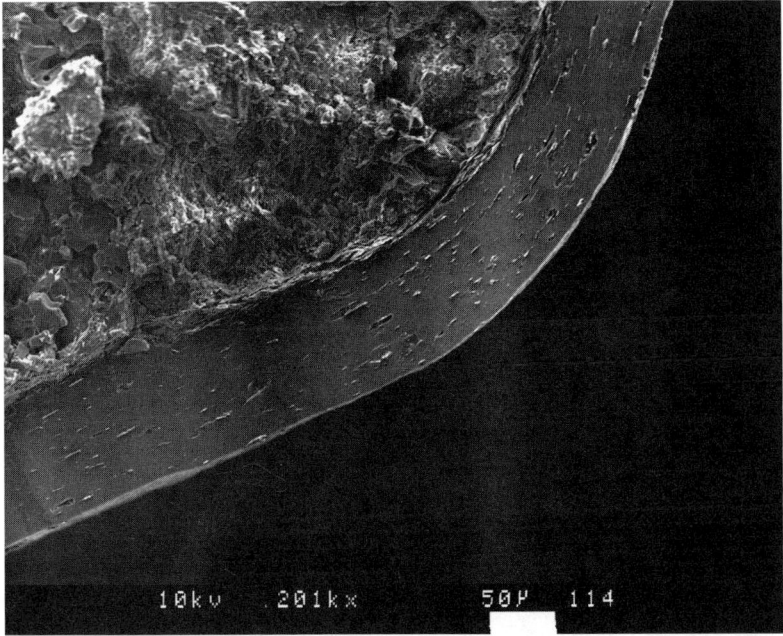

FIGURE 6 Scanning electron micrograph of the cross-section of a particle coated using a fluidized bed. *Source*: Courtesy of Glatt Air Techniques, Inc.

ROTOR OR CENTRIFUGAL PROCESSING

The rotary granulator is a later entry in fluidized bed processing. Though originally conceived as a granulator/dryer, it is now more widely used for the manufacture of core pellets. It is a relative newcomer in comparison to the top spray granulators and Wurster coaters that have been in existence for more than 30 years. The rotor product container incorporates a variable speed, solid spinning disc that may be height adjustable, depending on the variation offered by the vendors of such equipment. It may be configured as a totally enclosed insert to a fluid bed machine tower, a standalone version (for large scale production), or open and completely accessible from above. The enclosed version was initially introduced as a granulator capable of producing denser product than the traditional top spray fluidized bed processor. Probably due to its high capital cost and comparatively much smaller batch size (only up to about 30% of the volume of a production top spray granulator/dryer), it is not widely used for the granulation process. Subsequently, it is more commonly used for pelletizing and film coating.

Description of the Product Container

The rotor insert (Fig. 7) was conceived as a combination of a high shear mixer/granulator and fluidized bed dryer. In contrast with a traditional fluid bed dryer, the base of the product container is fitted with a solid rotating disc as opposed to a perforated air distribution plate and fine screen.[a] The disc height may be adjustable to allow the control of

---

[a] At least one supplier does provide perforated and screened segments in the disc to enhance drying.

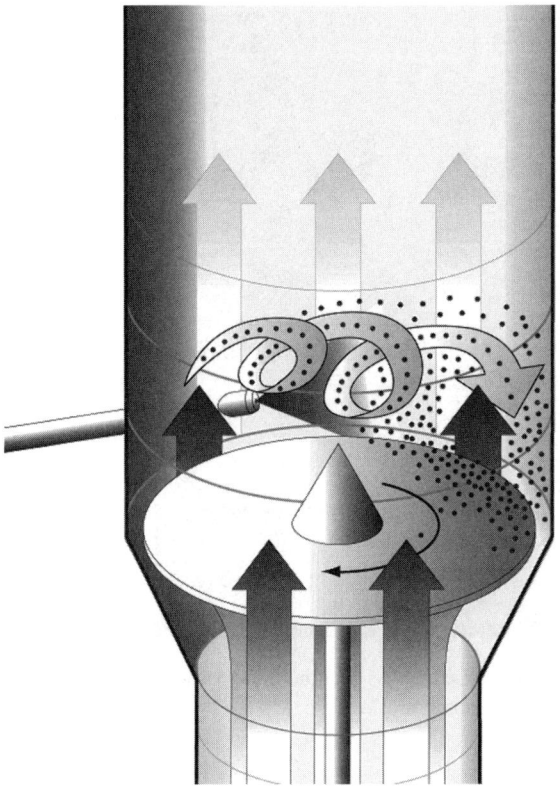

FIGURE 7 Diagram of a representative example of a rotary or centrifugal processor. *Source*: Courtesy of Glatt Air Techniques, Inc.

the air volume through the gap at the perimeter of the disc to be varied independently of air velocity (depending on the type of process being utilized). The fluidization pattern is formed by a combination of centrifugal force, air-flow (volume and velocity) upward at the perimeter of the disc, and gravity. A smooth disc surface is typically used for film coating, solution or suspension layering, and dry powder layering, to enhance the movement of the material past the spray nozzle.

The combination of mechanical energy imparted by the rotating disc, agglomerate growth control by atomization of the binder liquid, and drying efficiency via the fluidized bed, yield a high-density granulation in comparison with a traditional fluidized bed spray granulator. Although this was the original intent, this technique excels at producing high potency pellets by layering active materials onto some type of core or seed, which now dominates its use. In these types of operations, the smooth rotating disc plate is used only to enhance the pellets motion past the spray nozzles. This will allow a maximum spray rate without causing attrition.

A more aggressive surface, such as a waffle plate may be used in laboratory-sized equipment to impart a higher degree of energy into the tumbling particles. This configuration may be desirable for producing even higher density granules, spheronizing from a wet mass produced by wetting a bed of powders, or for spheronizing (rounding) as a step subsequent to a wet granulation/extrusion process.

The strength of pellets depends, to a great extent, on the physical forces that bond the primary particles together and their resulting interstitial porosity. The size of the gap at the perimeter of the disc is adjusted based on how much evaporation is desired. In some types of equipment and for certain operations in others, this air stream is used only to produce the fluidization pattern; the air volume and inlet temperature are kept at a minimum. For example, in certain pelletizing operations, mechanical forces such as tumbling, agitating, and compaction are needed to bring individual particles in close contact with one another. Liquid bridges may be critical to the formation of the desired product, and water can be sprayed into the bed to elevate the moisture content with the disc gap at a minimum. The corresponding air volume is set at a value adequate only to keep the material moving upward at the perimeter of the disc. To minimize evaporation, the low disc height is combined with a low process air temperature. The force transmitted by the rotating disc results in rounding and densification of the plastic mass. Elevation of the disc, reduction of its speed and a stepwise increase in process air temperature provide drying subsequent to the pelletizing steps.

Other types of processing (solution or suspension layering as well as film coating) in the rotor require that the evaporation rate be substantially higher. In these cases, the disc gap is increased significantly, as are the process air volume and temperature. Both parameters are adjusted in concert to retain a similar air velocity at the edge of the disc (measured indirectly by the product differential pressure).

The speed of the disc is also adjustable. In general, it is just enough to keep the substrate moving vigorously past the spray nozzles; slow speeds may lead to agglomeration and high speeds to attrition. However, for granulation or pelletizing from powders, increasing the disc speed will help to densify the forming agglomerates by increasing the mechanical energy transferred to the bed.

Three forces act on the product to produce a fluidization pattern best described as a spiraling helix. The rotation of the disc moves the substrate outward by centrifugal force. The fluidization air accelerates the product up the walls of the product container. Finally, gravity (and possibly turbulent air eddies) causes the particles to tumble inward toward the center of the disc. Typically the nozzle is immersed low in the product bed in a region of high substrate density and speed, and the liquid is sprayed concurrently with the flow of product, though at least one vendor locates the nozzle above the bed, spraying downward onto its surface.

A large expansion area above the product container is generally unnecessary because the air velocity is high only through the relatively narrow gap at the perimeter of the disc. Typically, the bed does not expand much above the product container. In most types of rotor processors, there is no screen at the base of the product container and any interruption in fluidization would probably result in loss of product below the disc (falling into the lower plenum). The filter housing is designed to allow for continuous fluidization. The outlet filters collect and retain fines, periodically returning them to the tumbling product bed (typically every 15–30 seconds).

Like the Wurster, the nozzle is immersed in the bed and is closely surrounded by product. This minimizes the distance that droplets must travel before contacting substrate and the resulting films are excellent. Using a scanning electron microscope, the films are seen to be smooth and dense. Core penetration is rarely a problem (or at least no more serious than with the other fluid bed techniques). Fluidization should be vigorous to avoid liquid bridges forming between particles during spraying.

Since spray rate is not necessarily limited by drying capacity, if agglomeration is occurring, the best way to improve application rate in larger equipment is to use more spray nozzles. In lab machines, 1 or 2 are used; production rotors may contain 5 or 6. It is recommended to maximize fluidization air volume to attain a high drying rate and particle velocity through the coating zone. Also, keeping the bed "aerated" will help assure that the particles are separated when sprayed, which will inhibit formation of liquid bridges between particles resulting in agglomeration. The disc speed for film coating is low (typical perimeter velocities range from 4 to 6 m/sec), used only to enhance particle motion. High speeds will expose the product to excessive shear, resulting in the potential for fracture of the pellet surface or the developing film.

The rotor is very flexible regarding batch size. Minimum batch size may be as low as 1/8 of working capacity. However, when applying films, the batch size should be selected such that the nozzle is immersed below the surface of the bed. This minimizes the potential that the high velocity atomization air will not blow some coating droplets through the bed where they may be spray dried and collected in the filter.

PERFORATED PAN PROCESSING

Film coating of tablets is commonplace, and the use of a perforated pan dominates this practice (Fig. 8). Tablets may be coated for a variety of reasons, including improved strength; identification; protection from the environment; organoleptic properties such as taste and mouth-feel; drug loading; and/or to modify their release characteristics (such as enteric or sustained release). In the vast majority of applications, pan coating is preferred to the fluidized bed method due to the lesser degree of mechanical stress imparted to the tablets. Most commonly supplied for handling product in a defined batch, they range in size from the lab scale of a few hundred grams (10–24 in. in diameter) to several hundred

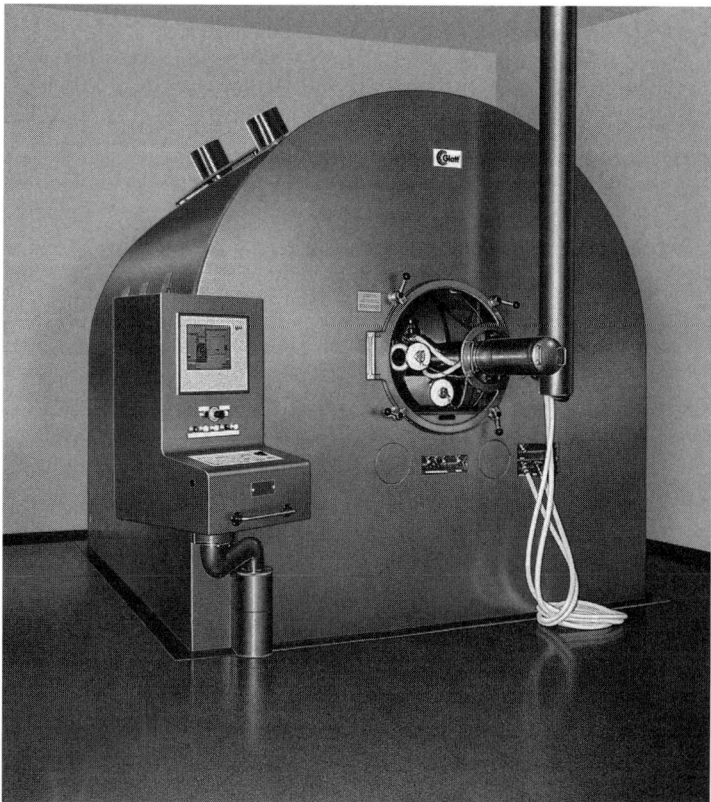

FIGURE 8 A representative example of a perforated pan coater. *Source*: Courtesy of Glatt Air Techniques, Inc.

kilograms in production machinery (up to 70 in. in diameter). The configuration of perforated pan coating equipment varies with the supplier, and there are several available. However, the product handling area has some common attributes. It is comprised of a perforated cylindrical section, oriented on a horizontal axis (Fig. 9). In most offerings the holes in this section of the pan or drum are round, in others they may be elongated. Additionally, the entirety of the cylindrical section may not be perforated—there may be some solid sections. The open area of the drum and the configuration and location of the process air and exhaust shoes or ducts also vary from vendor to vendor. The openings in the pan permit the process air to enter the interior of the drum and to draw air through the tablet bed and out. In most pans, the process air enters through the perforations and flows concurrent with the spray pattern. In other words, it is common for the air to enter the pan from its right side, behind the spray nozzles, flowing across them, towards the tablet bed surface. Its heat is exchanged for the moisture of the coating liquid, resulting in a drop in its dry bulb temperature, usually displayed as the exhaust air temperature. The exhaust shoe or duct, outside of the rotating drum and beneath the tablet bed, draws the air through the bed itself and evacuates it to a dust collector or other emission control devices. There are sufficient openings in the pan such that the distribution of airflow to the tablet bed and out of the pan may be more significantly governed by the bed itself and the configuration of the supply and exhaust air manifolds. It is important that the interface between the exhaust shoe and the perforated section of the pan be reasonably airtight. If not, the process air will "short-circuit" the tablet bed in favor of the "path of least resistance," the perforations in the pan outside of the tumbling bed. In this circumstance, drying of the tablet bed will be insufficient and product quality may be compromised.

On either side of the perforated segment of the drum are solid, truncated conical sections. A segment that encloses the rear of the pan is typically a vertical, solid wall, whereas the front conical section is enclosed by a glass door for visual observation of the process and for access to the tablets during the process (for sampling). To some degree,

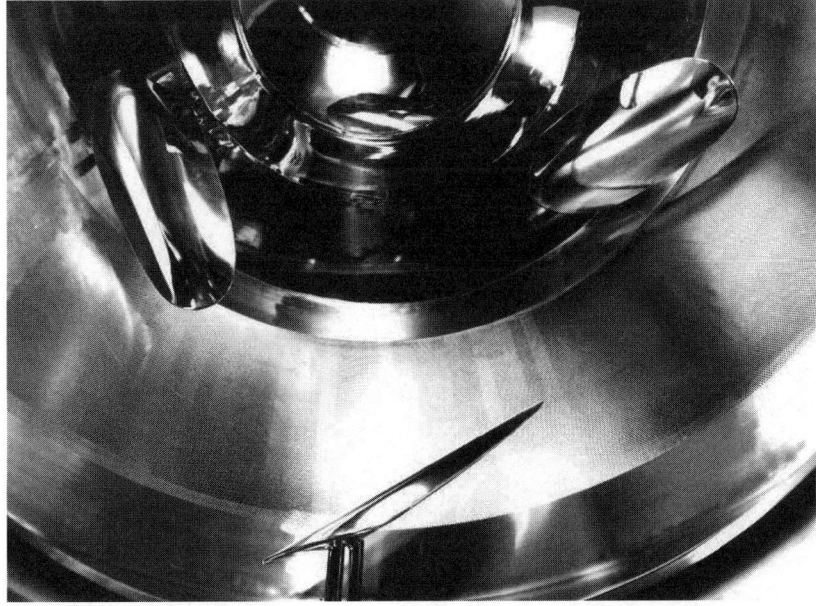

FIGURE 9 A representative example of a fully perforated drum in a pan coater. *Source*: Courtesy of Glatt Air Techniques, Inc.

the tapered sections of the pan assist with mixing by directing the outermost portions of the tumbling bed toward the perforated, cylindrical section of the drum. Rotation of the pan facilitates radial mixing of the tablet bed. Within the perforated section of the drum and along the tapered walls, baffles are located (Fig. 9). Their function is to enhance axial mixing of the tablet bed (front to rear). Radial and axial mixing is essential for ensuring the uniformity of distribution of the material being sprayed onto the tablet cores. Baffle geometry and positioning varies greatly with vendors. Combined with tablet geometry and the physical properties of the applied coating layer (particularly tackiness), these are often critical concerns, particularly during scale-up to production quantities. The ability to remove and replace the baffles to evaluate other geometries is desirable.

Typically in the front opening of the pan, some type of nozzle wand is anchored (in some versions it may enter through the rear pan wall). It contains one or more nozzles, depending on the horizontal depth of the pan. Small, laboratory machines usually have only one nozzle, whereas a production pan coater may contain as many as six. Air atomized nozzles predominate, though for applications using volatile organic solvents, a hydraulic, or pressure nozzle may be utilized. With solvents, the dry atomizing air is a significant contributor to evaporation as it shears the coating liquid to droplets often smaller than 20 µm. A consequent rapid rise in viscosity in the droplet may cause it to be incapable of spreading on contact with the tablet surface, yielding a porous coating. In the extreme case, some portion of the droplets will spray dry, negating their impact on the resultant product properties. This is particularly problematic for modified release coatings. The release behavior of all films should be governed by their intrinsic properties, and not by any degree of imperfection. This type of random porosity makes batch-to-batch and even tablet-to-tablet reproducibility a challenge. A hydraulic nozzle does not contribute to evaporation in this manner, and is worthy of consideration when the use of volatile solvents is mandated (due to a product's incompatibility with water).

Pneumatic nozzles prevail, but the spray pattern is somewhat different than found in a fluidized bed. In air suspension systems, the spray is usually a comparatively narrow, but solid cone of droplets. In a nozzle configured for perforated pan coating equipment, the initial spray pattern is also a solid cone. However, this pattern is flattened to an elliptical shape by the use of secondary atomizing air, delivered from openings adjacent to and angled slightly toward the primary atomized droplet stream (Fig. 10). In most nozzles, this secondary air is adjusted and controlled independently. The nozzle is

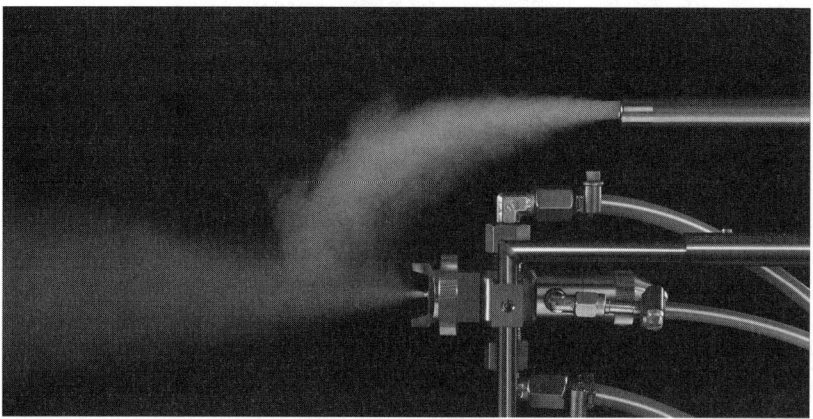

FIGURE 10 A traditional spray nozzle showing the influence of nozzle design on process air flow in the spray region. *Source*: Nozzle by Gustav Schlick Company and Glatt Air Techniques, Inc.

Coating Processes and Equipment

positioned such that the elliptical pattern covers as much of the horizontal width of the tablet bed as is practical, without spraying the exposed conical surfaces at the front and rear of the pan. As the horizontal depth of the pan increases in pilot and production sized coaters, additional nozzles are used to cover the front to rear surface of the tumbling bed. The width of the ellipse is adjusted such that there is minimal or no overlap of the spray patterns. The section of the wand inside the pan is further configured such that the nozzle's proximity to the surface of the cascading bed may be varied in two additional axes. The coating liquid is sprayed at essentially a right angle, or perpendicular (and at some distance) to the surface of the tumbling bed. In the second axis, it may be oriented such that the spray is applied high above the center of the downward angled cascading bed (dynamic angle of repose). In other words, in a pan coater rotating clockwise, the tablets climb the left, inner wall of the pan, finally reaching the zenith of the bed. They reverse direction, tumbling to the right, at a downward angle. Soon after beginning this cascade, as they approach or reach their peak velocity, they encounter the droplets of coating, having traveled less than half of the distance to the base of the bed. In this manner, the sprayed and now damp tablet surfaces are exposed to the dry process air for a longer duration before folding under at the far wall of the perforated section of the pan.

Process Considerations

Mixing

Several factors contribute to distribution uniformity of applied materials (coatings or layers), and several researchers have reported their findings. Pan speed, pan loading (vertical depth of the bed), tablet shape and size and the presence or absence of mixing baffles all have an impact on the movement of tablets in the pan (14). Axial mixing is also influenced by the geometry of baffles and the horizontal depth of the pan (front to rear), which varies with pan size, becoming of greater concern in production equipment. It is important that the equipment and process enable the tablets to appear in the spray zones with regularity and frequency.

Researchers have also reported on the influence of tablet shape on the distribution uniformity of applied materials. A spherical shape yields the best uniformity owing to the fact that there is no preferred spatial orientation—all surfaces are presented to the spray pattern over time. However, there are few products presented as spherical tablets, and as tablet shape becomes flatter, it is more likely that there will be a preferred spatial orientation in the tablet bed. The broader and flatter the tablet, the more likely it is to pass through the spray zone with its flat face exposed. Consequently, the face will have a thicker coating than the edges (15). A higher pan speed may mitigate this tendency to an extent and is worthy of investigation. Other researchers have found that tablet shape strongly affects distribution uniformity. Wilson and Crossman concluded that the most dramatic difference was shown by large oval tablets, followed by small oval tablets, then caplets. The round tablet showed the lowest relative thickness variation (16).

Spraying

Nozzle shape and geometry may contribute to processing challenges. In general, the atomizing air (primary and secondary) velocity is considerably higher than that of the concurrently flowing process air, in fact, approaching supersonic speeds. This may create a Venturi effect at the base of the spray pattern. The shape and size of the nozzle body and head or air cap (the nozzle itself may be an aerodynamic device), enhance the likelihood of turbulent eddies at or near the nozzle. The consequence is that droplets may backflow toward the head, depositing on the nozzle itself. The heated process air will dry them, and eventually a thin layer of film will coat the nozzle. As the film thickens, it is likely that its internal stresses will exceed its adhesion to the stainless steel surfaces of the nozzle, causing it to peel. If this occurs in the region of atomization or spray pattern formation, the pattern may become deformed, possibly concentrating it onto a smaller region of the tumbling tablets, or worse, causing incomplete atomization of the liquid. This will result in localized over-wetting, adversely affecting the coating properties and/or tablet appearance. Recently, nozzle and/or pan coating vendors have introduced nozzles with more streamlined profiles, particularly with respect to the air cap to avoid this type of 'over-spray' and its negative consequences (Fig. 11).

A second factor in nozzle fouling is related to process airflow. Thermodynamics dictate that the volume of process air impacts productivity. At a given temperature, the higher the flow, the greater the drying capacity. However, a high volume of air, flowing through the small openings in the pan or even at right angles to the bed, may cause significant turbulence inside of the pan. Again, this turbulence may adversely impact the behavior of the nozzles. In the extreme, over-spray will coat not only the nozzles, but also the wand and the exposed solid conical walls of the pan. It is also highly likely that the air leaving the pan is far from saturated—much of this capacity leaves the system unused. It is therefore prudent to select an air volume that is effective at heat and mass transfer, but minimizes the potential for turbulence in the region of the spray nozzles. It is also recommended to explore methods for enhancing the transit of tablets through the spray zone, and to maximize the interface between the tablets and coating droplets (to enlarge the coating "zone").

Using pneumatic nozzles, the droplet size is a function of the air to liquid mass ratio. The higher the atomizing air volume, the smaller the droplet size at a given spray rate. Tablet surface properties may be impacted by the droplet size. What is notable is that as atomizing air volume and pressure are raised, the velocity also increases. The distance between the nozzles and the tumbling bed is comparatively small, usually 6–12 in. If the droplets leave the nozzle at near supersonic speeds, their collision with the tablet surfaces may result in "bounce." A proportion of the spray liquid will bounce off of the surface of the tablets, and in the extreme, it may find its way to the walls of the pan or even become spray dried, decreasing the so-called coating efficiency. If it is possible, the exhaust shoe opening should be adjusted to create a velocity of process air through the

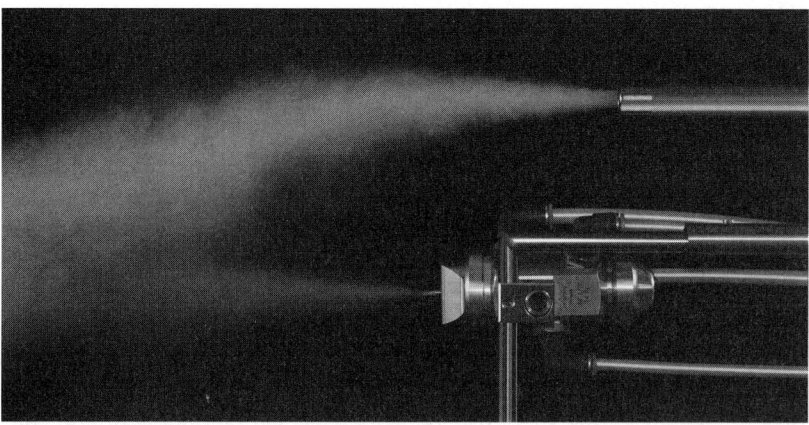

FIGURE 11 Spray nozzle designed to reduce turbulence in the spray region to prevent fouling. *Source*: Nozzle by Gustav Schlick Company and Glatt Air Techniques, Inc.

GENERAL PROCESSING CONSIDERATIONS FOR FILM COATING

The fluidized bed and perforated pan coating techniques described above have several process variables in common. A list of general process variables is shown in Table 1.

It is useful to examine each of the major categories listed in Table 1 and their influence on properties of the materials being processed.

Evaporation Rate

The rate of evaporation of the application media can significantly affect the properties of the applied layer or film using both aqueous and organic solvent systems (vendors of the coating material may recommend product temperatures for processing at which their materials will perform as intended). Process air volume, temperature, and dew point are the three components of this variable. In fluidized bed processing, the process air volume is a confounding variable. It not only delivers heat for evaporation of the application media and carries away the resultant vapor mass, it strongly impacts the fluidization pattern (pattern density and particle velocity). If possible, it should remain at the same value for the duration of the spray steps in the process. Any change in process airflow at the same temperature and absolute humidity (dew point) will also affect the product temperature. Unless the spray rate is also raised, the product temperature will drift upwards. If changes in the fluidization air volume are necessitated by an increasing batch weight or significant changes in the fluidization behavior of the substrate bed, these changes should be minor (usually not more than 10%), and at the same point in time for each batch.

In perforated pan coating, the process air volume does not materially influence the flow properties of the tablet bed. However, as described previously, it may impact turbulence in the region of the spray nozzles, increasing the potential for fouling. It is common that the process air volume remains the same for all of the spray steps in film coating. A further characteristic of pan coating is that the tumbling tablet bed may be considered to be a "dense phase" where the tablets are always in contact with each other. This is in contrast with the dilute phase behavior in the coating of substrates using a fluidized bed. As a consequence, there is not quite the intimate contact between the substrate and the drying medium for rapid evaporation. Contrasting the initial steps of a pan coating process with that of a fluidized bed may distinguish this. In both types of equipment, it is a common practice to pre-condition the machine's air-handling unit. This

TABLE 1 Process Variables Common to Coating Techniques

(A) Evaporation rate	Process air volume
	Process air temperature
	Process air dew point
(B) Droplet size	Atomization air pressure and volume
	Liquid spray rate
	Coating liquid properties
(C) Solids application rate	Liquid solution concentration
	Liquid spray rate

is done so that the process air temperature and dew point (where applicable) may come to equilibrium at a process air volume at or exceeding that to be used for the first step of the coating recipe. Just prior to loading the uncoated cores, the product-handling portion of the machine (the pan or fluid bed machine tower) is pre-heated. When the equipment is ready for use, the cores are loaded. Here is where the processes diverge. Fluidization is more mechanically stressful than tumbling in a perforated pan; therefore minimizing fluidization of uncoated core material is desirable. Taking advantage of the rapid and immediate capabilities for heat and mass transfer offered by dilute phase fluidization, the product warm-up step is usually limited to 1 minute. Spraying commences irrespective of the proximity of the product temperature to its ultimate target. Rapid heat and mass transfer by the warm fluidization air prevent penetration of the core by the coating material's application media. In the perforated pan, after loading of the cores, it is common practice to draw the conditioned process air through the static bed for a period of time to pre-heat the tablets to the desired product temperature. Intermittent jogging of the pan mixes the tablet bed to assure a reasonable distribution of heat in the bed. When the target product temperature is achieved, pan rotation becomes continuous and spraying is initiated.

In addition to the volume of the processing air, drying capacity for water-based systems is affected by the process air temperature and absolute humidity. Drying behavior for water-based materials for all types of processes may be illustrated using psychometrics. It should be noted that the data presented hereafter are for sea level conditions and have been derived using psychometry software. If processing is conducted in a location well above sea level, the input data should be adjusted accordingly.

In psychometry there are many properties representing the behavior of water in air, but only a few are important for this discussion. The temperature as we would normally measure it with a thermometer, but shielded from radiation or moisture is known as the dry bulb temperature. A dry bulb thermometer wrapped with cloth and wetted with water (by wicking) and exposed to air will reveal the wet bulb temperature. Air that is not saturated with moisture will evaporate water when passed over the cloth wick. This evaporative cooling will reduce the temperature of the thermometer in proportion to the drying capacity of the air. The larger the temperature difference between the dry and wet bulb temperatures, the lower the relative humidity of the air (defined as the percent of moisture in the air compared to how much would be in the air if it were saturated). Since this reflects the distance from saturation, it is related to the mass transfer driving force. The wet and dry bulb temperatures may be used to derive the dew point of the air, or the temperature at which the air is saturated, or at 100% relative humidity. Another term of interest is the absolute humidity, which is expressed as the weight of moisture over the weight of dry air. This is a good way to express humidity since it does not depend on the pressure or temperature of the air.

The example shown in Table 2 will illustrate the behavior of process air and a water-wet granulation for fluidized bed drying, assuming that water moves freely within the drying granules. Ambient air is drawn into the air-handling unit of the machine and dehumidified to a dew point temperature of 10 °C (7.6 g of water per kg of dry air). It is then heated to 60 °C for processing, and this drops its relative humidity to about 6%. Drawn through the batch of wet product, the process air exchanges heat for moisture and the product temperature, at steady state, drops to about 26 °C. The relative humidity of the exhaust air is essentially saturated, at about 99%, and the air now leaving the processor contains 21.2 g of water per kg of dry air for a water removal rate of 13.6 g of water per kg of dry air. Though this example ignores the process air volume, what it teaches is that each kg of air drawn through the batch will remove 13.6 g of water. Depending on its

TABLE 2 Illustration of Fluidized Bed Drying for a Granulation in which Water Moves Freely

Property	Process air	Process air dew point	Product/exhaust
Temperature (°C)	60	10	26.0
Absolute humidity (g/kg)	7.62	7.62	21.22
Relative humidity (%)	6.2	100	99.4

Note: Data derived using psychometry software.

temperature, a cubic meter of air weighs approximately 1.0 kg. In a production machine, if the process air volume is 5,000 m³/hr (about 3,000 ft³/min), under these conditions, the air can remove about 88 kg of water in 1 hour.

In fluidized bed drying, the process is isothermal. A few centimeters above the base of the product container, the speed of heat, and mass transfer is readily apparent. The temperature of the product bed is essentially the same radially and axially across the bed. At any elevation in the product container and the lower extremity of the expansion chamber, the temperature is the same. Similarly, the air leaving the processor is equally cooled and essentially saturated with moisture (during the constant rate zone of drying). Virtually the entirety of the product-handling volume of the processor is employed in the drying process. The mammoth surface area of contact between the drying air and product particles and the speed of their motion yield a process that may be referred to as being a "macro" state.

In the coating process, there is a significant difference to be considered. Coating starts with a substrate that is essentially dry, and takes place in a more finite or "micro" environment. While the process air's drying capacity is a consideration, maximizing the interface between the moving substrate particles and the atomized droplets—or "coating zone" is of paramount importance. Coating takes place on the surface of the substrate, and there is little if any penetration of the comparatively dry core by water. Contrary to the granule drying example, in film coating there is no reservoir of water to keep the surface of the substrate saturated with moisture. Consequently, a coating process never results in the exhaust air approaching a saturated condition, its relative humidity is always less than 100%. For sake of illustration, we will modify the previous example slightly (Table 3). Assume that the process air volume for the coating process is again 5,000 m³/hr with an air density of about 1.0 kg per cubic meter. It is dehumidified to 10 °C and heated to 60 °C for coating. The spray rate is 1000 g/min for a coating solution containing 10% solids (900 g/min based on water alone). The water addition (and removal) rate is 54 kg/hr, or 10.8 g of water per kg of dry air when distributed over the volume or mass of process air. Evaporative cooling drops the air/product temperature to 32.9 °C and elevates the relative humidity of the exhaust air to 58.3%.

One final illustration (Table 4) will show the influence of allowing the process air dew point to vary. All process conditions are replicated with one exception, the process

TABLE 3 Illustration of Drying Behavior for a Coating Process

Property	Process air	Process air dew point	Product/exhaust
Temperature (°C)	60	10	32.9
Absolute humidity (g/kg)	7.62	7.62	18.42
Relative humidity (%)	6.2	100	58.3

TABLE 4 Illustration of Drying Behavior for a Coating Process

Property	Process air	Process air dew point	Product/exhaust
Temperature (°C)	60	15	33.0
Absolute humidity (g/kg)	10.65	10.65	21.45
Relative humidity (%)	8.6	100	67.1

Note: Data derived using psychometry software. Dew point is elevated to 15°C.

air dew point is now at 15 °C. Examine the influence on product temperature and exhaust air relative humidity. In a coating process, the incidence of agglomeration (for multiparticulates) may be related to what is referred to as an "exit air relative humidity threshold." As the spray rate is increased and the process air temperature elevated to accommodate the moisture, the relative humidity of the process air moves toward saturation. The closer the air is to being saturated, the less is the driving force. In other words, the air begins to lose its ability to draw the moisture from the film, whose affinity for moisture will eventually dominate. At this threshold, there may be sufficient surface moisture to cause liquid bridges to form between particles, resulting in the formation of agglomerates. With some latex films, this surface "tackiness" may end in the partial or complete collapse of the batch (bed stalling). In the previous example, with the process air controlled to a dew point of 10 °C, the exhaust or exit air relative humidity was about 58%. Assume that the exit air humidity threshold for this product is 60%, beyond this value, either agglomeration begins to occur or the bed begins to stall. In the example that follows, nothing changes except that the process air dew point is raised to 15 °C, a seemingly minor difference. The relative humidity of the heated process air (at 60 °C) has risen from only 6.2% (with the dew point at 10 °C) to 8.6%. Superficially there is little impact on drying capacity. In fact, the slight increase in absolute humidity has almost no impact on the product temperature, which rises only 0.1 °C. A process operator would certainly not be alarmed by this insignificant difference. However, the exit air relative humidity has risen by 9% to 67.1%, well beyond the stated exit air humidity threshold.

As stated previously, the product temperature used during the coating process may significantly influence the behavior of an applied film. What is not as obvious is that the exhaust air relative humidity may also dramatically impact the release properties of the film. If the coating is applied to impart sustained release properties, the residual moisture in the film may alter its initial release profile, particularly with some latex films. A common problem is that the water is entrapped in the dense film and cannot be removed by a short drying step in the coating equipment, as a step subsequent to the spraying process. Its removal is not a heat and mass transfer problem, but is more likely related to diffusion through the coating membrane. Products such as this will likely need to be oven dried for a period of hours or days in an attempt to fully coalesce the film so that its release no longer changes.

Some equipment installations may not have process air handling units fitted with humidity control. It is evident that seasonal variations in absolute humidity can have an impact on productivity and product quality. However, if the product is robust and quality can be achieved under a relatively broad range of processing conditions, it is possible to adjust a few of the processing parameters to maintain equivalent drying conditions. An "environmental equivalency factor" (EEF) is described Novit (17). A computer model is used to calculate the mass and energy balances, characterizing the dryness or wetness of the coating pan environment. It then uses the exhaust air temperature and dew point to derive the EEF, a dimensionless number. Within a reasonable operating range, process variables such as air volume, temperature and spray rate may be adjusted in response to variation in ambient dew point. Under these circumstances, the EEF is replicated indicating that the water vapor environment inside the pan is similar.

Nearly all types of coating processes will benefit from a consistent process air dew point. Humidity control systems may be complex, incorporating dehumidifiers (for dew point reduction to about 5–10 °C), desiccant dryers (for products requiring low product temperatures and dew points below 0 °C), steam humidifiers (to increase dew point in cold, dry weather), etc. It is suggested that laboratory trials be conducted to evaluate product and process sensitivity to variations in inlet air dew point.

Droplet Size

A discussion on spraying is incomplete without a discourse on nozzle maintenance and testing. In any coating application, the spray nozzle is the single most critical component. Its performance dictates droplet size control, the quality of the applied film and the reproducibility of the resultant product properties. These include appearance, potency, film coating efficiency, and release characteristics. In retrospective process troubleshooting, spray nozzle performance is often the leading cause of product deviations.

Droplet size is governed by several factors, including the atomizing air pressure and volume, the liquid spray rate, and liquid properties such as the surface tension and viscosity. In general, irrespective of the process technique used, droplet size should be small relative to the particle size of product to be coated. For most coating equipment fitted with pneumatic nozzles, the qualified operating range for atomizing pressure is typically from about 1 bar (14.7 psi) to as much as 6 bar (nearly 90 psi). Irrespective of nozzle design, the lower the atomizing air pressure, the lower the atomizing air volume and velocity. For illustration, coating of tablets using 2 bar (30 psi) pressure may be sufficient to produce droplets yielding good film properties. Higher pressure and air volume will result in a higher atomization air velocity, increasing kinetic energy at the interface between the spray pattern and slower moving substrate. This would increase the potential for droplet "bounce" or spray drying, as mentioned earlier.

When coating small particles using a fluidized bed, a somewhat higher atomization air pressure may be necessary to achieve small droplet size and thereby avoid agglomeration. There is some risk, however, that the high shear associated with pressures in the 3–6 bar (45–90 psi) range, depending on the type and size of the spray nozzle, may cause breakage of fragile core material. This is especially true for production-sized nozzles that use significant quantities of compressed air to accommodate high spray rates. The Gustav Schlick Company, in Coburg, Germany, is a supplier of spray nozzles in widespread use in fluidized bed processing. The 970 series nozzle is found in small top spray (up to about 5 liters), small Wurster bottom spray coaters (3.5, 4, 6, 7, and 9 in.) and laboratory scale rotor or centrifugal processors (up to about 5 L). With water-like materials, it is useable in a spray rate range of approximately 0–100 g/min. Figure 12 is a graph that shows the influence of atomization air pressure on mean droplet size for water sprayed at 25 g/min (data by Schlick). Interestingly, increasing the pressure beyond 2 bar does little to decrease the droplet size. This is in part due to the fact that 25 g/min is well within the nozzle's ability to atomize. What should be noted is that if a process is being run in which agglomeration is a minor problem and increasing the atomization air pressure seems to improve the situation, it is likely a consequence of the increased air velocity and kinetic energy, not a smaller droplet size.

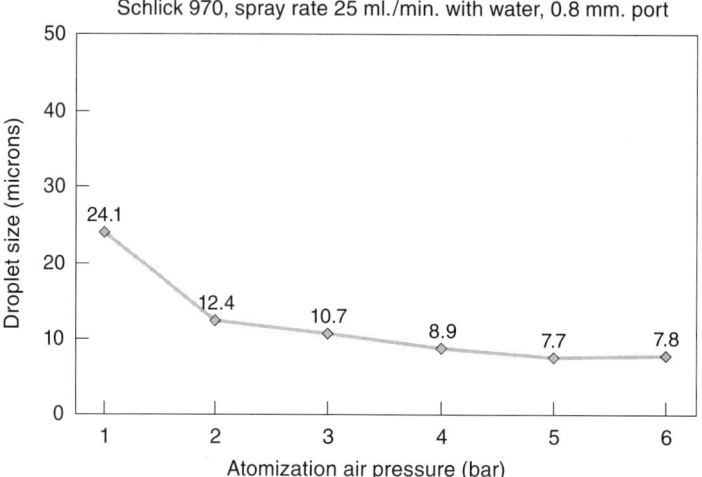

FIGURE 12 Droplet size and atomization air pressure for a Schlick 970 series nozzle.

Looking at the performance envelope of the Schlick 940 series nozzle (Fig. 13), which is used in pilot scale top spray, some intermediate Wursters and pilot/production scale rotors, it can be seen that droplet size increases with faster spray rates (at a constant atomization air pressure). In cases where the spray rate is 250 g/min or less, it is possible to increase atomization air pressure/volume/velocity to achieve droplets smaller than 20 μm. However, the data shown for the 500 g/min rate demonstrates that even at the highest practical atomization air pressure (6 bar), it is not possible to produce 20 μm droplets (for the small nozzle orifice size). This is an important consideration in larger capacity equipment where there may be significant drying capacity, and the rate limiting factor is the inability of the nozzle to atomize liquid (to a satisfactory droplet size) at the rate at which the process air may remove the resultant water vapor. The only possibility for taking advantage of the increased drying capacity is to enlarge the nozzle (use more compressed air at the same pressure) or to use multiple nozzles.

As shown, the 940 series nozzle is unable to produce droplets smaller than 20 μm at 500 g/min using water, even at very high atomization air pressures. A process that has excessive drying capacity but is limited by droplet size (e.g., fine particle coating) will result in unnecessarily hindered productivity. In a production Wurster processor,

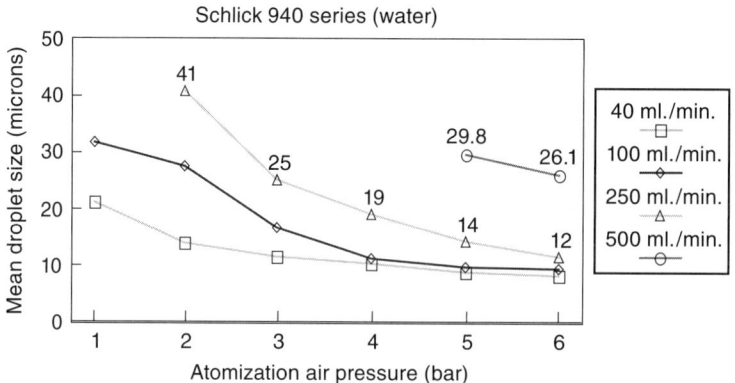

FIGURE 13 Droplet size and atomization air pressure for a Schlick 940 series nozzle.

upgrading to the HS (Schlick model 0/4) nozzle (Fig. 14), which uses substantially more compressed air at the same atomization air pressures (approximately three times the volume of the 940 series nozzle), will result in a dramatic improvement in drying capacity utilization. The graph depicts a droplet profile which is similar to the 940 series nozzle spraying at 250 g/min with the exception that the HS data is for 1000 g/min, a spray rate four times that of the 940 series nozzle. This permits the HS nozzle to be operated at low atomizing air volumes and pressures, limiting the potential for attrition due to high kinetic energy.

The surface tension and viscosity of the coating liquid also play a key role in product performance. Many of the available latex coating materials have very low surface tension and may be atomized to small droplets at low atomizing air pressures and volumes. The advantage is that the concomitant low kinetic energy assures that there will be a reduced potential for attrition of the substrate, particularly during the early stages of coating when the substrate is at highest risk. Of greater significance is the viscosity of the liquid. Pneumatic nozzles can atomize liquids with viscosities up to approximately 250 cP. However, at this high viscosity, the resultant droplets may not be ideal for film formation. Viscose liquids have a strong tendency to incorporate foam during their preparation. Forced or passive de-aeration prior to their use is strongly recommended. Formed droplets will have a high degree of surface area for evaporation and further concentration of solids as they travel through a heated air stream. With most liquids, the consequence is a further escalation in viscosity. Ultimately, the droplet may essentially retain its shape on contact with the substrate, resisting spreading, which is necessary for the formation of a continuous and defect-free film. Although the high solids content, leading to the thick liquid, could result in a faster process, if the film is imperfect its quality and reproducibility may be poor.

Solids Application Rate

Coated substrates are nearly universally stronger than uncoated cores. For this reason, it is incumbent to apply a protective layer as quickly as possible. To some extent this is governed by the initial process conditions (such as evaporation rate and the spray rate).

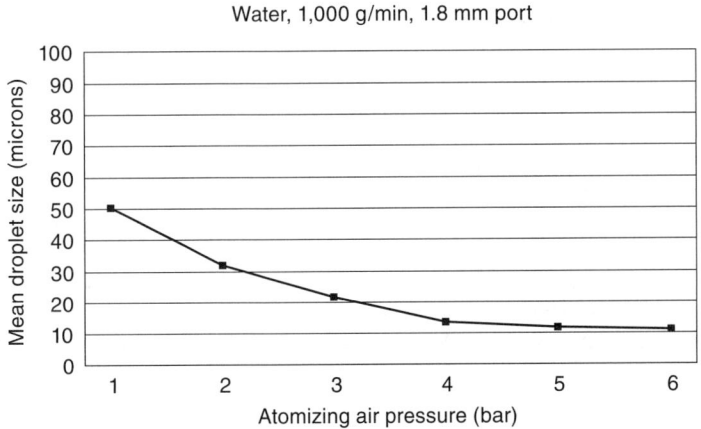

FIGURE 14 Droplet size and atomization air pressure for Schlick 0/4 (HS Wurster) series nozzles.

However, it is more dramatically influenced by the total solids content of the coating liquid. Though a high viscosity may compromise film quality, dilution of a coating material should not be a unanimous choice. Many latex materials possess a very low viscosity, even with the polymer solids content at 30% or more. If a plasticizer is necessary, it is prudent to add it to the coating liquid in its highest solids content to permit the highest uptake in the polymer (remaining plasticizer may stay in the water phase). Any dilution of the base liquid should involve only a quantity of water sufficient to externally incorporate other excipients such as anti-tacking agents, colorants, etc. This dispersion is then added to the polymer concentrate while mixing. Provided that the viscosity remains low, the optimized solids content will help to get a protective 'seal coat' onto the substrate quickly. Once a thin layer envelops the core, spraying may be accelerated to result in a rapid and economical process, irrespective of the type of process being utilized.

SUMMARY

Coating of substrates ranging from sub-100 μm particles to tablets is conducted widely in the pharmaceutical industry. Films may be applied using water or organic solvent-based liquids. The evaporative efficiency of fluidized bed equipment and the ability to apply a film to particles discretely suspended in an air stream have resulted in widespread use of this technique. The three fluidized bed methods are not functionally equivalent, but offer a broad variety of applications. These methods have some common features and process variables, but each has unique advantages and limitations. Tablet coating proliferates, with an increased interest in factors impacting the distribution uniformity of applied liquids in modified fluidized beds as well as in perforated pans. For the majority of applications, the perforated pan is the process of choice. Delivery of process air, liquids, and mixing of the substrate varies with suppliers. In the development of a product with commercialization as the ultimate goal, criteria such as economics, product, and process variables, and dosage form performance must be considered.

REFERENCES

1. Mehta A. Factors in the development of oral controlled release dosage forms. Pharm Manufact 1986; 31:23–29.
2. Jones DM, Percel PJ, Coating of multiparticulates using molten materials: formulation and process considerations. In: Ghebre-Sellassie I, ed. Multiparticulate Oral Drug Delivery. New York: Marcel Dekker, Inc., 1994; 113–42.
3. Jozwiakowski M, Franz R, Jones D. Characterization of a hot-melt fluid bed coating process for fine granules. Pharm Res 1990; 7(11):1119.
4. Geldart D. The effect of particle size and size distribution on the behaviour of gas fluidized beds. Powder Tech 1972; 6(4):201–15.
5. Darton RC, La Nauze RD, Davidson JF, Harrison D. Bubble growth due to coalescence in fluidised beds. Trans Inst Chem Engrs 1977; 55:274.
6. Davidson JF, Harrison D. Fluidization. New York: Academic Press, 1971; Chapters 2,4.
7. Harrison D, Leung LS. Bubble formation at an orifice in a fluidized bed. Trans Inst Chem Engrs 1961; 39:409.
8. Geldart D. Types of gas fluidization. Powder Tech 1973; 7(5):285–92.
9. Kunii D, Levenspiel O. Fluidization Engineering. Melbourne, FL: R.E. Krieger Publishing Co., 1984.

10. Vanecek V, Markvart M, and Drbohlav R. Fluidized Bed Drying. London: Lennard Hill, 1966.
11. Wurster DE. Air suspension technique of coating drug particles—a preliminary report. J Am Pharm Assoc 1959; 48:451.
12. Wurster DE. US patents 3,196,827; 3,241,520.
13. Jones DM. US patents 5,236,503; 5,437,889.
14. Pandey P, Turton R. Movement of different-shaped particles in a pan-coating device using novel video-imaging techniques. AAPS PharmSciTech 2005; 6(2):E237.
15. Frisbee SE, Mehta KA, McGinity JW. Processing factors that influence in vitro and in vivo performance of film-coated drug delivery systems. www.drugdeliverytech.com/cgi-bin/articles.cgi?idArticle=25, accessed July, 2007.
16. Wilson KE, Crossman E. The influence of tablet shape and pan speed on intra-tablet film coating uniformity. Drug Dev Ind Pharm 1997; 23(12):1239–43.
17. Novit ES. Understanding the effects of process-air humidity on tablet coating. Tablets and Capsules Magazine April 2006.

12
Aqueous Polymeric Film Coating

Dave A. Miller and James W. McGinity
College of Pharmacy, University of Texas at Austin, Austin, Texas, U.S.A.

BACKGROUND

Origins of Aqueous Film Coating

Film coating of pharmaceutical dosage forms has evolved from its rudimentary origins to become a sophisticated science that has contributed immeasurably to the advancement of drug delivery. The earliest application of pharmaceutical coating has been attributed to Rhazes (850–932 AD) who coated pills with the mucilage of psyllium seeds to mask unpleasant taste (1). Other early coating systems involved the application of gold and silver, talc, waxes, and gelatin to pills and tablets (2–4). These early coatings were typically applied to substrates individually by supporting them with forceps or mounting them on a needle and repeatedly dipping the articles into the coating fluid. The origin of large scale film-coating of pharmaceuticals began with the adoption of sugar coating from the candy industry which utilized the batch pan coating process. The first sugar-coated pills were made available in the United States in 1842 (5) and shortly thereafter were being manufactured in the United States in 1856 (6). Film coating with polymers emerged in the 1950s as a more efficient alternative to sugar coating due to a substantial reduction in drying time by the utilization of volatile organic solvents as the dispersion media. In addition, film coating offered the benefit of less rigid coats which reduced cracking and other coat defects and allowed for the successful coating of substrates other than tablets, i.e., powders, granules, pellets, and capsules. Although film coating with polymeric materials from organic solution offered many initial benefits, ultimately these coating systems lost their favor due to flammability, toxicity, environmental, and cost related issues. These problems regarding organic solvent-based film coating led pharmaceutical manufacturers to re-evaluate aqueous-based coating systems. By this time, coating equipment had substantially improved beyond the early pan coating systems, and thus drying efficiency with aqueous coating systems was no longer a prohibitive problem.

Latex vs. Pseudolatex Coating Dispersions

The movement of the pharmaceutical industry away from volatile solvents for coating applications coupled with advancements in coating equipment design led to an increase in the popularity of latex and pseudolatex coating systems. Latexes and pseudolatexes are both colloidal dispersions of polymer droplets in a continuous aqueous phase, the difference between them being that latex systems are formed by emulsion polymerization while pseudolatexes are produced by emulsifying a preformed polymer. The production procedure for latex dispersions involves emulsifying monomers in aqueous media by the use of surfactants and then introducing an initiator that catalyzes polymer chain growth within surfactant micelles typically by radical polymerization mechanisms. The resulting dispersion contains spherical polymer particles stabilized in the continuous aqueous phase by a surfactant shell.

Pseudolatexes are typically produced by dissolving the polymer in an organic solvent and then introducing this solution into aqueous media containing surfactants and stabilizers that limit particle aggregation by hydrophobic attraction of polymer droplets in aqueous media. This mixture is then homogenized and the organic phase is subsequently evaporated to yield a dispersion of stabilized, spherical polymer particles in a continuous aqueous phase. The solids content in latex and pseudolatex dispersions is commonly maximized at about 30% by weight. The average diameter of these polymer particles usually lies within the range of 0.1–0.3 µm. Maintaining a particle diameter within this range is important for colloidal stability as particles of larger diameter will have a greater tendency to settle on storage potentially resulting in particle aggregation and caking that would render the dispersion unsuitable for coating applications. Particle size is not only vital to colloidal stability, but to film formation as well.

Film Formation with Latexes and Pseudolatexes

The following description of the film formation mechanism for latexes and pseudolatexes is intentionally brief. The enquiring reader is referred to Wheatley and Steuernagel for a more in-depth discussion (7).

In general, continuous films are formed from latex and pseudolatex emulsions by fusion of the polymeric spheres contained in these aqueous colloidal dispersions. For the sake of brevity, the spherical polymeric particles contained in latex and pseudolatex dispersions will be referred in this section simply as latex particles. The process begins with the application of a thin film of the aqueous dispersion to the surface of a substrate which is typically accomplished by a spraying method. In this thin aqueous layer, the latex particles are held suspended throughout by electrostatic repulsion. As the dispersant liquid evaporates, the film volume is reduced, thus drawing latex particles into closer proximity until they ultimately make contact and form an ordered array of spherical polymeric particles on the substrate surface. Residual water from the dispersion remains entrapped within the interstitial spaces of this particle array. As this residual liquid evaporates, capillary action compresses adjacent particles causing them to deform while bringing them into intimate contact. This begins the process of neighboring particle coalescence and global fusion of polymer spheres on the substrate surface that ultimately produces a continuous film.

Complete fusion of the polymer particles entails interdiffusion of polymer chains contained within the latex spheres. However, for interdiffusion to occur the polymer chains must be sufficiently mobile on a molecular level such that chain ends are able to cross the interface between two merging particles to penetrate the neighboring polymer network and bridge the two particles. Plasticization is often required to impart sufficient molecular mobility and promote interdiffusion of polymer chains. The mechanism of plasticization involves interference with intermolecular interactions between polymer chains to reduce polymer cohesion and thus promote polymer chain mobility. The macroscopic result of plasticization is a reduction in the characteristic temperature at which a polymer transitions from a brittle, glassy state into a rubbery, malleable state.

This characteristic temperature is known as the glass transition temperature (T_g) of the polymer. The reduction in polymer T_g reduces the minimum temperature at which polymer interdiffusion can occur, thus decreasing the temperature at which continuous films can form. This critical temperature is known as the minimum film formation temperature (MFT) and in order for particle fusion to occur following latex particle contact and deformation, the temperature of the particles must exceed the MFT. Typically, for further coalescence of these particles to occur and a continuous film to form, post-treatment, or curing, is required. Curing involves storing the film coated articles in an environment that is heated above the MFT of the coating polymer and in some cases equilibrated at elevated humidity levels. During the curing process, sufficient energy is imparted on the polymer chains to promote molecular mobility and interdiffusion of polymers chains from adjacent latex particles. Therefore, following the curing process, complete coalescence of latex particles will have occurred and a continuous, equilibrated film will have formed over the surface of the substrate.

Substrates

Aqueous film coating has been applied to a variety of substrates for a number of different pharmaceutical applications. Tablets were the among the first film-coated substrates as film coating was a simple extension of early sugar coating applications by traditional pan coating processes. Today, pharmaceutical tablets are the most common substrates for film coating; however, pan coating is rarely used as the processing equipment has been substantially improved to provide better drying efficiencies and batch uniformity. As discussed above, the flexibility of film coating versus sugar coating brought about the possibility of applying coats to substrates other than tablets. Hence, film coating has expanded the list of commonly coated substrates to include multiparticulates such as pellets, non-pareils, granules, crystals, and powders as well as more delicate monolithic dosage forms such as hard and soft gelatin capsules.

FILM COATING FOR IMMEDIATE RELEASE APPLICATIONS

Initially, the applications of pharmaceutical film coating were similar to those of sugar coating; i.e., to mask the unpleasant taste or odors of active agents, to serve as a protective barrier to prevent degradation of the active initiated by environmental factors, to improve tablet chipping and dusting during handling, and to improve the pharmaceutical elegance of dosage forms. Although the applications of polymeric film coating of pharmaceutical dosage forms have become more varied and complex, these initial applications remain of the utmost importance to the design of solid dosage forms. In this section, the details of these immediate release applications of film coating are discussed along with the properties of the various coating systems utilized for each of these applications.

Taste Masking

When a medicament is delivered orally, particularly when the dosage form is designed for rapid drug release, taste can be a substantial problem as many drugs have unpleasant flavors. Eliminating an unpleasant flavor is essential to such dosage forms as poor patient compliance is expected when a dosage form is unpalatable. From a commercial perspective, an unpleasant flavor will result in reduced product sales as patients are likely to avoid a product with an unpleasant taste and show preference to a competing product that has been formulated to eliminate such flavor.

There are numerous strategies for masking the taste of active agents which include: the addition of flavoring agents, granulation, film coating, complexation with cyclodextrins, complexation with ion-exchange resins, spray congealing with lipids, freeze drying, emulsification, encapsulation in liposomes, as well as intimate mixing with taste masking excipients such as gelatin, gelatinized starch, lecithin, etc. (8). Of these techniques, polymeric film coating is one of the most often utilized because of its efficacy and simplicity. Additionally, film coating is a manufacturing process that is far more familiar to the pharmaceutical industry than some of these other techniques, and therefore is most often utilized.

Film coating masks the unpleasant tastes of drug molecules by acting as a physical barrier between the drug and taste buds. The film coat is designed to provide sufficient resistance to the permeation of saliva into the coated substrate to prevent dissolution of the active agent and eliminate the sensation of unpleasant taste. However, the film coat is only intended to serve as a barrier for a very brief time so as to not retard the rate of release of the active agent. Hence, polymers utilized in taste masking applications provide momentary resistance to the dissolution of the coated substrate while in the mouth of the patient, but dissolve rapidly and completely in the stomach.

Cosmetic Applications

Most solid oral dosage forms are colored not only to improve their appearance, but also to satisfy good manufacturing practices requirements that require products be differentiable at all stages during the manufacturing and distribution cycle (9). Therefore, film coating with pigments is essential in many cases to meet production regulations, and thus has vast importance to pharmaceutical manufacturing. Also, lustrous surfaces of solid pharmaceutical dosage forms are commonly recognized as more appealing to the consumer than a dull surface which often elicits an unfavorable impression as to the quality of its contents (10). Film coating is widely used to enhance the pharmaceutical elegance of dosage forms by increasing surface luster. Some active agents or excipients can cause a dosage form to appear spotted, mottled, or unpleasantly colored leading the consumer to believe the contents have degraded. In these cases, opaque coats are added to hide unsightly appearance. Brand recognition is also important with regard to the aesthetic appearance of pharmaceutical products. Particular colors and specific patterns on product surfaces are often utilized to render a dosage form more recognizable to consumers and to generate trademark protection opportunities. Therefore, with regard to the commercialization of pharmaceutical dosage forms, it is essential to consider appearance as it is an important factor with regard to consumer opinion and awareness.

Insulating/Protective Barrier

Film coating is often utilized to protect an active agent from environmental factors that may affect its physical and chemical stability, i.e., light, moisture, and air. The use of film coating as a moisture barrier can also protect the substrate from extensive moisture absorption that could lead to swelling and disintegration. Additionally, film coats can improve the mechanical integrity of tablets to reduce chipping and dusting during packaging and transport. With respect to tablet manufacturing, a protective film can increase productivity by reducing downtime required to clean tablet dust, and can reduce friction at the tablet surface to provide greater throughput by improving transport on high speed equipment. Thus, by simply providing a physical barrier surrounding a substrate, film coats can function in numerous ways to improve the stability, mechanical integrity, and processability of pharmaceutical dosage forms.

Improving Ease of Injestion/Swallowing

Film coated dosage forms have been reported to improve esophageal transit/swallowing over the uncoated counterpart (11). Film coatings can act as barriers to prevent adhesion of the dosage form to the esophagus and in this way act as a lubricant to improve the motility of dosage forms through the esophagus. Additionally, film coats can prevent disintegration of dosage forms in the esophagus that can lead to extensive adhesion of particulates to the esophagus. It is particularly important to avoid such adhesion with drugs such as aspirin, emepronium bromide, doxycycline, and potassium chloride as these are known irritants that can cause oesophagitis and possibly esophageal ulceration (12). Finally, film coatings can also be applied to cover sharp tablet edges and increase roundness such that the tablet will be easier and more comfortable to swallow.

Subcoats and Topcoats

Immediate release film coats are also used as subcoats that are applied to substrates prior to the addition of functional coatings. Subcoats are often necessary to improve the adhesion of functional films to the substrate. This not only improves continuous film formation but also increases coating efficiency by reducing the amount of the coating dispersion that must be applied to achieve the desired release profile. Subcoats are also applied to prevent the partitioning of active from the core into the outer coat as this can result in a burst release of drug and can impair film functionality. Immediate release film coats are also applied on top of functional coats to reduce adhesion of substrates caused by the tackiness of soft film coats after spraying. Topcoats can also be utilized to provide color or increase the gloss of film coated dosage forms.

Coating Materials for Immedite Release Applications

Water-Soluble Cellulose Ethers

Cellulose is the most abundant organic material found in nature (13). It is the primary component of plant cell walls and is therefore a large constituent of fruits and vegetables. Since cellulose is safe for human consumption, it is commonly used as an additive in food products. Cellulose and chemical derivatives of cellulose are also widely used as excipients in pharmaceutical applications. The biocompatibility of cellulose coupled with a molecular structure that is conducive to chemical modification, has made cellulose a staple of pharmaceutical formulations. Each anhydroglucose unit of the cellulose backbone contains three hydroxyl groups that provide reactive sites for chemical substitution. Thereby, cellulose can be chemically modified in a variety of ways to yield materials with differing properties useful for diverse pharmaceutical applications.

In the 1950s, patent literature began to emerge claiming the use of water-soluble cellulose ethers for film coating of pharmaceutical tablets intended for immediate release. The claimed utility of these coatings included: taste masking, odor sealing, protecting the substrate from oxidation and moisture, improving the appearance of the tablet, and improving the swallowability of tablets (14). The most commonly used water-soluble cellulose derivatives for film coating applications include hydroxyethyl cellulose (HEC), hydroxypropyl cellulose (HPC), and hydroxypropyl methylcellulose (HPMC). These materials are produced by reacting cellulose in alkaline solution with ethylene oxide, propylene oxide, and propylene oxide with methyl chloride to yield HEC, HPC, and HPMC, respectively. The different chemical substitutions on the cellulose backbone give these polymers their unique properties. The general structure of cellulose derivatives is shown in Figure 1 with the substitution corresponding to each polymer noted in the accompanying table. The degree of substitution can be varied for each of these polymers to yield different viscosity and solubility characteristics. Molecular weight can also be varied by partial hydrolysis during pretreatment to yield materials of

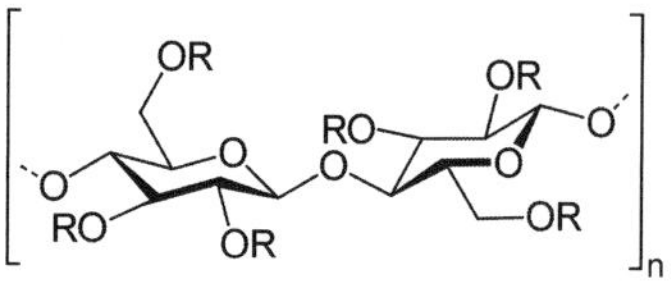

Polymer	Substituent groups (R)			
Ethyl cellulose (HEC)	—H	—CH$_2$CH$_3$		
Hydroxyethyl cellulose (HEC)	—H	—CHCH$_3$ | OH		
Hydroxypropyl cellulose (HPC)	—H	—CH$_2$CHCH$_3$ | OH		
Hydroxypropyl methylcellulose (HPMC)	—H	CH$_3$	—CH$_2$CHCH$_3$ | OH	
Cellulose acetate phthalate (CAP)	—H	CH$_3$C(=O)—	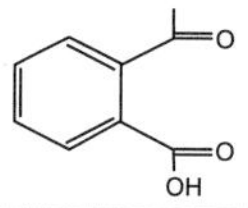 phthalate group	
Cellulose acetate succinate (CAS)	—H	CH$_3$C(=O)—	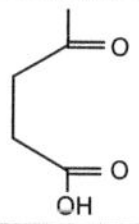 succinate group	
Cellulose acetate trimellitate (CAT)	—H	CH$_3$C(=O)—	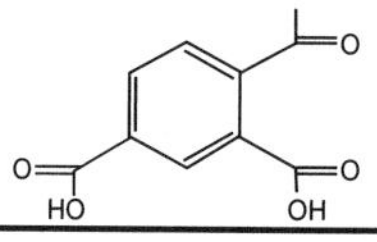 trimellitate group	
Hydroxypropylmethylcellulose phthalate (HPMCP)	—H	CH$_3$	—CH$_2$CHCH$_3$ | OH phthalate group 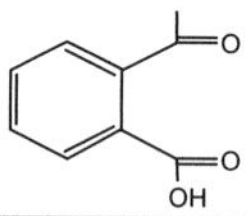	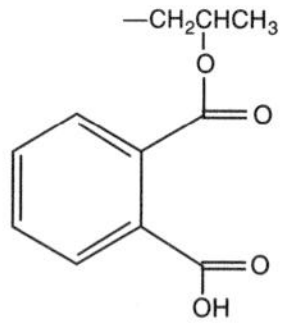 —CH$_2$CHCH$_3$ | O-phthalate
Hydroxypropylmethylcellulose acetate succinate (HPMCAS)	—H	CH$_3$C(=O)— CH$_3$	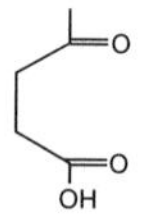 succinate group —CH$_2$CHCH$_3$ | OCOCH$_3$	—CH$_2$CHCH$_3$ | OH —CH$_2$CHCH$_3$ | OCOCH$_3$COO

FIGURE 1 Molecular structure of cellulose and its derivatives *Source*: From Ref. 37.

different viscosities and dissolution characteristics. Typically, low viscosity (<20 cP) grades of these polymers are used in film coating applications in order to facilitate the spraying process (15).

Of these water-soluble cellulose ethers, HPMC is the most commonly used cellulose for pharmaceutical film coating. The first published report demonstrating the use of HPMC for film coating applications appeared in 1962 in a patent by Singiser of Abbott Laboratories (16). However, widespread use of HPMC was not made possible until 1965 when low molecular weight grades (3, 6, and 15 mPa·s 2% solution in water at 20°C) were introduced by Shin-Etsu Chemical Co. Ltd., Tokyo, Japan (17). The advent of these low molecular weight grades, facilitated the spray application of HPMC from solutions with high polymer content (10–15%), thus improving the economy of coating with this polymer (18). HPMC is soluble in both aqueous media and some organic solvents which made it a popular polymer for early coating applications because it could be applied from organic solutions which gave excellent drying efficiency, yet would readily dissolve in gastrointestinal fluids. Even as concerns grew with the cost and health problems associated with the use of organic solvents, HPMC remained a popular coating material as high solids content aqueous solutions could also be used for coating applications.

HPMC is ideal for immediate release coating applications as it produces tough, yet flexible films that provide excellent protective barriers for coated substrates. With these properties, film coating with HPMC can increase the stability of the active, the mechanical integrity of the substrate, and provide a sufficient barrier for taste masking applications; yet is sufficiently soluble in gastrointestinal fluids so as not to retard drug release. HPMC films are clear but have excellent capacity for binding pigments, and thus can be easily colored and/or opacified. HPMC films are non-tacky, thus adhesion of coated dosage forms to each other and/or manufacturing equipment is not a problem.

The other water-soluble cellulose ethers used in film coating applications, HEC and HPC, have similar properties to HPMC with respect to aqueous solubility and general film functionality; however, some key distinctions exist that have limited the use of HEC and HPC in favor of HPMC. HEC is generally insoluble in organic solvents, and although it was one of the earliest water-soluble cellulose ethers used for film coating applications (14), its limited solubility in organic solvents restricted its industrial use as drying efficiency was a primary concern. Films produced from both HEC and HPC have a tendency to be tacky which limits production efficiency (18). Also, HEC and HPC films are more elastic and weaker in tension than HPMC films, and therefore are less resistant to breakage under mechanical stress (18–20). Therefore, HEC and HPC are most commonly used in conjunction with a primary film coating polymer, such as HPMC, to improve adhesion to the substrate and to improve film flexibility. Li et al. demonstrated the use of an HEC/HPMC combination for film coating of ibuprofen granules to be compressed into chewable tablets to mask the taste of the drug (19). To limit dissolution of the film in the patient's mouth, higher viscosity grades of HPMC were required; however, higher viscosity grades of HPMC formed more rigid films that were more susceptible to breakage. Therefore, HEC was included in the film to increase flexibility and breakage resistance under the forces of tablet compression and mastication of the final chewable tablet dosage form.

Commercial products based on these water-soluble cellulose ethers are readily available and in some cases are incorporated with additives as a complete prefabricated coating system. Opadry®, a product of Colorcon®, Inc., West Point, Pennsylvania, U.S.A., is a complete film coating system based on HPMC that contains both plasticizer as well as a customizable pigment and which can be used for both aqueous and organic coating. Numerous variations on the original Opadry formulation also exist containing various film forming materials. Bulk HPMC is available under a variety of brand names, but most notably as Methocel™ which is marketed by the Dow Chemical Company and Colorcon, Inc., and as Pharmacoat by the Shin-Etsu Chemical Company. A variety of HPMC grades are available that vary in molecular weight and degree of substitution to provide a range of viscosities and solubility characteristics to accommodate different applications. HPC is also available in a variety of grades of varying molecular weight and degrees of substitution. The leading commercial brand of HPC is Klucel® (Aqualon, Wilmington, Delaware, U.S.A.). HEC is available under the brand names Natrosol® and Cellosize™ (Aqualon, Wilmington, Delaware, U.S.A.) with different grades that vary similarly to HPC and HPMC. With each of these cellulose ethers, the low molecular weight grades are recommended for film coating applications.

Eudragit® E 100

Aminoalkyl Methacrylate Copolymer, known commercially as Eudragit E 100, (Röhm and Haas GmbH, Darmstadt, Germany) is a cationic copolymer produced by radical copolymerization of butyl methacrylate, dimethylaminoethyl methacrylate, and methyl methacrylate in a 1:2:1 ratio having an average molecular weight of 150,000 (21). The molecular structure of Eudragit E 100 is shown in Figure 2 with the corresponding substituent group noted in the accompanying table. The polymer is insoluble at pH greater than 5.5 (22), but becomes soluble at pH below 5.5 due to protonization of the dimethylaminoethyl pendant groups that results in a dense cationic charge on the polymer backbone that increases the hydrophilicity of the molecule. These solubility characteristics make Eudragit E 100 ideal for taste masking applications since the polymer is insoluble in saliva (pH 6.8–7.4), but readily soluble in gastric fluids (pH 1–1.5) (23). Thus, film-coated substrates will remain intact in the mouth of the patient protecting the taste buds from harshly flavored actives, but the film will disintegrate in the stomach allowing for rapid dissolution of the substrate. Hence, films of Eudragit E 100 function as taste masking barriers by a different mechanism than water-soluble cellulose ethers in that the pH dependence governs the disintegration of the film rather than a time lag to dissolution. Eudragit E 100 has been demonstrated to function as a protective film coat for moisture sensitive substrates and actives (24,25). As a protective barrier, Eudragit E

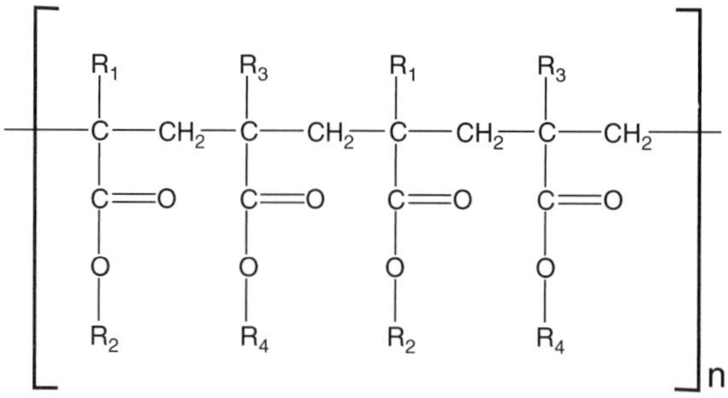

	R_1	R_2	R_3	R_4
EUDRAGIT® E	CH_3	$CH_2CH_2N(CH_3)_2$	CH_3	CH_3, C_4H_9
EUDRAGIT® L/S	CH_3	H	CH_3	CH_3
EUDRAGIT® FS	H	H, CH_3	CH_3	CH_3
EUDRAGIT® RL/RS	H, CH_3	CH_3, C_2H_5	CH_3	$CH_2CH_2N(CH_3)_3{}^+Cl^-$
EUDRAGIT® NE	H, CH_3	CH_3, C_2H_5	H, CH_3	CH_3, C_2H_5

FIGURE 2 Molecular structure of the EUDRAGIT® polymers.

100 can also shield actives from light and oxidation to improve the storage stability of dosage forms. Additionally, Eudragit E 100 provides a smooth glossy surface to coated substrates and exhibits high pigment binding capacity making it ideal for color coating applications to improve the pharmaceutical elegance and brand recognition of dosage forms. Eudragit E 100 has been claimed to improve the passage of dosage forms through the esophagus as well (26).

Kollicoat IR

Kollicoat® IR (BASF, Ludwigshafen, Germany) is a polyvinyl alcohol–polyethylene glycol (PEG) graft copolymer consisting of 75% polyvinyl alcohol units and 25% PEG units with an average molecular weight of 45,000 Da (27). Kollicoat IR is freely soluble in aqueous media over the entire range of physiological pH, and therefore is primarily used for instant release film coating applications. Films produced from Kollicoat IR are clear, have excellent pigment binding capacity, and can be easily printed; and thus are frequently utilized to improve the appearance of pharmaceutical dosage forms and to create brand trademarks (27). Kollicoat IR films are extremely flexible showing much greater elongation at break than cellulose derivatives (27), and therefore do not require the use of a plasticizer and in some cases may be more resistant to cracking or breaking than these more traditional coating alternatives. As a water-soluble film coat, Kollicoat IR is also useful for taste and odor masking applications, as well as to improve the stability of drugs that are sensitive to environmental perturbations.

Polyethylene Glycol and Povidone

Polyethylene glycol and povidone (PVP) are readily water-soluble polymers that are used in numerous pharmaceutical applications; however, their applications to film coating are limited by their hygroscopicity. Thus, films produced from these polymers are typically tacky, making coated dosage forms difficult to handle due to their adhesiveness. PEG and PVP are, however, used as additives to film coating formulations to stabilize pigments and to increase the gloss of film coatings (15). Low molecular weight PEGs (500–6000) are also commonly used as plasticizers in immediate release film coated formulations (15).

FILM COATING FOR MODIFIED RELEASE APPLICATIONS

In the previous section, film coating for immediate release applications was discussed at length with respect to its purposes and the principal film forming polymers. Common to each of the applications is that the film was not intended to interfere with the release of the drug. In this section, the discussion will focus on quite different applications of film coating in which the film coat is designed to alter drug release in a very specific way. The evolution of film coating into modifying the release of actives has led to very advanced delivery systems that have substantially expanded the complexity and capabilities of oral drug delivery. The different modes of modified drug delivery and the materials that enable these modes of delivery will be discussed in the following section.

Film Coating for Enteric Release

Enteric release refers to drug delivery that circumvents the stomach to release the delivered drug in the intestinal tract. Therefore, enteric-coated oral dosage forms remain intact in the stomach, releasing negligible amounts of drug, but dissolve rapidly in the intestinal tract. Polymers used for enteric film coating therefore resist dissolution in acidic media, yet dissolve readily in slightly acidic to neutral pH environments. There are a few reasons that enteric release is preferred for certain actives. If the active agent is irritating to the gastric mucosa, enteric delivery is preferred to avoid the discomfort and injury that may be experienced by the patient with an immediate release dosage form. Aspirin, for example, may cause ulceration of the gastric mucosa that can lead to internal bleeding if allowed to directly contact the gastric wall (28). Other drugs such as phenylbutazone, methyl salicylate, salicylic acid, and triamcinolone have also shown similar gastric irritation properties that would warrant oral delivery by means of an enteric system (29). With these drugs and others that inflame the gastric mucosa, an enteric release profile will avoid discomfort and possible injury to the patient.

If a drug molecule is acid labile or degraded by digestive enzymes in the stomach, enteric delivery is essential to maintaining its therapeutic activity as all or a portion of the dose may be degraded in the stomach thereby reducing bioavailability. Drugs such as pancreatin, erythromycin, pravastatin, omeprazole, dideoxyinosine, and digoxin are examples of those that are degraded in the gastric environment and should be delivered enterically to achieve maximum bioavailability.

Enteric delivery has also been demonstrated to improve the absorbance of some poorly water-soluble drugs. Since there is vastly more surface area for drug absorption in the small intestine than in the stomach, targeting the delivery of the maximum dissolved drug concentrations to the small intestine can substantially improve oral absorption. This mode of delivery has been demonstrated to be beneficial for poorly water-soluble drugs such as albendazole and itraconazole (30–32).

There are two types of materials that have been used for enteric coating of pharmaceutical dosage forms: (*i*) slowly eroding materials that provide enteric protection only if complete erosion does not occur before the dosage forms exits the stomach and (*ii*) pH-sensitive polymers (33). Erosion based enteric systems are highly dependent on gastric conditions and emptying times, and thus are not reliable. Therefore, pH sensitive polymers are more widely used for enteric coating as they provide greater consistency with respect to enteric drug release. Moreover, a variety of polymers exist with different pH solubility profiles to enable targeted drug delivery to specific areas of the intestinal tract.

All pH sensitive polymers used in enteric film coating exhibit enteric functionality as a result of free carboxyl groups contained on the polymer backbone. In acidic environments, these free carboxyl groups remain protonated (neutrally charged) and consequently the polymer remains hydrophobic and insoluble. As the acidity of the surrounding media is decreased, the free carboxyl groups become deprotonated and anionically charged rendering the polymer increasingly more hydrophilic up to a critical pH where there polymer becomes freely soluble. The pH at which this transition occurs depends on the degree of substitution of free carboxyl groups and the pKa of the substituent acid groups on the polymer chain. A greater degree of acidic functional group substitution corresponds to greater solubility of the enteric polymer.

Enteric polymers can be coated from aqueous latexes or from aqueous solutions that are produced by solubilizing the polymer via pH neutralization with the addition of an alkali or organic base. Typical neutralizing agents used to create aqueous solutions of enteric polymers include ammonia, sodium hydroxide, triethanolamine, 2-amino-2-methyl-1-propanol, and ammonium hydrogen carbonate. In most cases acid pretreatment is required to convert the enteric polymer from its salt state back to the neural state to achieve enteric functionality of the polymer; however, it has been reported that acid post-treatment is not required when ammonium hydrogen carbonate is used as the neutralizing agent. The plasticizer requirement is usually less when enteric coats are produced from neutralized aqueous solutions versus latex dispersions since the process of particle coalescence to achieve film formation is avoided. Plasticizer is only required in sufficient concentrations to improve film flexibility to avoid splitting or cracking. When enteric coating is conducted with latex formulations, in most cases, curing at elevated temperatures and relative humidity is required to complete film formation and ensure gastro-protection of the enteric coat.

Enteric Cellulose Derivatives

In 1940, Eastman Kodak Company published a U.S. patent that provided one of the earliest descriptions of enteric coating of medicaments. The patent claimed the use of a cellulose derivative containing free carboxyl groups as an enteric film forming polymer. Specifically, the claimed enteric polymer was cellulose acetate phthalate (CAP) (34). Numerous enteric cellulose derivatives have been developed since this early account and these polymers remain as some of the most widely used for enteric coating applications. In addition to CAP these derivatives include: cellulose acetate trimellitate (CAT), cellulose acetate succinate (CAS), hydroxypropyl methylcellulose phthalate (HPMCP), and hydroxypropyl methylcellulose acetate succinate (HPMCAS). The molecular structure of these polymers is depicted in Figure 1 with their respective substituent groups listed in the caption.

CAP is produced by reacting the partial acetate ester of cellulose with phthalic anhydride in the presence of a tertiary organic base or a strong acid (35). The USP specifies that CAP must contain 21.5–26.0% acetyl groups and 30–36% phthalyl groups on the cellulose backbone as calculated on an anhydrous basis. This degree of substitution equates to acylation of about half of the available hydroxyl groups and about one quarter esterified with one of the two free carboxyl groups of phthalic anhydride. With only one carboxyl group on the phthalic moiety involved in the substitution, the other remains free to form salts and thus provides the enteric functionality to the polymer (18). At this degree of substitution, i.e., free carboxyl group concentration on the cellulose backbone, CAP shows aqueous solubility around pH 6 (33,36). Degree of substitution is key to complete film dissolution in intestinal fluids. It has been determined that CAP has a threshold of approximately 20% phthalyl substitution to ensure rapid dissolution at intestinal pH (37).

The glass transition temperature (T_g) of CAP ranges from 160°C to 175°C (37,38), and therefore the addition of plasticizer is required to reduce the T_g of the polymer so as to improve film flexibility and robustness, and to achieve complete film formation. The formation of a continuous film is essential to achieving adequate protection of the dosage form in the gastric environment. Therefore, plasticization of enteric polymers, particularly cellulose-based polymers, is recommended to ensure the formation of a continuous film and to eliminate incidences of cracking or splitting of the film. Typically, 25–35% plasticizer based on dry polymer weight is sufficient. CAP is compatible with most water-soluble and insoluble plasticizers with diethyl phthalate (DEP), tributyl citrate (TBC), triethyl citrate (TEC), tributyrin, and triacetin being the most commonly used (13,37). It has been demonstrated that the T_g of CAP was reduced from 175°C to 100°C and 95°C by the addition of 25% DEP and triacetin, respectively (37). Obara and McGinity reported MFTs for a CAP pseudolatex coating system known as Aquateric® (now known as Aquacoat® CPD) in the range of 32–42°C with the addition of 25–45% of either TEC or DEP, with TEC producing MFTs 2–4°C lower than DEP (39).

Williams and Liu evaluated the influence of plasticizer and heat/humidity post treatment (curing) on film formation with Aquacoat CPD coated beads (40). In this study, it was determined that without the addition of plasticizer continuous CAP films were not formed, and hence rapid drug release was observed in acidic media irrespective of the post-treatment conditions. TEC was found to be a more efficient plasticizer for CAP than DEP. It is seen in Figure 3 that 10% TEC was insufficient for complete film formation while continuous films were formed with 25% TEC. Heat and humidity curing conditions were observed to improve film formation and acid protection of CAP films when sufficient plasticizer was incorporated into the film. A minimum plasticizer content of 15% was found to produce enteric release profiles following heat/humidity curing.

CAT has similar properties to those of CAP, but is not commonly used and does not currently have USP/NF compendial status. CAT is formed by the same synthesis process as CAP with trimellitic anhydride as the substituent group in place of phthalic anhydride. Typical values for timellityl and acetyl substitution are 29% and 22%, respectively. Trimellitic anhydride contains an additional free carboxyl group over that of phthalic anhydride, and hence CAT contains a greater concentration of acidic groups for a given degree of substitution than CAP rendering it more soluble in aqueous media. Also, the pKa of CAT is between 4.1 and 4.3 which is slightly lower than CAP (37). With a relatively low pKa value and greater functional group concentration, CAT is the most soluble enteric cellulose derivative with the onset of dissolution occurring at pH 4.7–5.0 (37). This pH solubility makes CAT ideal for targeted drug release to the proximal regions of the small intestine. Plasticizer considerations for CAT are identical to that of CAP.

CAS is another cellulose derivative with enteric characteristics which is produced by reacting cellulose acetate with succinic anhydride according to the same synthesis

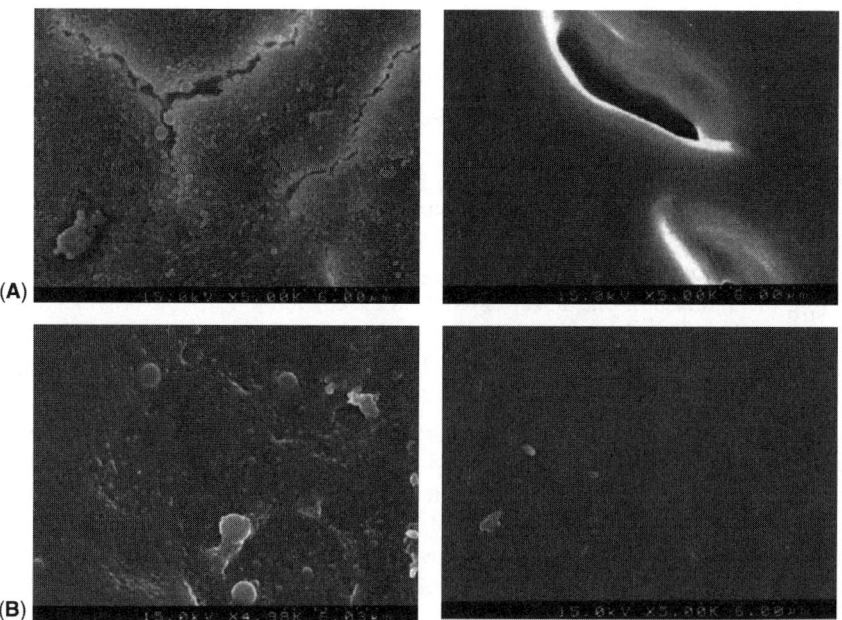

FIGURE 3 Surface morphology of beads coated with Aquacot® CPD containing TEC as the plasticizer. (**A**) 10% TEC; (**B**) 25% TEC; 1: Heat-only cured (50°C); 2: Heat-humidity cured (50°C/75% RH). Abbreviation: TEC, triethyl citrate. *Source:* From Ref. 39.

process as CAP and CAT. CAS is not a compendial excipient and is currently considered an experimental polymer. The properties of CAS are also similar to the previously discussed enteric cellulose derivatives. Butyric anhydride is the substituent group that provides the enteric functionality for this polymer. CAS has compendial status, but is not often used for pharmaceutical film coating.

HPMCP is a derivative of HPMC that is produced by the transesterification of HPMC with phthalic anhydride (13). HPMCP was first introduced in 1971 by the Shin-Etsu Chemical Company as a cellulose derivative for enteric coating. HPMCP has been admitted in the European and Japanese pharmacopeias and included in the USP/NF under the name hypromellose phthalate. Depending on the degree of phthalyl substitution, HPMCP is soluble in aqueous media in a pH range of 5–5.5. There are three primary grades of HPMCP produced by Shin-Etsu: HP-50, HP-55, and HP-55S. The HP-50 grade has a 24% nominal phthalyl content and dissolves at pH ≥ 5.0, while the HP-55 and HP-55S grades have a 31% nominal phthalyl content and dissolve at pH ≥ 5.5. The HP-55S grade has a greater molecular weight than the HP-55 grade which results in higher solution viscosity, greater film strength, and increased resistance to simulated gastric fluid (41). The HP-55S grade therefore requires less applied coating for enteric functionality and exhibits greater cracking resistance than the HP-55 grade. One of the benefits of HPMCP over CAP is that HPMCP is soluble in water/ethanol cosolvent systems which allows for improved drying efficiency and eliminates the need for neutralization to produce an aqueous-based solution coating system. Additionally, solutions and film coats prepared from HPMCP show greater thermal stability compared to CAP and CAT (37).

HP-50 and HP-55 have glass transition temperatures of 137 and 133°C, respectively, and hence plasticizers are required to improve film flexibility and film formation from latex systems. Although HPMCP can be applied to substrates without plasticizer from neutralized solutions, the addition of plasticizer will reduce film cracking and thus improve acid resistance. Effective plasticizers include: TEC, diacetin, triacetin, diethyl and dibutyl phthalate, castor oil, acetyl monoglyceride, and PEGs (42). Muhammad et al. reported that a HP-50 dispersion without added plasticizer did not form a continuous film by casting (43). The addition of 30% plasticizer was found to be sufficient for the formation of a continuous HPMCP film from pseudolatex dispersions, and TEC was determined to be a more efficient plasticizer than DEP. For coating of HPMCP from neutralized aqueous solutions, TEC concentrations from 2.5% to 5% have been reported to be sufficient (44). Thoma et al. reported that the particle size of HP-55 also substantially affected film formation as larger particles (10 μm) required a 33% film coat to impart gastro-resistance, whereas for smaller particles (5 μm) a 20% film coat was sufficient to achieve acid resistance (45).

HPMCAS, or hypromellose acetate succinate as it is known in the USP/NF, is derived from HPMC by the esterification of free hydroxyl groups on the polymer backbone with acetic anhydride and succinic anhydride. The chemical structure of HPMCAS is shown in Figure 1. HPMCAS was developed by Shin-Etsu Chemical Company Tokyo, Japan, and marketed as AQOAT®, a redispersible powder form of the polymer. It was first approved in Japan in 1985, and has sense been approved in Europe and the United States (17). HPMCAS, like the previously described enteric polymers, is insoluble in acidic media, yet soluble in neutral pH according to ionization of free carboxyl groups on the polymer backbone. Shin-Etsu produces three grades of AQOAT; AS-LF, AS-MF, AS-HF; which differ according to the percent of acetyl and succinoyl substitution. These three grades are available in both a granular and a micronized powder form. The onset of aqueous solubility of HPMCAS is in a pH range of 5.5–6.8 according to the polymer grade where the determining solubility factor is the ratio of succinoyl to acetyl group substitution (46). The AS-LF grade has the highest ratio, and thus dissolves at the lowest pH, followed by the AS-MF and the AS-HF grades. HPMCAS has been demonstrated to be more chemically stable than CAP and HPMCP as indicated by a substantial reduction in the evolution of free acid when stored at 60°C and 100% relative humidity (RH) (17).

The T_g of HPMCAS lies in the range of 120–135°C according to polymer grade. Since HPMCAS is a relatively rigid polymer, plasticization is utilized to improve film flexibility and reduce cracking as well as to promote film formation from HPMCAS aqueous dispersions. Nagai et al. demonstrated that TEC, triacetin, and propylene carbonate formed clear, continuous films from an HPMCAS dispersion at concentrations in the range of 30–50% by weight of HPMCAS; however, due to evaporation during the spraying process propylene carbonate was found to be unsuitable for film coating applications (17). Triacetin content in films on coated tablets was seen to decrease by about 30% on storage at 40°C/75% RH, whereas TEC showed no change on storage. As a result, it was concluded that of the investigated plasticizers TEC was the most suitable for HPMCAS. Siepmann et al. demonstrated the importance of plasticizer level and post-treatment conditions on the enteric functionality of HPMCAS produced from an aqueous dispersion (47). Theses results are shown in Figure 4. It can be seen from the figure that 30% TEC followed by 24 hours (curing) at 40°C/75% RH resulted in the greatest acid resistance.

Methacrylic Acid Copolymers

Methacrylic acid copolymers are widely used for enteric coating applications. These acrylic copolymers were first introduced for enteric coating applications by Lehmann and Dreher in the mid-1960s (48). Today, these enteric polymers are marketed most notably by Degussa Röhm America (Parsippany, New Jersey, U.S.A.) under the proprietary Eudragit brand name. There are four types of Eudragit polymers with enteric release capabilities: Eudragit L 100-55 (also marketed by BASF as Kollicoat MAE 100P), Eudragit L 100, Eudragit S 100, and Eudragit FS 30 D. The molecular structure of each of these polymers is shown in Figure 2 with their corresponding substituent group indicated in the accompanying table. Each of these polymers is produced by a radical emulsion polymerization synthesis process in water.

Eudragit L 100-55, or methacrylic acid copolymer Type C USP/NF, is an anionic copolymer of methacrylic acid and ethyl acrylate having an average molecular weight of approximately 250,000 (49). The ratio of free carboxyl groups to ester groups is approximately 1:1. The molecular structure of Eudragit L 100-55, most importantly the functional group ratio, gives the polymer its characteristic pH-dependant aqueous solubility profile. The onset of dissolution begins at or above pH 5.5 according to the ionization of free carboxyl groups. The polymer is available from Degussa as an aqueous dispersion known as Eudragit L 30 D-55 and in a spray-dried powder form known as Eudragit L 100-55.

The T_g of Eudragit L 100-55 has been reported to be in the range of 123–129°C, and thus films formed from this polymer require plasticizer to facilitate film formation and to improve the mechanical properties of films. With the addition of 10–20% plasticizer, the MFT of Eudragit L 100-55 is reduced to about 15°C, and thus continuous films are formed from this material under typical coating conditions (50). In their evaluation plasticizers for use with Eudragit L 30 D-55, Schimdt and Niemann found that the greatest enteric protection of coated pellets was achieved with the addition of 20% dibutyl phthalate (51). TEC is a commonly used plasticizer for Eudragit L 100-55.

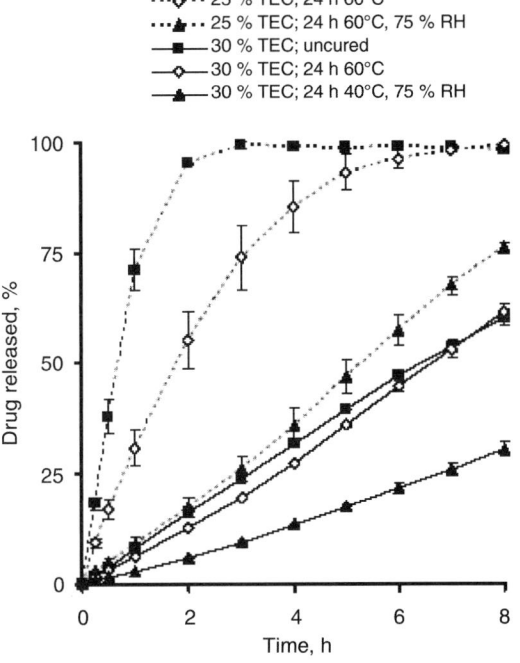

FIGURE 4 Effects of the plasticizer level and curing conditions (indicated in the figure) on theophylline release from pellets coated with HPMCAS in 0.1 M HCl (20% coating level). *Abbreviation*: HPMCAS, hydroxypropyl methylcellulose acetate succinate. *Source*: From Ref. 46.

Triacetin and low molecular weight PEGs have also been successfully utilized (50). Hydrophobic plasticizers tend to be less effective in reducing the MFT of Eudragit L 100-55.

As mentioned above, Eudragit L 30 D-55 is a 30% polymeric dispersion in water which following the addition of plasticizer, other functional additives, and dilution with deionized water is ready for spray application to substrates. Eudragit L 100-55, the spray dried form of the coating material, can be easily redispersed in water to solids contents of 30–40% with the addition of 3–5 mol % of a neutralizing agent such as an alkali or organic base (50). The addition of a neutralizing agent increases the dispersion pH, ideally to a pH of about 5, which improves the wetting of latex particles and facilitates the dispersion of agglomerates as primary particles in the aqueous medium. The mean particle diameter of such redispersed latexes is about 250 nm which is comparable to the original latex (50). The gastroresistance of films produced from redispersed powders are also comparable to that of the original latex.

Acryl-Eze® MP, a product of Colorcon, Inc., is a complete pre-formulated enteric coating system based on methacrylic acid copolymer Type C. Acryl-Eze MP is a powder mixture of Eudragit L 100-55 along with neutralizing agents, plasticizers, and pigments that is easily redispersed in water. This complete coating system eliminates several of the production steps required for the preparation of the coating dispersion, and thus improves coating efficiency particularly for large-scale production.

Eudragit L 100 and S 100, or methacrylic acid copolymer Types A and B as they are respectively titled in the USP/NF, are anionic copolymers of methacrylic acid and methyl methacrylate having an average molecular weight of approximately 135,000 (52). The molecular structure of these polymers is illustrated in Figure 2. The ratio of methacrylic acid to methyl methacrylate units is approximately 1:1 for Eudragit L 100 and 1:2 for Eudragit S 100. Thus, Eudragit L 100 has a greater concentration of free carboxyl groups on the polymer backbone than Eudragit S 100. Consequently, the dissolution of Eudragit L 100 begins at about pH 6.0 while Eudragit S 100 begins to dissolve at pH 7 (50). Both polymers provide enteric protection to coated substrates; however, with Eudragit S 100 the onset of drug release is further delayed and will occur in the more distil regions of the intestinal tract as compared to Eudragit L 100.

The T_gs of Eudragit L 100 and S 100 have been reported to be about 160°C and the MFT has been reported to be about 85°C. Thus, continuous film formation is problematic at typical coating conditions and resulting films are brittle. Therefore, relatively large amounts of plasticizer (40–50% based on dry polymer weight) are required to achieve complete film formation and to improve film flexibility (50). Plasticizers such as triacetin, poloxamer, and TEC at a concentration of about 50% have been demonstrated to produce film coats with sufficient gastric resistance (53). The addition of 30% TEC has been demonstrated to reduce the MFT of Eudragit L 100 and S 100 to 37 and 41°C, respectively (50). Thereby, with the addition of a compatible plasticizer, enteric coats with Eudragit L 100 and S 100 can be achieved under typical film coating conditions that provide sufficient acid resistance.

Eudragit FS 30 D is a 30% (w/w) aqueous dispersion of a copolymer produced by the polymerization of methacrylic acid, methyl acrylate, and methyl methacrylate monomers. The free carboxyl to ester group ratio of this polymer is approximately 1:10, and thus this polymer is less soluble than the previously discussed Eudragit polymers. The onset of dissolution for Eudragit FS 30 D with increasing pH occurs above pH 7. With this pH solubility profile, Eudragit FS 30 D leads to drug release very late in the intestinal tract and is therefore most commonly used for colon-targeted drug delivery. For example, Gupta et al. reported the use of Eudragit FS 30 D as a top coat on sustained release pellets to target extended release of 5-aminosalicylic acid to the colon (54,55). The MFT of Eudragit FS 30 D is 14°C, and thus no plasticizer is required for film coating applications (56).

Polyvinyl Acetate Phthalate

According to the USP/NF, polyvinyl acetate phthalate (PVAP) is the reaction product of phthalic anhydride and partially hydrolyzed polyvinyl acetate (PVAc) that contains no less than 55.0% and no more than 62.0% phthalyl groups. The onset of aqueous dissolution of PVAP begins at a pH of about 5.0 allowing for enteric release as well as the potential for targeted drug release to the proximal small intestine (46). The glass transition temperature of PVAP was reported by Porter et al. to be 42.5°C (57) and later by Colorcon Inc. as approximately 78°C (58). Although the T_g of PVAP is relatively low, plasticizers are typically incorporated for film coating applications to facilitate film formation and to reduce splitting and cracking. PVAP is compatible with several of the most common plasticizers; namely glyceryl triacetate, TEC, acetyl triethylcitrate, DEP, and PEG 400 (59). Sureteric®, a product of Colorcon Inc., is a complete preformulated coating system consisting of a powder blend of PVAP, plasticizers, and other functional ingredients intended for reconstitution in water for rapid coating dispersion production.

Film Coating for Sustained Release

The overall goal in designing sustained release oral dosage forms is to provide systemic drug concentrations that remain within the therapeutic concentration range for a prolonged time period. The primary benefit of sustained release dosage forms is the reduction of the daily dosing regime for drug therapies requiring several daily doses. In many cases sustained release delivery systems can reduce dosing to a twice or once-daily schedule. By reducing the number of required daily doses, the convenience of the drug therapy is improved resulting in better patient compliance and often reduced cost. Additionally, a well-designed sustained release dosage form can stabilize systemic drug concentrations by providing a constant rate of drug release (and absorption), as opposed to the peaks and valleys of systemic drug levels seen with multi-dosing. Therefore, modified release dosage forms can improve drug therapy by reducing fluctuations of systemic drug levels that could lead to toxicity and/or poor efficacy. For certain applications, such as pain therapy, therapeutic drug action must be sustained for prolonged intervals such that the patient is able to sleep throughout the night without incidences of pain breakthrough. For applications such as these, modified release dosage forms substantially improve a patient's quality of life.

Polymeric film coating and matrix tablet systems are the principal technologies utilized in the production of sustained release dosage forms. However, film coating offers some distinct advantages over matrix tablets stemming from the ability to produce multi-particulate dosage forms. In comparison to monolithic dosage forms, multi-particulates exhibit less variable gastrointestinal transit times and are more sparsely distributed over the intestinal tract, thus providing greater uniformity of drug absorption and reduced potential for mucosal irritation (60–62). Also, combining fractions of multiparticulates that are coated to produce different drug release profiles within a single capsule provides flexibility in tailoring overall drug release. This kind of multi-phase release profile can be difficult to achieve with matrix tablets. In addition to matrix tablets, coated multiparticulates are also distinctly more desirable for sustained release applications than coated tablets because the dose is distributed throughout a multitude of individually coated particles. Therefore, coat failure of a few particulates does not have the catastrophic dose-dumping effect as would coat failure of a monolithic dosage form. Multiparticulates also provide greater surface area for drug release over matrix or film coated tablets which is typically necessary to achieve the desired rate and extent of drug release. As a result of these advantages, multiparticulate film coating has become the preferred method for the production of sustained release dosage forms.

Sustained release polymeric film coating is based upon a generic reservoir device design in which the release of active from a concentrated core is controlled by an encompassing semi-permeable membrane. The membrane controls the rate of water permeation into the drug core, thereby controlling the dissolution and subsequent outward diffusion of the active agent. The semi-permeable membrane, in almost all modern oral sustained release coating formulations, is primarily composed of a polymer which is insoluble in water over the entire range of gastrointestinal pH. The insolubility of the membrane is crucial to maintaining the film's integrity and preserving the film properties that control drug release over the length of the gastrointestinal tract. Therefore, insoluble cellulose derivatives, insoluble polymethacrylates, as well as polyvinylacetate are the most commonly used polymers for sustained release film coating owing to their water-insolubility as well as other desirable properties for film coating that will be discussed in this section.

Membrane permeability is a function of thickness, porosity, tortuosity, and composition. Therefore, film formation is a substantial determinant of drug release rate through a sustained release film coat. Drug release through an insoluble polymeric membrane produced from a latex dispersion will decrease with the evolution of film formation owing to decreasing porosity and increasing tortuosity of the polymer film. Therefore, a sustained drug release profile that is stable with time depends almost entirely on the formation of a complete polymeric film and the static nature of that film over time and under various storage conditions. In the following sections, the utilization of appropriate plasticizers as well post-treatment of coated substrates will be discussed as they are essential to complete and stable film formation with sustained release polymers.

Ethylcellulose

Ethylcellulose is one of the most commonly used polymers for sustained release film coating. The polymer is insoluble, but permeable in water over the range of gastro-intestinal pH, and thus can be utilized to produce semi-permeable membranes that control the rate of drug release from coated substrates. Ethylcellulose is derived from cellulose via a reaction with ethyl chloride in alkaline solution followed by purification of crude ethylcellulose. The resulting molecular structure is shown in Figure 1. The USP/NF dictates that ethylcellulose must contain not less than 44.0% and not more than 51.0% ethoxy groups as calculated based on dry polymer weight. Bulk ethylcellulose is produced by the Dow Chemical Company primarily with a "Standard" ethoxy content of 48.0–49.5% (63). Ethylcellulose is available in a variety molecular weights corresponding to 5% solution viscosities in a range of 3–385 cP (63). Ethylcellulose is soluble in alcohols, chlorinated solvents, and natural oils. Therefore, solvent coating with ethylcellulose is commonly conducted from ethanolic solutions, while pseudolatex systems must be used for aqueous film coating.

Aquacoat ECD and Surelease® are two commercially available ethylcellulose pseudolatex dispersions. Aquacoat ECD, a product of FMC Corporation, is produced by an emulsification/solvent evaporation process that utilizes sodium lauryl sulfate and cetyl alcohol as colloid stabilizers (64). The Aquacoat ECD dispersion contains approximately 27% ethylcellulose and 30% total solids. The dispersion does not contain plasticizer, and therefore an appropriate plasticizer must be added to the dispersion prior to coating. The dispersion is typically diluted to a final solids content in the range of 15–20% prior to spray coating. Although, intended to be a pH-independent sustained release coating system, the content of sodium lauryl sulfate in the Aquacoat ECD dispersion has been demonstrated to cause reduced drug release rates in acidic media versus media of neutral pH (65,66).

Surelease, a product of Colorcon, is produced by first melt extruding ethylcellulose with oleic acid and dibutyl sebacate (DBS) (or fractionated coconut oil) to form a molten plasticized polymeric blend. This molten blend of plasticized ethylcellulose is then introduced into an ammoniated water solution under high shear and pressure to disperse small droplets of plasticized ethylcellulose into the water phase (67). Ammonium oleate is produced in situ during this emulsification process to stabilize the colloidal ethylcellulose particles (67). Additional purified water is then added to reduce the final solids content of the pseudolatex dispersion to 25%. The Surelease coating system does not contain an ionic surfactant, and therefore does not exhibit the pH-dependent drug release observed with Aquacoat ECD (66).

The T_g of bulk ethylcellulose is in the range of 129–133°C, and therefore at ambient conditions films of ethylcellulose are substantially brittle. To be used in film coating applications, ethylcellulose requires the addition of plasticizer to improve film flexibility and toughness. The T_g of dried latex particles of Aquacoat ECD has been reported to be 89°C (7). The reduced T_g of ethylcellulose particles dried from a pseudolatex is the result of the temporary plasticizing effects of water. Although the T_g of ethylcellulose pseudolatex particles is less than that of bulk ethylcellulose, additional plasticizer is required to reduce the internal stress of latex particles and facilitate their coalescence during film formation. Figure 5 illustrates the effect of plasticizer type and concentration on the T_g of Aquacoat ECD latex particles (7). It is evident from this figure that TEC is the most efficient plasticizer of ethylcellulose as a T_g value of about 36°C is achieved at a plasticizer concentration of 20%. Although not as efficient as TEC, DBS is often used to plasticize ethylcellulose as it has been shown to provide greater sustained drug release profiles over TEC owing to its hydrophobic nature (68). It has been reported by several researchers that complete film formation with Aquacoat ECD does not occur when less than about 18–20% DBS is incorporated as a plasticizer (69,70). Consequently, the onset of linear drug release from beads coated with Aquacoat ECD begins at 20% DBS concentration with reducing rates of drug release up to 24% (7). Below 24% DBS, major flaws are present in the ethylcellulose coat which cause accelerated rates of drug release (69). Since plasticization of ethylcellulose occurs during the melt extrusion phase of the Surelease process, additional plasticization of the dispersion prior to coating is not necessary.

Ideally, drug release rates from sustained release film coated dosage forms can be easily modulated by varying film thickness. Porter demonstrated that for the Surelease coating system, a broad range of chlorpheniramine maleate release rates from coated pellets (fast to near-zero order) could be achieved in a range of 6–20% applied coat weight (71). This represents an ideal distribution of drug release versus coat weight as drug release rate is only mildly dependant on coat weight and thus the desired release profile can be obtained easily by coating to a specific weight of applied polymer. For Aquacoat ECD plasticized with 24% DBS, Wheatley and Steuernagel demonstrated that in the range of 2–8% of applied polymer weight the release of theophylline from beads ranged from near-immediate (2% and 4% weight gain) to sustained (6% and 8% weight gain) with a substantial disparity in drug release rates between 4% and 6% applied coat weights (7). These results are shown in Figure 6. These findings represent a substantial

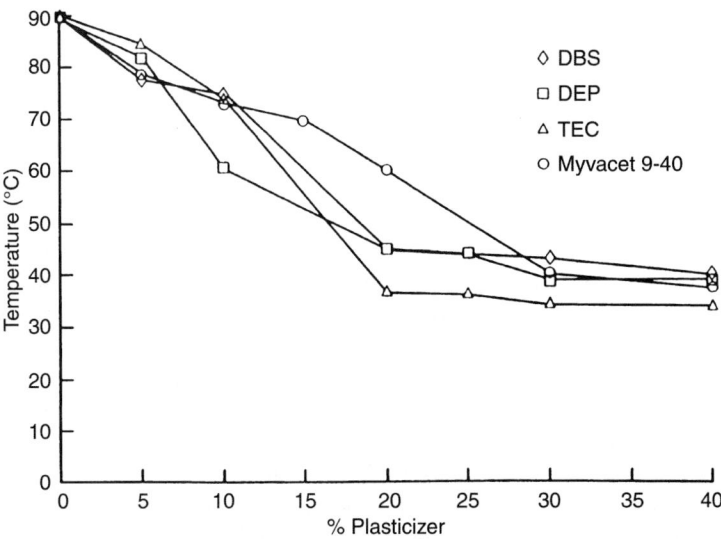

FIGURE 5 Glass transition temperature of plasticized ethylcellulose latex as a function of plasticizer type and concentration. *Source*: From Ref. 69.

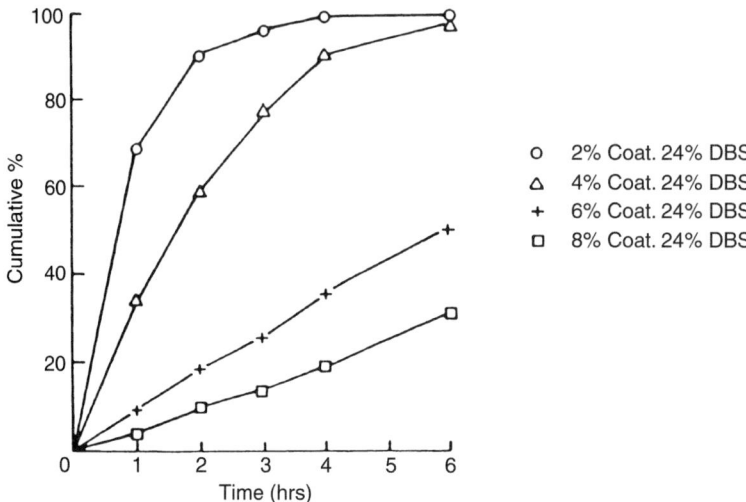

FIGURE 6 Effect of coat level on release rate of theophylline from pellets coated with ethylcellulose plasticized with 24% DBS. *Abbreviation*: DBS, dibutyl sebacate. *Source*: From Ref. 7.

problem to sustained release coating systems as thin film coats often result in a large degree of variability in drug release, and the range of coat thicknesses that produced the desired range of release rates is too narrow to precisely achieve a particular release rate. To improve the permeability of films produced with Aquacoat ECD, Wheatley and Steuernagel incorporated HPMC as a pore forming agent. Consequently, thick ethylcellulose film coats could be applied to theophylline beads without shutting down drug release. These results are shown in Figure 7. This figure illustrates that HPMC was able to increase the rate of drug release through thick ethylcellulose film coats and that the rate of release could be precisely controlled by varying the concentration of HPMC in the film. Similar results were also achieved with Surelease using methylcellulose as a pore forming agent. Thus, these studies demonstrate that in some cases altering coat thickness is sufficient to modulate the drug release profile; however, when this technique cannot be applied, altering film permeability by the addition of additives is an alternative means of controlling drug release rates.

When coating with rigid polymers such as ethylcellulose, depending on the level of plasticization, film formation can be incomplete following the film spraying process. Incomplete film formation leads to further gradual latex particle coalescence and film densification on storage causing a decrease in drug release rate with time. Thermal treatment, known as curing, is often required to ensure complete film formation and static drug release profiles on storage. During the curing process, coated substrates are stored at temperatures above the glass transition temperature of the polymer to promote mobility of polymer chains, and consequently accelerate film formation. Bodmeier et al. demonstrated the effect of curing on drug release from chlorpheniramine maleate beads coated with Aquacoat ECD plasticized with different levels of TEC (72). These results are shown in Figure 8. From these results, it is seen that 10% plasticizer was insufficient for complete film formation irrespective of curing conditions and with higher levels of plasticizer curing had a dampening effect on drug release. At intermediate plasticizer concentrations (20–25%), curing is recommended for ethylcellulose pseudolatex dispersions to achieve a stable drug release profile. Thermal treatment of coated substrates at

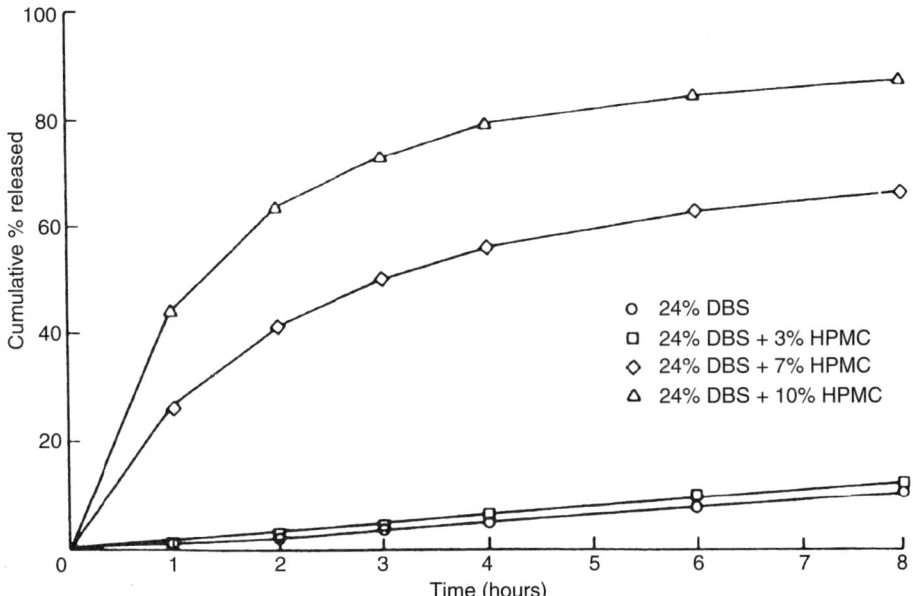

FIGURE 7 Effect of water-soluble additive HPMC on the release rate of theophylline from pellets coated with ethylcellulose. *Abbreviation*: HPMC, hydroxypropyl methylcellulose. *Source:* From Ref. 7.

60°C for 1–2 hours is typically sufficient to force complete film formation. Higher plasticizer levels may be used to avoid curing steps; however, excessive tackiness of the substrates could result.

Polymethacrylates

Polymethacrylate latex coating systems are also used for sustained release film coating. These latexes are produced by Degussa and marketed under the Eudragit brand name. The different grades include Eudragit RL 100, Eudragit RS 100, and Eudragit NE 30 D. The Eudragit RL 100 and RS 100 polymers are available as fine powder (PO), granules (100), 12.5% w/w organic solution (12.5), and as a 30% (w/w) aqueous colloidal dispersion in water (30 D). Eudragit NE 30 D is only available as a 30% (w/w) aqueous colloidal dispersion. These systems are composed of polymers that are water insoluble, but swellable over the range of physiological pH, and thus are ideal for sustained release film coating applications.

Eudragit RL 100 and RS 100, also known as ammonio methacrylate copolymers Types A and B USP/NF, respectively are produced by radical copolymerization of ethyl acrylate, methyl methacrylate, and trimethyl-ammonioethyl methacrylate chloride in a 1:2:0.2 ratio (RL 100 grade) and 1:2:0.1 (RS 100 grade). The molecular structures of these polymers are illustrated in Figure 2. The ammonio methacrylate content of Types A (Eudragit RL 100) and B (Eudragit RS 100) polymers is 8.85–11.9% and 4.48–6.77%, respectively. In aqueous media, the quaternary ammonium groups on the Eudragit RL 100 and RS 100 polymers become ionized causing films to swell by ionic repulsion resulting in controlled permeation of the surrounding medium. Eudragit RL 100 has a greater concentration of ammonio methacrylate pendant groups, and hence films

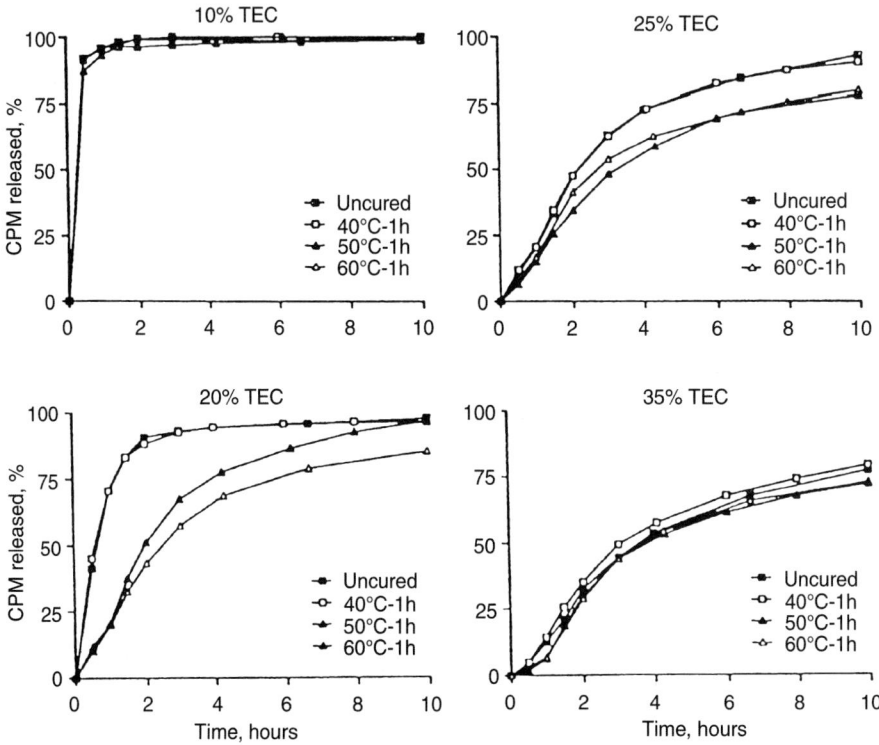

FIGURE 8 Effect of TEC concentration and curing conditions (curing temperature-curing time) on the chlorpheniramine maleate release in 0.1 M pH 7.4 phosphate buffer. *Abbreviation*: TEC, triethyl citrate. *Source*: From Ref. 72.

produced from this polymer are substantially more permeable than films produced from Eudragit RS 100. Therefore, drug release rates through Eudragit RL 100 membranes are much greater than that of Eudragit RS 100 membranes. Blending of these two polymers is a common method to achieve intermediate sustained drug release rates.

The MFTs of Eudragit RL 100 and RS 100 polymers range between 40°C and 50°C, and thus plasticizer is required to form continuous films at typical coating and curing temperatures. Amighi and Moës reported that initial film formation with Eudragit RS 30 D is substantially improved with increasing amounts of plasticizer (TEC) up to 30% (73). Moreover, further gradual coalescence was found to be more pronounced for films with lower plasticizer content as 7 months storage time at 40°C/50% RH was required for films containing 10% TEC to reach equilibrium, versus 7 days for films containing 20% TEC. No change on storage was observed for films containing 30% TEC.

Eudragit RL 100 and RS 100 coating systems have been used in a variety of different sustained release film coating applications. Gupta et al. utilized a blend of Eudragit RL/RS 100 along with an Eudragit FS 30 D topcoat to produce sustained release pellets of 5-aminosalicylic acid targeted specifically to the colon (54,55). The drug release profile of the pellets is shown below in Figure 9. Zhang et al. utilized a blend of Eudragit RL 100 and RS 100 as a semi-permeable rate-controlling membrane for a pulsed-release osmotic tablet system (74). Plasticized Eudragit RL/RS 100 blends have also been demonstrated to be sufficiently flexible for utilization as a sustained release film coat for

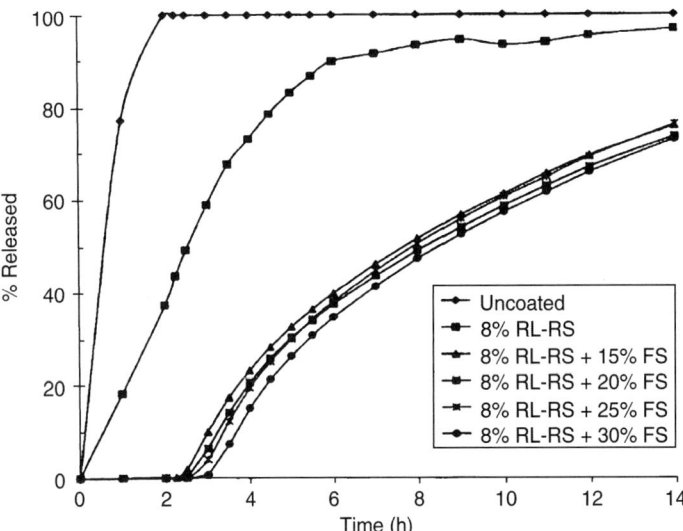

FIGURE 9 Dissolution of 5-aminosalicylic acid pellets for the first 2 hour at pH 1.2 followed by pH 7.0 USP phosphate buffer. *Source*: From Ref. 74.

multiparticulates intended for subsequent tablet compression (50). Chang and Bodmeier demonstrated the use of Eudragit RS 30 D for the production of sustained release drug-containing microspheres (75).

Eudragit NE 30 D is another polymethacrylate-based coating system used for sustained release film coating. Eudragit NE 30 D is a latex dispersion of a neutral polymer produced by emulsion polymerization of ethyl acrylate and methyl methacrylate. The molecular structure of the polymer is illustrated in Figure 2. The ratio of ethyl acrylate to methyl methacrylate on the polymer chain is 2:1, and the average molecular weight of the polymer is 800,000 (50). Eudragit NE 30 D is similar to the Eudragit RL 100 and RS 100 polymers in that it is insoluble in aqueous media over the entire range of physiological pH, but is swellable independent of media pH. Therefore, Eudragit NE 30 D is used in film coating applications as a drug release rate-controlling membrane to sustain release of active over the entire length of the gastrointestinal tract. With respect to permeability, the Eudragit NE 30 D films are moderately permeable producing drug release rates between that of Eudragit RL 100 and Eudragit RS 100. The MFT of Eudragit NE 30 D is 5°C, and therefore plasticization is not required for the formation of continuous, flexible films (50). However, despite its low MFT, significant reductions in the release rate of diphenhydramine HCl from pellets coated with Eudragit NE 30 D were seen following curing at 45 and 60°C (76). This result indicates that despite the low MFT of Eudragit NE 30 D, films produced from this latex dispersion undergo further gradual coalescence. Therefore, substrates coated with Eudragit NE 30 D should be heat treated following the coating process to accelerate the formation of a stable film and ensure static drug release profiles on storage.

Polyvinyl Acetate

Kollicoat SR 30 D is a sustained release coating dispersion marketed by BASF based on PVAc. Kollicoat SR 30 D is a 30% (w/w) dispersion of PVAc (27%) in water stabilized by povidone (2.7%) and sodium lauryl sulfate (0.3%) prepared by an emulsification polymerization method (77). PVAc is insoluble in aqueous media and therefore provides sustained release of active agents from coated substrates by controlling the rate of media diffusion through the film. The Kollicoat SR dispersion has an MFT of 18°C and therefore can be utilized for film coating without the need for plasticization or curing; however, plasticization will enhance film formation and flexibility (78). Recommended plasticizer concentration is in the range of 0–10% based on dry PVAc weight. TEC has been shown to be an efficient plasticizer reducing the MFT to 1°C at a concentration of 10% (78). As a result of the low MFT, sticking commonly occurs with substrates coated with Kollicoat SR, and therefore anti-tacking agents such as talc should be added to the coating dispersion or the coated substrates should be mixed with colloidal silica after coating. The addition of talc at a concentration of 35% (based on dry polymer mass) was observed to have an insignificant effect on drug release in 0.1 N HCl from coated pellets (78).

Dashevsky et al. and Shao et al. reported on the effects of process and formulational parameters of film coating with Kollicoat SR on drug release from non-pareil pellets layered with actives (78,79). In both reports it was found that the rate of drug release could be easily modulated by varying the coating level without changing the mechanism of release. Dashevsky et al. reported that plasticization and curing did not affect the release of propranolol HCl from film coated pellets (Fig. 10). However, contrasting results were reported by Shao et al. as plasticization and curing were seen to reduce drug release rates. In these two studies, different aging effects were also reported as Dashevsky et al. saw no effect of storage on drug release while Shao et al. demonstrated a stepwise decrease in dissolution rate with storage at 40°C/75% RH. Shao et al. speculated these differences could be the result of different drug candidates and/or different properties of the substrates. Finally, Dashevsky et al. demonstrated that drug release rates from Kollicoat SR coated pellets was minimally affected by the pH and ionic strength of dissolution media (78). Although, these reports give conflicting conclusions regarding some details of film coating with Kollicoat SR, they both demonstrate the sustained release functionality of the coating system and establish its place as a sustained release film coating system.

Combined Coated Multiparticulates for Extended Release

For numerous drug therapies, a sustained release coating system alone is therapeutically insufficient as an extended release product does not produce an immediate onset of action. In these cases, mixed coated multiparticulate systems with bimodal drug release

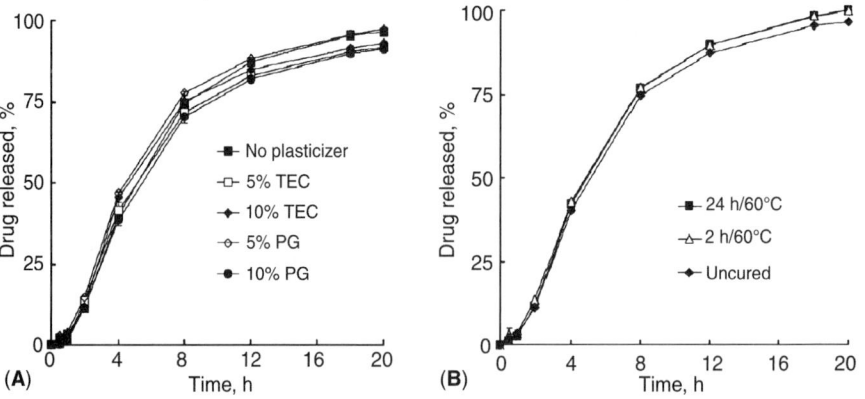

FIGURE 10 Effect of: (**A**) plasticizers and (**B**) curing on the propranolol HCl release in 0.1 N HCl from Kollicoat® SR 30 D-coated pellets (15% coating level). *Source*: From Ref. 78.

profiles are an ideal solution as they provide an initial burst release of drug followed by either a secondary delayed burst release or a secondary sustained drug release profile. These systems are produced by filling a capsule with two or more fractions of film coated multiparticulates. The immediate release fraction can be produced by either incorporating the drug into the pellet core, or layering the drug onto the surface of a non-pareil with the use of an excipient binder. In either case, the immediate release fraction is typically coated with polymers such as HPMC or Eudragit E to serve as a protective layer and/or taste masking barrier. The secondary (and possibly tertiary) fractions of multiparticulates are coated with either a pH-sensitive, or sustained release film former to provide the delayed or sustained component of the bimodal release profile.

The Spheroidal Oral Drug Absorption System (SODAS™) is a multiparticulate extended release drug delivery system, which is proprietary to Elan Corporation (Dublin, Ireland). In one application, this delivery system was utilized to produce an extended release capsule of morphine sulfate known as Avinza®. Each Avinza capsule contains both immediate and controlled release morphine sulfate beads (1–2 mm in diameter) in a 9:1 w/w ratio with respect to drug content (80). With this combination of beads, plateau morphine levels are achieved within 30 minutes via the immediate release portion while the extended release beads maintain these blood levels for the 24 hours dosing interval. The system is produced by first coating sugar spheres with a morphine sulfate/excipient layer followed by the application of an ammonio-methacrylate copolymer coat, i.e., Eudragit RL 30 D and/or RS 30 D (80). The immediate release beads are formed by the same process; however, they do not contain the ammonio-methacrylate sustained release polymer coating. These two bead fractions are then combined in the appropriate ratio and filled into hard gelatin capsules to produce the final dosage form.

Once ingested, the gelatin capsule rapidly dissolves releasing the beads into the gastric fluid. As there is no rate-controlling polymer on the immediate release beads, the drug contents are rapidly dissolved and subsequently absorbed, hence providing and immediate therapeutic effect. The ammonio-methacrylate copolymer layer is permeable to gastrointestinal fluids, which allows the fluid to enter the bead at a controlled rate. Fumaric acid contained in the core acts as both an osmotic agent and as a local acidifier, thus mediating the rate at which the gastrointestinal fluid permeates the insoluble film and solubilizes the drug (80). The resultant morphine solution then diffuses out of the core through the film at a predetermined rate, thereby prolonging in vivo drug release and extending absorption for 24 hours.

In another aspect of the SODAS design, the secondary pellet fraction is produced as described above; however, the delayed release beads are produced by coating the IR beads with an enteric polymer (methacrylic acid copolymer) rather than a sustained release polymer (81). This bi-modal release system was used in the formulation of Ritalin LA® and was demonstrated to produce two distinct plasma concentration peaks separated by approximately 4 hours (81). This bi-modal pulsed release system was demonstrated to be bioequivalent to two immediate release tablet doses administered four hours apart.

A similar extended release combined coated multiparticulate capsule system is described in U.S. patent 6,344,215. The delivery system is capable of immediately releasing a portion of the dose to provide rapid onset of action followed by release of the remainder of the dose for a period of about 12 hours (82). The dosage form is composed of a multitude of film coated beads with two distinct populations; one fraction provides immediate drug release while the second fraction provides extended release portion. The immediate release beads are produced by layering the drug and polyvinylpyrrolidone onto sugar spheres from an aqueous solution and then applying a seal coat. The extended release beads are produced by applying an ethylcellulose coat to the immediate release beads.

These three systems described above demonstrate the benefit of combining coated multiparticulates with different drug release characteristics into a single dosage form. The combination of immediate release and modified release coated multiparticulates has been demonstrated to produce extended release dosage forms with an immediate and prolonged onset of therapeutic action. Therefore, this type of dosage form is ideal for extended release delivery systems for drug therapies which also require an immediate onset of therapeutic action.

INFLUENCE OF ADDITIVES TO FILM COATING FORMULATIONS

It is a rare circumstance when a coating formulation contains only the primary film-forming polymer. Most often, film coating formulations contain one or more functional additives included to facilitate the spraying process, improve film coat appearance, improve post-process handling, and/or to modify drug release characteristics. In this section, the various classes of functional additives for film coating will be reviewed with respect to the different excipients and their particular functionality.

Plasticizers

Most polymers used in pharmaceutical film coating are mechanically weak and therefore brittle at ambient conditions owing to glass transition temperatures which are substantially greater than room temperature. The brittle nature of these polymer films results in cracking, edging, and splitting of films on the coated substrate. Therefore, increasing the elasticity and mechanical toughness of polymer films by the addition of plasticizers is essential to film coating to increase coat toughness, reduce breakage, and improve film continuity. Moreover, when film coating with latex dispersions, complete film formation would not occur in many cases without the addition of an effective plasticizer to facilitate the coalescence of latex polymer spheres. Since film discontinuities caused by cracks or incomplete film formation would preclude coat functionality, plasticizers are essential additives to film coating formulations.

Plasticizers are most often incorporated into coating formulations by dissolution, dispersion, or emulsification in the liquid phase of the coating solution or dispersion. With polymeric solutions, a compatible plasticizer is directly incorporated into the polymer film upon formation owing to its low volatility and affinity for the polymer. With latex coating dispersions, plasticizer must partition from the water phase into the latex droplets in order to exert is plasticizing effects on the polymer. The rate and extent of plasticizer partitioning into latex particles during plasticization is dependant upon the water solubility of the plasticizer and its affinity for the polymer phase (68). Once inside a latex polymeric particle, the plasticizer acts to soften and swell the particle reducing internal stress and the resistance to deformation, thereby facilitating the initial phases of latex particle coalescence. On a molecular level, an effective plasticizer interferes with cohesive intermolecular forces between polymer chains and increases molecular mobility. Plasticization decreases polymer T_g, and in the case of latex dispersions decreases the MFT. The MFT of a latex dispersion should be reduced by plasticization to below the coating temperature so as to produce a continuous film during the spraying process. Improved molecular mobility also accelerates the interdiffusion of polymer chains of adjacent fusing latex particles to facilitate the final phase in latex particle coalescence and complete film formation.

It is essential to efficient polymer plasticization for both aqueous solution and latex coating systems that the plasticizer be compatible/miscible with the polymer. Compatibility of the plasticizer with the polymer is essential to ensure that the plasticizer will readily partition into the latex particles during plasticization, and also ensures that the plasticizer will not leach from the polymer following film formation, on storage, or in aqueous media. Leaching will cause a change in the mechanical properties of films that often results in splitting of the film and loss of functionality. Compatibility arises from a molecular attraction between the plasticizer and the polymer, and can be recognized by a concurrent decrease in polymer T_g with increasing plasticizer concentration. A plasticizer is compatible with a polymer up to the concentration at which no further reduction in T_g is achieved. A compatible plasticizer can also be identified if it is a good solvent for the polymer of interest (18). Plasticizer compatibility has been extensively evaluated for most of the commonly used coating polymers.

Numerous molecules have been utilized as plasticizers for pharmaceutical film coating applications. Wheatley and Steuernagel have defined a plasticizer to be a non-volatile, high boiling, non-separating substance that is able to modify certain physical, and mechanical properties of the polymer to be plasticized (7). Plasticizers are commonly classified as water soluble or insoluble. The most commonly used water-soluble plasticizers include: TEC, triacetin, low molecular weight polyethylene glycol, propylene glycol, and glycerol. The most commonly used water-insoluble plasticizers include: acetyltriethyl citrate, acetyltributyl citrate, dibutyl phthalate, DBS, DEP, and TBC. Castor oil, coconut oil, and acetylated monoglycerides are less commonly used insoluble plasticizers. The criteria for selecting an optimum plasticizer for a particular polymer includes: miscibility with the polymer, ability to effectively reduce the T_g of the polymer, the minimum concentration required to achieve the MFT, required plasticization time, and affect on film functionality.

Plasticization generally results in substantial changes in the mechanical properties of polymer films. By interposing itself between polymer molecules and disrupting cohesive bonds, a plasticizer acts as a molecular lubricant reducing the internal friction between polymer chains and decreasing the resistance to segmental movement. Therefore, when under tensile stress, a plasticized polymer film will be less resistant to elongation than the unplasticized film. Specifically, plasticization results in reduced tensile strength and elastic modulus and increased percent elongation of polymer films. Several authors have demonstrated such changes in the tensile properties of polymer films that are commonly used in film coating applications. Gutierrez-Rocca and McGinity demonstrated a reduction in tensile strength and elastic modulus for films of Eudragit L 100-55 following plasticization with different water-soluble and insoluble plasticizers (83). Honary and Orafai reported a decrease in tensile strength of HPMC by plasticization with low molecular weight PEG (84). Hutchings et al. evaluated the effects of 10 different plasticizers on the mechanical properties of free films produced from Aquacoat ECD (85). In this study, a general trend of increasing film elongation and decreasing modulus and stress with increasing plasticizer content was observed with the extent of plasticization correlating to molecular structure of the plasticizer. These studies, along with the theoretical analysis of polymer plasticization, reveal the benefit of plasticizer addition for improving the workability of polymer films and their application to pharmaceutical film coating.

Since plasticizers are typically incorporated into film coating formulations in significant concentrations, their inclusion commonly affects the permeability of polymer films and consequently drug release from coated substrates. Therefore, plasticizer selection for film coating applications must be carefully considered as plasticizers substantially influence permeability. Specifically, the hydrophilicity/hydrophobicity of a plasticizer will determine if the plasticizer will accelerate or impede water permeation, and consequently drug release through a polymer film. Water-soluble plasticizers will typically diffuse out of polymeric films in aqueous media generating void spaces in the film through which diffusion occurs more readily. The result being accelerated dissolution of the substrate and accelerated release of the active. Hydrophobic plasticizers tend to remain in polymer films and decrease film wettability, typically resulting in reduced permeation of the film and slower drug release rates. The release of hydrophobic plasticizers from polymeric films will depend on the solubility of the agent in aqueous media. Increased film permeability by the incorporation of hydrophilic plasticizers is often detrimental to film functionality for many film coating applications; specifically taste masking, enteric release, and sustained release. Lin et al. reported that permeability of Eudragit E films was substantially greater when plasticized with triacetin than with DEP, dibutyl phthalate, or tributyl citrate owing to the greater hydrophilicity of triacetin over these hydrophobic plasticizers (86). Al-Omaran et al. reported greater taste masking with ethylcellulose-based microcapsules when the hydrophobic plasticizer DEP was utilized versus polyethylene glycol due to the reduced permeability of the ethylcellulose coat (87).

Increased permeability of enteric films with water-soluble plasticizers has also been reported. Raffin et al. reported that CAP films plasticized with DEP provided superior gastroresistance than triacetin owing to its hydrophobicity (88). Similar results were reported by Bechard et al. where tablets coated with CAP plasticized with TEC (water-soluble plasticizer) absorbed 40–50% by tablet weight of the 0.1 N HCl dissolution medium during acid phase testing of the enteric tablets (89). Although < 1% of the active agent was released during acid phase dissolution testing with TEC plasticized CAP, the authors concluded that the CAP/TEC film did not provide adequate protection of acid labile drugs due to the extent of acid absorption by the tablet core.

Sustained release film coating is perhaps the application most significantly affected by plasticizer selection. The rate of drug release through a retardant polymer film is controlled by the water permeation rate of the film. As discussed above, the permeability of a polymeric film depends on its physical characteristics; i.e., porosity, tortuosity, and surface morphology; which are strongly influenced by plasticizer due to the effects on film formation. Additionally, plasticizers can substantially alter the permeability of a polymer film by affecting its affinity for aqueous media. Therefore, by these two mechanisms plasticizer choice can drastically affect the rate of drug release from substrates with sustained release coatings.

In a study by Bodmeier et al., it was demonstrated that plasticizer selection strongly influenced the rate of theophylline release in 0.1 N HCl from beads coated with Aquacoat ECD (68). The results of this study are shown in Figure 11. From this figure it can be seen that incomplete film formation resulted from plasticization with triacetin as a result of incompatibility between the hydrophilic plasticizer and the hydrophobic ethylcellulose latex particles. Complete film formation was achieved with all other investigated plasticizers: TEC, Myvacet, tributyl citrate, DBS, and acetyl tributyl citrate; however, faster drug release was seen with TEC due to the water solubility of TEC versus the water-insolubility of the other investigated plasticizers.

Pore Forming Agents

Water-soluble molecules are often incorporated into sustained release film coats as pore forming agents to increase coat permeability. Pore forming agents thus provide a simple and precise means of controlling drug release rates through an insoluble film. Water-soluble molecules dispersed in an insoluble film will dissolve when the coated substrate is placed in aqueous media resulting in the formation of cavities throughout the film coat that act as channels for water permeation. A film will become increasingly more porous and water permeable with increasing concentrations of water-soluble additives. These additives allow for the use of thicker coats in sustained release applications and more precise control of drug release rates. Without the addition of additives to modulate the permeability of a film, typically release rates from sustained release systems can be either too fast or too slow. Often, the desired release rates fall somewhere between these two extremes, and thus alternative formulation approaches must be utilized to achieve these rates. The incorporation of pore forming agents in film coating formulations is perhaps the best technique for altering the permeability of polymeric films to achieve a range of sustained drug release rates.

As discussed previously, Wheatley and Steuernagel demonstrated that the incorporation of HPMC into an ethylcellulose film increased permeability of thick coats and allowed for direct modulation of drug release by adjusting the concentration of HPMC in the film (7). Bussemer et al. also demonstrated the use of HPMC as a water-soluble pore forming agent that acted to increase water absorption of Eudragit RS 30 D and ethylcellulose films (90). Appel and Zentner demonstrated the use of urea as a pore forming agent to increase the permeability of films produced from an ethylcellulose pseudolatex and a cellulose acetate latex to increase drug release rates from osmotic tablets (91,92). Bodmeier and Paeratakul reported increased permeability of aqueous latexes with the use of a pH-dependant pore former, dibasic calcium phosphate (93).

Anti-Taking Agents/Glidants

Most film coats exhibit a certain degree of tackiness due to the adhesive nature of the material. Tackiness of film coats often leads to adhesion and agglomeration of coated substrates to each other or to the equipment surfaces during the coating or curing processes. Adhesion of polymeric films has been shown to be directly proportional to the concentration of plasticizer in the film, coating and curing temperatures, and inversely proportional to the MFT (94). Since high plasticizer content, low MFT, and elevated coating and/or curing temperatures are often required to achieve complete film formation

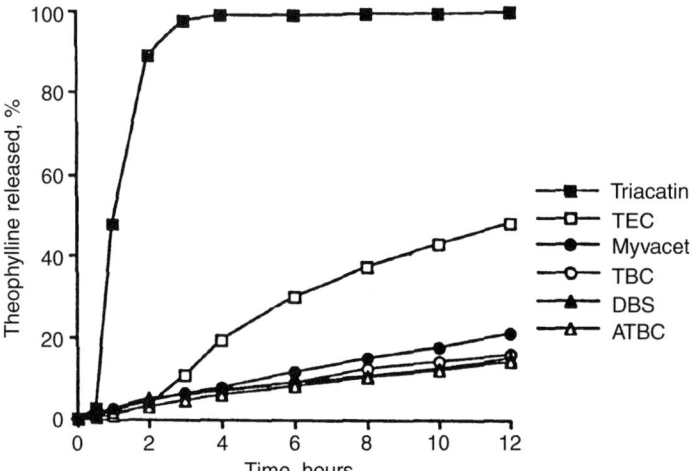

FIGURE 11 Effect of plasticizers on the theophylline release from beads coated with Aquacoat ECD in 0.1 M HCl. *Source*: From Ref. 68.

from latex coating systems; adhesion is a common problem facing aqueous film coating. Adhesion causes substantial problems with respect to handling of the coated product. Sticking of coated substrates can also result in coating defects and in some cases irreversible fusion of multiparticulate substrates.

Adhesion of polymeric films is the result of intermolecular forces that arise when film surfaces make intimate contact and is exacerbated by deformation of the film surfaces while in contact (95). Additionally, if intimate contact is maintained for extended time, interdiffusion of polymer chains can occur that bridges contacting surfaces. Hence, it can be understood that plasticizer content, low MFT, and high temperatures exacerbate adhesion as each of these conditions increases molecular mobility of polymers and renders films soft and deformable.

A common solution to this adhesion problem is the addition of glidants or anti-taking agents to film coating formulations to decrease film tackiness. Talc is one of the most commonly used additives to reduce sticking and agglomeration of coated substrates. However, high levels of talc are often required (up to 100% of polymer mass) to reduce sticking which can lead to sedimentation and nozzle clogging during the coating process (96). Magnesium stearate and kaolin have also been used as glidants with similar efficacy to talc. Colloidal silicon dioxide has also been used as an anti-taking agent and has been shown to be effective at substantially lower concentrations than talc; however, colloidal silicon dioxide has been shown to affect drug release owing to its hygroscopic nature (97). Petereit et al. reported excellent anti-tack efficiency with glyceryl monostearate, a non-ionic surfactant, at concentrations of 2–10% (98). Wesseling et al. reported similar results with GMS finding 5% to be equally as effective as 50% talc for reducing the tackiness of films produced with Eudragit RL, RS, NE 30 D, and Aquacoat ECD coating systems (94). Nimkulrat et al. also reported efficient anti-tack effects with the non-ionic surfactants Span 40 and 60 at a concentration of 5% (w/w) for Eudragit NE 30 D and RS 30 D films without adversely affecting film flexibility (99). These authors showed that Span and GMS function to reduce film tack by decreasing the proportion of exposed polymer at film surfaces thereby reducing contact area for adhesion. These studies indicate that although tackiness of film coated substrates can be problematic, with the addition of anti-tacking agents the complications of substrate adhesion can be eliminated.

Coloring Agents and Opacifiers

The benefits of coloring agents and/or opacifiers to pharmaceutical film coating formulations were discussed in detail previously in this chapter. Briefly, opacifiers are added to film coating formulations to protect photolytic drugs from degradation and to hide imperfections of the substrate such as mottled or unpleasantly colored cores. Coloring agents are added to film coating formulations for a variety of reasons including: to improve the aesthetic appeal of a coated dosage form, improve product identification, create trademark protection of branded products, and to inhibit counterfeiting. Opacifying agents and coloring agents are water-insoluble additives that most commonly include aluminum lakes of water-soluble dyes and inorganic pigments like titanium dioxide and iron oxide. The degree to which an insoluble additive is able to render a polymeric film opaque is dependent on the difference in the indices of refraction of the polymer film and the additive, as well as the dispersed state of the additive in the film. Greater amounts of light will be reflected at the polymer-additive interface with increasing difference in refractive index of the two phases. Additionally, a finer dispersion leads to greater interfacial area of the two phases. Hence, an insoluble additive in sufficient concentration, with a refractive index substantially different than the polymer film and that is finely dispersed in the film will impart significant opacity to the film coat. If the refractive indices of the insoluble additive and the polymer film are near in value, the resulting film will appear transparent. Since aluminum lakes typically have indices of refraction near that of most polymer films, they do not function well as opacifying agents. On the other hand, red iron oxide and titanium dioxide have substantially greater refractive indices than most common polymer films, and are therefore excellent opacifying agents.

Coloring agents currently used in pharmaceutical film coating applications are almost exclusively aluminum lakes. Aluminum lakes are water-insoluble complexes of organic dyes with hydrated alumina. The production process of aluminum lakes essentially involves creating the hydrated alumina substrate by a reaction of aluminum chloride with sodium carbonate, followed by the adsorption of an organic dye to the hydrated alumina substrate (18). There are several advantages to using these water-insoluble pigments over water-soluble dyes for film coating applications. These include: reduced color migration, increased film opacity, improved color stability, decreased film permeability, and reduced film tackiness (18).

It has been suggested that the addition of pigment to a film coating formulation in the amount of 2–3 mg/cm^2 is sufficient to mask the underlying substrate surface (50). Greater amounts may be desired to improve the richness of the color; however, the concentration must remain below the critical pigment volume concentration (CPVC). The CPVC is the point at which there is insufficient polymer to surround the pigment particles in the dry film and is characteristic to the specific polymer-additive combination. If the CPVC is exceeded, marked changes to the appearance, mechanical properties, and permeability of the polymeric film occur (100). Below the CPVC, the presence of pigment decreases film permeability, but once the CPVC is exceeded an increase in film permeability occurs with increasing pigment concentration (101). With respect to the mechanical properties of polymeric films, pigments typically reduce tensile strength, decrease elongation in tension, and increase the elastic modulus. These effects increase with increased concentration of the insoluble additive, and with increased particle size of the additive. Therefore, the effects of colorants and opacifiers on the properties of polymeric films must be carefully considered during formulation to avoid problems concerning the permeability and toughness of the film coating.

Other Notable Additives

Flavoring agents can be included in coating formulations to improve the taste masking functionality of a film coat. Waxes have been utilized to enhance the pharmaceutical elegance of film coated dosage forms by enhancing the gloss of a polymeric film coat. Saccharides such as polydextrose, maltodextrin, and lactose have also been incorporated into film coating formulations to improve adhesion of polymeric films to substrates (102). Surfactants and other excipient stabilizers are included in coating formulations to improve the stability of colloidal dispersions and to emulsify water-insoluble plasticizers. For example, sodium lauryl sulfate and cetyl alcohol are included in the Aquacoat ECD formulation to stabilize the colloidal ethylcellulose dispersion. Sorbitan esters are used to stabilize latex formulations with methacrylic acid copolymers and to aid in the redispersion of spray dried powder forms of these polymers. Povidone has also been used as a stabilizer to prevent latex particle agglomeration with the addition of pigments to coating dispersions (50). The addition of surfactants to coating dispersions often causes the evolution of foam during the coating process, and consequently anti-foaming agents, such as dimethicone, are typically added to eliminate this problem. Thus, there are numerous different auxiliary additives to a coating formulation that can be utilized to improve the coating process and the final product.

PROBLEMS OF POLYMERIC FILM COATING

Physical Aging

Amorphous polymers cooled below their glass transition temperatures are essentially frozen polymeric liquids in a state of thermodynamically disequilibrium owing to an excess of free volume for the solid material (103). Since this is an energetically unfavorable state, the polymer chains in a glassy film will over time reorient themselves to achieve equilibrium. The rate at which this reorientation of polymer chains occurs depends upon the difference between the T_g of the polymer and the temperature of the storage conditions as molecular mobility will be greater when the storage temperature is nearer to and above the T_g of the polymer. The reorientation of polymer chains leads to the elimination of excess free volume and the contraction/densification of the film. Permeability is reduced as the film contracts owing to reduced porosity and increased tortuosity. Hence, drug release rates from substrates coated with amorphous polymers are often seen to decrease with time due to physical aging. Physical aging with respect to film coating with latex and pseudolatex systems involves the additional mechanism of further coalescence of latex particles by continued interdiffusion of polymers over time. The interdiffusion of polymers from adjacent fusing latex particles leads to the reduction void space within the film with time, thus decreasing film permeability and drug release rate through the film.

The incorporation of high plasticizer levels has been reported to control the problem of physical aging by substantially reducing the T_g of the coating polymer to accelerate equilibrated film formation (104). Extensive plasticization promotes the formation of more stable polymeric films and static drug release profiles on storage; however, excessive tackiness can result causing agglomeration and handling problems. It has also been reported that curing film coated substrates at elevated temperatures following coating can be utilized to reduce physical aging by increasing polymer mobility to accelerate further particle coalescence and complete film formation (104). The addition of additives to film coating formulations has also been utilized to reduce or eliminate the effects of physical aging and to stabilize drug release profiles on storage. Maejima and McGinity reported that high levels of talc (200% based on polymer mass) stabilized drug release profiles from pellets coated with Eudragit RS/RL 30 D for 3 months when stored at 40°C/75% RH (105). Different polymeric additives and blends have also been reported to reduce physical aging of polymethacrylate coating systems. Zheng et al. demonstrated the use of hydroxyethyl cellulose to stabilize theophylline release on storage from pellets coated with Eudragit RS 30 D according to a "coalescence blocking" mechanism (106). Zheng and McGinity reported that blending Eudragit NE 30 D with Eudragit L 30 D-55 in a 5:1 ratio reduced the effects of physical aging on pellets coated with Eudragit NE 30 D alone (107). Similarly, Wu and McGinity utilized Eudragit L 100-55 to eliminate the effects of physical aging of theophylline pellets coated with Eudragit RS 30 D (108). These studies thus indicate that the effects of physical aging can be minimized by formulation and post processing strategies.

Coating Defects

Polymeric film coats are usually quite thin with typical thickness ranging from 10 to 100 μm. Thin film coats are advantageous in many respects as discussed previously; however, thin film coats can be disadvantageous as even minor defects can substantially affect film continuity and functionality. There are numerous types of film coat defects that result from processing factors, formulational factors (both film and substrate), or a combination of the two. Visual inspection of coat defects is often sufficient to diagnose the underlying cause and make the necessary adjustments to reduce further defects.

Cracking, chipping, and splitting of film coats are the three common coating defects with a few potential causes. If film breakage is not excessive and occurs primarily at the edges of the tablet, the underlying cause is likely to be attrition resulting from the coating process (109). This can be eliminated by simply decreasing the rotational speed of the drum in pan coating systems or decreasing the fluidizing air pressure in fluid bed coating systems. If cracking, chipping, or splitting is excessive, it typically indicates incomplete film formation or poor film toughness. Insufficient plasticization can be the cause of this problem and may be eliminated by increasing the concentration of plasticizer in the film or utilizing a more compatible plasticizer for the polymer. Finally, poor film toughness attributable to the grade of the coating polymer can cause these types of coating defects as well which can be remedied by utilizing a higher molecular weight grade of the coating polymer (110). Peeling and flaking are coating defects whereby large potions of the film coat peel back or flake off exposing relatively large sections of the tablet surface. These coating defects are extensions of cracking, chipping, or splitting and can be eliminated by the process or formulation adjustments described above.

Film defects known as picking and cratering can occur when the application rate of the coating solution or suspension is too great or if the substrate bed is excessively wet. Cratering occurs when the coating liquid is applied too quickly at the start of a coating process causing the surface of the substrates to partially disintegrate. This causes the formation of craters on the substrate surface that will be subsequently covered by the film coat. This problem can be solved by spraying the coating dispersion at a reduced rate to begin the coating run. After a sufficient coat has been applied to the surface of the substrates (~2% by bed weight), the spray rate of the coating dispersion can then be increased without damaging the substrates. If the bed temperature is too low or the inlet air flow rate is insufficient to force evaporation of the coating dispersion liquid phase, moisture will accumulate within the substrate bed. Often, under these conditions substrates will momentarily agglomerate and then be forced apart by the movement of the coating bed. As the substrates are forced apart, portions of the film coat pull away from the surface forming large and small voids in the surface of the film which is known as picking. Picking can be eliminated by ensuring that the substrate bed remains sufficiently dry during coating either by reducing the dispersion spray rate, increasing the inlet air flow rate, or increasing the bed temperature by increasing the temperature of the inlet air.

Although it is important to ensure the substrate bed remain sufficiently dry during coating, it is also important to ensure that the substrate bed not become excessively hot as pitting and film blistering can occur. Pitting involves the melting substrate components such as stearic acid and polyethylene glycol during the coating process (109,111). This defect does not interrupt the film coat, but does diminish the pharmaceutical elegance of the dosage form by creating small indentations in the surface of the coated substrate. If the substrate formulation cannot be altered to eliminate this problem, pitting can be reduced by avoiding preheating of tablets prior to coating, particularly if this process elevates the bed temperature above the melting points of core constituents. The temperature of the inlet air can be also be adjusted to avoid pitting. Wrinkling of a polymeric film can also result from elevated bed temperatures. This defect occurs when gasses trapped beneath a film coat cause the film to expand, detach from the substrate surface, and then collapse forming a wrinkle on the surface. This is typically caused by overheating the substrate bed and can be intensified by poor adhesion of the film to the substrate. Therefore, this problem can also be diminished by reducing the bed temperature and/or altering the film or substrate formulation to ensure adequate adhesion. Surface roughness can also occur if the coating temperature is excessive. In this case, liquid from the coating suspension evaporates in flight causing atomized droplets of the coating dispersion to become viscous or dry. This prevents spreading and coalescence of the coating polymer resulting in a rough surface texture.

Mottling or inadequate color uniformity is another common film coating defect that can arise from a variety of causes. Inhomogeneous color dispersion can result from failure to adequately disperse pigment particles throughout the coating suspension. Therefore, when applied to substrates, the film coat will appear to be spotted where larger agglomerates are present. Dye migration can also occur resulting in an accumulation of dye at the film surface. The use of water-soluble dyes in coating formulations can cause this problem as the dye will remain in the evolving water phase, eventually depositing on the film surface and leaving a mottled appearance. Also, desorption of dye from pigments has been observed to occur particularly in the presence of certain plasticizers in which the dye is soluble (112). These problems can be avoided by avoiding the use of water-soluble dyes and lakes of poor quality, as well as ensuring adequate dispersal of pigments during the production of the coating suspension.

Other coat defects such as blushing, blooming, and bridging are somewhat common and the inquiring reader is referred to the review by Rowe for more information on these and the above mentioned coat defects (109).

SUMMARY

Aqueous-based film coating was developed to circumvent the limitations of preceding technologies and has since become one of the most important pharmaceutical processes utilized today. The applications of aqueous polymeric film coating to oral drug delivery are vast and span simple cosmetic enhancements to modifying drug release for improved oral drug therapies. Each application of aqueous polymeric film coating to drug delivery is unique with regard to its underlying principles, associated materials, and processing considerations. This chapter has provided a detailed discussion of the fundamentals of aqueous polymeric film coating with respect to its specific purposes in oral drug delivery with particular emphasis on materials and their properties. Understanding these fundamentals of aqueous polymeric film coating is essential to the successful development of pharmaceutical film coating formulations. Moreover, these fundamentals will serve as a basis for the continued development and expansion of pharmaceutical coating technology.

REFERENCES

1. Porter SC. Coating of pharmaceutical dosage forms. In: Gennaro AR, ed. Remington: The Science and Practice of Pharmacy. 20th ed. Baltimore, MD: Lippincott Williams & Wilkins, 2000.
2. Kremmers E, Urdang G. History of Pharmacy. Philadelphia: Lippincott, 1940.

3. Urdang G. What's new. J Am Pharm Assoc 1943; 34(135):5–14.
4. White RC. J Am Pharm Assoc 1922; 11:345.
5. Weigand TS. Am J Pharm 1902; 74:33.
6. Warner WR. The sugar coated pill. Am J Pharm 1902; 74:32.
7. Wheatley TA, Steuernagel CR. Latex emulsions for controlled drug delivery. In: McGinity JW, ed. Aqueous Polymeric Coatings for Pharmaceutical Dosage Forms. 2nd ed. New York: Marcel Dekker, 1997:15.
8. Sohi H, Sultana Y, Khar R. Taste masking technologies in oral pharmaceuticals: Recent developments and approaches. Drug Dev Ind Pharm 2004; 30(5):429–48.
9. Jones BE. Colours for pharmaceutical products. Pharm Technol Int 1993; 5:14–20.
10. Cheiken AH, Bavitz JF, inventors; Merck & Co., Inc., assignee. Method for Applying High Luster Coating to Tablets. US Patent No. 3,576,665. 1971.
11. Perkins AC, Wilson CG, Frier M, et al. Oesophageal transit, disintegration and gastric emptying of a film-coated risedronate placebo tablet in gastro-oesophageal reflux disease and normal control subjects. Aliment Pharmacol Ther 2001; 15(1):115–21.
12. Anonymous. Tablets and capsules that stick in the oesophagus. Drug Ther Bull 1981; 19(9):33–4.
13. Wallace JW. Cellulose derivatives and natural products utilized in pharmaceutics In: Swarbrick J, Boylan JC, eds. Encyclopedia of Pharmaceutical Technology. New York: Marcel Dekker, Inc., 1990: 319–37.
14. Doerr DW, Serles ER, Deardorff DL, inventors; University of Illinois Foundation, assignee. Hydroxyethyl cellulose tablet coating. US Patent No. 2,816,062. 1957.
15. Lehmann K, Brogmann B. Tablet coating. In: Swarbrick J, Boylan JC, eds. Encyclopedia of Pharmaceutical Technology. New York: Marcel Dekker, Inc., 1996.
16. Singiser RE, inventor Abbott Laboratories, assignee. Japanese Patent 37-12294. 1962.
17. Nagai T, Obara S, Kokubo H, Hoshi N. Application of HPMC and HPMCAS to aqueous film coating of pharmaceutical dosage forms. In: McGinity JW, ed. Aqueous Polymeric Coatings for Pharmaceutical Dosage Forms. 2nd ed. New York: Marcel Dekker, Inc., 1997; 177–225.
18. Hogan JE. Film-coating materials and their properties. In: Cole G, ed. Pharmaceutical Coating Technology. Bristol, PA: Taylor & Francis Inc., 1995.
19. Li SP, Martellucci SA, Bruce RD, Kinyon AC, Hay MB, Higgins JD. Evaluation of the film-coating properties of a hydroxyethyl cellulose/hydroxypropyl methylcellulose polymer system. Drug Dev Ind Pharm 2002; 28(4):389.
20. Technical literature: Klucel EF Pharm Hydroxypropylcellulose. Aqualon, 2000. (Accessed February 27, 2007, at http://www.herc.com/aqualon/product_data/brochures/250_49.pdf#hpc.)
21. Specifications and test methods for Eudragit® E 100, Eudragit® E PO and Eudragit® E 12,5. degussa, 2004. (Accessed February 27, 2007, at http://www.eudragit.com/pharmapolymers/en/downloads/.)
22. Lehmann K. Acrylic resin coatings for drugs: relation between their chemical structure, properties and application possibilities. Drug Made Germany 1968; 11:34–41.
23. Ishikawa T, Watanabe Y, Utoguchi N, Matsumoto M. Preparation and evaluation of tablets rapidly disintegrating in saliva containing bitter-taste-masked granules by the compression method. Chem Pharm Bull 1999; 47:1451–4.
24. Chowhan ZT, Amaro AA, Chi LH. Comparative evaluation of aqueous film coated tablet formulations by high humidity aging. Drug Dev Ind Pharm 1982; 8:713–37.
25. Thoennes CJ, McCurdy VE. Evaluation of a rapidly disintegrating, moisture resistant laquer film coating. Drug Dev Ind Pharm 1989; 15:165–85.
26. Guidelines for Formulation Development and Process Technology for Protective Coatings. degussa, 2006. (Accessed February 27, 2007, at http://www.eudragit.com/pharmapolymers/en/downloads/.)
27. Kollicoat IR Technical Information. BASF, 2004. (Accessed February 27, 2007, at http://www.pharma-solutions.basf.com/.)
28. Babb RR, Wilbur RS. Asprin and Gastrointestianl Bleeding. Calif Med 1969; 110(5):440–1.

29. Strom JG, Jun HW. Gastric irritation and bleeding after drug administration. J Pharm Sci 1974; 63(11):1812–3.
30. Overhoff KA, Moreno A, Miller DA, Johnston KP, Williams Iii RO. Solid dispersions of itraconazole and enteric polymers made by ultra-rapid freezing. Int J Pharm 2007; 330(1–2): 61–72.
31. Kohri N, Yamayoshi Y, Xin H, et al. Improving the oral bioavailability of albendazole in rabbits by the solid dispersion technique. J Pharm Pharmacol 1999; 51:159–64.
32. Miller DA, McConville JT, Yang W, Williams III RO, McGinity JW. Hot-melt extrusion for enhanced delivery of drug particles. J Pharm Sci 2007; 96(2):361–76.
33. Chambliss WG. Enteric coatings. In: Swarbrick J, Boylan JC, eds. Encyclopedia of Pharmaceutical Technology. New York: Marcel Dekker, Inc., 1992; 189–200.
34. Hiatt GD, inventor Eastman Kodak Company, assignee. Enteric Coating. US Patent No. 2,196,768. 1940.
35. Miller LA. Cellulose acetate phthalate. In: Rowe RC, Sheskey PJ, Owen SC, eds. Pharmaceutical Excipients. Pharmaceutical Press and American Pharmacists Association, 2006.
36. Edgar KJ. Cellulose esters in drug delivery. Cellulose 2006; 14:49–64.
37. Wu SHW, Wyatt DM, Adams MW. Chemistry and applications of cellulosic polymers for enteric coatings of solid dosage forms. In: McGinity JW, ed. Aqueous Polymeric Coatings for Pharmaceutical Dosage Forms. New York: Marcel Dekker, Inc., 1997.
38. Sakellariou P, Rowe RC, White EFT. The thermomechanical properties and glass transition temperatures of some cellulose derivatives used in film coating. Int J Pharm 1985; 27:267–77.
39. Obara S, McGinity JW. Influence of processing variables on the properties of free films prepared from aqueous polymeric dispersions by a spray technique. Int J Pharm 1995; 126(1–2):1–10.
40. Williams RO, Liu J. The influence of plasticizer on heat-humidity curing of cellulose acetate phthalate coated beads. Pharm Dev Technol 2001; 6(4):607.
41. Anonymous. Hypromellose phthalate NF enteric coating material. Shin Etsu Chemical Company Technical Literature
42. Gaskonda S, Lee J. Hypromellose phthalate. In: Rowe RC, Sheskey PJ, Owen SC, eds. Pharmaceutical Excipients 5. Pharmaceutical Press and American Pharmacists Association 2005.
43. Muhammad NA, Boisvert W, Harris MR, Weiss J. Evaluation of hydroxypropyl methylcellulose phthalate-50 as film forming polymer from aqueous dispersion-systems. Drug Dev Ind Pharm 1992; 18(16):1787–97.
44. Rafati H, Ghassempour A, Barzegar-Jalali M. A new solution for a chronic problem; Aqueous enteric coating. J Pharm Sci 2006; 95(11):2432–7.
45. Thoma K, Bechtold K. Influence of aqueous coatings on the stability of enteric coated pellets and tablets. Eur J Pharm Biopharm 1999; 47(1):39–50.
46. Felton L, McGinity J. Enteric film coating of soft gelatin capsules. Drug Deliv Technol 2003; 3(6):34–9.
47. Siepmann F, Siepmann J, Walther M, MacRae R, Bodmeier R. Aqueous HPMCAS coatings: Effects of formulation and processing parameters on drug release and mass transport mechanisms. Eur J Pharm Biopharm 2006; 63(3):262–9.
48. Lehmann K, Dreher D. Permeable acrylic resin coatings for the manufacture of depot preparation of drug. Pharm Ind 1969; 31:319–22.
49. Anonymous. Specifications and test methods for Eudragit L 100-55. In: Degussa Pharma Polymers; 2004, www.eudragit.com.
50. Lehmann KOR. Chemistry and application properties of polymethacrylate coating systems. In: McGinity JW, ed. Aqueous Polymeric Coatings for Pharmaceutical Dosage Forms. 2nd ed. New York: Marcel Dekker, Inc., 1997: 101–76.
51. Schmidt PC, Niemann F. The miniwid-coater 2. Comparison of acid resistance of enteric-coated bisacodyl pellets coated with different polymers. Drug Dev Ind Pharm 1992; 18(18):1969–79.

52. Anonymous. Specifications and test methods for Eudragit L 100 and Eudragit S 100. In: Degussa Pharma Polymers; 2004, www.eudragit.com.
53. Lehmann K, Petereit H-U. Film coats based on polymethacrylate dispersions with retarded decay within the intestinal tract. Drug Made Germany 1993; 55:615–8.
54. Gupta VK, Assmus MW, Beckert TE, Price JC. A novel pH- and time-based multi-unit potential colonic drug delivery system. II. Optimization of multiple response variables. Int J Pharm 2001; 213(1–2):93–102.
55. Gupta VK, Beckert TE, Price JC. A novel pH- and time-based multi-unit potential colonic drug delivery system. I. Development. Int J Pharm 2001; 213(1–2):83–91.
56. Rudolph MW, Klein S, Beckert TE, Petereit H-U, Dressman JB. A new 5-aminosalicylic acid multi-unit dosage form for the therapy of ulcerative colitis. Eur J Pharm Biopharm 2001; 51(3):183–90.
57. Porter SC, Ridgway K. An evalutation of the properties of enteric coating polymers: measurement of glass transition temperature. J Pharm Pharmacol 1983; 35:341–4.
58. Mehuys E, Remon J-P, Vervaet C. Production of enteric capsules by means of hot-melt extrusion. Eur J Pharm Sci 2005; 24(2–3):207–12.
59. Cable C. Polyvinyl acetate phthalate. In: Rowe RC, Sheskey PJ, Owen SC, eds. Pharmaceutical Excipients 5. Pharmaceutical Press and American Pharmacists Association, 2005.
60. Hogan JE. Coating of tablets and multiparticulates In: Aulton ME, ed. Pharmaceutics: The Science of Dosage Form Design. New York: Churchill Livingstone; 2001: 441–8.
61. Collett J, Moreton C. Modified release peroral dosage forms In: Aulton ME, ed. Pharmaceutics: The Science of Dosage Form Design. New York: Churchill Livingstone; 2001: 289–305.
62. Abrahamsson B, Alpsten M, Jonsson UE, et al. Gastro-intestinal transit of a multiple-unit formulation (metoprolol CR/ZOK) and a non-disintegrating tablet with the emphasis on colon. Int J Pharm 1996; 140(2):229–35.
63. Anonymous. Ethocel. In: Ethylcellulose Polymers Technical Handbook. The Dow Chemical Company: Dow Cellulosics; 2005, www.ethocel.com
64. Onions A. Films from water-based colloidal dispersions. Manufact Chem 1986; 57(4):66–7.
65. Bodmeier R, Paeratakul O. Process and formulation variables affecting the drug release from chlorpheniramine maleate-loaded beads coated with commercial and self-prepared aqueous ethyl cellulose pseudolatexes. Int J Pharm 1991; 70(1–2):59–68.
66. Iyer U, Hong WH, Das N, Gherbre-Sellassie I. Comparative evaluation fo three organic solvent and dispersion-based ethylcellulose coating formulations. Pharm Technol 1990; September:68–86.
67. Leng DE, Sigelko WL, Saunders FL, inventors; The Dow Chemical Company, assignee. Aqueous dispersions of plasticized polymer particles US Patent No. 4,502,888. 1985.
68. Bodmeier R, Guo X, Paeratakul O. Process and formulational factors affecting the drug release from pellets coated with the ethylcellulose-pseudolatex aquacoat. In: McGinity JW, ed. Aqueous Polymeric Coatings for Pharmaceutical Dosage Forms. 2nd ed. New York: Marcel Dekker, Inc., 1997: 55–80.
69. Ozturk AG, Ozturk SS, Palsson BO, Wheatley TA, Dressman JB. Mechanism of release from pellets coated with an ethylcellulose-based film. J Control Release 1990; 14(3):203–13.
70. Goodhart FW, Harris MR, Murthy KS, Nesbitt RU. An evaluation of aqueous film-forming dispersions for controlled release. Pharm Technol 1984; 8:64–71.
71. Porter SC. Use of opadry, sureteric, and surelease for the aqueous film coating of pharmaceutical oral dosage forms. In: McGinity JW, ed. Aqueous Polymeric Coatings For Pharmaceutical Dosage Forms. 2nd ed. New York: Marcel Dekker, Inc., 1997: 327–83.
72. Bodmeier R, Paeratakul O. The effect of curing on drug-release and morphological properties of ethylcellulose pseudolatex-coated beads. Drug Devel Indl Pharm 1994; 20(9):1517–33.

73. Amighi K, Moes A. Influence of plasticizer concentration and storage conditions on the drug release rate from Eudragit® RS30D film-coated sustained-release theophylline pellets. Eur J Pharm Biopharm 1996; 42(1):29–35.
74. Zhang Y, Zhang ZR, Wu F. A novel pulsed-release system based on swelling and osmotic pumping mechanism. J Control Release 2003; 89(1):47–55.
75. Chang CM, Bodmeier R. Organic solvent-free polymeric microspheres prepared from aqueous colloidal polymer dispersions by a w/o-emulsion technique. Int J Pharm 1996; 130(2):187–94.
76. Lin AY, Muhammad NA, Pope D, Augsburger LL. Study of the effects of curing and storage conditions on controlled release diphenhydramine HCl pellets coated with Eudragit® NE30D. Pharm Develop Technol 2003; 8(3):277–87.
77. Anonymous. Technical information: Kollicoat SR 30 D. In: BASF Pharma Solutions; 2006, www.pharma-solutions.basf.com.
78. Dashevsky A, Wagner K, Kolter K, Bodmeier R. Physicochemical and release properties of pellets coated with Kollicoat® SR 30 D, a new aqueous polyvinyl acetate dispersion for extended release. Int J Pharm 2005; 290(1–2):15–23.
79. Shao ZJ, Morales L, Diaz S, Muhammad NA. Drug release from Kollicoat SR 30D-coated nonpareil beads: Evaluation of coating level, plasticizer type, and curing condition. AAPS PharmSciTech 2002; 3(2):87–96.
80. Anonymous. Package insert. Avinza (morphine sulfate). San Diego: Ligand Pharmaceuticals, February 2003.
81. Anonymous. Package insert: Ritalin LA (methylphenidate hydrochloride). East Hanover, NJ: Novartis Pharmaceuticals Corporation 2006.
82. Bettman MJ, Percel PJ, Hensley DL, Vishnupad KS, Venkatesh GM, inventors; Eurand America, Inc., assignee. Methylphenidate modified release formulations US patent 6,344,215. 2002.
83. Gutierrez-Rocca JC, McGinity JW. Influence of water-soluble and insoluble plasticizers on the physical and mechanical properties of acrylic resin copolymers. Int J Pharm 1994; 103:293–301.
84. Honary S, Orafai H. The effect of different plasticizer molecular weights and concentrations on mechanical and thermomechanical properties of free films. Drug Develop Ind Pharm 2002; 28(6):711–5.
85. Hutchings D, Clarson S, Sakr A. Studies of the mechanical properties of free films prepared using an ethylcellulose pseudolatex coating system. Int J Pharm 1994; 104(3):203–13.
86. Lin S, Chen K, Run-Chu L. Organic esters of plasticizers affecting the water absorption, adhesive property, glass transition temperature, and plasticizer permanence of Eudragit acrylic films. J Control Release 2000; 68:343–50.
87. Al-Omran MF, Al-Suwayeh SA, El-Helw AM, Saleh SI. Taste masking of diclofenac sodium using microencapsulation. J Microencapsul 2002; 19(1):45–52.
88. Raffin F, Duru C, Jacob M, et al. Physico-chemical characterization of the ionic permeability of an enteric coating polymer. Int J Pharm 1995; 120(2):205–14.
89. Bechard SR, Levy L, Clas S-D. Thermal, mechanical and functional properties of cellulose acetate phthalate (CAP) coatings obtained from neutralized aqueous solutions. Int J Pharms 1995; 114(2):205–13.
90. Bussemer T, Peppas NA, Bodmeier R. Time-dependent mechanical properties of polymeric coatings used in rupturable pulsatile release dosage forms. Drug Develop Ind Pharm 2003; 29(6):623–30.
91. Appel LE, Zentner GM. Use of modified ethylcellulose lattices for microporous coating of osmotic tablets. Pharm Res 1991; 8(5):600–4.
92. Appel LE, Clair JH, Zentner GM. Formulation and optimization of a modified microporous cellulose-acetate latex coating for osmotic pumps. Pharm Res 1992; 9(12):1664–7.
93. Bodmeier R, Paeratakul O. Constant potassium-chloride release from microporous membrane-coated tablets prepared with aqueous colloidal polymer dispersions. Pharm Res 1991; 8(3):355–9.

94. Wesseling M, Kuppler F, Bodmeier R. Tackiness of acrylic and cellulosic polymer films used in the coating of solid dosage forms. Eur J Pharm Biopharm 1999; 47(1):73–8.
95. Anand JN. Contact theory of adhesion. Reply to comments. J Adhesion 1973; 5:265–7.
96. Felton LA, McGinity JW. Influence of insoluble excipients on film coating systems. Drug Develop Ind Pharm 2002; 28(3):225–43.
97. Vecchio C, Fabiani F, Gazzaniga A. Use of colloidal silica as a separating agent in film forming processed performed with aqueous dispersion of acrylic resins. Drug Dev Ind Pharm 1995; 21:1781–7.
98. Petereit HU, Abmus M, Lehmann K. Glyceryl monostearate as a glidant in aqueous film-coating formulation. Eur J Pharm Biopharm 1995; 41:219–28.
99. Nimkulrat S, Suchiva K, Phinyocheep P, Puttipipatkhachorn S. Influence of selected surfactants on the tackiness of acrylic polymer films. Int J Pharm 2004; 287(1–2):27–37.
100. Okhamafe AO, York P. Effect of Solids polymer interactions on the properties of some aqueous-based tablet film coating formulations 2. Mechanical characteristics. Int J Pharm 1984; 22(2–3):273–81.
101. Chatfield HW. The science of surface coatings. New York: Van Nostrand, 1962.
102. Jordan MP, Easterbrook MG, Hogan JE. In: Proceedings in 11th International Pharmaceutical Technology Conference, Manchester, 1992.
103. Guo JH. Aging processes in pharmaceutical polymers. Pharm Sci Technol Today 1999; 2(12):478–83.
104. Amighi K, Moes AJ. Influence of plasticizer concentration and storage conditions on the drug release rate from Eudragit RS 30 D film-coated sustained-release theophylline pellets. Eur J Pharm Biopharm 1996; 42(1):29–35.
105. Maejima T, McGinity JW. Influence of film additives on stabilizing drug release rates from pellets coated with acrylic polymers. Pharm Develop Technol 2001; 6(2):211–21.
106. Zheng W, Sauer D, McGinity JW. Influence of hydroxyethylcellulose on the drug release properties of theophylline pellets coated with Eudragit® RS 30 D. Eur J Pharm Biopharm 2005; 59(1):147–54.
107. Zheng WJ, McGinity JW. Influence of Eudragit® NE 30 D blended with Eudragit® L 30 D-55 on the release of phenylpropanolamine hydrochloride from coated pellets. Drug Develop Ind Pharm 2003; 29(3):357–66.
108. Wu CB, McGinity JW. Influence of an enteric polymer on drug release rates of theophylline from pellets coated with Eudragit® RS 30D. Pharm Develop Technol 2003; 8(1):103–10.
109. Rowe RC. Defects in aqueous film-coated tablets. In: McGinity JW, ed. Aqueous Polymeric Coatings for Pharmaceutical Dosage Forms. 2nd ed. New York: Marcel Dekker, Inc., 1997: 419–40.
110. Rowe RC. The effect of molecular weight on the properties of films prepared from hydroxypropyl methylcellulose. Pharm Acta Helv 1976; 51(11):330–4.
111. Rowe RC, Forse SF. Pitting-a defect on film coated tablets. Int J Pharm 1983; 13:347.
112. Proter SC. Tablet coating-problems with film coating Drug Cosmet Ind 1981; 129(9):50.

13
The Application of Thermal Analysis to Pharmaceutical Dosage Forms

Duncan Q. M. Craig
School of Chemical Sciences and Pharmacy, University of East Anglia, Norwich, U.K.

INTRODUCTION: WHAT IS THERMAL ANALYSIS AND WHY IS IT USED?

The term "thermal analysis" refers to a family of techniques whereby the structure and properties of a sample are studied by means of observing what happens when they are heated or cooled. There are now a very wide variety of such methods available and only the most widely used will be covered here, along with a discussion of how and why they are used. Nevertheless, there are some general comments that can be made at the outset that put the techniques and their uses in a pharmaceutical context.

The first point is the distinction, which may admittedly often become blurred, between physical and chemical measurements. Chemical analysis addresses issues such as the identification of the elements present and the structure of the molecules present in a sample, the measurement of the quantity of that material, the identification of degradation products, and the identification of molecular interactions between the molecules and other components of the sample. A classic pharmaceutical example would be the development of a high performance liquid chromatography assay for a new drug so that its quantity and integrity within a formulation may be assessed. Physical analysis, however, is usually applied to systems whereby we already know the chemical composition but we are instead interested in how those molecules are assembled together and the energies required to separate them. A pharmaceutical example would be the identification of different polymorphs of the same drug molecule via differences in their melting points, an issue that will be discussed in more detail later in the chapter. The vast majority of thermal methods give the operator physical rather than chemical information as these approaches essentially yield information on the nature of how molecules interact with each other, hence the problems that are addressed using these methods tend to relate to physical arrangements rather than chemical structure.

The measurement of temperature is one of the fundamental means of assessing the properties of a system, going back to the simple method of putting one's hand on or in a system such as a pool of water. It is useful to consider this apparently trivial example in more detail as many of the principles of thermal analysis may be understood in this way. In reality, what is being performed is a comparison of the "hotness" of the water to that of the body (or more specifically that of the skin). This leads to two of the underpinning concepts of thermal analysis. The first is that we make measurements of thermal properties by comparison, not by absolute measurements. All thermal methods work in this way in one form or another and that is why suitable calibration or referencing is so essential, as we are measuring differences in properties in, for example, heat content or flow compared to a known standard.

The second issue is that it is necessary to be clear with regard to the difference between heat content and temperature. The heat content (almost invariably expressed in terms of the enthalpy H) is a measure of the energy contained by the molecular motions within a system and is an extremely useful parameter, for reasons that will be explained later. It is, therefore, dependent on the number of molecules in the system, i.e., if one doubles the number of molecules, one doubles the enthalpy, hence it is often expressed per unit mass of material. Temperature is a scale where the heat exchange properties of a system are compared to a known standard, in other words the temperature measures the propensity of heat to move from one object to another. For example, the mercury in a thermometer expands in a predictable manner as its heat content changes and its heat content is related to that of its immediate environment, hence we are able to derive scales such as the centigrade scale whereby we are able to relate the heat content of the environment to the volume of the mercury. This in turn allows us to measure, for example, body temperature at 37°C. The temperature is not dependent on the volume of the system; 100 mL of water at 50°C has the same temperature as 200 mL of water at 50°C as both have the same propensity to give heat energy to materials they come into contact with that have a lower temperature (e.g., heat going into your immersed hand). There is, of course, an absolute (Kelvin) temperature scale where 0K represents the complete absence of molecular motion for a perfect crystal, although this scale is itself used by conversion from comparative methods such as the centigrade scale as we have no method of making direct comparisons with a sample at 0K. A further key point is that temperature is much easier to measure than heat content as all that is required is some form of thermometer such as a thermocouple with which the heat flow to or from a standard is assessed by looking at the temperature difference between them, hence all thermal methods involve the measurement of temperature in some form.

Turning these principles to thermal methods, the first type of thermal analysis, other than simple temperature measurement, was to measure the melting point of a sample. This would be (and still is) performed by heating a crystalline sample while also measuring the temperature. The temperature at which the sample turns to liquid is then noted, either visually (for early instruments) or more recently via changes in heat flow properties, as will be described below. The melting point is a key parameter and is one of the first properties of a new drug to be measured, as it gives information on the crystal form, the intermolecular bond strength and the purity of the material.

Melting point measurements are still the most widely used application of thermal analysis within the pharmaceutical field, as described in more detail in the following section. However, a range of other properties may also be measured, some of which are outlined below. Nevertheless, the basic principles of thermal methods are universal. All such methods involve heating (or cooling) a sample so causing heat flow into (or out of) it which in turn changes some property of a sample, all involve temperature measurement in some form and the majority of applications are associated with assessing the physical rather than chemical structure of a sample. The information yielded by these methods is so fundamental to drug development that virtually all pharmaceutical companies possess thermal instrumentation, the most common being differential scanning calorimetry (DSC) and thermogravimetric analysis (TGA) but with other methods also being found in a significant number of companies.

Application of Thermal Analysis to Pharmaceutical Dosage Forms

The field of thermal analysis is extremely wide due to versatility of the methods and hence there is a considerable body of literature available on the topic. The interested reader is referred to texts that outline the fundamentals of thermal methods in more detail (1–4) and also two books that deal specifically with thermal analysis of pharmaceutical systems (5,6).

THERMOANALYTICAL METHODS

Differential Scanning Calorimetry and Modulated Temperature

DSC is the most widely used method of thermal analysis at the present time and is likely to remain so for the foreseeable future. In essence, the method involves subjecting a small sample (in the order of a few milligrams) to a heating programme and measuring both the temperature and energy associated with a thermal event such as melting. Modern instruments are simple to use yet highly accurate and are able to give the formulator a wealth of information on an extremely wide range of samples, hence it is an essential component of any physical characterization laboratory.

The instrument is a derivation of an earlier approach known as differential thermal analysis (DTA). It involves the placing thermocouples in a sample and an inert reference and subjecting the assembly to a heating programme (usually one that means the temperature plotted against time gives a straight line) (Fig. 1A). As the sample undergoes a thermal event (again using melting as an example), the temperature of the sample will change in comparison to the reference. It is this temperature difference that is measured as its occurrence allows the operator to identify the temperature at which the transition starts and the range over which it occurs. The reason why the temperature difference occurs is because when a sample goes through an event such as melting (endothermic) or crystallization (exothermic), heat will be absorbed or evolved, respectively. This means that the sample and reference will no longer be at the same temperature and, as stated in the introduction, it is this difference that is measured.

DSC works on a similar principle but has several advantages over DTA, not least of which being the ability to easily measure the energy associated with the transition as well as the temperature at which it occurs. There are two main forms of DSC, power compensation and heat flux. Power compensation DSC involves the use of two furnaces (rather than the one used for DTA), one placed under the sample and the other under the reference (Fig. 1B). The system operates on the basis of keeping the sample and reference at the same temperature. This therefore means that energy must be supplied to the reference in order to make it follow the predetermined temperature programme and

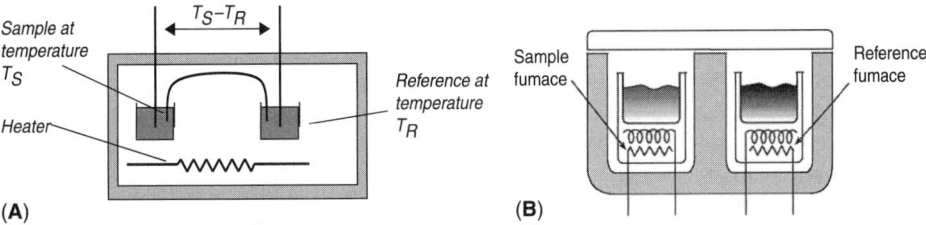

FIGURE 1 (A) Schematic diagram of a DTA apparatus. (B) Schematic diagram of a power compensation DSC cell. *Abbreviations*: DTA, differential thermal analysis; DSC, differential scanning calorimetry. *Source*: From Refs. 1, 6, 7.

to the sample to keep its temperature the same as the reference even if it goes through a thermal event. For example, as a sample melts the temperature will be fractionally lower than the reference for the reasons stated above. The system compensates for this by supplying additional energy to the sample furnace to maintain a zero temperature difference. This, in turn, means that not only will the temperature range of the event be known, as for DTA, but the energy associated with that event will also be identified because it is related to the difference in electrical energy supplied to the sample and reference furnaces. The second type of DSC, known as heat flux DSC, works on a similar principle in that the system comprises a sample and reference but these are both placed in the same furnace. Instead of compensating for the temperature difference, the heat flow difference to the two pans is measured from this temperature difference as a function of temperature. In practice, the outputs from the two types of DSC are extremely similar.

The output of a typical DSC experiment is shown in Figure 2. Typically, the power output of the instrument is plotted against temperature. Strictly speaking, it is preferable to plot heat capacity rather than power and the temperature should be given in Kelvin rather than degree Celsius, but in practice many operators in the pharmaceutical field use the former system due largely to familiarity. Before the thermal event occurs a flat baseline is seen, indicating that no thermal events are taking place. In fact this baseline is more significant than it may first appear, as while no melting or crystallization is taking place the sample is still absorbing heat as the temperature increases, according to

$$dQ/dt = C_p . dT/dt \tag{1}$$

where dQ/dt is the power output (energy per unit time), dT/dt is the heating rate, and C_p is the heat capacity. This last parameter is the energy required to raise the temperature of a sample by a unit amount and is a fundamental property of the sample, hence the more correct use of heat capacity on the ordinate as the power is dependent on both the properties of the system (heat capacity) and the heating rate. Indeed, this is why events appear larger in terms of power output when using higher heating rates even if the same sample is used.

When the thermal event takes place (in this case melting) the power output will change to reflect the endothermic event as described earlier. One might reasonably expect the melting process to be effectively instantaneous, as when one reaches the melting point all the intermolecular bonds holding the molecules in the crystal lattice should break

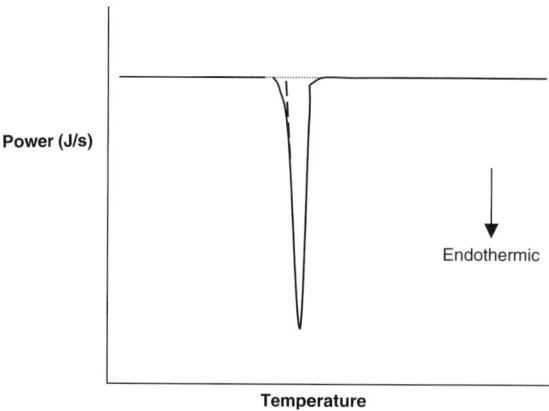

FIGURE 2 Typical melting endotherm for a low molecular weight, high purity material. *Source*: Adapted from Ref. 6.

together as they should all be of the same strength. In practice one always sees a finite width to the melting process for two principal reasons. First, there will always be thermal lags within the system, hence there will always be a finite amount of time required for the heat to travel from the furnace to the sample and for the temperature difference to be measured by the thermocouples, hence some peak broadening will always take place. Second, the samples are never in practice perfect crystals and hence there will be some element of there being a range of bond strengths within the material. This then leads to questions as to what exactly one should take as the melting point. The obvious answer may appear to be to use the peak temperature. However, the vast majority of operators use the onset at which the melting process starts (or the extrapolated onset whereby a line is drawn between the leading peak slope and the baseline) as this removes effects associated with thermal conductivity and so this value changes little with heating rate (whereas peak temperature can change significantly). With reference to Figure 2, if the sample was undergoing crystallization then the peak would be seen to point upwards to reflect the exothermic nature of the event. It should be noted that some instruments show endothermic (melting) peaks going up while others have these peaks pointing down, so some care is required to avoid confusion.

The energy associated with event may also be derived by measuring the area under the peak. In practice the operator uses standards such as indium whereby not only the temperature may be calibrated (from the known melting temperature) but, as the energy of melting (heat of fusion) is known for these standard materials, a calibration graph can be constructed so the heat of melting of an unknown can be found by measuring the area under its melting peak. In terms of practicalities, the DSC comprises a furnace with a removable lid, under which two positions are clearly marked on which the sample and (usually empty) reference plans and placed. The pans are usually composed of aluminium and may be completely sealed such that no vapor escape is possible (hermetically sealed) or may be crimped closed such that the pan forms a tight but not hermetic seal around the sample, thereby allowing gas to escape as the sample is heated. A third possibility that is widely employed is the use of pans which have a small hole drilled in the lid. These are sealed such that the hole is the only escape point for any vapor generated. The advantage of these "pinhole" pans is that the dimensions of the hole are controlled and hence the gas escape route is uniform. The choice of pan is highly significant as pharmaceutical samples very often contain water. This water may significantly alter the thermal properties of the system (outlined in more detail below), hence the operator must decide whether to allow the water to escape (in which case a crimped or pinhole pan is used) or whether the water should remain entrapped with the sample.

Sample sizes are typically in the 2–10 mg range. Smaller samples have the advantage of reducing temperature gradients through the sample (i.e., the measured temperature closely matches what the sample is experiencing) but if one is looking for very small thermal events then these may be difficult to see. Larger samples allow these events to be visualized more easily but care is required in interpreting the results as larger temperature gradients within the sample will lead to peak broadening. In terms of heating rates, typically one uses a range between approximately 5 and 20°C/min, although faster and slower rates may be used depending on the applications.

Brief mention must also be made of modulated temperature DSC (MTDSC). This is an extension of conventional DSC whereby, in addition to the linear temperature programme, a modulation in heating rate is applied. This may typically take the form of a sine wave. The principles of the method are described in much more detail in Ref. 8, but in brief the use of the modulation allows much more information to be obtained from the data. If we consider Equation (1) in terms of what happens during a thermal event, we can see that there to be two contributions to the heat flow, one relating to the heat capacity and one relating to the heat associated with the event itself such that

$$dQ/dt = C_p.dT/dt + f(t,T) \qquad (2)$$

where $f(t,T)$ represents some function of time and temperature associated with the event itself. The use of the modulation allows, in many cases, these two components to be separated, hence one obtains the total heat flow (equivalent to the conventional DSC response), the reversing heat flow (equivalent to the $C_p.dT/dt$ term) and the non-reversing heat flow [equivalent to the $f(t,T)$ term]. In other words, one obtains three curves for each run rather than the one that is obtained using conventional DSC. The significance of this will be explained in "Glassy Systems" section, but in essence the method is extremely useful for measuring glass transitions and characterization of polymeric systems, amongst others.

Thermogravimetric Analysis

TGA is a method whereby the mass of a sample is measured as a function of temperature. Along with DSC, it is a standard technique within the pharmaceutical field as the measurements are rapid, simple to interpret (at least on a basic level) and yield highly important information, for reasons outlined below. The instrumentation itself comprises a furnace containing a microbalance in which a pan containing the sample (usually 2–10 mg) is suspended. The furnace applies a heating programme to the sample, usually a linear function of time in the range of 5–10°C/min. As the sample loses vapor, the mass decreases and this is recoded as a function of temperature. The instrument may be interfaced with mass spectroscopy in order to allow the vapor to be chemically analyzed, but in most cases the operator makes a judgement with regard to the nature of the evolved gas based on prior knowledge of the sample and the temperature at which the loss of volatiles is detected; arguably this lack of chemical specificity represents one of the most significant weaknesses of the method and caution is always required when making such assumptions. The output of the instrument is usually expressed in terms of percentage weight against temperature, with the initial reading being considered to be 100%. This allows the percentage loss to be easily assessed as the sample is heated. A typical result is shown in Figure 3 for trehalose monohydrate, showing the weight loss associated with the evaporation of the water of hydration.

The basic uses of the technique for pharmaceutical applications fall into three broad categories. In the first instance, the technique may be used to detect the presence and amount of trace solvents, particularly water. For example, if a sample has undergone a process such as freeze or spray drying whereby extensive solvent content is involved then it is usual to run the sample through the TGA to assess the level of residual water or other solvents. For more accurate and specific measurements a technique such as Karl Fischer is preferable for measuring water contents, although such studies are longer and arguable more cumbersome than TGA. Similarly, the sensitivity of the instrument is such that if one is concerned with trace levels of potentially toxic organic solvents then TGA is unlikely to be sufficiently sensitive to pick up these solvents. However, when the loss is of the order of a few percent of the total weight then TGA is perfectly adequate.

TGA may also be used to characterize hydrates and solvates, as outlined in more detail below. This represents one of the major uses of the technique, as the operator may not only detect the hydrate but may also determine both the stoichiometry of the binary system and the binding strength of the solvent within the matrix. The third basic use of

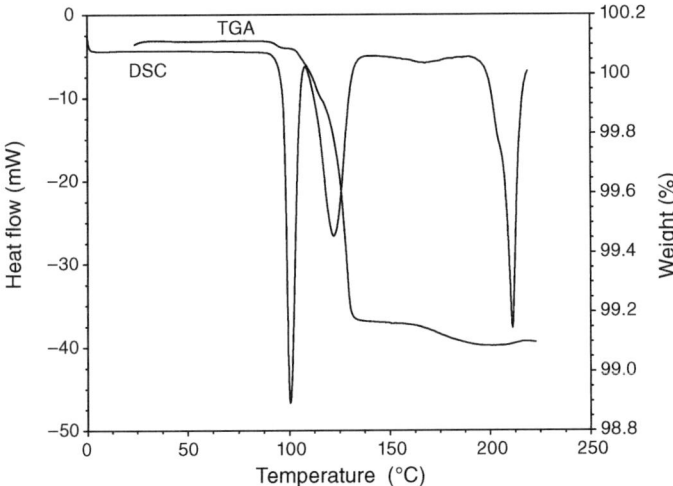

FIGURE 3 TGA data for trehalose monohydrate alongside equivalent DSC data, showing the weight change associated with the loss of the water of hydration. *Source*: From Ref. 9.

the method is to study decomposition. Any drug will decompose on heating and TGA allows the temperature range and potentially the nature (if used with mass spectroscopy) of the decomposition to be assessed. Again, caution is required when interpreting TGA data in the absence of such spectroscopic information as it is often difficult to determine when solvent loss ends and decomposition begins, with both processes being seen simply as weight loss processes.

Information may also be obtained by observing not simply the absolute amounts of weight loss but also the temperature profile itself. For example, residual water is likely to be lost at a temperature range of approximately 60–100°C, while loss of organic solvents may be lost at temperature well below that, depending on the vapor pressure of the solvent and the binding to the solid substrate. Loss of water of hydration tends to occur over a narrow temperature range (Fig. 3) and may therefore be distinguished from residual solvent loss which tends to be more gradual. A sudden change of gradient of loss may indicate a second process occurring such as decomposition, while complex samples such as creams in which water may be bound in several different states can be effectively characterized by observing the sequential nature of the water loss corresponding to water present in different locations within the sample. It is also possible to apply kinetic analysis to the loss process, both by heating the sample at different rates and also by holding the sample at a stated temperature and measuring weight loss as a function of time.

Hot Stage Microscopy

Hot stage microscopy is a highly useful, semi-quantitative technique whereby an optical microscope is fitted with a temperature controlled stage, thereby allowing the operator to visually observe the morphology of the sample as a function of temperature. While it is possible to derive the temperature of transitions by simple observation, the real strength of the technique lies in the ability visualize structural changes as a function of temperature. The instrument may be run in a range of modes, including polarized light, differential interference contrast, and others. In general, it is used as a supplement to DSC as it may provide invaluable assistance to the interpretation of thermal events, particularly for complex samples. An example of this is the study of different crystal structures in lipids or the transitions between different polymorphic forms, as shown in Figure 4 for the transition between Forms II and I caffeine.

Microcalorimetry

Microcalorimetry is widely used within the pharmaceutical industry for applications ranging from the detection of amorphous material through to excipient compatibility. A typical instrument comprises a reaction vessel housed in a water bath which acts as a heat sink. The enthalpy of the process taking place within the reaction vessel is measured via means of a thermopile that measures temperature differences between the reaction vessel and the heat sink. Modern instruments are able to detect extremely small heat fluctuations, rendering microcalorimetry one of the most accurate and sensitive methods for detecting subtle or long-term (i.e., very slow) reactions. The instrument is almost invariably run in isothermal mode, which means that the temperature of the heat sink is maintained constant and the reaction followed as a function of time as opposed to being used to apply a ramped temperature programme to a sample, as was the case for the previous techniques. It is also possible to control the environment within the reaction vessel such that the humidity and gas content may be varied, thereby allowing exploration of the effects of water and oxygen on reaction rates.

The sensitivity of the instrument has attracted interest for a wide range of pharmaceutical systems. These include the monitoring of slow chemical reactions, a highly important issue within the industry due to the need to predict drug stability at non-elevated temperatures in the presence and absence of excipients. Buckton (11) provides a useful discussion of the strengths and weaknesses of the approach. He differentiates

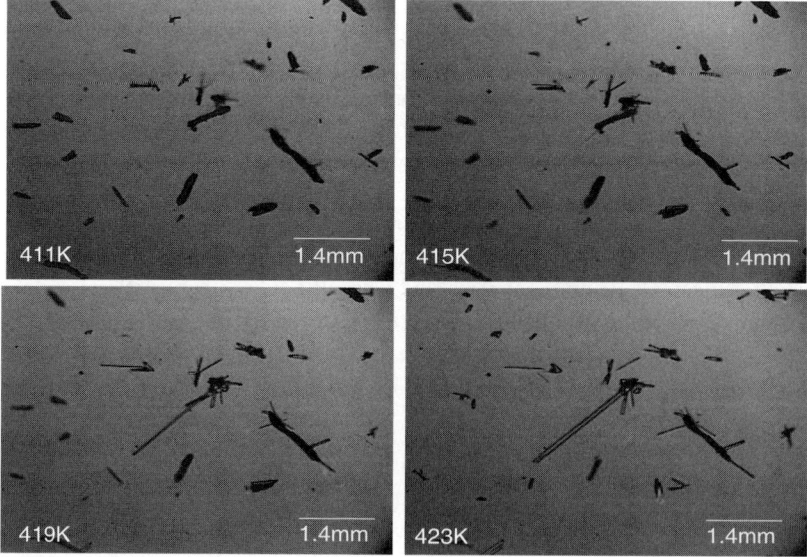

FIGURE 4 Hot stage microscopy images of caffeine Form II undergoing transformation to the needle-shaped Form I crystals on heating. *Source*: From Ref. 10.

between the possibilities associated with solution and solid state reactions in that in order to provide a meaningful kinetic analysis of the reaction it is essential to know the quantity of material reacting. This may be obtained for solutions as it is reasonable to assume that the reaction occurs homogeneously through the system, hence the quantity available to react will be known from the initial concentrations. For solids, however, such reactions occur at points of contact between the drug and environment or excipient rather than throughout the sample mass, hence it is extremely difficult to relate the measured enthalpy to the amount of material undergoing the reaction in question. However, other applications are uncontroversial in their usefulness, notably the use of the technique to detect small quantities of amorphous material which will be discussed the "Glassy systems" section.

Emerging Thermal Techniques

As mentioned in the introduction, there are a wide range of techniques available and it is not appropriate to attempt to cover all of these approaches here. However there are a number of new methods that are generating considerable interest within the field. These include fast scan or high speed DSC (sometimes referred to as Hyper DSC™), whereby scanning rates of several hundred degrees per minute are used. The perceived advantages of this approach include the obvious increase in throughput, but perhaps more importantly the use of such speeds sometimes allows greater sensitivity for very subtle reactions such as small glass transitions. This may be related back to the arguments presented earlier in which it was noted with reference to Equation (1) that sensitivity increases when faster scan rates are used. However, it is also true that sensitivity increases as the sample mass is increased; in both cases, increasing heating rate and increasing sample mass, larger temperature gradients are created within the sample with consequent distortion of the results. It follows that, if there is a problem in detecting a low energy transition with a 2-mg sample at 20°C/min. the experimenter can increase sensitivity by 10 × either by using a 20-mg sample or a 200°C/min heating rate; in both cases peak broadening will occur due to increasing temperature gradients. Increasing both sample size and heating rate increases sensitivity further and this can be appropriate in some cases but this combination should be used with care as very large temperature gradients within the sample can be produced. A further very interesting possibility is that one of the problems associated with conventional DSC is that the operator has to be aware of the possibility of changes to the sample taking place during the scan itself, hence the data may reflect these changes rather than reflecting the structure of the system prior to the experiment starting. By using very high heating rates, it is argued that there is insufficient time for these changes to take place during the run and the data may, therefore, more closely reflect the original structure of the sample.

A further technique that has attracted great interest is microthermal (now nanothermal) analysis. This represents a derivative of atomic force microscopy, whereby a fine probe is moved across a sample surface to give extremely detailed surface profiling. In the microthermal technique the conventional probe is replaced by a small thermal one, allowing the operator to heat very specific regions of complex samples. This in turn opens up the possibility of characterizing drugs while they are still embedded in dosage forms, this having been extremely difficult to achieve to date.

In its simplest mode, the technique uses the principle of localized thermomechanical analysis whereby the probe position is monitored as a function of temperature. As the sample immediately underneath the probe softens due to, for example, melting the probe penetrates into the sample and the movement detected. Figure 5A shows a crystalline indomethacin surface after it has been subject to nano-thermal analysis. The ringed region highlights the very precise melting region seen as the small indentation in the centre (in the order of 600 nm in diameter), with Figure 5B showing the corresponding melting profile. Here the probe is at first raised due to the thermal expansion of the sample and then penetrates into the material at the melting point, seen as the rapid inflexion in the probe position profile. Again, the technique is gaining interest at the time of writing and is being seen as a method of obtaining site-specific information on complex pharmaceutical samples.

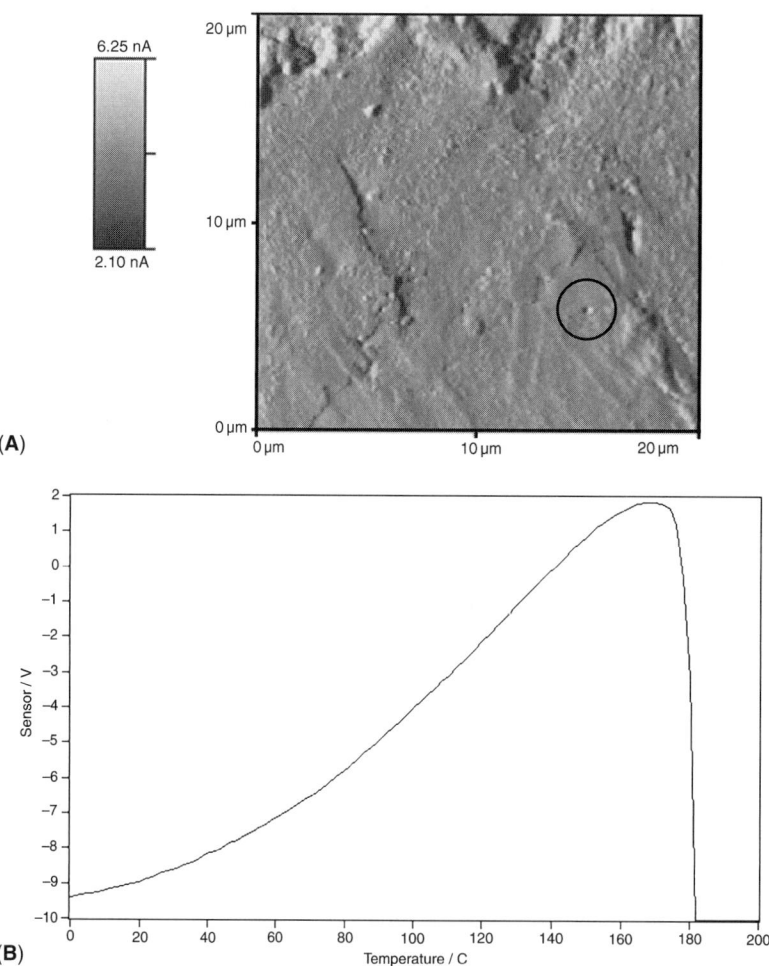

FIGURE 5 (**A**) Internal sensor image of crystalline indometacin following localized thermomechanical analysis, showing a typical indentation caused by the measurement (*circled*). (**B**) Localized thermomechanical analysis of the amorphous indometacin surface, showing an initial rising in probe position caused by thermal expansion followed by penetration of the probe as the sample melts. *Source*: From Ref. 12.

THERMAL ANALYSIS FOR PREFORMULATION AND FORMULATION STUDIES

The Study of Polymorphism

Polymorphism is the term used to describe the existence of more than one unit cell structure for a particular drug molecule. It is an extremely widespread phenomenon and is of fundamental importance for pharmaceutical development for several reasons. In the first instance, only one polymorphic form is stable under given conditions of temperature and pressure, hence an unstable form will convert over a period of time which may vary from minutes to years. Second, polymorphs exhibit different physical properties with respect to each other. In particular, the solubility is greater and melting point lower for the unstable (metastable) forms, the latter being particularly significantly for thermal analysis. Finally, there are regulatory and registration issues associated with polymorphism, not least of which being the possibility of patenting different forms as well as the need to establish the stability of the formulation for the market in order to obtain regulatory approval.

In thermodynamic terms, polymorphs may be considered to be enantiotropic or monotropic. Two forms that are enantiotropic may both be stable depending on the temperature (assuming constant pressure), with a transition temperature between the two. Below this temperature one form will be stable and the other metastable with the opposite applying above this temperature. Monotropic systems only have one stable form irrespective of temperature, i.e., one will always be metastable with respect to the other. That is not to say that only one form may exist at any point in time. A form may be metastable thermodynamically but relatively stable kinetically, meaning that while eventually it will convert to the stable form that conversion process may be very slow so as to be very difficult to detect. This represents a very significant problem for the pharmaceutical industry as it is often by no means obvious whether one has the stable or metastable form. Similarly, by changing a drug manufacturing process on, for example, scaling up it is possible to accidentally generate a new polymorphic form. Furthermore, it is very much in the interests of a company to obtain a robust profile of the conversion processes undergone by a new chemical entity. The interested reader is referred to a thorough article by Giron (13) for a more detailed discussion of polymorphic interconversion, while Hilfiker (14) has produced an excellent book on the relevance of polymorphism to the pharmaceutical industry.

The study of polymorphic forms represents the most common use of DSC within the industry. Companies tend to use the method as a means of screening drugs to detect any changes in melting point compared to a previous batch, to detect any features in the DSC profile that would lead them to believe that more than one polymorph may be present and to temperature cycle drugs so as to attempt to induce the generation of different polymorphic forms. All of these approaches work on the basis that the polymorphs will have different melting points, with the less stable forms having lower values. Indeed, a common method of nomenclature of these polymorphs is to assign them numbers (or letters) in order of their melting point as this also corresponds to their stability. In addition, DSC is almost invariably used in conjunction with X-ray diffraction which is able to both detect and structurally characterize the different forms.

Several examples of such characterization studies are available in the literature, although a significant proportion of these studies are not published due to the commercial sensitivity of the information. Figure 6 shows a typical pair of profiles for two forms of a

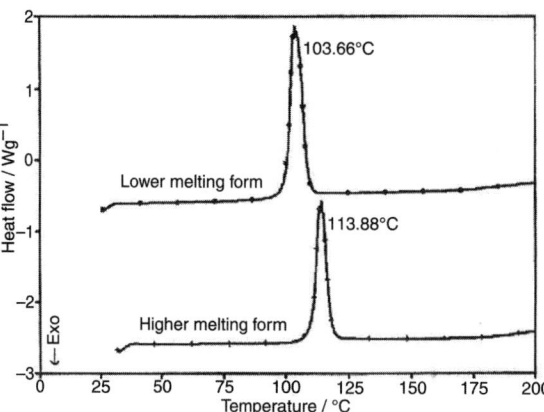

FIGURE 6 Differential scanning calorimetry (DSC) curve for two crystal forms of developmental drug. *Source*: Ref 15, courtesy of Springer Science and Business Media.

developmental drug, where one form has a clearly lower melting point than the other more stable form (note that this is an example of where endothermic events are shown as peaks pointing upwards). However, this information does not in itself guarantee that the higher melting form is stable, as it merely indicates that it is more stable than the other, lower melting form.

The above example shows a fairly unequivocal profile for a pair of polymorphic forms. In many other cases, however, the profile may be more complex and the interpretation correspondingly more complex. In particular, it may be possible to observe transitions between the forms that occur during the DSC scan itself. This is both an advantage and a disadvantage, as with correct interpretation it may be possible to use such observations to detect new polymorphs and to gain information on the relationship between the forms. However, without a knowledge of the basic tenets of the polymorph thermal profiles such observations are prone to misinterpretation. To use an example, caffeine exists in two enantiotropic polymorphic forms, Form I which is stable above the transition temperature of circa 140°C and Form II which is stable below it and is therefore the form commonly found at room temperature. As one heats Form II the material undergoes a solid-solid transition to Form I which is seen as a small endotherm at around 140°C. Form I then melts at 235°C. The significance of this is that the melting points that are quoted for caffeine are for Form I, not the room temperature material (Form II) for which the melting point is not in fact known as the material converts before melting of this form can occur (10).

Returning to the question of whether forms are monotropic or enantiotropic has been addressed by the group of Burger (16,17), who developed a series of rules based on the free energy diagrams of the two types of polymorphic system. These are summarized in Table 1. Interestingly, it is remarkably simple to identify whether a pair of polymorphs are enantiotropic or monotropic by, for example, comparing their heats of fusion (obtained without due difficulty using DSC) or assessing whether any observed transition between polymorphs is endothermic or exothermic.

An example of a more complex system is shown in Figure 7 for premafloxacin (18). Here the unstable Form I melts and converts into Form II which itself melts and converts to Form III which subsequently melts to enter the liquid state, as shown by comparison with pure Form III. Indeed, it is common practice to attempt to generate different polymorphs and run DSC profiles on each, using the melting data of the more stable forms to interpret the progressively more complex unstable forms.

Application of Thermal Analysis to Pharmaceutical Dosage Forms

TABLE 1 Summary of Means of Differentiating Between Monotropic and Enantiotropic Polymorphism, with Form I Being the Higher Melting Form

Enantiotropy	Monotropy
I Stable > transition	I Always stable
II Stable < transition	II Not stable at any temperature
Transition reversible	Transition irreversible
Solubility I higher < transition	Solubility I always lower than II
Transition II to I endothermic	Transition II to I exothermic
$\Delta H^I_F < \Delta H^{II}_F$	$\Delta H^I_F > \Delta H^{II}_F$ [b]
IR Peak I before II	IR Peak I after II
Density I < Density II	Density I > Density II

Source: Adapted from Refs. 13, 16, 17.

Mention should be made of the use of techniques other than DSC for the characterization of polymorphs, as given the importance of this issue the pharmaceutical industry is, not surprisingly, constantly looking for novel methods of characterising these systems. A study by Lehto and Laine (19) has used microcalorimetry to monitor the conversion of Form I to Form II caffeine, allowing the heat flow associated with the conversion to be measured in real time. Similarly, Manduva et al. (10) have used microthermal analysis to differentiate between polymorphs of caffeine, demonstrating that the conversion to Form I may be detected as a discontinuity in the localized thermomechanical analysis response at the temperature corresponding to the conversion. This in turn means that Form II (showing the discontinuity) and Form I (showing no discontinuity) may be differentiated. These authors then demonstrated that it is possible to map the conversion between polymorphs on a tablet surface by performing a series of experiments at different locations across the tablet surface.

High speed DSC techniques are also attracting considerable interest as a means of characterising polymorphism. An interesting example of this is the study by McGregor

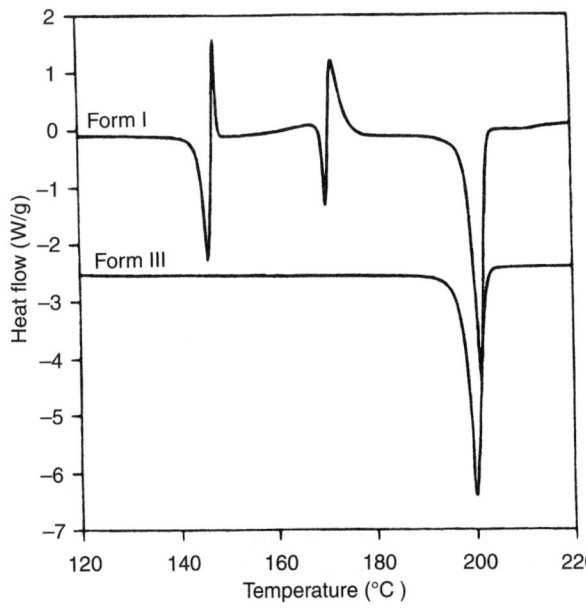

FIGURE 7 DSC curves of Forms I and III premafloxacin samples. *Source*: From Ref. 18.

et al. (20) whereby the authors were able to characterize the temperature and enthalpy of melting of the unstable Form III carbamazepine. Conventional DSC rendered this extremely difficult due to the overlapping transformation to the more stable Form I during the heating run. By using much higher heating speeds it was possible to kinetically inhibit the recrystallization process (i.e., the scan was too fast to allow the transformation to take place), hence the melting endotherm of the Form III could be seen in its entirety (Fig. 8). At the time of writing the technique is being studied by a number of groups and companies and the merits and disadvantages of the approach will undoubtedly become clearer in the near future.

Pharmaceutical Hydrates

While DSC may be used to study pharmaceutical hydrates, the most useful thermal method is undoubtedly TGA. Hydrates are materials whereby molecules of water are incorporated into the lattice structure of that solid at specific ratios, hence a monohydrate has one molecule of water for each molecule of drug, a dihydrate two molecules of water etc. The stoichiometry may also be fractional. Hydrates are again extremely important pharmaceutically as the physical properties differ from the anhydrous form, the former having, for example, a lower water solubility. Many drugs are marketed as hydrate forms, often due to their greater physical stability than the anhydrous form which may convert to the hydrate over a period of time if exposed to water vapor.

There are numerous examples in the literature of the use of TGA for hydrate characterization, notably from the group of Grant which performed much of the seminal work in the area. An example of this is given in Figure 9 which shows the TGA profiles of a range of hydrates of nedocromil magnesium, showing the different temperatures at which the water may be lost (21). This study demonstrates several important principles associated with hydrate characterization. In the first instance it may be seen that by assessing the percentage water loss and converting to molar ratios it is possible to calculate the stoichiometry of the hydrate [most clearly seen in curve (C)]. Second, the study

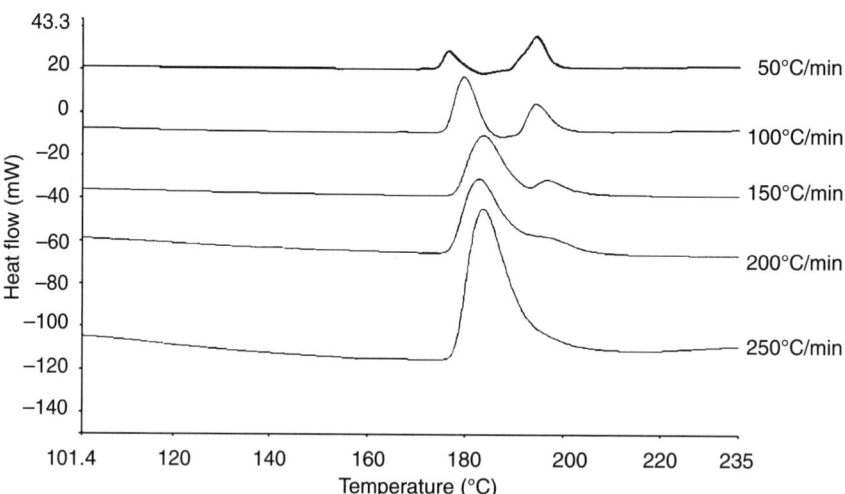

FIGURE 8 High speed DSC profile of carbamazepine Form III, showing that at high scanning speeds the melting endotherm of Form III may be seen in isolation from the conversion to Form I. *Source*: From Ref. 20.

Application of Thermal Analysis to Pharmaceutical Dosage Forms

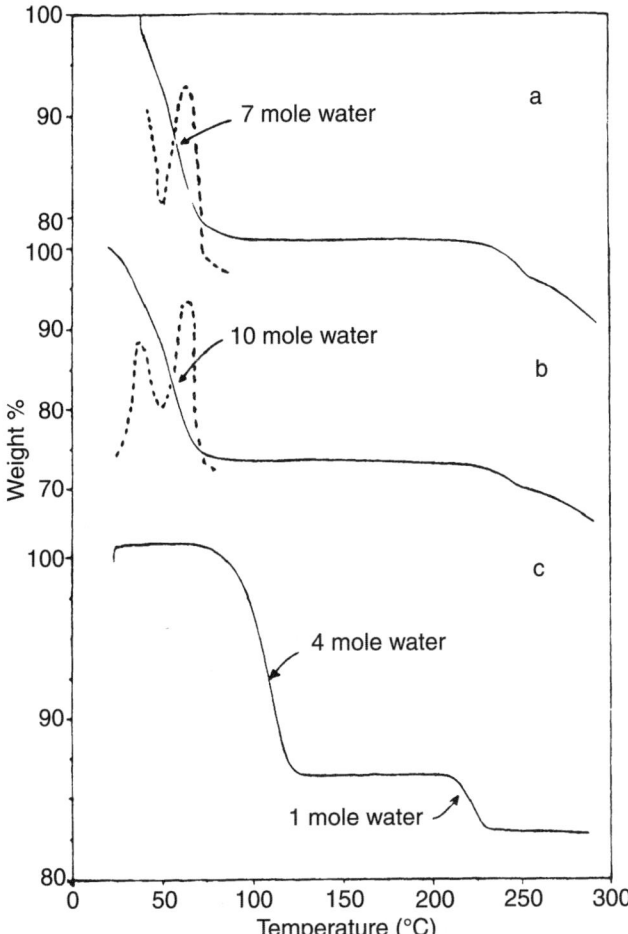

FIGURE 9 Thermogravimetric analysis (TGA) curves (*full line*) and derivative TGA curves (*dotted line*) of the nedocromil magnesium hydrates: (**A**) heptahydrate, (**B**) decahydrate, and (**C**) pentahydrate. *Source*: From Ref. 21.

demonstrates the differences in water binding that may occur; again curve (C) shows that the four water molecules of the pentahydrate are bound in a different manner to the final, fifth molecule which is bound more tightly into the lattice (as indicated by the higher temperature at which it is lost, indicating a greater temperature requirement). Finally the figure illustrates the use of a simple but very effective technique whereby overlapping water losses may be identified. This is shown by the dotted line in curves (A) and (B) which represents the derivative (or gradient) of the TGA curve. While this does not generate new data as such compared to the original weight loss curve, it does illustrate how it is possible to identify two partially overlapping loss processes, particularly in curve (B).

Glassy Systems

The discussions so far have focused on the characterization of crystalline drug systems. However there is considerable interest in the use of thermal methods for the characterization of amorphous or glassy systems. These are materials for which there is no long-range order, this being in contrast to crystalline systems which are composed of repeating ordered lattice structures. Amorphous systems are important for several reasons. In the first instance, their dissolution rates tend to be more rapid that their counterpart crystalline systems due to the absence of lattice energy which needs to be overcome prior to dissolution. Second, many materials or processes inevitably result in amorphous material generation; these include many polymeric materials which are unable to crystallize (dealt with in the "Use of Polymers in Dosage Form Design" section). In addition, however, processes such as freeze drying and spray drying tend to result in the formation of amorphous materials. Finally, amorphous materials may be accidentally generated by processes such as grinding or compression. Such disordered material tends to be present at the surface of the otherwise crystalline material, thereby having a potentially profound effect on particle-particle interactions and agglomeration behaviour. The realization of the prevalence and potential uses of amorphous material has led to very considerable interest in developing methods for characterising glassy systems, with thermal methods being at the forefront of such considerations. In order to aid understanding of how thermal methods may be used in this regard, a brief summary of the basic principles of the amorphous state will be given here, although the interested reader is referred to any one of a number of texts for further information (22,23).

A glass may be formed via a number of routes including rapid cooling from the melt, precipitation from solvents or processing as outlined above, but for simplicity it is best to focus on cooling from the melt. Figure 10 shows a typical phase diagram which shows the possible outcomes for a material cooled from the liquid state, expressed in terms of volume against temperature. If one considers the top right hand corner in the first instance, as the material is cooled it may undergo crystallization to the solid state, with an accompanying reduction in volume as the molecules form ordered arrays from the previously highly mobile state. However, if cooling is sufficiently rapid the material may supercool below the crystallization temperature and simply continue to reduce in volume as the temperature is lowered. For thermodynamic reasons (known as the Kauzmann paradox) the sample is not able to simply continue to reduce in volume and a temperature

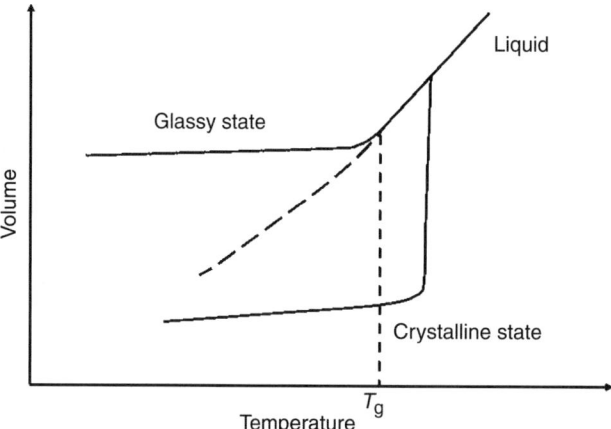

FIGURE 10 Phase diagram of an amorphous system, showing the volume change as a material cools from the liquid state. The sample may crystallize or alternatively may supercool and form a glass at the glass transition temperature T_g.

is reached whereby a sudden decrease in molecular mobility (and hence increase in rigidity) is seen. This temperature, the glass transition temperature or T, is seen visually as the point where a material becomes brittle or glassy as opposed to rubbery (in the polymer sciences the states below and above T_g are referred to as glassy and rubbery, respectively). Indeed, it appears to the naked eye as though the material has suddenly changed from a liquid to a solid as it cools through T_g. In fact both states are technically liquid as both are disordered, the material below the glass transition being essentially a highly viscous supercooled liquid. The difficulty as far as glassy pharmaceuticals are concerned is that the glassy state is thermodynamically unstable with respect to the crystalline state and glasses will tend to recrystallize over time. This may take such a long period so as to be effectively irrelevant, volcanic rock being potentially millions of years old yet still amorphous, but unfortunately glassy drugs tend not to be anything like as stable and there is a significant danger of recrystallization within the lifetime of the product.

There are some general rules with regard to stability that assist the formulator in maintaining the integrity of the amorphous drug. The first and most important is that glasses are considerably more stable below T_g than above this value due to the lower molecular mobility of the glassy state. There is considerable interest in determining to what extent a system below T_g is indeed stable, the clear evidence being that amorphous systems may still recrystallize well below this temperature. Indeed, Hancock and Zografi (22) have suggested that in order to be guaranteed stability it is necessary to store the material at 50 °C or more below T_g. However this then leads to the second complication; many (typically low molecular weight) materials, notably including water, may act as plasticizers whereby the presence of this second component results in a lowering of the T_g. This effectively means that an amorphous drug with a supposedly high T_g may, on adsorbing water, have that T_g lowered such that the resultant value is close to or below the temperature of storage, with accompanying stability problems. On this basis, it is essential to have effective means of measuring T_g and also to have an understanding of the basic principles of glassy systems in order to formulate amorphous products or to be able to characterize partially amorphous systems.

The measurement of T_g has traditionally been conducted using DSC. The measurement is not difficult as such but at the same time is non-trivial for two reasons. First, glass transitions are changes in molecular mobility rather than highly energetic bond making or breaking processes. Consequently, the T_g is not represented by a large, energetic and obvious peak in the DSC profile but rather by a shift in the baseline, as indicated in Figure 11. The reason for this, in thermodynamic terms, is that the glass transition is a change in the heat capacity of the sample. If one then reconsiders the arguments given in the "Differential Scanning Calorimetry and Modulated Temperature Differential Scanning Calorimetery" section with regard to the nature of the DSC measurement [with particular reference to Equation (2)] it becomes clear that the glass transition will in its pure form be represented by a shift in the baseline in turn reflecting a shift in C_p. Consequently, if one does not have a very stable (flat) baseline it may be very difficult to see the T_g response. The second complication is that superimposed on the glass transition may be a response known as an endothermic relaxation. In essence, as one stores a glass its volume will decrease; the same applies to its heat content (enthalpy). This process is known as relaxation. Consequently as one heats a stored glass back through the T_g to the liquid state it must regain that lost enthalpy. This is achieved by absorbing heat energy during the DSC run in a similar manner to the way in which energy is absorbed in order to melt a crystalline sample, hence the process will be seen as an endotherm superimposed on the T_g. This endotherm may be used to calculate the

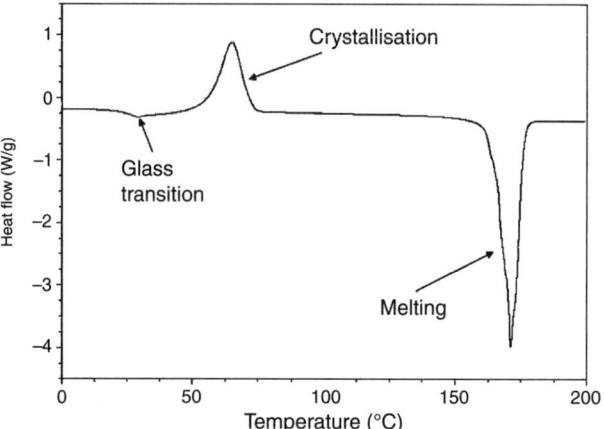

FIGURE 11 Typical thermal profile for an amorphous drug, showing the glass transition as a shift in the baseline, crystallisation of the material as it is heated above T_g and melting of that crystalline material.

molecular mobility of the sample but its presence also complicates interpretation of the DSC profile for those not familiar with this possibility.

There are a number of solutions to both these problems, but probably the most widely used and elegant is to use MTDSC rather than conventional DSC. Figure 12 gives the response of a glassy drug (saquinavir), showing the three responses (total heat flow, reversing heat flow, and non-reversing heat flow). The total heat flow is equivalent to the conventional DSC response. One may see the endothermic relaxation peak but, by comparing the baseline before and after the transition, it is also possible to see that there has been shift in baseline through this transition, representing the glass transition itself. The splitting of the response into the reversing and non-reversing signals allows the operator to separate these two components of the response. The reversing signal shows

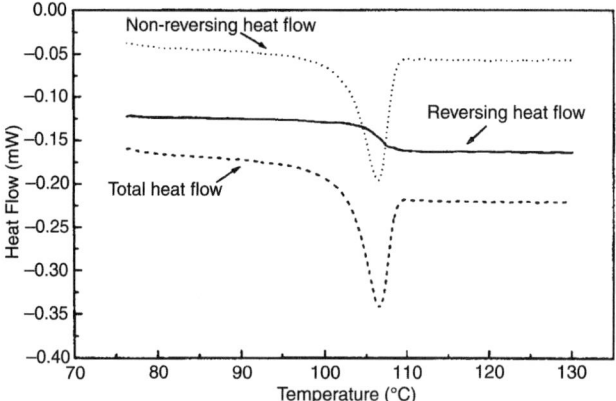

FIGURE 12 Modulated temperature differential scanning calorimetry (MTDSC) response of amorphous saquinavir, showing the total heat flow (equivalent to conventional DSC), the non-reversing heat flow showing the endothermic relaxation and the reversing heat flow showing the glass transition in isolation. *Abbreviation*: DSC, differential scanning calorimetry. *Source*: From Ref. 24.

the T_g in isolation from the endothermic response, which is in turn seen in isolation in the non-reversing signal. The full explanation for this is beyond the scope of this text, but very simply if one inspects Equation (2) it can be seen that total response is composed of the heat capacity term (containing the glass transition, see in the reversing heat flow) and the thermal event term (or more correctly kinetically hindered thermal event, which includes the endothermic relaxation which is seen in the non-reversing curve). In this way the glass transition and the endothermic relaxation can be seen separately and clearly. As most glassy drugs show this relaxation endotherm this represents a major advantage in terms of characterization and it is now common practice to use MTDSC to study the T_g.

However, measurement of T_g is not the only important consideration when dealing with amorphous systems. It is also often necessary to quantify the amount of amorphous material in partially crystalline systems; this is particularly important in, for example, inhalation systems whereby powders are often ground to obtain a size fraction that shows suitable lung penetration. In this respect, the method that has attracted most interest has been microcalorimetry. The group of Buckton in particular have worked extensively on the development of humidity-induced recrystallization as a means of quantifying amorphous components of otherwise crystalline materials (25,26). This approach is based on the premise that if water vapor is introduced to the microcalorimetry cell, the amorphous material will become plasticized such that the T_g will fall to below that of the calorimeter, at which point crystallization will occur. This is a relatively energetic event and is easily detected by the calorimeter, as indicated in Figure 13. This method has been shown to be able to detect amorphous material in otherwise crystalline samples to a few percent or better.

Drug Excipient Compatibility

It is well recognized that the presence of certain excipients may accelerate the degradation of drugs, hence there is a very considerable need to develop means of predicting which excipients will induce instability. There have been a number of suggestions revolving around thermal methods. Classically, it has been suggested that by heating a drug and excipient together in a DSC pan then one may detect instability by observing

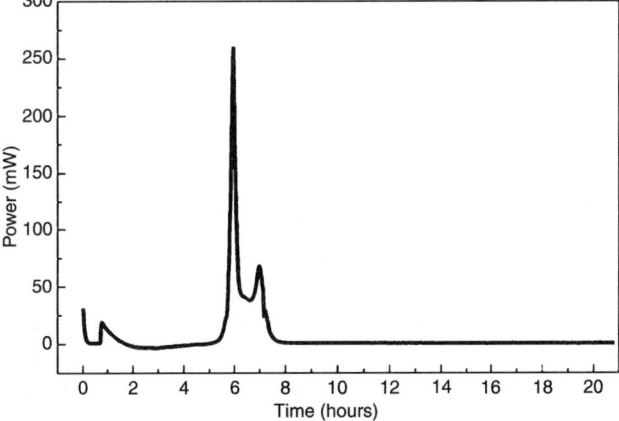

FIGURE 13 Power-time response obtained using isothermal microcalorimetry for a sample of amorphous lactose held at 53% RH at 25°C. *Source*: From Ref. 26.

changes in the melting behavior of the two individual components (27), the well-known example of this being magnesium stearate and aspirin whereby the presence of the lubricant leads to an energetic response when heated (28). As well as DSC, microcalorimetry has also been used as a means of detecting the presence of a thermal signal on mixing the drug and excipient in turn indicating incompatibility (29). Similarly, high sensitivity DSC (HSDSC) has been used. This is a technique that is similar to conventional DSC but allows measurements of greater sensitivity to be made over a more limited temperature range. Wissing et al. (30) showed that by holding the mixtures at a series of temperature intervals and measuring the energy output as a function of time at each step it is possible to detect interactions with greater sensitivity than conventional DSC.

The use of thermal methods for excipient compatibility testing is to some extent controversial, with many companies believing that these methods are not sufficiently reliable to be used extensively. On reflection it could be argued that their greatest use is as a screening method whereby "dangerous" combinations may be identified quickly rather than as an absolute predictive method. By discarding certain combinations of drugs and excipients early on in the development process it may be possibly to save a great deal of cost and effort by performing real time studies which later show there to be a problem.

THERMAL ANALYSIS OF POLYMERIC SYSTEMS

The Use of Polymers in Dosage Form design

Polymers have always been a vital component of pharmaceutical formulations, ranging from naturally occurring molecules such as alginates to synthetic polymers such as polyethylene glycols. However, the prominence of polymers in dosage form design has increased steadily in recent years, ranging from controlled release devices to polymer-based drugs. This has in turn led to a greater need to develop effective characterization methods, both for the polymer alone and also for that polymer when incorporated in the dosage form. Thermal methods play a key role in this respect and indeed are a vital component of characterization strategies in the polymer science field (which is in many ways the key market for thermal approaches). In this respect, virtually all the comments and techniques outlined above are applicable to polymers used in pharmaceutical science. Nevertheless, there are some general points that are pertinent to performing such characterization studies which need to be highlighted.

In the first instance, polymeric solids may be intrinsically crystalline, semi-crystalline, or amorphous, the last two categories being the most relevant to pharmaceutical systems. Polyethylene glycols (PEGs) in the molecular weight range of 4,000–20,000 are semicrystalline solids at room temperature, while polyvinylpyrrolidone (PVP), hydroxypropyl methylcellulose (HPMC) and many of the polymers derived from lactic acid (polylactides, PLA) are amorphous. This means that one may have to consider both melting and glass transitional behavior when dealing with polymeric samples, although most commonly used polymers are amorphous. The amorphous nature of these materials is a function of the high molecular weight and molecular flexibility which in turn results in a lower propensity to form an organized lattice structure. Second, polymers are almost invariably polydispersed, meaning that not every molecule in a batch will have the same molecular weight. This results in a considerable degree of interbatch variation as well as many physical properties presenting as a range rather than a specific value, the classic example being melting whereby the endothermic peaks tend to be considerably broader than those found for low molecular weight drugs. The problem is compounded for substituted polymers (whereby groups are attached intermittently along the length of the main chain) as such substitution is rarely completely uniform and hence also adds to the complexity of the chemical structure. Nevertheless, effective characterization is both possible and highly desirable, with examples of polymeric systems found in pharmacy and their corresponding thermal characterization given below.

Mention should be made here of a technique that is particularly well suited to the study of polymeric systems (especially polymer films), namely dynamic mechanical analysis (DMA). This was not outlined in the section on "Thermoanalytical Methods" as it arguably does not form part of the most widely used arsenal of techniques commonly used by industry, but is very widely used within the polymer sciences. The technique essentially is a combination of rheology and thermal analysis, whereby a film is subjected to a mechanical force as a function of temperature. As the film goes through a glass transition the mechanical properties change for the reasons outlined above, this may then be detected in the rheological properties to a high degree of sensitivity. The interested reader is referred to the thorough chapter by Jones (31) for more details of how the technique may be used for pharmaceuticals and also to the comprehensive treatise edited by Turi (32) on the use of thermal methods in the polymer sciences.

Characterization of Polymer Films

The fundamental characteristic of polymer systems is usually the glass transition temperature. This has been particularly important for the study of film coats on tablets (or more accurately films composed of film coating materials) as the mechanical properties of the film are crucial to the performance. As outlined previously, the T_g indicates the temperature at which the material undergoes a radical change in mechanical properties. However, the usefulness of knowledge of the T_g goes beyond simply identifying this softening temperature per se as manipulation of the T_g by the inclusion of plasticizers allows the flexibility of the film to be controlled in a general sense. There are predictive models available regarding how mechanical properties alter around the T_g but in essence if one lowers the T_g of a polymer such as HPMC by inclusion of a plasticizer such as a low molecular weight PEG then one sees an increase in flexibility of the film. This in turn renders the film less brittle and more suitable for filling subtle surface features such as logo lettering or breaklines on the tablet.

The measurement of the film T_g may be performed using a number of techniques, although dynamic mechanical analysis (DMA) and DSC (and MTDSC) are the most widely studied. The interested reader is referred to the body of work by Rowe (33,34) who performed much of the fundamental characterization of pharmaceutical film coating systems. In practice, there are now a wide range of proprietary film coating systems available whereby the film characterization has been performed by the manufacturing company, hence it is not routine practice to remove and thermally characterize the coat when preparing finished dosage forms. However, such studies may be extremely useful in terms of both developing new film coats and also understanding on a fundamental level how and why coating problems may occur. There have several studies outlining how thermal methods may be of use in this regard, particularly using MTDSC. McPhillips (35) performed an analysis of HPMC films using MTDSC, highlighting some of the difficulties associated with studying this material in film form. In the first instance, the sample weight of a single layer of the film was so small that measurement of the T_g proved difficult in terms of sensitivity, necessitating the preparation of several film layers within the pan. However, the authors also found that the sorbed water needed to be carefully considered, given that HPMC is a highly hygroscopic material. The use of pinholed pans allowed the water to escape prior to the T_g, although it proved necessary to examine the reversing (heat capacity) signal in order to visualize the very subtle T_g that this material exhibits. The authors also made the interesting observation that even when using hermetically sealed pans whereby the water could not escape, an endotherm for water evaporation was still seen due to the vaporization of bound water within the headspace of the pan itself.

A further issue is the study of the miscibility of films with both plasticizers and other high molecular weight polymers. This is highly significant as the base polymer is almost invariably used in conjunction with other materials which confer favorable coating, mechanical or dissolution properties, hence it is essential to have knowledge of whether these materials are mixing at a molecular level or whether they exist in phase separated domains. Nyamweya and Hoag (36) studied the miscibility and phase behavior of blends of HPMC with other commonly used polymers including hydroxypropyl cellulose (HPC), methyl cellulose (MC), and polyvinylpyrrolidone (PVP). These authors were able to demonstrate that HPMC was miscible with PVP and MC but not HPC via examination of the glass transition (measured using MTDSC). In brief, a miscible pair of polymer will demonstrate a glass transition intermediate between that of the two component materials while an immiscible blend will show two distinct T_gs, indicating the presence of phase separated regions, each responding to the heating signal independently. The authors were also able to model the change in T_g with composition so as to gain an idea of the ideality of the mix between the various components.

Polymeric films may of course be used as dosage forms in their own right rather than being used as coating materials. For example, Kranz et al. (37) used a combination of mechanical and thermal methods to characterize biodegradable polylactide (PLA) and polylactide-co-glycolide (PLGA) films. Interestingly, these authors studied the effect of exposure to an aqueous medium on the plasticized films, finding that the water-soluble plasticizer triethyl citrate (TEC) was leached out from the film, resulting in an increase in T_g, while the unplasticized films and those plasticized with the water-insoluble acetyltributyl citrate (ATBC) showed no change in T_g after 28 days immersion in pH 7.4 buffer. Over and above the data obtained for these particular systems, the study very effectively demonstrates the need to relate the physicochemical properties of the films to the behavior in a simulated biological environment.

Polymeric Dosage Forms

There are now an extremely wide range of polymeric dosage forms either on the market or in development. Indeed, polymers form one of the basic tools for the design of controlled release dosage forms due to their ability to release drugs at specific rates. Given their pivotal role in the performance of the corresponding dosage forms, effective physical characterization is clearly essential and thermal methods once again play a major role in this respect. One of the earliest polymer-based dosage forms are known as solid dispersions, whereby a poorly soluble drug is dispersed in a water soluble carrier such as polyethylene glycol via either melting or dispersion in a common solvent followed by evaporation. These systems were found to result in much faster dissolution rates than the drug alone. A number of explanations having been submitted for this increase, including changes in drug particle size, particle separation and enhanced wetting and solubilization by the polymer in the aqueous layer immediately adjacent to the dissolving surface (38). It has proved remarkably difficult to ascertain the exact physical nature of the drug within the dispersion, given that there are typically only two components present. DSC in particular has been widely used in characterising the dispersions, particularly as the early thinking within the field was that the systems may be forming solid solutions (whereby the drug is dispersed on a molecular basis) or eutectics (microfine dispersions of the two components), both of which have characteristic phase diagrams that may be ascertained by DSC. In fact the characterization process proved more complex, particularly because the melting of the drug could be influenced by the presence of the molten polymer. More specifically, the PEGs used for solid dispersions tend to melt at circa 60°C, hence above this temperature the drug would dissolve into the molten polymer, thereby giving the impression of an alteration in drug melting behavior which was in fact an artefact of the heating process.

Emphasis now has been placed on preparing dispersions by melt extrusion (39), a process well known within the polymer sciences but which has recently gained considerable prominence. The method consists of heating the polymer/drug mix and forcing the molten or softened material through some form of orifice, thereby allowing a solid dispersion to be formed rapidly and reproducibly without the use of excessive heat or organic solvents. There is currently considerable industrial interest in this method of dosage form production.

While solid dispersions are primarily focused on improving the dissolution properties of poorly soluble drugs, the majority of polymeric dosage forms are associated with slowing or controlling the release of materials to improve the therapeutic profile of the drug. For example, there is a very considerable body of literature describing polymeric microspheres composed of polymers such as PLA and PLGA. Interestingly, there are numerous studies outlining either the manufacture or the biological fate of these spheres but arguably fewer dealing with the characterization of these dosage forms in a physical sense. This is arguably unfortunate as both the means by which the drug is distributed within the spheres and the effect of the drug on the T_g of the constituent polymer could be extremely important in determining the subsequent release behavior. Studies that have addressed this issue include Blanco et al. (40) who studied the degradation of PLA and PLGA microspheres on immersion in an aqueous environment over a period of months as a means of simulating their fate in a biological environment. The authors noted that PLA showed limited change in molecular weight due to hydrolytic ester cleavage and showed a similarly small decrease in T_g over the storage period (Fig. 14). The more hydrophilic PLGA systems, however, showed a much more extensive decrease in molecular weight and accompanying T_g, with marked mass loss also noted. The authors suggested that as the T_g of the PLGA spheres was lowered to that approaching the temperature of incubation, the physical integrity of the spheres was compromised, resulting in the formation of what they term a solid elastic mass which in turn accelerated the mass loss profile.

CONCLUDING COMMENTS

Thermal analysis has been and will continue to be widely used for pharmaceutical formulation, due both to its versatility and also the ability to present key information on the physical (and sometimes chemical) structure and behavior. Modern thermal methods tend to be simple to use and, for basic measurements, the amount of training required is often fairly limited. This is clearly an advantage in most respects, although this simplicity of use leads to a danger of underestimating the wealth of information that may be obtained

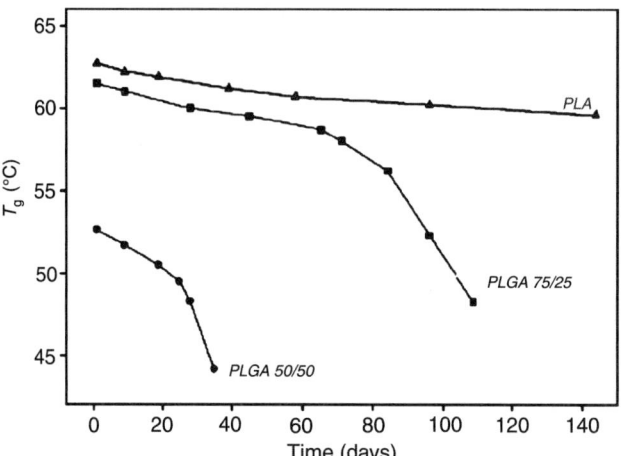

FIGURE 14 Glass transition temperature (T_g) of poly (DL-lactide) (PLA) and poly (DL-lactide-co-glycolide) (PLGA) microscospheres as a function of incubation time in phosphate buffer (pH 7.4) at 37°C. The rank order of hydrophilicities of the polymers studied were PLA, 75/25 PLGA and 50/50 PLGA. *Abbreviations*: PLA, poly (DL-lactide); PLGA, poly (DL-lactide-co-glycolide). *Source*: From Ref. 40.

by the appropriate choice of instrument and judicious use of experimental design and application of basic principles to the interpretation of data. It should also be appreciated that there is a growing emphasis on fundamental understanding of the relationship between processing, structure and behavior of dosage forms, hence the need for these techniques is likely to increase as the demand for more detailed information on the physical characteristics of the delivery systems continues to rise.

ACKNOWLEDGEMENT

The author would like to express gratitude to Professor Mike Reading for his helpful comments and corrections to the chapter.

REFERENCES

1. Wendlandt W. Thermal Analysis. 3rd edn. New York: Wiley-Interscience, 1986.
2. Wunderlich B. Thermal Analysis. San Diego, USA: Academic Press, 1992.
3. Brown M, ed. Handbook of Thermal Analysis. Amsterdam, Holland: Elsevier, 1998.
4. Mathot VBF. Calorimetry and Thermal Analysis of Polymers. Munich, Germany: Hanser Publishers, 1994.
5. Ford JL, Timmins P. Pharmaceutical Thermal Analysis. Chichester, UK: Ellis Horwood, 1989.
6. Craig DQM, Reading M. Thermal Analysis of Pharmaceuticals. Boca Raton, USA: CRC Press, 2007.
7. Hobbs CB. Thermal Properties of Polymers Part 1: Industrial Guide to Measurement by Differential Scanning Calorimetry (DSC). (http://midas.npl.co.uk/midas/content/mn058.html)
8. Reading M, Hourston DJ. Modulated Temperature Differential Scanning Calorimetry, Theory and Practical Applications in Polymer Characterisation. Dordrecht, Holland: Springer, 2006.

9. McGarvey OS, Kett VL, Craig DQM. An investigation into the crystallisation of α, α-trehalose from the amorphous state. J Phys Chem B 2003; 107:6614–20.
10. Manduva R, Kett VL, Banks SR, et al. Calorimetric and spatial characterisation of polymorphic transitions in caffeine using quasi-isothermal MTDSC and localised thermomechanical analysis. J Pharm Sci 2007; 97(2008):1285–1300.
11. Buckton G. Principles and Pharmaceutical Applications of Isothermal Microcalorimetry. In: Craig DQM, Reading M, eds. Thermal Analysis of Pharmaceuticals. Boca Raton, USA: CRC Press, 2007: 265–86.
12. Harding L, King WP, Craig DQM, et al. Nanoscale characterisation and imaging of partially amorphous materials using local thermomechanical analysis and heated tip AFM. Pharm Res 2007; 24:2048–2054.
13. Giron D. Thermal analysis and calorimetric methods in the characterization of polymorphs and solvates. Thermochim Acta 1995; 248:1–59.
14. Hilfiker R, ed. Polymorphism in the Pharmaceutical Industry. Wenheim: Wiley-VCH, 2006.
15. Vitez IM. Utilization of DSC for pharmaceutical crystal form quantitation. J Therm Anal Calorim 2004; 78:33–45.
16. Burger A, Ramberger R. On the polymorphism of pharmaceuticals and other molecular crystals. I. Theory of thermodynamic rules. Mikrochim Acta 1979; 2:259–71.
17. Burger A, Ramberger R. On the polymorphism of pharmaceuticals and other molecular crystals. II. Applicability of thermodynamic rules. Mikrochim Acta 1979; 2:273–316.
18. Schinzer WC, Bergren MS, Aldrich DS, et al. Characterization and interconversion of polymorphs of premafloxacin, a new quinolone antibiotic. J Pharm Sci 1997; 86:1426–31.
19. Lehto VP, Laine E. A kinetic study of polymorphic transition of anhydrous caffeine with microcalorimeter. Thermochim Acta 1988; 317:47–58.
20. McGregor C, Saunders MH, Buckton G, et al. The use of high-speed differential scanning calorimetry (hyper-DSC™) to study the thermal properties of carbamazepine polymorphs. Thermochim Acta 2004; 417(2):231–7.
21. Zhu H, Khankari RK, Padden BE, et al. Physicochemical characterization of nedocromil bivalent metal salt hydrates.1. Nedocromil magnesium J Pharm Sci 1996; 85:1026–34.
22. Hancock BC, Zografi G. Characteristics and significance of the amorphous state in pharmaceutical systems. J Pharm Sci 1997; 86:1–12.
23. Coleman NJ, Craig DQM. Modulated temperature differential scanning calorimetry: A novel approach to pharmaceutical thermal analysis. Int J Pharm 1996; 135:13–29.
24. Royall PG, Craig DQM, Doherty C. Characterisation of the glass transition of an amorphous drug using modulated DSC. Pharm Res 1998; 15:1117–21.
25. Samra RM, Buckton G. The crystallisation of a model hydrophobic drug (terfenadine) following exposure to humidity and organic vapours. Int J Pharm 2004; 284:53–60.
26. Dilworth SE, Buckton G, Gaisford S, et al. Approaches to determine the enthalpy of crystallisation, and amorphous content, of lactose from isothermal calorimetric data. Int J Pharm 2004; 284:83–94.
27. Venkataram S, Khohlokwane M, Wallis SH, Differential scanning calorimetry as a quick scanning technique for solid state stability studies. Drug Dev Ind Pharm 1995; 21:847–55.
28. Mroso PV, Po ALW, Irwin WJ. Solid state stability of aspirin in the presence of excipients—kinetic interpretation, modeling and prediction. J Pharm Sci 1982; 71:1096–101.
29. Schmitt EA, Peck K, Sun Y, et al. Rapid, practical and predictive excipient compatibility screening using isothermal microcalorimetry. Thermochim Acta 2001; 380:175–83.
30. Wissing S, Craig DQM, Barker SA, Moore WD. An investigation into the use of stepwise isothermal high sensitivity DSC as a means of detecting drug-excipient incompatibility. Int J Pharm 2000; 199:141–50.
31. Jones DS. Thermorheological (dynamic oscillatory) characterization of pharmaceutical and biomedical polymers. In: Craig DQM, Reading M, eds. Thermal Analysis of Pharmaceuticals. Boca Raton: CRC Press, 2007: 311–58.
32. Turi EA, ed. Thermal characterization of polymeric materials Vols 1 and 2, Second Edition. San Diego, USA: Academic Press, 1997.

33. Sakellariou P, Rowe RC, White EFT. The thermomechanical properties and glass-transition temperatures of some cellulose derivatives used in film coating. Int J Pharm 1985; 27:267–77.
34. Sakellariou P, Hassan A, Rowe RC. Plasticization of aqueous poly(vinyl alcohol) and hydroxypropyl methylcellulose with polyethylene glycols and glycerol. Eur Polym J 1993; 29:937–43.
35. McPhillips H, Craig DQM, Royall P, et al. Characterisation of the glass transition behaviour of HPMC using modulated differential scanning calorimetry. Int J Pharm 1999; 180:83–90.
36. Nyamweya N, Hoag SW. Assessment of polymer-polymer interactions in blends of HPMC and film forming polymers by modulated temperature differential scanning calorimetry. Pharm Res 2000; 17:625–31.
37. Kranz H, Ubrich N, Maincent P, et al. Physicomechanical properties of biodegradable poly (D, L-lactide) and poly(D, L-lactide-co-glycolide) films in the dry and wet states. J Pharm Sci 2000; 89:1558–66.
38. Serajuddin ATM. Solid dispersion of poorly water-soluble drugs: Early promises, subsequent problems, and recent breakthroughs. J Pharm Sci 1999; 88:1058–66.
39. Breitenbach J. Melt extrusion: from process to drug delivery technology. Eur J Pharm Biopharm 2002; 54:107–17.
40. Blanco MD, Sastre RL, Teijon C, et al. Degradation behaviour of microspheres prepared by spray-drying poly(D, L-lactide) and poly(D, L-lactide-co-glycolide) polymers. Int J Pharm 2006; 326:139–47.

14

Preformulation Studies for Tablet Formulation Development

Raghu K. Cavatur and N. Murti Vemuri
Sanofi-Aventis, Bridgewater, New Jersey, U.S.A.

Raj Suryanarayanan
University of Minnesota, Minneapolis, Minnesota, U.S.A.

INTRODUCTION

Orally administered tablets are expected to be robust enough to withstand the rigors of manufacturing, packaging, and shipping, but readily disintegrate in the GI tract, and present the drug substance for rapid and complete dissolution and absorption from the GI tract. Additionally, the tablets should have an acceptable shelf-life. The tablet manufacturability and performance are dependent, among other things, on the physicochemical properties of the drug substance. A comprehensive characterization of the drug substance is necessary rational formulation development. The characterization of the physicochemical and mechanical properties of the active pharmaceutical ingredient (API) is referred to as preformulation. Preformulation also includes the evaluation of the compatibility of the API with potential excipients. During the drug development process, a general evaluation of physicochemical properties of a chemical compound is performed, with a goal of ascertaining its druggability. Additional studies, related to tablet dosage form development, are focused on specific properties relevant to this dosage form. The desired properties, from a commercial manufacture and product usage, include: (*i*) ease of manufacture, (*ii*) hardness with very low friability, (*iii*) long shelf-life, (*iv*) rapid disintegration, and (*v*) rapid dissolution. The physicochemical properties of the drug substance will be the predominant determinant of the shelf-life as well as the dissolution behavior of the dosage form. In dosage forms where the API is not the major formulation component, the ease of manufacture, hardness, and friability can usually be controlled through excipients.

The focus of this chapter is a discussion of various preformulation studies related to tablet dosage form development. The physicochemical properties of interest can be divided into two broad categories: (*i*) molecular properties which are intrinsic to the drug substance and cannot be modified without chemical modification of the API, and (*ii*) physical properties, which are amenable to modification to suit the needs of formulation. The molecular and the physical properties are listed in Table 1.

A thorough discussion of the molecular and physical properties, with the appropriate theoretical background, is beyond the scope of this chapter. The information is also extensively available in literature. Instead, the discussion will focus on properties that can

TABLE 1 Physicochemical Properties of the API that Can Influence the Performance of a Tablet Dosage Form

Physicochemical parameter/property	Classification	Effect on tablet performance
pKa	Molecular	Solubility, dissolution rate, stability
Aqueous solubility	Molecular	Dissolution rate
Crystal habit	Physical	Powder flow, tabletability
Particle size distribution	Physical	Powder flow, tabletability, dissolution rate
Wettability	Physical/molecular	Granulation during wet massing; dissolution rate
Solid-state properties	Physical/molecular	Powder flow, tabletability, solubility, dissolution rate, stability

Abbreviation: API, active pharmaceutical ingredient.

be modified so as to have a significant impact on tablet formulation development as well as the performance of the finished product.

Early on in product development, the potential for the successful development of a solid oral dosage form is assessed, based on the physicochemical properties of the API (1). Prior to solid dosage form development, it is necessary to anticipate the physicochemical properties that can have a major influence on product manufacture and performance. The early development (preformulation and early formulation development) studies should focus on these properties so as to avoid problems at later stages of development. While the molecular properties dictate the intrinsic solubility and the chemical stability of the compound, by controlling the physical form of the compound and by modifying physical properties (e.g., particle size), the dissolution rate can be enhanced with the potential for improving bioavailability. This chapter will focus on physical properties including particle characteristics, and most importantly, the physical form (i.e., solid state) of the API.

INFLUENCE OF PHYSICOCHEMICAL PROPERTIES ON TABLET FORMULATION PROCESS

The formulation and manufacture of tablets involves many processing steps during which the drug substance and excipients are exposed to a variety of stresses. The physical and chemical properties of the API influence the selection of excipients as well as the processing conditions chosen for manufacture. Table 2 contains the typical processing steps in the manufacture of tablets. The possible phase transformations of the API and their implications on product performance are also listed in Table 2. The latter two issues will be discussed in detail later.

Particle Size and Shape

The dissolution of drug substance from tablets involves a series of steps starting with disintegration of the tablet to granules, which further deaggregate into individual particles, which undergo dissolution. The series of events are shown in Figure 1.

The dissolution rate (dC/dt) described by the Noyes–Nernst equation [Equation (1)], is dependent on the equilibrium solubility (C_s) of the compound as well as the surface area (A) of the dissolving particles.

Preformulation Studies for Tablet Formulation Development

TABLE 2 Possible Phase Transformations During Tablet Manufacture

Processing step	Purpose of processing step	Possible solid-state phase transformations	Implications on tablet formulation
Milling	Size reduction; to improve powder flow and content uniformity	Polymorphic conversion; dehydration; amorphous phase formation	Chemical stability; dissolution rate; bioavailability
Roller compaction	Dry granulation	Polymorphic conversion; dehydration; amorphous phase formation	Chemical stability; dissolution rate; bioavailability
Wet massing	Wet granulation	Polymorphic conversion; hydrate formation; salt to free acid/base conversion; amorphous phase formation	Chemical and physical stability; dissolution rate
Drying of granules	Solvent removal	Polymorphic conversion; dehydration	Chemical stability; dissolution rate; tablet hardness

$$\frac{dC}{dt} = A \cdot \frac{D}{h} \cdot \frac{(C_s - C)}{V} \qquad (1)$$

In this equation, D is the diffusion coefficient of the solute, h is the hydrodynamic layer thickness, V is the volume of medium, and C is the solute concentration in the bulk of the solution. Water is the usual solvent used for these studies.

At an early stage of drug development, it is necessary to thoroughly evaluate the impact of particle size and shape on the processing steps of tablet manufacture, and ultimately on the content uniformity. Content uniformity can be a challenging issue in low dose formulations. A recent review has a comprehensive discussion on the principles, terminology, and instrumentation pertaining to particle size analysis (2). The International Conference on Harmonization guideline has particle size specifications in the form of an algorithm (Fig. 2).

Crystal shape (habit) can influence many processing steps including wetting, powder flow, mixing, and dissolution. Spherical particles tend to have the least contact surface area and exhibit good flow, whereas acicular particles tend to have poor flow (3). Crystal shape has been demonstrated to have a significant impact on mixing and tabletability. L-lysine monohydrate, with plate-shaped crystals exhibited greater tabletability than the prism-shaped crystals (4). This difference was attributed to the favorable orientation of slip plane of plate-shaped crystals. Crystal habit appears to have an influence on the amount of disordered phase formed upon micronization (5). The degree of lattice disorder induced by milling of plate-shaped p-succinic acid was higher than that of needle-shaped crystals.

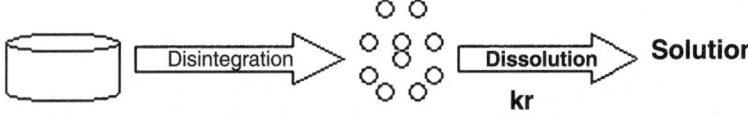

FIGURE 1 Schematic of release of drug substance from a tablet.

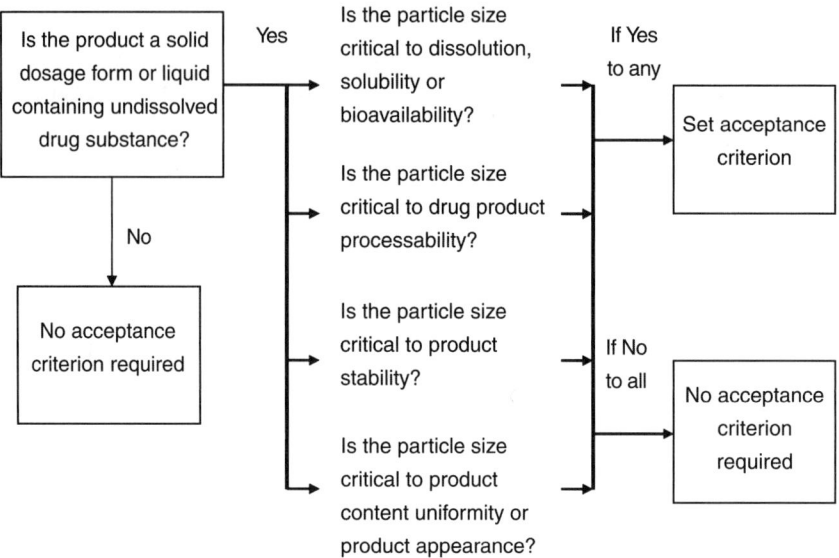

FIGURE 2 Algorithm for setting specifications (ICH Q6A) for particle size distribution. *Source*: From Ref. 44.

SOLID-STATE PROPERTIES

Compounds of pharmaceutical interest can exist in different solid forms. Broadly, they can be classified as being in the amorphous or in the crystalline state. In crystalline pharmaceuticals, solvates are formed when the solvent molecule is incorporated, either stoichiometrically or non-stoichiometrically, in the crystalline lattice. Hydrates are a subclass of solvates, wherein the incorporated solvent is water. Because of regulatory considerations, non-aqueous solvates find limited use as pharmaceuticals. Our discussions will, therefore, be restricted to hydrates. If the solvent is non-volatile, co-crystals are obtained, and this is an emerging field in solid-state pharmaceutics. In case of weakly acidic and basic compounds, salt forms are prepared with the goal of obtaining the desired biopharmaceutical properties. Figure 3 is a schematic representation of the various types of solid forms of interest in pharmaceuticals (6).

The issues related to preparation and screenings of salts have been discussed elsewhere. We will also not be discussing co-crystals in this chapter. This topic has received excellent attention in the literature (7). Similarly, mesophases, which exhibit partial order between the crystalline and amorphous states, will not be discussed. Drug substances are occasionally known to exist as liquid crystals (8).

From a formulation perspective, it is desirable to use the thermodynamically stable form of the API in dosage forms. Biopharmaceutical and processability considerations may dictate the deliberate selection of a metastable form for processing.

Crystalline Pharmaceuticals

A considerable fraction of APIs used in solid dosage forms exist in a highly crystalline state. Polymorphism is the ability of a compound to have two or more arrangements and/or conformations of the molecules in the crystal lattice (9). Polymorphism is an important issue since the different polymorphs of a substance can exhibit differences, sometimes

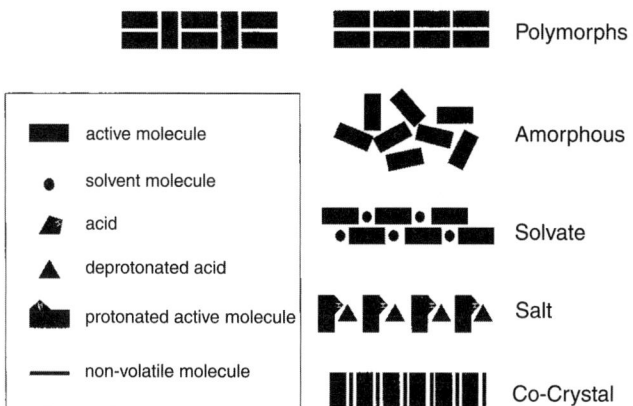

FIGURE 3 Schematic representation of the different types of solid forms of pharmaceuticals. *Source*: From Ref. 6.

pronounced, in their physical properties. The physical properties that can differ among the polymorphs are presented in Table 3.

Grant has comprehensively discussed the thermodynamics of polymorphs (9). The stability of polymorphs and the driving force for polymorphic transitions is governed by the difference in Gibbs free energy, ΔG, between two polymorphs:

$$\Delta G = \Delta H - T\Delta S, \tag{2}$$

where H and S refer to enthalpy and entropy, respectively. The temperature dependence of G and H for two polymorphs, 1 and 2, is shown in Figure 4, and for the purpose of this discussion, we will assume that forms 1 and 2 are solids in the entire temperature range, and the experiments are conducted at ambient pressure. At the transition temperature (T_t), the two forms are in equilibrium, while form 1 is stable below the transition temperature ($G_1 < G_2$), while form 2 is stable above the transition temperature ($G_2 < G_1$). When form 1 is heated, and it is transforms to form 2 at T_t, the enthalpy of transition, $H_t = T_t\Delta S$. A differential scanning calorimeter can be used to determine this enthalpy value.

From Figure 4, it is evident that one polymorph is stable over one temperature range, while the second polymorph is stable over a different temperature range, and the

TABLE 3 List of Physical Properties that Differ Among Various Polymorphs

Packing properties	Molar volume and density, refractive index, electrical and thermal conductivity, hygroscopicity
Thermodynamic properties	Melting and sublimation temperatures, internal energy (i.e., structural energy), enthalpy (i.e., heat content), heat capacity, entropy, free energy and chemical potential, thermodynamic activity, vapor pressure, solubility
Spectroscopic properties	Electronic, vibrational, rotational, and nuclear spin transitions
Kinetic properties	Dissolution rate, solid-state reactivity, stability
Surface properties	Surface free energy, interfacial tensions, habit (i.e., shape)
Mechanical properties	Hardness, tensile strength, tableting, handling, flow, and blending

Source: Adapted from Ref. 9.

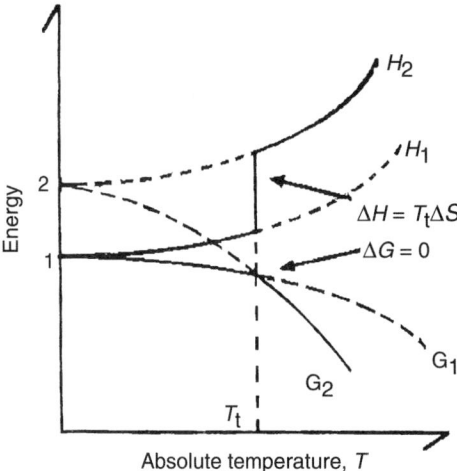

FIGURE 4 Temperature dependence of the Gibbs free energy (G) and the enthalpy (H), at constant pressure, for two polymorphs, 1 and 2. T_t is the transition temperature and S is the entropy. *Source*: From Ref. 9.

transition temperature is below the melting point of both the polymorphs. This is referred to as an enantiotropic polymorphic system, and Figure 5 (upper panel) is a detailed plot of this system. In contrast, in a montropic system, only one polymorph is stable over the entire temperature range with the other polymorph being metastable (lower panel of Fig. 5).

To aid in the identification of the type of transition in a polymorphic pair, Burger and Ramberger (10) formulated four thermodynamic rules. Two of these rules have been extensively used by the pharmaceutical community. According to the heat of transition rule, if an endothermic polymorphic transition is observed (typically, the sample is subjected to a controlled temperature program in a differential scanning calorimeter), the two forms are enantiotropically related, and if an exothermic polymorphic transition is observed, they are monotropic. According to the heat of fusion rule, if the polymorph with the higher melting point has the lower heat of fusion, it is an enantiotropic pair. These rules are evident from Figure 5.

Amorphous Pharmaceuticals

In contrast to crystalline solids, which are characterized by three-dimensional long-range lattice periodicity, amorphous materials exhibit, at best, short-range molecular order. While some pharmaceuticals are intrinsically amorphous (e.g., polymers, proteins), others (e.g., sugars) are rendered amorphous by pharmaceutical processing steps, such as milling. In drugs exhibiting dissolution rate limited absorption, the amorphous state may enhance bioavailability, and the feasibility of this approach has been documented (11). However, the amorphous state, in light of its higher free energy when compared with its crystalline counterpart, confers increased chemical as well as physical instability. This can pose serious challenges when the API in a solid dosage form is amorphous.

The characterization of amorphous materials is intrinsically more challenging than that of crystalline solids. Wide angle X-ray diffractometry is of limited utility in light of the lack of long-range lattice periodicity. However, thermoanalytical techniques, specifically differential scanning calorimetry, find widespread application for the determination of the glass transition temperature, T_g (Fig. 6 and Table 4). Figure 6 is a schematic representation of the specific volume (V_{sp}) or enthalpy (H) as a function of

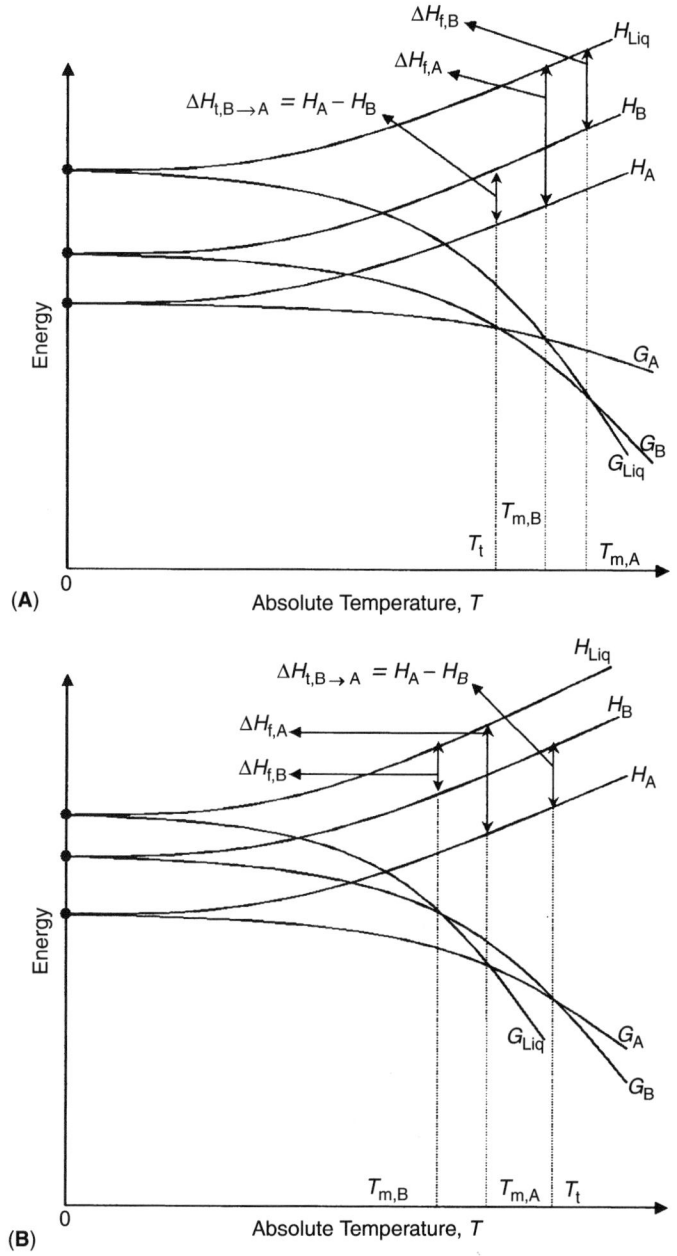

FIGURE 5 Energy-temperature and enthalpy-temperature plots (at constant pressure) for (**A**) enantiotropic and (**B**) monotropic systems of two polymorphs, A and B. G, H and T are the free energy, enthalpy, and temperature, respectively. The subscripts f, m, and t, respectively refer to fusion, melting, and transition, respectively. *Source*: From Ref. 45.

temperature. When a crystalline material is heated, there is a discontinuity in both H and V at the melting temperature. When the melt is rapidly cooled, instead of crystallization at T_m, the system enters the supercooled liquid region, followed by the glass transition event, eventually yielding Glass 1. Above T_g, the material exists as a supercooled liquid (rubber) while below T_g it is a frozen glass. In contrast to the melting temperature (T_m),

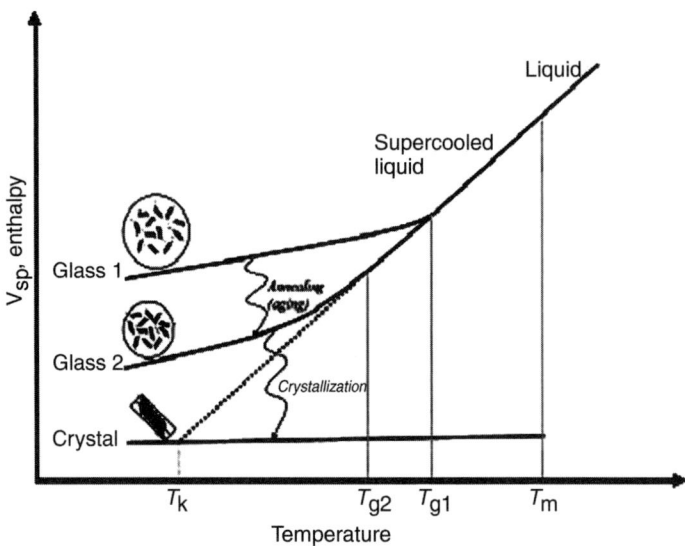

FIGURE 6 Schematic representation of changes in specific volume and enthalpy with temperature. The effect of annealing of a glass, and the associated molecular reorientation is also shown; in addition to the melting (T_m) and Kauzmann (T_k) temperatures, the two glass transition temperatures (T_{g1} and T_{g2}) are pointed out. *Source*: From Ref. 16.

T_g is a kinetic property, dependent both on the thermal history and the cooling (or heating) rate used in the DSC run. If the melt is cooled at a slower rate, the system is characterized by a lower glass transition temperature (T_{g2} in Fig. 6). The Kauzmann temperature (T_K) can be thought of as the lower limit of T_g, attained at an infinitely slow cooling rate.

The effect of enthalpic relaxation, brought about by annealing (or aging), is also shown in Figure 6. In a freshly formed glass (Glass 1), annealing causes a decrease in specific volume (or enthalpy) to yield Glass 2. The possible crystallization of Glass 2 is also shown.

Several excellent reviews have been published on the relevance, characteristics, significance, and stabilization of amorphous materials of pharmaceutical interest (12–15).

TABLE 4 Techniques for Characterization of Amorphous Pharmaceuticals

Technique	Information
XRD	DOC
Molecular spectroscopy	DOC, SR, LM (solid-state NMR)
DSC	DOC, SR, T_g, LM
Isothermal calorimetry	SR, DOC
Solution calorimetry	DOC
DEA	T_g, SR, LM
Solubility	Difference in free energy from the crystalline form
TSDC	SR, DOC, LM
Water sorption	DOC, crystallization

Abbreviations: DEA, dielectric analysis; DOC, degree of crystallinity; DSC, differential scanning calorimetry; LM, local mobility (secondary relaxations) SR, structural relaxation; T_g, determination of glass transition temperature; TSDC, thermally stimulated depolarization current spectroscopy; XRD, X-ray diffractometry. *Source*: Adapted from Ref. 15.

Here, we will exclusively focus on issues relating to the physical stability of amorphous pharmaceuticals. If an amorphous API is used in a solid dosage form, what are the stability implications? The prediction of chemical stability can be reasonably straightforward, since the degradation kinetics generally exhibit Arrhenius temperature dependence. However, the physical instability, manifested as crystallization, is not amenable to accelerated studies since our interest is the onset of crystallization (i.e., the detection of a crystalline phase) (16).

The factors affecting crystallization from the amorphous state have been comprehensively reviewed (16). From a preformulation perspective, in addition to thermodynamic and kinetic factors, it is important to consider the effect of additives and the sample preparation method. At any temperature, the free energy difference between the metastable (i.e., amorphous) and the crystalline state will be the thermodynamic driving force for crystallization. A detailed analysis is outside the scope of this chapter, but can be found in the literature (16).

The physical as well as chemical instability observed in the amorphous state, may be attributable to the molecular mobility in the amorphous state. Conventionally, T_g has been considered an indicator of molecular mobility, and therefore, the stability of an amorphous material. However, this approach neglects several other factors including thermal history and fragility of the glass (16).

One measure of molecular mobility is the structural relaxation time (τ), and there appears to be a correlation between crystallization tendency and τ. The strength of hydrogen bonding in the amorphous matrix may influence the structural relaxation time, and hence the tendency for crystallization (17). The differences in the hydrogen bonding properties between an amorphous phase and its crystalline counterpart may be an important determinant of the tendency to crystallize (17). This conclusion was based on comparing the hydrogen bonding tendencies of seven dihyropyridine anaologs in the crystalline and amorphous states (18). An understanding of these interactions may provide a mechanistic basis for both processing effects (e.g., annealing) and formulation (e.g., use of additives) approaches for amorphous phase stabilization. Table 4 lists some of the experimental techniques used to measure structural relaxation.

Dielectric analysis (DEA) is being increasingly used to characterize amorphous pharmaceuticals. It has an advantage in measuring molecular mobility over DSC in that it provides direct information about relaxation times. Moreover, it is an excellent complement to DSC and vibrational spectroscopy. For example, while we can easily study glass transition and crystallization in an amorphous system using DSC, DEA could be used to characterize the secondary relaxations and also the distribution of relaxation times for both the primary and secondary relaxations.

Amorphous pharmaceuticals have been prepared by several methods including, quench-cooling of melt, precipitation from solution, mechanical processing (milling, compression), and drying (freeze-drying, spray-drying, dehydration of a hydrate). The differences, both in thermal history and the processing-induced stress, can lead to pronounced differences in both the chemical and physical stability of the product phase. Moreover, even when glasses are stored at temperatures far below their T_g, there can be sufficient molecular mobility to result not only in relaxation but also nucleation. Therefore, both the method of preparation, and the storage history of the sample, will have to be monitored and controlled as a part of the preformulation screening (19,20). While emphasis in the literature has been placed on the correlation between mobility associated with alpha relaxation (glass transition) and crystallization, secondary (or beta) relaxations have been shown to be directly coupled to physical stability (21–25) as well as chemical stability (26). Secondary relaxation is attributed to motions on much smaller length scale than alpha, and the two may not be coupled. Even if the secondary relaxations are not directly responsible for the physical or chemical instability in an amorphous matrix, it is extremely important to characterize these non-cooperative motions in a system since some secondary relaxations, also called the Johari–Goldstein relaxations, are thought to be the precursors of glass transition (27,28). Consequently, factors promoting such relaxations could also facilitate the cooperative α-relaxations eventually leading to physical or chemical instability. There may also be multiple secondary relaxations in a system having different temperature dependences that may indirectly influence the physical and chemical stability.

Although the existence of "polyamorphism" is debatable, heterogeneity is inherent in an amorphous system (29–31). Amorphous systems, in addition to exhibiting cooperative primary or α-relaxations and non-cooperative secondary or β-relaxations, may reveal multiple secondary relaxations (32). These different relaxation processes are likely to have different temperature dependences, e.g., α-relaxations are generally described by the VTF or WLF models whereas the Johari–Goldstein relaxations are usually described by Arrhenius model (27).

Hydrates

A large number of APIs exist as hydrates. Hydrates may recrystallize when water or a water–organic solvent mixture is used during the manufacture of the API, typically in the final step of recrystallization. In addition to the potential use of water as the solvent for recrystallization, anhydrous compounds can interact with water vapor in the atmosphere to form a hydrate, and a hydrate may be the stable form under ambient conditions. Over 150 compounds listed in the USP exist as hydrates.

The use of a hydrate poses some unique challenges. Dehydration during processing or storage, will not only result in the liberation of water, but may also yield an amorphous anhydrous phase which may be chemically reactive, as has been demonstrated in case of cephradine dihydrate (33).

We will restrict our discussion to stoichiometric hydrate. The thermodynamics of hydrate formation has been discussed by Lohani and Grant (45). Assuming that a drug D, forms a hydrate with m moles of water of crystallization, the equilibrium can be expressed as:

$$D\text{(solid)} + mH_2O \overset{K_{h,m}}{\Longleftrightarrow} D \cdot mH_2O \text{(solid)} \tag{3}$$

The equilibrium constant can be expressed as:

$$K_{h,m} = \frac{\alpha[D \cdot mH_2O\text{(solid)}]_{eq}}{\alpha[D\text{(solid)}]_{eq}(\alpha[H_2O]_{eq.m})^m} \tag{4}$$

where $\alpha[D \cdot mH_2O\text{(solid)}]_{eq}$, $\alpha[D(solid)]_{eq}$, and $\alpha[H_2O]_{eq,m}$ are respectively the activities of the hydrate, anhydrate and water. The hydrate will be stable when

$$\alpha[H_2O] > (K_{h,m})^{-1/m} \tag{5}$$

The water activity is often expressed as relative humidity (RH) which is the ratio of water vapor pressure (P) to the saturated water vapor pressure (P_0), expressed in percentage (at a fixed temperature).

Preformulation Studies for Tablet Formulation Development

The stability of a hydrate will be dictated by the temperature as well as water vapor pressure. During pharmaceutical processing and storage, the drug substance may experience a range of temperatures and water vapor pressures. The potential to form a hydrate, and the hydrate stoichiometry should therefore be evaluated over a range of temperatures and water vapor pressures. In addition to the potential to form a hydrate with m moles of water of crystallization, let us assume that the D, can form second hydrate, with n moles of water ($n > m$) of crystallization. The phase diagram indicates the conditions of temperature and pressure under which each of the three solid phases—D, D.mH$_2$O, and D.nH$_2$O is stable (Fig. 7). In the case of APIs with a propensity to form hydrate phases, such a phase diagram should be generated over the range of temperatures and water vapor pressures of interest.

Morris (33) has classified hydrates based on their structure. In the first type, referred to as isolated site hydrates, the water molecules in the lattice are isolated and do not come into direct contact with other water molecules. Cephradine dihydrate is a representative example. The second type is channel hydrates, wherein the water molecules of adjoining unit cells are in close proximity. This is subdivided into (*i*) expanded channels which have the propensity to form non-stoichiometric hydrates (e.g., cromolyn sodium hydrate), (*ii*) planar hydrates (e.g., nedocromil zinc; capable of existing in different hydration states), and (*iii*) dehydrated hydrates, wherein dehydration results in a structure very similar to the hydrate, but with a lower density. The third type is ion associated hydrates which contain metal ion coordinated water, and the hydrates of calteridol sodium are examples of this type.

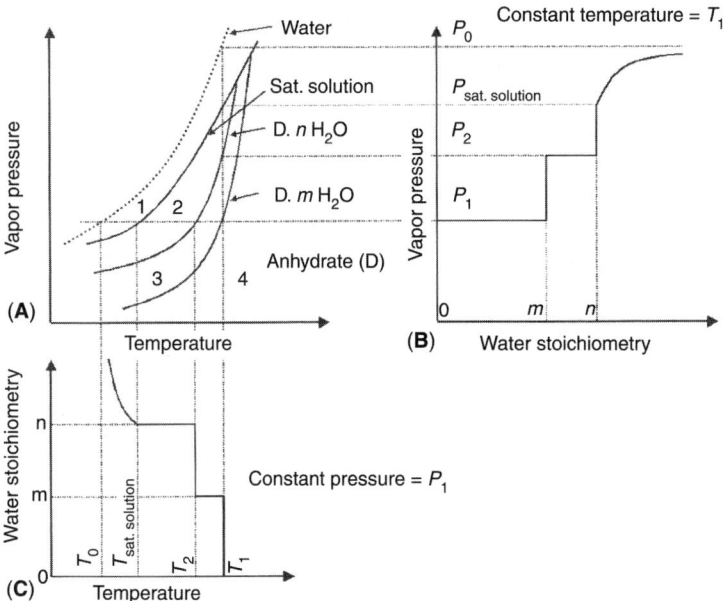

FIGURE 7 (**A**) Water vapor pressure–temperature diagram of a drug D, capable of existing as an anhydrate (D), and as two stoichiometric hydrates, D.nH$_2$O and D.mH$_2$O (45). Regions 1–4 represent the range of pressure–temperature values wherein solution of D in water, D.nH$_2$O, and D.mH$_2$O and D are the equilibrium stable phases. (**B**) Dependence of hydrate stoichiometry on vapor pressure at a constant temperature, T_1. (**C**) Dependence of hydrate stoichiometry on temperature at a constant pressure, P_1. *Source*: From Ref. 45.

Figure 8 shows the solubility of the anhydrous and monohydrate forms of theophylline as a function of temperature (34). Just as the free energy difference between polymorphs can be calculated from the solubility difference, the free energy of hydration can be obtained from the solubility difference.

As pointed out by Morris (33), it is important to recognize the difference between polymorphs and hydrates. If we are dealing with polymorphism in an anhydrous compound, the free energy is specified by the temperature and pressure. A crystalline hydrate being a two-component system is described by the temperature, pressure and water activity. However, if we assume atmospheric pressure, then the free energy can be described by the temperature and water activity.

Interaction with Water

Evaluation of the interaction of the API with water is an important and essential preformulation activity. For the purposes of our discussion, we will assume (*i*) the API of interest is a non-porous solid, (*ii*) the API does not form a non-stoichiometric hydrate, and (*iii*) non-aqueous solvates of the API will not be considered for development. If these issues are of interest, they are addressed in the literature (35).

The tendency of a solid to take up water from the atmosphere, as it is subjected to a controlled RH program under isothermal conditions, is referred to as hygroscopicity (35). The hygroscopicity of a solid can be classified based on the amount or rate of water uptake when a solid is exposed to controlled RH values at a specified temperature (Table 1 from Ref. 35). The RH of a saturated solution of the API, RH_0, can also be of importance. From a preformulation perspective, it is important to know the effect of water sorption on the pharmaceutically relevant properties of the API.

The interaction of water with crystalline solids is fundamentally different from that with amorphous phases (36). In crystalline solids, water can be adsorbed on the surface.

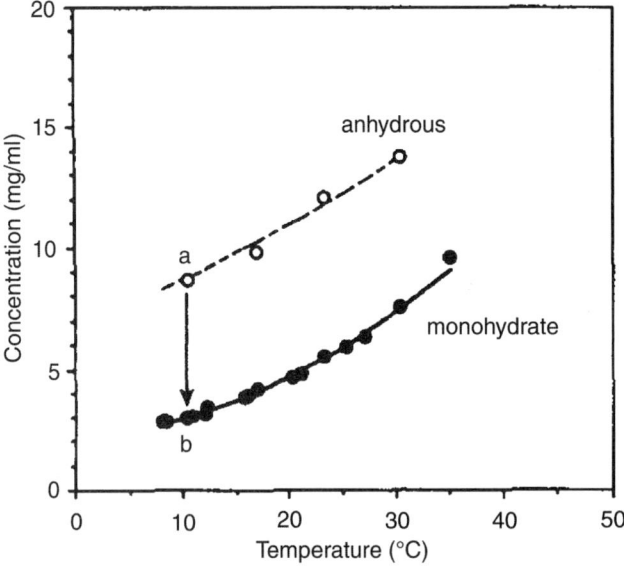

FIGURE 8 Solubility of anhydrous and monohydrate forms of theophylline as a function of temperature. In the concentration range represented by points a and b, the phase transition was studied. *Source*: From Ref. 34.

Adsorption can bring about changes in surface properties, thereby affecting particle aggregation and flow with minimal effects on bulk properties (35). Water can also be incorporated into the lattice to form a hydrate, and this is expected to occur at defined water vapor pressures. As discussed elsewhere, the anhydrous and hydrated forms of a drug can exhibit pronounced differences in properties. In case of amorphous materials, the water is absorbed into the bulk, and the amount absorbed can change progressively with the RH. This can bring about pronounced changes in properties, including an increase in molecular mobility. This is brought about by an increase in free volume and a decrease in glass transition (36). The resulting increase in reactivity can lead to a decrease in physical as well as chemical reactivity.

The heterogeneity of pharmaceutical solids poses some unique challenges. For example, even in highly crystalline solids, there can be small regions of high lattice disorder. These "disordered regions" with a high potential for sorbing water, are likely to be much more reactive than the rest of the highly ordered lattice. Thus, even in chemically pure phases, the physical heterogeneity can be a source of chemical instability as well as batch-to-batch variations in properties.

The uptake as well as loss of water from pharmaceutical solids, as a function of RH, is typically measured gravimetrically. The conventional approach was to store the solid in chambers maintained at different RH values (using saturated salt solutions), usually at room temperature. The use of automated water vapor sorption instruments has now become quite common. In these instruments, the sample weight is monitored continuously while the sample is subjected to controlled RH. Figure 9 is a representative example, wherein the water sorption behavior of amorphous trehalose prepared by different methods is plotted (20). It is evident that the water sorption behavior is strongly influenced by the method of preparation of the amorphous phase. While panel (a) provides the extent of water uptake, from the perspective of handling and manufacture of both the raw material and the drug product, the rate of uptake is of importance. This information is also available in the automated water sorption instruments (Fig. 9, panel b).

Newman et al. (35) have developed a flow-chart that can be used to evaluate the water uptake behavior of pharmaceuticals (Fig. 10). In addition to the determination of the extent of water sorption, it is also necessary to characterize the solid using suitable physical characterization techniques. This can form an excellent starting point during the preformulation screening of APIs.

PROCESSING-INDUCED PHASE TRANSFORMATION STUDIES

Even when the appropriate physical form of the API has been selected, it may not be retained in the finished tablet. The mechanical and thermal stresses experienced during processing, and the interaction with formulation components, can result in phase transitions (37). The possible phase transformations during tablet manufacture and their implications on product performance were presented earlier (Fig. 2). This subject has also been comprehensively reviewed recently (38). While the phase transformations of active ingredients have been extensively investigated, such changes in excipients can have implications on the physical and chemical stability of the API and also affect product quality. Figure 11 is a comprehensive representation of processing-induced phase transformations. It must be recognized that, during conventional tablet manufacture, the formulation components will not undergo all of the processes listed in Figure 11.

The schematic representation (Fig. 12), based on the stress-relaxation concept, shows how stress (thermal/mechanical) or interaction with formulation components, can

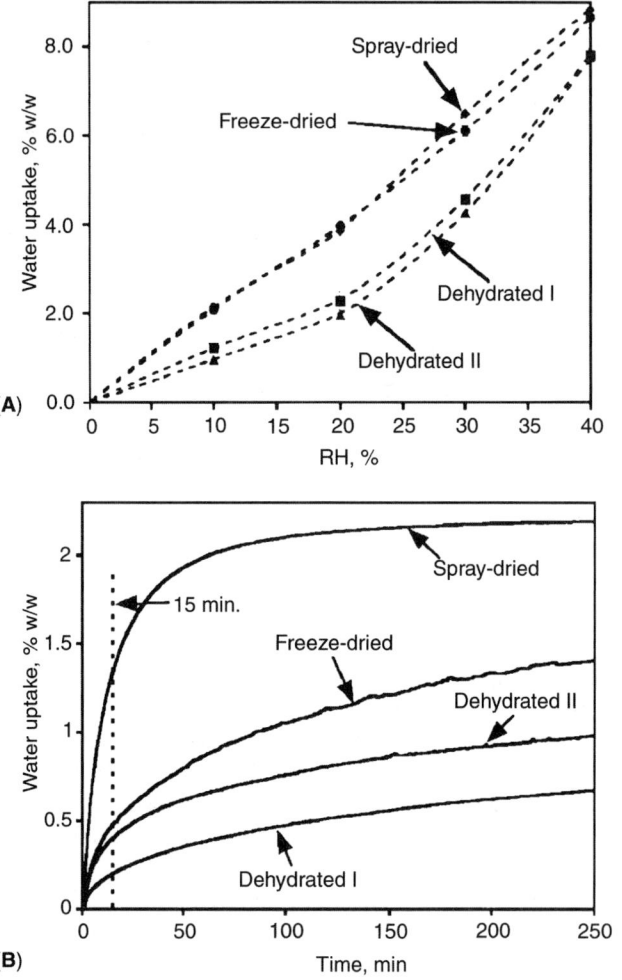

FIGURE 9 Water vapor sorption behavior (at 25°C) of amorphous trehalose prepared by different methods — freeze-drying, spray-drying and dehydration of trehalose dihydrate. (**A**) Extent of uptake from 0% to 40% RH. Replicate analyses were performed at selected RH values (mean ± SD; n 3). (**B**) Kinetics of uptake at 10% RH. Dehydration was carried out under two conditions — at 100°C under vacuum (50 Torr) for 24 hours (*dehydrated I*) or at 97°C under partial vacuum (~400 Torr) for 24 hours (*dehydrated II*). *Abbreviation*: RH, relative humidity. *Source*: From Ref. 20.

induce phase transformations (37,39). Under the stress, the transition may be thermodynamically favored resulting in a stable product phase. Examples are as follows: (1) anhydrate→hydrate transition during the wet massing stage of granulation, and (2) kinetically stable amorphous form produced by milling. When the stress is removed, the system which was trapped under the stress may relax back to the original state.

Otsuka et al. demonstrated a reduction in crystallinity on milling of several drugs including cephalothin and nitrofurantoin (40,41). An amorphous product can be obtained if the processing temperature is substantially below the T_g of the product phase. Since amorphous phases in general tend to be less chemically stable when compared to their crystalline counterparts, the stability of micronized drug substance in presence of excipients has to be assessed prior to formulation development.

Preformulation Studies for Tablet Formulation Development

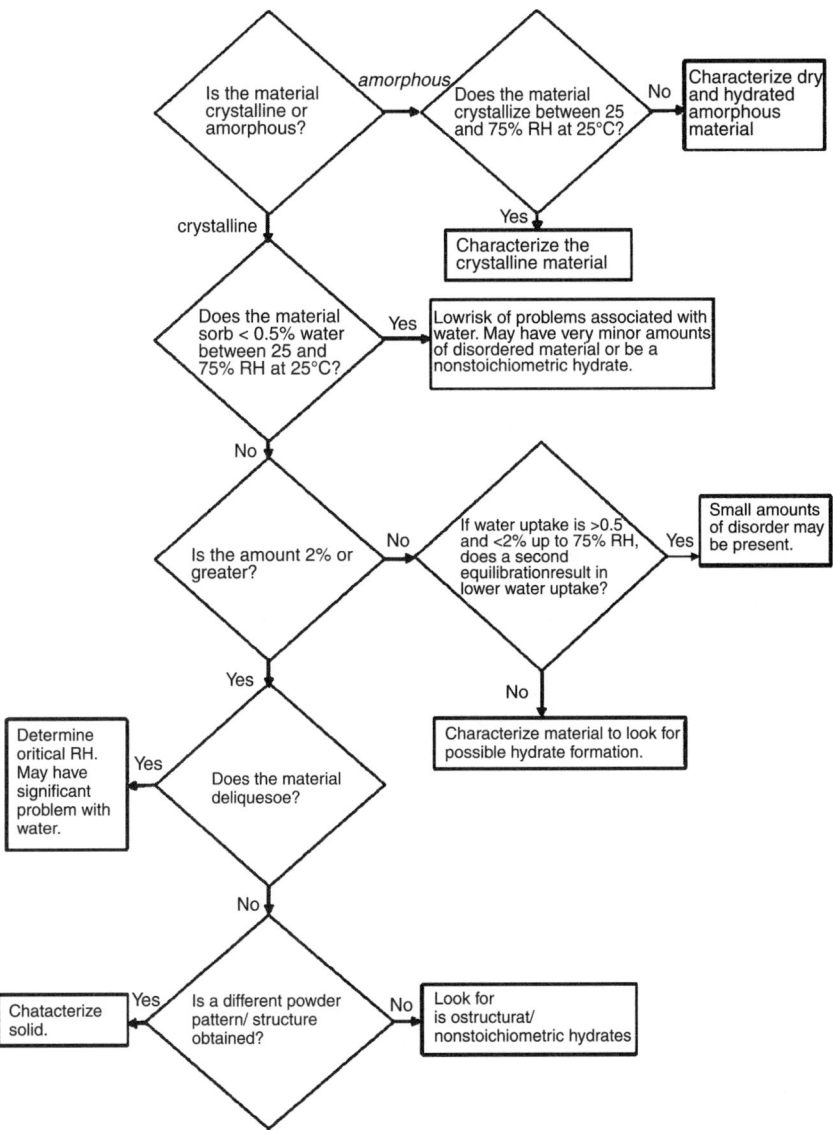

FIGURE 10 Evaluation of water sorption behavior of solids. *Source*: From Ref. 35.

Chan and Deolker studied the compression-induced conversion of unstable crystal forms of several drugs including caffeine and sulfabenzamide into their corresponding stable forms (42). They evaluated the effect of particles size and compression pressure and concluded that nucleation of the stable form can be initiated at the crystal defect sites. While investigating the influence of excipients, it was observed that the compression-induced dehydration of theophylline monohydrate and crystallization of amorphous indomethacin were minimized in presence of carrageenan (43). The effect was attributed to the pronounced elastic recovery of carrageenan during decompression.

Milling and compression studies on API will help in identifying any issues related to phase transformation prior to formulation development and should be integrated into

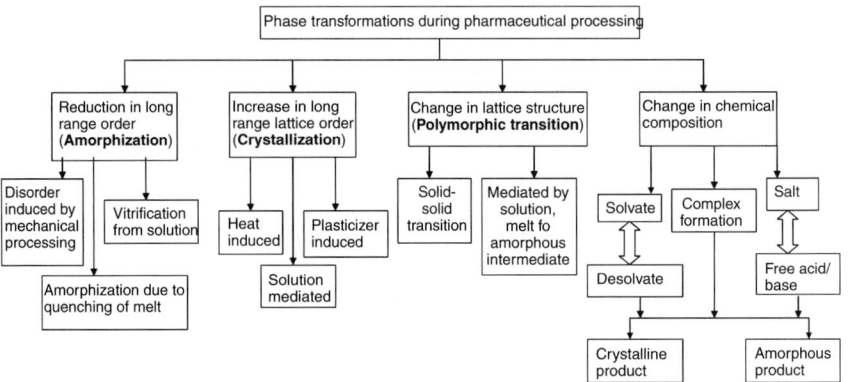

FIGURE 11 Schematic representation of processing-induced phase transformations. *Source*: From Ref. 37.

preformulation screening procedures. Similarly, hydrate→anhydrate transformation during wet massing and drying have to be evaluated. In some cases, biopharmaceutical considerations may necessitate the use of the unstable physical forms prone to solid-state transformation. In such cases, the judicious selection of excipients and careful monitoring

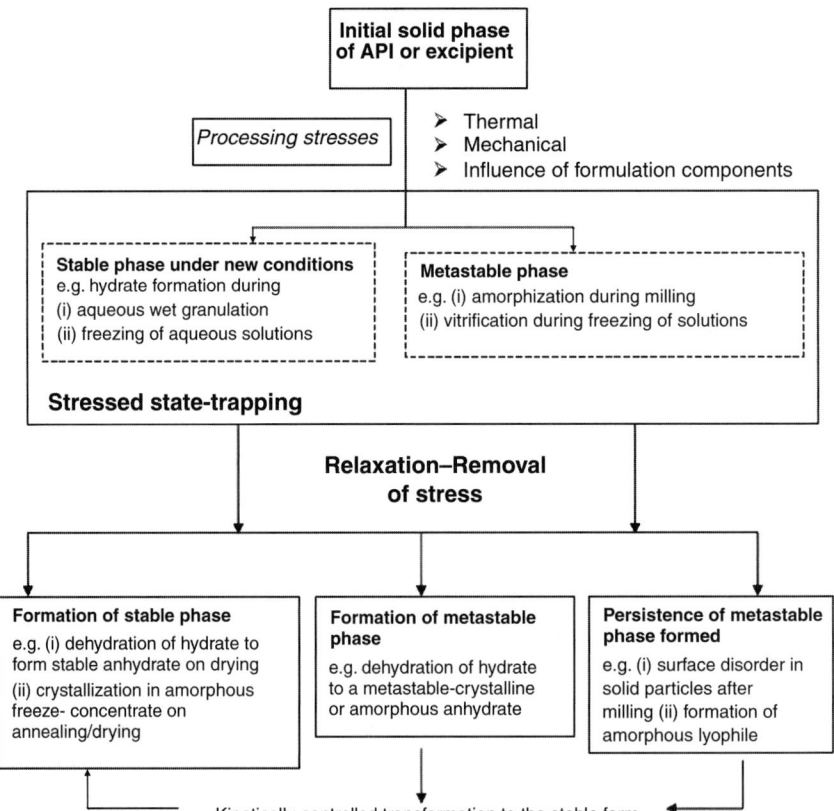

FIGURE 12 A schematic representation of the mechanism of phase transformations as a result of processing stresses. *Source*: From Ref. 37.

of processing will be necessary to control the physical form of the API during product manufacture and subsequent storage.

SUMMARY

Pharmaceutical preformulation studies are generally aimed at assessing physicochemical properties of the API so as to obtain the desirable in vitro and biopharmaceutical performance of the dosage form. Tablet preformulation studies also have to take into account the influence of these properties on manufacturability. The aim is to provide the formulator with information regarding the properties that might pose challenges in dosage form design and manufacture. For example, characterizing particle shape can provide important information on powder flow and potential for desegregation during mixing. The information can be used either to adapt the process so as to avoid flow and content uniformity issues, or to alter the particle shape so as to avoid these problems. While there are numerous physicochemical properties that warrant consideration, this chapter has focused on the physical form of the API.

ACKNOWLEDGEMENTS

The assistance provided by Sisir Bhattacharya, Paroma Chakravarty, and Prakash Sundaramurthi is gratefully acknowledged.

REFERENCES

1. Lipinski CA, Lombardo F, Dominy BW, et al. Experimental and computational approaches to estimate solubility and permeability in drug discovery and development settings. Adv Drug Delivery Rev 2001; 46:3–26.
2. Shekunov BY, Chattopadhyay P, Tong HHY, et al. Particle size analysis in pharmaceutics: principles, methods and applications. Pharm Res 2007; 24:203–27.
3. Venables HJ, Wells JI. Powder mixing. Drug Development and Industrial Pharmacy 2001, 27: 599–612.
4. Sun C, Grant DJW. Influence of crystal shape on the tableting performance of L-lysine monohydrochloride dihydrate. J Pharm Sci 2001; 90:569–79.
5. Chikhalia V, Forbes RT, Storey RA, et al. The effect of crystal morphology and mill type on milling induced crystal disorder. Eur J Pharm Sci 2006; 27:19–26.
6. Hilfiker R, Blatter F, von Raumer M. Relevance of solid-state properties for pharmaceutical products. In: Hilfiker R, ed. Polymorphism in the Pharmaceutical Industry, Weinheim, Germany: Wiley-VCH, 2006: 1–19.
7. Vishweshwar P, McMahon JA, Zaworotko MJ. Crystal engineering of pharmaceutical co-crystals. In: Tiekink ERT, Vittal JJ, eds. Frontiers in Crystal Engineering. New Jersey: John Wiley Ltd, 2006: 25–49.
8. Stevenson CL, Bennett DB, Lechuga-Ballesteros D. Pharmaceutical liquid crystals: The relevance of partially ordered systems. J Pharm Sci 2005; 94:1861–80.
9. Grant DJW. Theory and origin of polymorphism. In: Brittain HG, ed. Polymorphism in Pharmaceutical Solids. New York: Marcel Dekker, 1999: 1–34.
10. Burger A, Ramberger R. On the polymorphism of pharmaceuticals and other molecular crystals. I. Theory of thermodynamic rules. Mikrochim Acta 1979; 2:259–71.
11. Zheng X, Yang R, Zhang Y, et al. Bioavailability in Beagle dogs of nimodipine solid dispersions prepared by hot-melt extrusion. Drug Dev Ind Pharm 2007; 33:783–9.

12. Craig DQM, Royall PG, Kett VL, et al. The relevance of the amorphous state to pharmaceutical dosage forms: glassy drugs and freeze dried systems. Int J Pharm 1999; 179:179–207.
13. Hancock BC, Zografi G. Characteristics and significance of the amorphous state in pharmaceutical systems. J Pharm Sci 1997; 86:1–12.
14. Hilden LR, Morris KR. Physics of amorphous solids. J Pharm Sci 2004; 93:3–12.
15. Yu L. Amorphous pharmaceutical solids: preparation, characterization and stabilization. Adv Drug Del Rev 2001; 48:27–42.
16. Bhugra C, Pikal MJ. Role of thermodynamic, molecular, and kinetic factors in crystallization from the amorphous state. J Pharm Sci 2008; 97:1329–49.
17. Gunawan L, Johari GP, Shanker RM. Structural relaxation of acetaminophen glass. Pharm Res 2006; 23:967–79.
18. Marsac PJ, Konno H, Taylor LS. A comparison of the physical stability of amorphous felodipine and nifedipine Systems. Pharm Res 2006; 23:2306–16.
19. Gupta P, Thilagavathi R, Chakraborti AK, et al. Role of molecular interaction in stability of celecoxib-PVP amorphous systems. Mol Pharm 2005; 2:384–91.
20. Surana R, Pyne A, Suryanarayanan R. Effect of preparation method on physical properties of amorphous trehalose. Pharm Res 2004; 21:1167–76.
21. Alie J, Menegotto J, Cardon P, et al. Dielectric study of the molecular mobility and the isothermal crystallization kinetics of an amorphous pharmaceutical drug substance. J Pharm Sci 2004; 93:218–33.
22. Alig I, Braun D, Langendorf R, et al. Simultaneous ageing and crystallization processes within the glassy state of a low molecular weight substance. J Non-Cryst Solids 1997; 221:261–4.
23. Hikima T, Hanaya M, Oguni M. Microscopic observation of a peculiar crystallization in the glass transition region and beta-process as potentially controlling the growth rate in triphenylethylene. J Mol Struct 1999; 479:245–50.
24. Vyazovkin S, Dranca I. Physical stability and relaxation of amorphous indomethacin. J Phys Chem B 2005; 109:18637–44.
25. Vyazovkin S, Dranca I. Effect of Physical aging on nucleation of amorphous indomethacin. J Phys Chem 2007; 111:7283–7.
26. Yoshioka S, Miyazaki T, Aso Y. Beta-relaxation of insulin molecule in lyophilized formulations containing trehalose or dextran as a determinant of chemical reactivity. Pharm Res 2006; 23:961–6.
27. Ngai KL. Relation between some secondary relaxations and the alpha relaxations in glass-forming materials according to the coupling model. J Chem Phys 1998; 109:6982–94.
28. Ngai KL. Correlation between the secondary beta-relaxation time at T_g with the Kohlrausch exponent of the primary alpha relaxation or the fragility of glass-forming materials. Phys Rev E 1998; 57:7346–9.
29. Hancock BC, Shalaev EY, Shamblin SL. Polyamorphism: a pharmaceutical science perspective. J Pharm Pharmacol 2002; 54:1151–2.
30. Mishima O, Calvert LD, Whalley E. 'Melting ice' I at 77 K and 10 kbar: a new method of making amorphous solids. Nature 1984; 310:393–95.
31. Mishima O, Calvert LD, Whalley E. An apparently first-order transition between two amorphous phases of ice induced by pressure. Nature 1985; 314:76–8.
32. De Gusseme A, Carpentier L, Willart JF, et al. Molecular mobility in super-cooled trehalose. J Phys Chem B 2003; 107:10879–86.
33. Morris KR. Structural aspects of hydrates and solvates. In: Brittan HG, ed. Polymorphism in Pharmaceutical Solids, New York: Marcel Dekker, 1999: 125–81.
34. Rodriguez-Hornedo N, Lechuga-Ballesteros D, Wu HJ. Phase transition and heterogeneous/epitaxial nucleation of hydrated and anhydrous theophylline crystals. Int J Pharm 1992; 85:149–62.
35. Newman AW, Reutzel-Edens SM, Zografi G. Characterization of the hygroscopic properties of active pharmaceutical ingredients. J Pharm Sci 2008; 97:1047–59.
36. Zografi G. States of water associated with solids. Drug Dev Ind Pharm 1988; 14:1905–26.

Preformulation Studies for Tablet Formulation Development

37. Govindarajan R, Suryanarayanan R. Processing-induced phase transformations and their implications on pharmaceutical products quality. In: Hilfiker R, ed. Polymorphism in the Pharmaceutical Industry. Weinheim: Wiley-VCH, 2006: 333–64.
38. Zhang GGZ, Law D, Schmitt EA, et al. Phase transformation considerations during process development and manufacture of solid oral dosage forms. Adv Drug Del Rev 2004; 56:371–90.
39. Morris KR, Griesser UJ, Eckhardt CJ, et al. Theoretical approaches to physical transformations of active pharmaceutical ingredients during manufacturing processes. Adv Drug Delivery Rev 2001; 48:91–114.
40. Otsuka M, Kaneniwa N. Effect of grinding on the crystallinity and chemical stability in the solid state of cephalothin sodium. Int J Pharm 1990; 62:65–73.
41. Otsuka M, Matsuda Y. Effect of environmental humidity on the transformation pathway of nitrofurantoin modifications during grinding and the physicochemical properties of ground products. J Pharm Pharmacol 1993; 45:406–13.
42. Chan HK, Doelker E. Polymorphic transformation of some drugs under compression. Drug Dev Ind Pharm 1985; 11:315–32.
43. Schmidt AG, Wartewig S, Picker KM. Potential of carrageenans to protect drugs from polymorphic transformation. Eur J Pharm Biopharm 2003; 56:101–10.
44. http://www.ich.org.
45. Lohani S, Grant DJW. Thermodynamics of polymorphs. In: Hilfiker R, ed. Polymorphism in the Pharmaceutical Industry. Weinheim, Germany: Wiley-VCH, 2006: 21–42.

15
Stability Kinetics

Robin Roman
GlaxoSmithKline, R&D, King of Prussia, Pennsylvania, U.S.A.

INTRODUCTION

The purpose of stability testing is to provide evidence on how the quality of the dosage form varies with time under the influence of a variety of environmental factors, such as temperature, humidity and light, and to establish a shelf life for the product and recommended storage conditions. The attributes that are monitored during stability studies are assay, degradation products, dissolution or disintegration, description and, if present, antioxidant content. Any of these attributes can define the shelf life and storage conditions for the product. The shelf life should not exceed that predicted for any single attribute.

REGULATORY REQUIREMENTS

In the United States, the Current Good Manufacturing Practices Regulations (CGMPs) published in the Federal Register (21 part 211) state that "There shall be a written testing program designed to assess the stability characteristics of drug products. The results of such stability testing shall be used in determining appropriate storage conditions and expirations dates." It further states "to assure that a drug product meets acceptable standards of identity, strength, quality, and purity at the time of use, it shall bear an expiration date determined by appropriate stability testing." Similar CGMP regulations are in place in Europe, Japan, and most other countries. Thus, stability testing is a legal requirement for pharmaceutical products intended for human consumption.

In the United States, dietary supplements, which include vitamins and minerals are not considered pharmaceutical products but are considered as a special category under the general umbrella of foods. Although the Food and Drug Administration (FDA) has long had the authority to promulgate CGMP regulations for dietary supplements it only did so in 2007. The regulations in 21 CFR part 111 are based on those for food rather than drugs and only provide general information on stability testing. Because of the large range of dietary supplements, including botanical products, the FDA has concluded that generally available methods to determine expiration dating are not currently in place for some products. As a result, expiration dating is not required for dietary supplements. Because the final rule does not require that an expiration date needs to be established, the FDA has declined to offer guidance on the type of data that are acceptable to support an expiration date should a manufacturer choose to establish one other than to indicate that any expiration date placed on a product (including a "best if used by" date) should be supported by data.

COMPENDIAL REQUIREMENTS

The United States Pharmacopeia/National Formulary (USP/NF) chapter on Pharmaceutical Stability, <1150>, provides general guidance on stability studies needed to establish a product's shelf life (1). This chapter also defines the term "controlled room temperature" in terms of the mean kinetic temperature of the region where the products is being distributed. Since the term "room temperature" is used in different ways in different countries, for products shipped outside the United States, it is recommended that product labeling refers to a maximum storage temperature or temperature range in degrees Celsius.

The USP/NF also has a chapter, <2750>, on Manufacturing Practices for Dietary Supplements (2). Unlike the FDA regulations on CGMPs for dietary supplements, the principles in the chapter are derived from the CGMPs for drugs. However, the practical application of these principles to dietary supplements may be different. The chapter states "Dietary supplements should bear a date indicative of its shelf life, determined by appropriate testing, to ensure that they meet applicable standards of identity, strength, quality, and purity at or before the labeled shelf life date. Shelf life should be related to any storage conditions stated on the labeling." It further states "There should be a written protocol designed to assess the stability characteristics of dietary supplements. The results of such testing should be used in determining appropriate storage conditions and shelf life."

REGULATORY GUIDELINES

In 1991, the Commission of European Communities, the FDA, the Japanese Ministry of Heath and Welfare, the International Federation of Pharmaceutical Manufacturers Associations, the European Federation of Pharmaceutical Manufacturers Associations, the U.S. Pharmaceutical Manufacturers Association and the Japanese Pharmaceutical Manufacturers Association organized the first International Conference on Harmonization (ICH). The goal of the conference was to begin to harmonize requirements for regulatory submissions in the United States, Europe and Japan in the areas of quality, safety, and efficacy. One of the quality topics was stability testing.

In subsequent years, a number of guidance documents related to stability of pharmaceutical products have been issued. The guidance documents are based on the concept of climatic zones (1). There are four zones based on Mean Kinetic Temperature and Mean Annual Relative Humidity (RH): Zone I (temperate climate), e.g., Canada and Northern European, Zone II (subtropical), e.g., the United States and Southern Europe, Zone III (hot and dry), e.g., Egypt and Zone IV (hot and humid), e.g., Brazil. The United States, Europe, and Japan are all in Zones I and II so the ICH guidelines are applicable for these zones.

The guidance documents that are directly relevant to stability testing are: Q1A (R2) Stability Testing of New Drug Substances and Products; Q1B Photostability Testing of New Drug Substances and Products; Q1C Stability Testing for New Dosage Forms; Q1D Bracketing and Matrixing Designs for Stability Testing of New Drug Substances and Products and Q1E Evaluation of Stability Data (3). These guidance documents all describe requirements for New Drug Applications (NDAs) in the United States and Japan and Marketing Authorisation Applications (MAAs) in Europe.

The guidance documents provide very specific information on the design of stability studies for NDAs and MAAs including temperatures and humidities used for storage conditions as well as testing intervals. For products intended for storage at room temperature, the long term storage conditions are 25°C/60% RH or 30°C/65% RH, intermediate storage conditions are 30°C/65% RH and accelerated storage conditions are 40°C/75% RH. Testing is conducted on three batches of product and should be conducted on every individual strength and container size unless bracketing or matrixing is applied.

Contrary to the specific guidance given for studies to support NDAs and MAAs, the guidance for stability studies to support clinical supplies is very general. The FDA has issued the Guidance for Industry entitled INDs for Phase 2 and Phase 3 Studies Chemistry, Manufacturing and Controls Information May 2003 (3). There is also a draft Guidance for Industry entitled INDs—Approaches to Complying with CGMP During Phase 1(3). The European Medicines Agency (EMEA) issued a Guideline on the Requirements to the Chemical and Pharmaceutical Quality Documentation Concerning Investigational Medicinal Products in Clinical Trails in October 2006 (4). Both the FDA and EMEA guidance acknowledge that incomplete stability knowledge will be available for Phase 1 studies with stability testing often being conducted concurrently with the clinical study. Extrapolation of data to establish a shelf life is allowed. More stability data is collected as the compound progresses through Phases 2 and 3 clinical studies and this stability information is used to design the stability protocols for the NDA and MAA submissions.

CHEMICAL STABILITY

Solution Kinetics

Solution kinetic studies are frequently used as the first step in understanding the stability of solid dosage forms. Solutions are simpler systems than solid dosage forms where excipients can complicate the stability assessment. Thus, it is more straightforward to establish the potential reaction mechanism(s) in solution. It is also often easier to identify reaction products in solutions as recovery of these products is not complicated by the presence of excipients. Finally, forced degradation in solution is used to establish the stability-indicating assay that is required to assess the stability in dosage forms. ICH Q3B (R2) Impurities in New Drug Products indicates that validation of the analytical procedure should include samples stored under relevant stress conditions: light, heat, humidity, acid/base hydrolysis, and oxidation (3).

Reaction Order

The order of a chemical reaction is the mathematical relationship between the concentration of the reactants and the time course of the reaction. Most chemical reactions fall into three categories: zero, first, or second order.

A zero-order reaction is one in which the rate does not depend on the concentration of any of the reactants. The reaction can be expressed by the differential equation:

$$-\mathrm{d}(A)/\mathrm{d}t = k,$$

where $\mathrm{d}(A)/\mathrm{d}t$ is the rate of change in concentration for reactant A and k is the rate constant. A plot of concentration versus time is a straight line with a slope of k. The half-life for the reaction is given by the following equation:

$t_{1/2} = 0.5(A_0)/k$,

where (A_0) is the concentration of reactant A at time zero.

Zero-order reactions are rare for pharmaceutical products. Photochemical reactions can be zero order since the driving force for the reaction is the intensity and wavelength of light rather than concentration of the reactant. Suspension formulations can also exhibit zero-order kinetics since the concentration of the reactant is constant as long as excess solid is present.

A first-order reaction can be expressed by the following equation:

$-d(A)/dt = k(A)$

Integrating from $t = 0$ to $t = t$ where the concentration of A at $t = 0$ is A_0 results in the equation:

$\ln(A) = \ln(A_0) - kt$

A plot of $\ln(A)$ versus t results in a straight line with slope of k. The half-life for the reaction is given by the following equation:

$t_{1/2} = 0.693/k$

When a reaction depends on the concentration of two reactants but where the concentration of one reactant is far greater than the other, the result is a pseudo–first-order reaction. Hydrolysis reactions in aqueous solutions are a good example of this phenomenon. Because water is typically present at much higher concentration than the other reactant, the water concentration is relatively unchanged during the course of the reaction and the reaction appears to be first order.

When the rate of a reaction is proportional to the concentration of two reactants or to the square of the concentration of a single reactant, e.g., a dimerization reaction, the reaction is second order. A second-order reaction can be expressed by the equation

$-d(X)/dt = k(A_0 - X)(B_0 - X)$

for a reaction between A and B or

$-d(X)/dt = k(A_0 - X)^2$

for a reaction where the rate is proportional to the square of (A), where (X) is the concentration that reacts in time t and (A_0) and (B_0) are the concentrations at t equals zero. Integrating the differential equation leads to the following equation:

$kt = 1/(A_0 - B_0) \ln[B_0(A_0 - X)/A_0(B_0 - X)]$

A plot of $\ln[B_0(A_0 - X)/A_0(B_0 - X)]$ versus t results in a straight line with slope k $(A_0 - B_0)$.

Complex Reactions

In real life, reaction kinetics are often more complex that the simple zero-, first- and second-order reactions described above. For example, two or more reactions can proceed in parallel, an initial reaction product can further react and a reaction can proceed to a certain point and level off because an equilibrium between species is established. Rate equations can be written for all these reactions, but it become difficult to understand the kinetics by just measuring loss of the drug. For this reason, it is common practice to

Stability Kinetics

measure not only drug loss but also the formation of degradation products. In an ideal situation, it is possible to establish a mass balance so that loss of the drug can be accounted for by the formation of degradation products. Under these circumstances, losses of drug that are too small to be measured directly can be calculated by measuring the formation of low levels of degradation products.

Role of Temperature on the Reaction Rate

The rate of all chemical reactions increases with increasing temperature. In solution, there is a well known relationship between the rate constant (k) and absolute temperature (T) called the Arrhenius equation,

$$k = A \, e^{-E_a/RT}$$

where E_a is the activation energy for the reaction, A is the frequency factor, and R is the gas constant. If a plot of the logarithm of k versus the reciprocal of T yields a linear relationship then A and E_a can be assumed to be independent of temperature and the activation energy can be used as a measure of the temperature dependence of the rate constant. For most drugs, the activation energy is in the range 10–30 kcal/mol which results in a two to fivefold increase in rate for every 10°C increase in temperature. The advantage of using the Arrhenius equation is that it is possible to extrapolate from short-term high temperature studies to lower temperatures where it would take much longer to measure the rate of the reaction. However, these extrapolations must be treated with caution. If the degradation mechanism changes with temperature the relationship may not be linear at the lower temperatures. Additionally, if more than one reaction is proceeding in parallel, it is likely that each reaction will have a different activation energy resulting in two or more Arrhenius relationships.

Role of pH on the Reaction Rate

The rate of many reactions varies as a function of pH. For this reason, it is common to measure the reaction rate as a function of pH. Typically, a pH rate profile is conducted over a pH range of 1–10, but minimally it should be conducted over the physiological pH range 1–8. There are a number of benefits from conducting a pH rate profile. The profile allows the assessment of the pH of maximum stability. This information is not only valuable in formulation development, but also of value in selecting an optimal salt form for a drug candidate. For example, if a basic drug is unstable in acid conditions it is probably best to avoid salts of strong acids. The converse would be true for acidic drugs. The profile also aids understanding the stability of the drug under in vivo conditions. An orally administered drug can encounter a pH range of 1–8 during passage from the stomach through the large intestine. If a drug is unstable in acidic conditions or if a toxic degradation product is formed it may be necessary to develop an enteric coated product to bypass the stomach.

Types of Chemical Reactions

A wide variety of chemical reactions have been reported for drugs. The most common reactions are hydrolysis, oxidation, elimination, isomerization, and dehydration along with more complex reactions involving excipients, or impurities in excipients, and other drugs.

The most common hydrolysis reactions involve drugs that have ester or amide functional groups. Esters are most commonly those of carboxylic acids but can also include those of phosphoric acid and sulfuric acid. Drugs that have hydrolyzable ester groups include aspirin (5), enalapril (6), benzocaine (7), procaine (8), atropine (9), scopolamine (10), methylphenidate (11), mepiridine (12), and numerous esters of the steroids cortisone (13), estradiol (14), hydrocortisone (15), methyl prednisolone (16), and testosterone (17). Cyclic esters of carboxylic acids, lactones, such as pilocarpine (18), warfarin (19,20), and camptothecin (21) also undergo hydrolysis.

Amides are typically more stable to hydrolysis than are esters and are frequently stable in solid dosage forms. An exception is the beta-lactam antibiotics which are cyclic amides, lactams, that are susceptible to hydrolysis. Hydrolysis has been reported for the penams, such as ampicillin (22), amoxicillin (23), carbenicillin (24), and penicillin G (25,26) and the cephems, such as cefaclor (27), cefadroxil (28), cefotaxime (29), cefazolin (30), cefoxitin (31), ceftazidime (32), cefuroxime (33), and cephalexin (34).

The rate of hydrolysis for most esters and amides varies as a function of pH. When the hydrolysis rate results in unacceptable stability it is sometimes possible to improve stability by modulating the microenvironment pH in the dosage form (35). If this is insufficient, moisture resistant packaging and desiccants can be used.

Oxidation reactions are more complex than hydrolysis reactions. The main reason is that while molecular oxygen is ubiquitous in the environment it is not reactive with the majority of organic compounds. The typical autoxidation reaction observed with most drugs involves peroxy radicals, formed from the reaction of oxygen with an organic free radical, reacting with susceptible chemical moieties in the drug. The formation of the organic free radical requires an initiator, which in solid dosage forms is often a transition metal impurity. Initiators only need to be present at trace levels to catalyze oxidation reactions. Once initiated, a chain reaction can occur unless a "chain breaking" substance is included in the dosage form. In addition to molecular oxygen, many excipients also contain low levels of hydroperoxides as impurities (36). Hydroperoxides can generate peroxy radicals that can initiate the chain reactions described above. They can also generate alcoxyl radicals that can react directly in a non-chain reaction with amines to form N-oxides and sulfides to form sulfoxides or sulfones. Predicting the reaction rate of oxidation reactions in solid dosage forms is difficult since the rate is often a function of low levels of transition metals, often in the excipients, that can vary from supplier to supplier and even batch to batch from the same supplier. Levels of hydroperoxides in excipients can also vary from batch to batch (36).

The most common functional groups that are susceptible to oxidation are alkenes, substituted aromatic groups, such as phenols, ethers, thioethers, sulfides, and amines (37). The conjugated alkene simvastatin has been shown to be susceptible to peroxy radical addition resulting in oligomers up to pentomers (38). Excipients that contain alkene groups, such as the partially unsaturated fatty acids, can also undergo oxidation resulting in active species that can initiate the oxidation of drugs. The oxidation of the catechol epinephrine has been studied in detail (39). The antifungal micronazole can undergo oxidation of its ether functional group (40). Excipients with ether functional groups such as polyethylene glycol and polysorbate can also be oxidized with the formation of peroxides and aldehydes that can react with drugs (41,42). Thioethers such as phenothiazines are also susceptible to oxidation (43). Sulfides such as captopril can be oxidized to disulfides in a reaction analogous to than observed in peptides and proteins (44). The tertiary amine functional group in raloxifene has been reported to be oxidized to the N-oxide by the peroxide impurities in povidone and crospovidone (45).

Unlike moisture, it is more difficult to protect solid dosage forms from oxygen. Oxygen scavengers are commercially available but have had only limited use with pharmaceuticals (46). One difficulty with the oxygen scavengers is that they create a vacuum in the container as they react with oxygen. For products in high-density polyethylene (HDPE) bottles, this can cause the bottles to buckle inward. A blanket of inert gas over the product is used for parenteral products but it is not common for solid dosage forms. Thus, the approaches generally used to minimize oxidation include the addition of "chain-breaking" antioxidants (47), oxygen scavengers (48), and chelators to sequester transition metals (49). However, care must be taken with these approaches since some antioxidants can react to produce actives species that can actually exacerbate the oxidation reaction and even chelated transition metals can still initiate hydroperoxide formation (50). If oxygen scavengers are used, then compounds that are not "prooxidants" such as methionine should be used (37).

A number of elimination reactions have been reported for drugs including the elimination of the hydroxymethyl group from trimelamol (51), and the iodine from levothyroxine (52). Perhaps the most common elimination reaction is decarboxylation which has been reported for drugs such as etodolac (53) and foscarnet (54).

Isomerization of drugs typically involves racemization or epimerization of optical isomers or *cis–trans* isomerization of compounds containing an alkene functional group. Examples of epimerization include pilocarpine (55), rolitetracycline (56), and ergotamine (57). Drugs susceptible to racemization include benzodiazepines, penicillins, and cephalosporins. The rearrangement of amphotericin B is an example of *cis–trans* isomerization (58).

Dehydration reactions are as not common in solid dosage forms. However, the angiotensin converting enzyme inhibitors enalapril maleate (59) and moexipril hydrochloride (60) undergo facile dehydration to form a diketopiperazine in the presence of common excipients used in solid dosage forms.

Interaction with Excipients

Drugs in solid dosage forms are typically less stable than the pure crystalline drug substances. This is the case since many excipients in solid dosage forms or the gelatin shells for capsules contain free moisture that can facilitate chemical instability. In addition to moisture, excipients can contain impurities that can either react with the drug or catalyze drug degradation. Most mechanistic studies indicate that drug degradation in solid dosage forms take place at amorphous regions or crystal defect sites on the drug particles (61). These disordered regions can absorb water leading to increased molecular mobility and hence increased rates of reaction. Excipients can induce disorder in the drug crystals at the surface contact points between the drug and excipient. Decreasing the particle size of either the drug or the excipient will increase the number of surface contact points. As an example, the hydrolysis rate for aspirin was found to be five times faster when formulated with dibasic calcium phosphate having a particle size of $10\,\mu m$ versus $40\,\mu m$ (62).

The most common reaction between drugs and excipients is the reaction between aldehydes and primary or secondary amines. The reaction with reducing carbohydrates is called the Maillard or browning reaction. Examples of reducing carbohydrates found in solid dosage forms are lactose, glucose, maltose, maltodextrins, starch, and cellulose. In addition, aldehyde impurities have been identified in polyethylene glycol (42), polysorbate (41), hydroxyethlycellulose (63), and mannitol (64). Despite the numerous publications on the reaction between amines and aldehydes, a survey of generic formulations of fluoxetine hydrochloride, a secondary amine, found lactose as the most common excipient (65). All of these formulations were less stable that a starch-based formulation and contained measurable levels of lactose-related degradation products. Even polysaccharides such as starch and cellulose have terminal glucose units that are capable of reacting with amines. The reaction of hydralazine hydrochloride with starch to form a high molecular weight polysaccharide-bonded degradation product has been reported (66).

Although much less common than the aldehyde–amine reaction, the formation of amides from an amine containing drug has been reported (67). Duloxetine hydrochloride tablets coated with the enteric polymer hydroxypropyl methylcellulose phthalate were found to contain a duloxetine phthalamide degradation product whereas duloxetine hydrochloride pellets coated with hydroxypropyl methylcellulose succinate were found to contain a duloxetine succinamide degradation product. The authors propose that phthlalic anhydride and succinic anhydride present as either impurities or degradation products in the enteric polymers resulted in the formation of the degradation products.

The excipient-mediated degradation of seproxetine maleate is an interesting example of the role that different excipients can have on the degradation mechanism for a drug (68). Seproxetine is a primary amine that is structurally related to fluoxetine. Stability studies on a capsule formulation with pregelatinized starch as a filler indicated that the degradation product was the 1,4 Michael addition product with maleic acid. The Michael addition product was also observed in solutions of seproxetine maleate suggesting that the "free" water in starch and the gelatin capsule is acting like liquid water. Excipient compatibility studies were subsequently conducted with lactose and talc. With lactose a new degradation product was observed. While not identified, it was postulated to be the product of the Maillard reaction between lactose and the drug. Surprisingly, the study with talc resulted in a different degradation product, the maleic acid amide of seproxetine. Amide formation is not favored in aqueous solution. Thus, the degradation of seproxetine maleate in the presence of talc is via a different mechanism than that in the presence of starch.

Impact of Processing

As mentioned previously, available data suggest that the bulk of chemical instability occurs in amorphous regions or crystal defects in the drug. In addition, to surface contact points with the excipients, processing can also lead to disordered regions in the crystalline drug. Amorphous drug can form during wet granulation if the drug dissolves or partially dissolves in the granulating liquid and does not recrystallize on drying. Milling has been demonstrated to generate partially amorphous regions for a number of drugs (69). Milling also reduces the particle size of the drug allowing more surface contact points with excipients. Compression can also lead to increased disorder and increased rates of degradation. Higher compression forces led to a more rapid reaction between lactose and metoclopramide (70).

Role of Temperature and Moisture on Stability

Unfortunately, the effect of temperature on solid dosage forms is more complex than that for solutions since the reaction rate is a function of both temperature and RH. Samples stored at 50°C and ambient conditions may be more stable than those stored at 25°C and 75% RH since the higher temperature can remove "free" water from the dosage form whereas the lower temperature and high humidity allow ample water to either react with the drug or facilitate the reaction. As indicated previously, current regulatory guidelines indicate that stability studies for marketed products are to be conducted at controlled temperature and humidity. In some cases, it is possible to establish an Arrhenius relationship for solid dosage forms at controlled RH. Vitamin C and aspirin tablets adhered to the Arrhenius equation over the temperature range 20–70°C and humidity range 10–75% RH (71). A linear relationship was also observed for a plot of ln k versus % RH. The authors conclude that this linear relationship results from the increased mobility of the reacting species as the RH increases. To add to the complexity of predicting reaction rates, regulatory stability studies are conducted in sealed packs. The equilibration of the humidity in the pack to the external storage conditions can take considerable time depending on the moisture permeability of the pack. As this equilibration is occurring, the rate of the reaction is likely changing.

Moisture increases the rate of most reactions in solid dosage forms. A good example of this is provided by the study of oxidative degradation in formulated granules stored at different RHs and headspace oxygen concentrations (72). Oxygen concentrations were varied from 21% (air) to 0% (oxygen scavengers) while humidities were varied from 20% RH to 65% RH by the use of pre-equilibrated silica desiccants in sealed containers. The highest level of degradation was observed at the high oxygen concentration and high RH condition. However, somewhat surprisingly, the level of degradation was very low and relatively independent of oxygen concentration at the 20% RH condition. Oxygen levels only led to a significant improvement in stability when reduced to very low levels (<0.025%). The study also looked at the effect of drug load on the degradation rate. Granules containing 31.6% and 3.3% drug load were stored under the same conditions. The granules with the low drug load were about a factor of four less stable than those with a high drug load. The authors suggest that this observation could be due to the presence of oxidative initiators or catalysts in the excipients or to increased levels of amorphous drug in the low drug load granules resulting from the wet granulation process used to manufacture the granules. Finally, while degradation was observed to increase with time under most conditions, the degradation rate appeared to slow down at higher extents of degradation. The authors point out that this slowing in the degradation rate is consistent with depletion of either initiation sites where the drug and excipients are in close contact or amorphous drug regions that eventually slows down the reaction.

The source of moisture in dosage forms can be either from the atmosphere, in the case of open containers or semipermeable packs, or from the excipients. Some excipients in solid dosage forms contain significant levels of water. However, it is "free" water rather than the tightly bound water or water of hydration that is available to facilitate chemical reactions. For example, the stability of aspirin and niacinamide tablets manufactured with anhydrous lactose and lactose monohydrate were found to be the same demonstrating that the water in the lactose monohydrate crystals was not contributing to the reaction (73). Cellulose and starch-based excipients can absorb significant amounts of water at relatively low RHs (74). At low RHs this water is tightly bound but at higher RHs the properties approach those of pure liquid water and it is available to facilitate chemical reactions.

If moisture levels are causing unacceptable levels of instability in solid dosage forms, there are a number of approaches that can be used to minimize the problem. One approach would be to select fillers that contain low levels of "free" water such as lactose or dicalcium phosphate. Unfortunately, all of the super disintegrants used in formulations are quite hygroscopic and can pick up large amounts of water. However, they are typically present at much lower levels than the fillers so the overall impact on moisture levels is lower. If excipient selection is not sufficient, protective packaging can be used. Different packaging materials have significantly different water vapor transmission rates. Studies on a moisture sensitive compound indicated that the rate of moisture permeation for a polyvinyl chloride (PVC) blister pack was 260 times faster than for a aluminum foil blister (75). After storage for 6 months at 40°C/75% RH, the tablets in the PVC pack had degraded 16% whereas those in the aluminum foil blister were 100% intact. One disadvantage of moisture impervious packs is that any moisture in the dosage form when it is packaged is trapped in the pack and is available to facilitate chemical degradation at elevated temperatures. If it is necessary to reduce the level of moisture in a formulation, desiccants are frequently used. The most commonly used desiccants in pharmaceutical products are based on silica gel, clay or molecular sieves. Silica gel and clay can achieve RH levels of 10–20% RH while molecular sieves can achieve RH levels below 10% (76). Desiccants are most commonly used in bottle packs but desiccant blister packs are available. An alternative to the use of desiccants is the manufacture of products under low humidity conditions followed by packaging in moisture impervious containers as is done for some effervescent products.

Role of Microenviromental pH on Stability

As was mentioned previously, the rates of most hydrolysis reactions are pH sensitive. In addition, the rate of many oxidation, elimination, isomerization, and dehydration reactions also vary as a function of pH. Although the concept of pH is well understood for aqueous solutions, it is much more complex in solid dosage forms. The terms surface acidity or microenvironmental pH have been used to describe pH at the surface of a drug or excipient. The modulation of microenvironmental pH in solid dosage forms has been the subject of a recent review (35). Although the authors conclude that there are few rules to predict a priori how a pH modifier would modulate the microenvironmental pH and subsequently the performance of a formulation, significant improvements in stability have been observed in some cases. The use of wet granulation to bring the pH modifier into intimate contact with the drug surface improved the stability of moexipril hydrochloride (58) and the experimental drug DMP 754 (77) compared to dry processing approaches.

Photostability

Although a large number of drugs are susceptible to photodegradation in solution, these reactions are much less common in solid dosage forms since only the drug at the surface of the dosage form is exposed to light. If photodegradation at the tablet or capsule surface is a problem, the reaction can be minimized by an opaque coating on the tablet or an opaque capsule shell. If the opaque coating is insufficient, packs that protect the dosage form from light such as foil/foil blisters can be used.

The ICH Guidance Document Q1B Photostability Testing of New Drug Substances and Products provides detailed instructions for conducting photostability studies on dosage forms being submitted for marketing approval (3). The types of light sources that are acceptable for conducting the tests are defined in the guideline as is the total amount of light required (not < 1.2 million lux hours and an integrated near ultraviolet energy of not < 200 Whr/m^2). The tests to assess the photostability of formulated products are carried out in a sequential manner starting with testing the fully exposed product, the unpackaged tablets or capsules, then progressing as necessary to the product in the immediate pack and then in the marketing pack. The testing should progress until the results demonstrate that the product is adequately protected from exposure to light. Samples are tested for changes in appearance, dissolution/disintegration, assay and degradation products. Depending on the extent of any change, special labeling or packaging may be needed to mitigate exposure to light. A decision flow chart for conducting photostability testing is shown in Figure 1.

Stability Kinetics

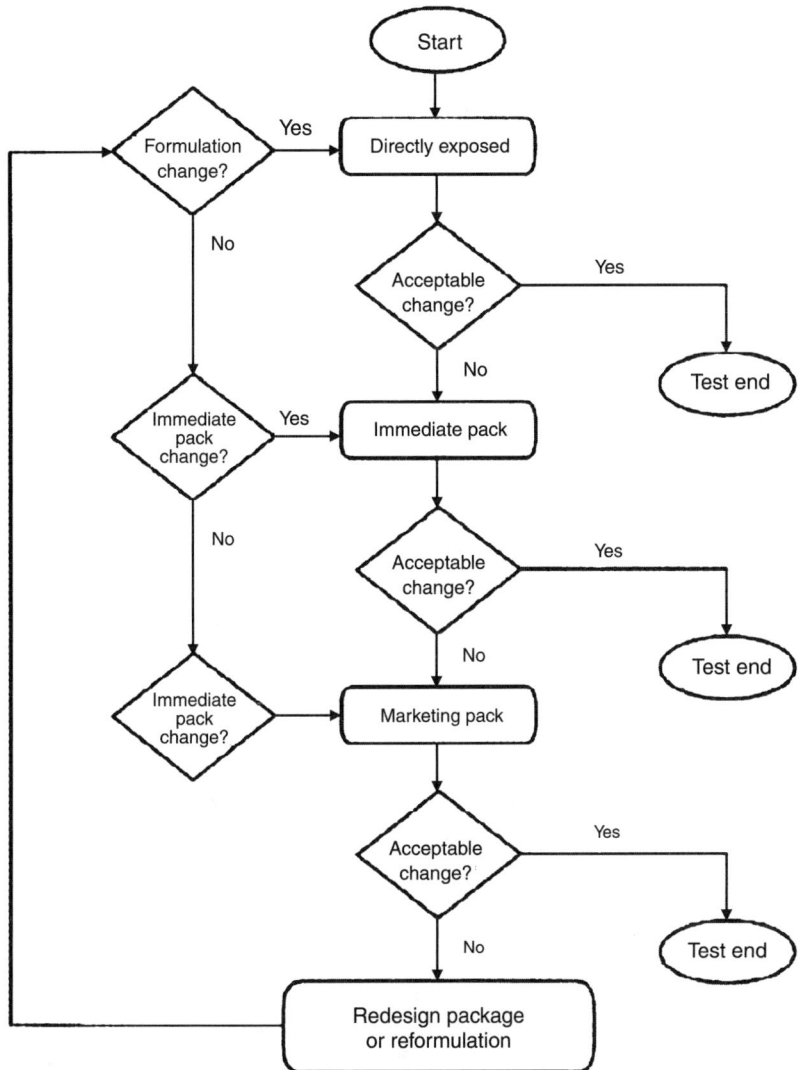

FIGURE 1 Decision flow chart for photostability testing of dosage forms.

PHYSICAL INSTABILITY

There are several physical changes that can occur to solid dosage forms on storage including changes in dissolution rate/disintegration time, tablet hardness, capsule brittleness, and color change. Dissolution or disintegration and identification are normal tests on a shelf life specification. Thus, changes in test results for these attributes over time can limit the shelf life or storage conditions for the product. Additionally, in some cases dissolution rate is correlated with bioavailability so that changes in dissolution could result in changes in the in vivo performance of the product.

There have been numerous reports of tablet dissolution rate slowing on stability but few systematic studies have been performed. Perhaps, the most comprehensive study is that of Gordon et al. who investigated the effect of aging on wet granulated tablets containing super disintegrants (78). The authors investigated croscarmellose sodium, crospovidone, and sodium starch glycolate incorporated both intragranulary and extragranularly with both soluble and insoluble fillers. In addition to dissolution rate, moisture content, tablet dimensions and tablet hardness were measured. In all 90 tablet batches were manufactured and then stored at room temperature and 37°C/80% RH. Dissolution slowing was observed for all of the tablet formulations over time. The three super disintegrants showed different extents of dissolution slowing with formulations containing croscarmellose sodium exhibiting greater slowing than the other two disintegrants. For the fillers, lactose exhibited greater dissolution slowing than dibasic calcium phosphate or naproxen. Tablet hardness increased for all batches on storage but there was no correlation with dissolution rate. There was no substantial swelling for tablets stored at 37°C/80% RH. The authors conclude that the dissolution slowing was due to loss of the disintegrant functionality and, for the lactose formulations, case hardening of the tablets due to exposure to the high humidity conditions.

A study on the dissolution slowing for benazepril hydrochloride also concluded that "preactivation" of the disintegrant, crospovidone, resulted in the dissolution slowing observed at 40°C/75% RH (79). The authors found that there was a critical moisture content in the tablets above which there was a good correlation between moisture content and dissolution slowing. Dissolution slowing was reduced but not eliminated for tablets stored in HDPE bottles containing a desiccant. A model was developed that provided a good prediction of tablet moisture content and hence dissolution rate based on the water vapor transmitted through the HDPE bottle and the capacity of the desiccant.

Dissolution slowing in tablets containing a highly water soluble investigational drug was shown to be due to physical changes in the binder used in the formulation (80). Decreased dissolution rates were seen after 24 weeks storage at 40°C/75% RH but not at 50°C/5% RH, 25°C/60% RH, 30°C/60% RH and 40°C/20% RH. The authors demonstrated that the glass transition temperature of polyvinylpyrrolidone (PVP) was reduced from 170°C to below 40°C at high RHs. This allowed the binder to convert from the glassy to the rubbery state resulting in dissolution slowing.

A different mechanism for dissolution slowing was reported for delavirdine mesylate tablets (81). In this direct compression formulation, the methane sulfonic acid from the drug was shown to react with the disintegrant croscarmellose sodium to form the free acid of croscarmellose and the poorly soluble delavirdine free base. The authors conclude that similar reactions could occur for any acid salt of a basic drug.

Carbamazepine is an example where changes in dissolution rate resulted in changes in bioavailability. An investigation of commercial products was initiated following a product recall of carbamazepine tablets due to clinical failures of the product (82). Pharmacokinetic analyses of the innovator's product and three generic products indicated that the mean areas under the plasma concentration–time curves for the generic products ranged from 60 to 113% that of the innovator product. A good relationship was found between the in vivo parameters and the dissolution results for the four products. A more detailed study of multiple lots of carbamazepine tablets from six manufacturers indicated that all products showed dissolution slowing when tablets were stored at high humidity for 6–7 days (83). However, there were large differences in dissolution slowing from product to product. The authors suggest that the dissolution slowing at high humidity may be due to the formation of less soluble dihydrate form of carbamazepine.

The dissolution rate of a dosage form can be impacted by a number of factors during manufacture including the drug substance and excipient physical properties, manufacturing method and process variables. The stability of dissolution on storage is complex to predict as it depends on the factors at the time of manufacture and the packaging and storage conditions. The available literature indicates that moisture plays a large role in dissolution slowing on storage and that some protection from moisture ingress is needed for most dosage forms. Open container studies at the standard accelerated stability conditions of 30°C/65% RH and 40°C/75% RH can often provide an early prediction of potential dissolution slowing but these data need to be confirmed by long term storage of packaged products at room temperature conditions.

Many of the mechanisms for dissolution slowing in tablets also apply to capsules. However, for capsules, the main cause of dissolution slowing is the cross-linking of the gelatin shells (84). Cross-linking converts soluble gelatin to a rubbery insoluble form that can dramatically slow the capsule dissolution rate. Cross-linking can be induced by reaction of the gelatin with aldehydes, storage of the capsules at high humidities and temperatures above 30°C or exposure to ultraviolet light for prolonged periods (85). Formaldehyde levels as low as 20 ppm are able to cross-link gelatin shells in 6 days at room temperature (86). Trace level aldehydes can be present in a number of excipients used in hard and soft gelatin capsules formulations, such as starch, polyethylene glycols and polysorbates (87). Trace levels of aldehyde in a rayon coil in a HDPE bottle has also resulted in capsule cross-linking (88). Bioavailability studies of cross-linked and non-cross-linked capsule formulations for etodolac (89), amoxicillin (90), and acetaminophen (86) have been reported. In all cases, the dissolution slowing observed for capsules having moderate cross-linking did not result in a difference in bioavailability. All three studies investigated alternate dissolution media containing enzymes, either pepsin or pancreatin, and indicated that such media were better predictors of in vivo performance of the capsule formulations than media without enzymes. The current USP/NF chapter on dissolution, <711>, indicates that if hard or soft gelatin capsules or gelatin coated tablets fail the dissolution specification then the test can be repeated using the same medium containing either pepsin or pancreatin (91).

For immediate release dosage forms the dissolution rate may sometimes be directly linked to the bioavailability of the product but this is the exception rather than the rule. However, for modified release formulations an in vitro–in vivo correlation or relationship is often established. In this situation, significant changes in dissolution rate will have a direct effect on the in vivo performance of the product. Changes in dissolution rate for modified release formulations are more complex than for immediate release formulations since in most cases, the drug release rate is controlled by a polymer or wax whose properties can change with aging. Unlike immediate release formulations where dissolution slowing is the norm on aging, the dissolution rate for modified release formulations can either increase or decrease over time. The wide variety in the types of modified release products and associated polymers and waxes puts review of the dissolution stability of these products outside the scope of this chapter. However, stability of these products has been reviewed elsewhere (92).

Although assessment of the appearance or color of a dosage form is a physical test, a change in color on aging usually has a chemical basis. The Maillard reaction between reducing sugars and primary and secondary amines usually leads to brown or yellow colored degradation products. Discoloration of tablets containing lactose and amines was reported as early as 1962 (93). A number of drug classes are known to degrade to form colored products. Catechols such as epinephrine oxidize to red colored products and beta-lactam antibiotics degrade to form yellow/brown products. Some colorants in tablets and in coating materials can fade when exposed to light.

STABILITY STUDY DESIGN

The design of stability studies to support submission of NDAs and MAAs are described in the ICH Guidance Q1A (R2) Stability Testing of new Drug Substances and Products (3). The sections relevant to solid dosage forms are described below.

Batch Selection and Storage Conditions

The design of the formal stability studies for the drug product should be based on knowledge of the behavior and properties of the active ingredient, results from stability studies on the active ingredient, and experience gained from clinical formulation studies.

Data from stability studies should be provided on at least three primary batches of the drug product. The primary batches should be of the same formulation and packaged in the same container closure system as proposed for marketing. The manufacturing process used for primary batches should simulate that to be applied to production batches and should provide product of the same quality and meeting the same specification as that intended for marketing.

Two of the three batches should be at least pilot scale batches, and the third one can be smaller if justified. Where possible, batches of the dosage form should be manufactured by using different batches of the active ingredient.

Stability studies should be performed on each individual strength and container size of the drug product unless bracketing or matrixing is applied.

For long term studies, frequency of testing should be sufficient to establish the stability profile of the drug product. For products with a proposed shelf life of at least 12 months, the frequency of testing at the long term storage condition should normally be every 3 months over the first year, every 6 months over the second year, and annually thereafter through the proposed shelf life.

At the accelerated storage condition, a minimum of three time points, including the initial and final time points (e.g., 0, 3, and 6 months), from a 6-month study is recommended. Where an expectation (based on development experience) exists that results from accelerated testing are likely to approach significant change criteria, increased testing should be conducted either by adding samples at the final time point or by including a fourth time point in the study design.

When testing at the intermediate storage condition is called for as a result of significant change at the accelerated storage condition, a minimum of four time points, including the initial and final time points (e.g., 0, 6, 9, 12 months), from a 12-month study is recommended.

In general, a drug product should be evaluated under storage conditions (with appropriate tolerances) that test its thermal stability and its sensitivity to moisture. The storage conditions and the lengths of studies chosen should be sufficient to cover storage, shipment, and subsequent use.

The long term testing should cover a minimum of 12 months' duration on at least three primary batches at the time of submission and should be continued for a period of time sufficient to cover the proposed shelf life. Data from the accelerated storage condition and, if appropriate, from the intermediate storage condition can be used to evaluate the effect of short term excursions outside the label storage conditions (such as might occur during shipping). Long term, accelerated, and, where appropriate, intermediate storage conditions for drug products are detailed in Tables 1 and 2. Alternative storage conditions can be used if justified.

Stability Kinetics

TABLE 1 Drug Product Intended for Storage at Room Temperature

Study	Storage condition	Minimum time period covered by data at submission
Long term[a]	25°C ±2°C/60% RH ±5% RH or 30°C ±2°C/65% RH ±5% RH	12 months
Intermediate[b]	30°C ±2°C/65% RH ±5% RH	6 months
Accelerated	40°C ±2°C/75% RH ±5% RH	6 months

[a]It is up to the applicant to decide whether long term stability studies are performed at 25°C ±2°C/60% RH ±5% RH or 30°C ±2°C/65% RH ±5% RH.
[b]If 30°C ±2°C/65% RH ±5% RH is the long term condition, there is no intermediate condition.
Abbreviation: RH, relative humidity.

TABLE 2 Drug Product Intended for Storage in a Refrigerator

Study	Storage condition	Minimum time period covered by data at submission
Long term	5°C ±3°C	12 months
Accelerated	25°C ±2°C/60% RH ±5% RH	6 months

Abbreviation: RH, relative humidity.

If long term studies are conducted at 25°C ±2°C/60% RH ±5% RH and significant change occurs at any time during 6 months' testing at the accelerated storage condition, additional testing at the intermediate storage condition should be conducted and evaluated against significant change criteria.

In general, significant change for a drug product is defined as one or more of the following:

- A 5% change in assay from its initial value
- Any degradation product's exceeding its acceptance criterion
- Failure to meet the acceptance criteria for appearance
- Failure to meet the acceptance criteria for dissolution for 12 dosage units

If significant change occurs between 3 and 6 months' testing at the accelerated storage condition, the proposed shelf life should be based on the real time data available from the long term storage condition.

If significant change occurs within the first 3 months' testing at the accelerated storage condition, a discussion should be provided to address the effect of short term excursions outside the label storage condition (e.g., during shipment and handling). This discussion can be supported, if appropriate, by further testing on a single batch of the drug product for a period shorter than 3 months but with more frequent testing than usual.

Bracketing and Matrixing

Bracketing and matrixing can considerably reduce the amount of stability testing required to be submitted in an NDA or MAA. However, there are situations where the use of these approaches is not appropriate. Guidance on the use of bracketing and matrixing in the stability study design are given in ICH Q1D Bracketing and Matrixing Designs for Stability Testing of New Drug Substances and Products (3). The sections relevant to solid dosage forms are described below.

A full study design is one in which samples for every combination of all design factors are tested at all time points. A reduced design is one in which samples for every factor combination are not all tested at all time points. A reduced design can be a suitable alternative to a full design when multiple design factors are involved. Any reduced design should have the ability to adequately predict the shelf life. Before a reduced design is considered, certain assumptions should be assessed and justified. The potential risk should be considered of establishing a shorter shelf life than could be derived from a full design due to the reduced amount of data collected.

Whether bracketing or matrixing can be applied depends on the circumstances, as discussed in detail below. The use of any reduced design should be justified. In certain cases, the conditions described in the guidance are sufficient justification for use, while in other cases, additional justification should be provided. The type and level of justification in each of these cases will depend on the available supporting data. Data variability and product stability, as shown by supporting data, should be considered when a matrixing design is applied.

Bracketing and matrixing are reduced designs based on different principles. Therefore, careful consideration and scientific justification should precede the use of bracketing and matrixing together in one design.

Bracketing

Bracketing is the design of a stability schedule such that only samples on the extremes of certain design factors (e.g., strength, container size, and/or fill) are tested at all time points as in a full design. The design assumes that the stability of any intermediate levels is represented by the stability of the extremes tested.

The use of a bracketing design would not be considered appropriate if it cannot be demonstrated that the strengths or container sizes and/or fills selected for testing are indeed the extremes.

Bracketing can be applied to studies with multiple strengths of identical or closely related formulations. Examples include but are not limited to (*i*) capsules of different strengths made with different fill plug sizes from the same powder blend and (*ii*) tablets of different strengths manufactured by compressing varying amounts of the same granulation.

With justification, bracketing can be applied to studies with multiple strengths where the relative amounts of drug substance and excipients change in a formulation. Such justification can include a demonstration of comparable stability profiles among the different strengths of clinical or development batches.

In cases where different excipients are used among strengths, bracketing generally should not be applied.

Bracketing can be applied to studies of the same container closure system where either container size or fill varies while the other remains constant. However, if a bracketing design is considered where both container size and fill vary, it should not be assumed that the largest and smallest containers represent the extremes of all packaging configurations. Care should be taken to select the extremes by comparing the various characteristics of the container closure system that may affect product stability. These characteristics include container wall thickness, closure geometry, surface area to volume ratio, headspace to volume ratio, water vapor permeation rate or oxygen permeation rate per dosage unit or unit fill volume, as appropriate. With justification, bracketing can be applied to studies for the same container when the closure varies. Justification could include a discussion of the relative permeation rates of the bracketed container closure systems.

Before a bracketing design is applied, its effect on the shelf life estimation should be assessed. If the stability of the extremes is shown to be different, the intermediates should be considered no more stable than the least stable extreme (i.e., the shelf life for the intermediates should not exceed that for the least stable extreme).

An example of a bracketing design is given in Table 3. This example is based on a product available in three strengths and three container sizes. In this example, it should be demonstrated that the 15 and 500 mL HDPE container sizes truly represent the extremes.

TABLE 3 Example of a Bracketing Design

Strength		50 mg			75 mg			100 mg		
Batch		1	2	3	1	2	3	1	2	3
Container size	15 mL	T	T	T				T	T	T
	100 mL									
	500 mL	T	T	T				T	T	T

Abbreviation: T, sample tested.

Matrixing

Matrixing is the design of a stability schedule such that a selected subset of the total number of possible samples for all factor combinations would be tested at a specified time point. At a subsequent time point, another subset of samples for all factor combinations would be tested. The design assumes that the stability of each subset of samples tested represents the stability of all samples at a given time point. The differences in the samples for the same drug product should be identified as, for example, covering different batches, different strengths, different sizes of the same container closure system, and possibly, in some cases, different container closure systems.

When a secondary packaging system contributes to the stability of the drug product, matrixing can be performed across the packaging systems.

Each storage condition should be treated separately under its own matrixing design. Matrixing should not be performed across test attributes. However, alternative matrixing designs for different test attributes can be applied if justified.

Matrixing designs can be applied to strengths with identical or closely related formulations. Examples include but are not limited to (*i*) capsules of different strengths made with different fill plug sizes from the same powder blend and (*ii*) tablets of different strengths manufactured by compressing varying amounts of the same granulation.

Other examples of design factors that can be matrixed include batches made by using the same process and equipment, and container sizes and/or fills in the same container closure system.

With justification, matrixing designs can be applied, for example, to different strengths where the relative amounts of drug substance and excipients change or where different excipients are used or to different container closure systems. Justification should generally be based on supporting data. For example, to matrix across two different closures or container closure systems, supporting data could be supplied showing relative moisture vapor transmission rates or similar protection against light. Alternatively, supporting data could be supplied to show that the drug product is not affected by oxygen, moisture, or light.

A matrixing design should be balanced as far as possible so that each combination of factors is tested to the same extent over the intended duration of the study and through the last time point prior to submission. However, due to the recommended full testing at certain time points, as discussed below, it may be difficult to achieve a complete balance in a design where time points are matrixed.

In a design where time points are matrixed, all selected factor combinations should be tested at the initial and final time points, while only certain fractions of the designated combinations should be tested at each intermediate time point. If full long term data for the proposed shelf life will not be available for review before approval, all selected combinations of batch, strength, container size, and fill, among other things, should also be tested at 12 months or at the last time point prior to submission. In addition, data from at least three time points, including initial, should be available for each selected combination through the first 12 months of the study. For matrixing at an accelerated or intermediate storage condition, care should be taken to ensure testing occurs at a minimum of three time points, including initial and final, for each selected combination of factors.

Examples of matrixing designs on time points for a product in two strengths (S1 and S2) are shown in Tables 4 and 5. The terms one-half reduction and one-third reduction refer to the reduction strategy initially applied to the full study design. For example, a one-half reduction initially eliminates one in every two time points from the full study design and a one-third reduction initially removes one in every three. In the examples shown in Table 4 and 5, the reductions are less than one-half and one-third due to the inclusion of full testing of all factor combinations at some time points as discussed previously. These examples include full testing at the initial, final, and 12-month time points. The ultimate reduction is therefore less than one-half (24/48) or one-third (16/48), and is actually 15/48 or 10/48, respectively.

Additional examples of matrixing designs for a product with three strengths and three container sizes are given in Tables 6 and 7. Table 6 shows a design with matrixing on time points only and Table 7 depicts a design with matrixing on time points and factors. In Table 6, all combinations of batch, strength, and container size are tested, while in Table 7, certain combinations of batch, strength and container size are not tested. The key to Tables 6 and 7 is shown in Table 8.

TABLE 4 Example of One-Half Reduction Matrixing Design on Time Points for a Product with Two Strengths

Time point (months)			0	3	6	9	12	18	24	36
Strength	S1	Batch 1	T	T		T	T		T	T
		Batch 2	T	T		T	T	T		T
		Batch 3	T		T		T	T		T
	S2	Batch 1	T		T		T		T	T
		Batch 2	T	T		T	T	T		T
		Batch 3	T		T		T		T	T

Abbreviation: T, sample tested.

Stability Kinetics

TABLE 5 Example of One-Third Reduction Matrixing Design on Time Points for a Product with Two Strengths

Time point (months)			0	3	6	9	12	18	24	36
Strength	S1	Batch 1	T	T		T	T		T	T
		Batch 2	T	T	T		T	T		T
		Batch 3	T		T	T	T	T	T	T
	S2	Batch 1	T		T	T	T	T	T	T
		Batch 2	T	T		T	T		T	T
		Batch 3	T	T	T		T	T		T

Abbreviation: T, sample tested.

TABLE 6 Example of a Matrixing Design on Time Points for a Product with Three Strengths and Three Container Sizes

Strength	S1			S2			S3		
Container size	A	B	C	A	B	C	A	B	C
Batch 1	T1	T2	T3	T2	T3	T1	T3	T1	T2
Batch 2	T2	T3	T1	T3	T1	T2	T1	T2	T3
Batch 3	T3	T1	T2	T1	T2	T3	T2	T3	T1

Note: The key for Table 6 is given in Table 8.

TABLE 7 Example of a Matrixing Design on Time Points and Factors for a Product with Three Strengths and Three Container Sizes

Strength	S1			S2			S3		
Container size	A	B	C	A	B	C	A	B	C
Batch 1	T1	T2		T2		T1		T1	T2
Batch 2		T3	T1	T3	T1		T1		T3
Batch 3	T3		T2		T2	T3	T2	T3	

Note: The key for Table 7 is given in Table 8.

TABLE 8 Key to Tables 6 and 7

Time-point (months)	0	3	6	9	12	18	24	36
T1	T		T	T	T	T	T	T
T2	T	T		T	T		T	T
T3	T	T	T		T	T		T

S1, S2, and S3 are different strengths.
A, B, and C are different container sizes.
T, sample tested.

The following, although not an exhaustive list, should be considered when a matrixing design is contemplated:

- Knowledge of data variability
- Expected stability of the product
- Availability of supporting data

- Stability differences in the product within a factor or among factors
- Number of factor combinations in the study

In general, a matrixing design is applicable if the supporting data indicate predictable product stability. Matrixing is appropriate when the supporting data exhibit only small variability. However, where the supporting data exhibit moderate variability, a matrixing design should be statistically justified. If the supportive data show large variability, a matrixing design should not be applied.

A statistical justification could be based on an evaluation of the proposed matrixing design with respect to its power to detect differences among factors in the degradation rates or its precision in shelf life estimation.

If a matrixing design is considered applicable, the degree of reduction that can be made from a full design depends on the number of factor combinations being evaluated. The more factors associated with a product and the more levels in each factor, the larger the degree of reduction that can be considered. However, any reduced design should have the ability to adequately predict the product shelf life.

Due to the reduced amount of data collected, a matrixing design on factors other than time points generally has less precision in shelf life estimation and yields a shorter shelf life than the corresponding full design. In addition, such a matrixing design may have insufficient power to detect certain main or interaction effects, thus leading to incorrect pooling of data from different design factors during shelf life estimation. If there is an excessive reduction in the number of factor combinations tested and data from the tested factor combinations cannot be pooled to establish a single shelf life, it may be impossible to estimate the shelf lives for the missing factor combinations.

A study design that matrixes on time points only would often have similar ability to that of a full design to detect differences in rates of change among factors and to establish a reliable shelf life. This feature exists because linearity is assumed and because full testing of all factor combinations would still be performed at both the initial time point and the last time point prior to submission.

SHELF LIFE DETERMINATION

Specifications

Guidance for specifications are given in ICH Q6A Test Procedures and Acceptance Criteria for New Drug Substances and New Drug Products: Chemical Substances (3). The sections relevant to solid dosage forms are described below. The tests that are conducted during stability studies and that are typically included in the specification are assay, degradation products, dissolution or disintegration, description and, if present, antioxidant content. Tests such a content uniformity and identity are also included on the specification but are only tested at batch release and not on stability.

A specification is defined as a list of tests, references to analytical procedures, and appropriate acceptance criteria that are numerical limits, ranges, or other criteria for the tests described. It establishes the set of criteria to which a dosage form should conform to be considered acceptable for its intended use. Specifications are critical quality standards that are proposed and justified by the manufacturer and approved by regulatory authorities as conditions of approval.

The following tests and acceptance criteria are considered generally applicable to solid dosage forms.

Description. A qualitative description of the dosage form should be provided (e.g., size, shape, and color). If any of these characteristics change during manufacture or storage, this change should be investigated and appropriate action taken. The acceptance criteria should include the final acceptable appearance. If color changes during storage, a quantitative procedure may be appropriate.

Assay. A specific, stability-indicating assay to determine strength (content) should be included for all dosage forms. In many cases, it is possible to employ the same procedure (e.g., HPLC) for both assay of the active ingredient and quantitation of impurities.

Impurities. Organic and inorganic impurities (degradation products) and residual solvents are included in this category. Organic impurities arising from degradation of the new active ingredient and impurities that arise during the manufacturing process of the dosage form should be monitored. Acceptance limits should be stated for individual specified degradation products, which may include both identified and unidentified degradation products, as appropriate, and total degradation products. Process impurities from the active ingredient synthesis are normally controlled during its testing, and therefore are not included in the total degradation product limit. However, when a synthesis impurity is also a degradation product, its level should be monitored and included in the total degradation product limit. When it has been conclusively demonstrated via appropriate analytical methodology that the active ingrediant does not degrade in the specific formulation, and under the specific storage conditions proposed in the new drug application, degradation product testing may be reduced or eliminated upon approval by the regulatory authorities.

ICH Q3B Impurities in New Drug Products defines three thresholds for degradation products: reporting level, identification level, and qualification level. The reporting threshold is a limit above which a degradation product should be reported, the identification threshold is a limit above which the chemical structure of a degradation product should be identified and the qualification threshold is a limit above which a degradation product should be qualified. Qualification is the process of acquiring and evaluating data that establishes the biological safety of an individual degradation product or a given degradation profile at the levels specified. The levels for reporting, identification and qualification vary as a function of the daily dose for the drug and are presented in Table 9.

TABLE 9 Thresholds for Degradation Products in New Drug Products

Threshold	Maximum daily dose[a]	Level[b,c]
Reporting	<1 g	0.1%
	>1 g	0.05%
Identification	<1 mg	1.0% or 5 ug TDI, whichever is lower
	1–10 mg	0.5% or 20 ug TDI, whichever is lower
	>10 mg – 2 g	0.2% or 2 mg TDI, whichever is lower
	>2 g	0.1%
Qualification	<10 mg	1.0% or 50 ug TDI, whichever is lower
	10–100 mg	0.5% or 200 ug TDI, whichever is lower
	>100 mg – 2 g	0.2% or 3 mg TDI, whichever is lower
	>2 g	0.15%

[a]The amount of drug substance administered per day.
[b]Thresholds for degradation products are expressed either as a percentage of the drug substance or as TDI of the degradation product. Lower thresholds can be appropriate if the degradation product is unusually toxic.
[c]Higher thresholds should be scientifically justified.
Abbreviation: TDI, total daily intake.

Figure 2 shows a decision tree that addresses the extrapolation of meaningful limits on degradation products from the body of data generated during development. At the time of filing it is unlikely that sufficient data will be available to assess process consistency. Therefore, it is considered inappropriate to establish acceptance criteria that tightly encompass the batch data at the time of filing.

Dissolution. The specification for solid oral dosage forms normally includes a test to measure release of the active ingredient from the dosage form. Single-point measurements are normally considered to be suitable for immediate-release dosage forms. For modified-release dosage forms, appropriate test conditions and sampling procedures should be established. For example, multiple time-point sampling should be performed for extended-release dosage forms, and two-stage testing (using different media in succession or in parallel, as appropriate) may be appropriate for delayed-release dosage forms. In these cases, it is important to consider the populations of individuals who will be taking the dosage form (e.g., achlorhydric elderly) when designing the tests and acceptance criteria. In some cases, dissolution testing may be replaced by disintegration testing as shown in the decision tree in Figure 3.

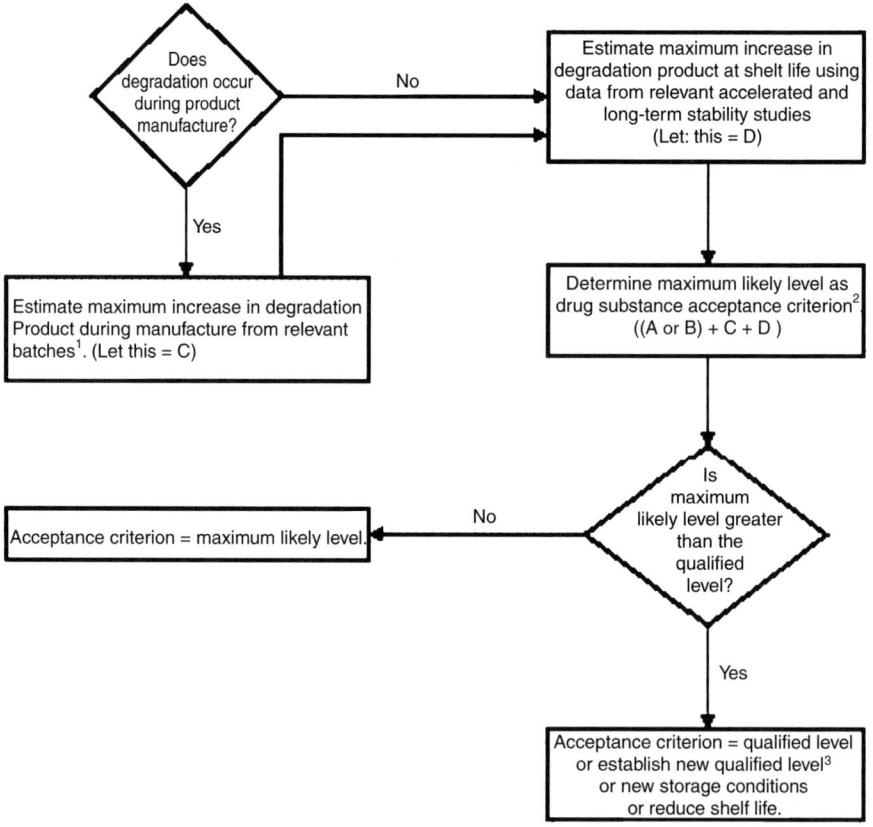

[1] Relevant batches are those from development, pilot and scale-up studies.
[2] Refer to Decision tree 1 for information regarding A and B.
[3] Refer to ICH Guideline on impurities in New Drug Products.

FIGURE 2 Decision tree establishing acceptance criterion for degradation products in a dosage form.

Stability Kinetics

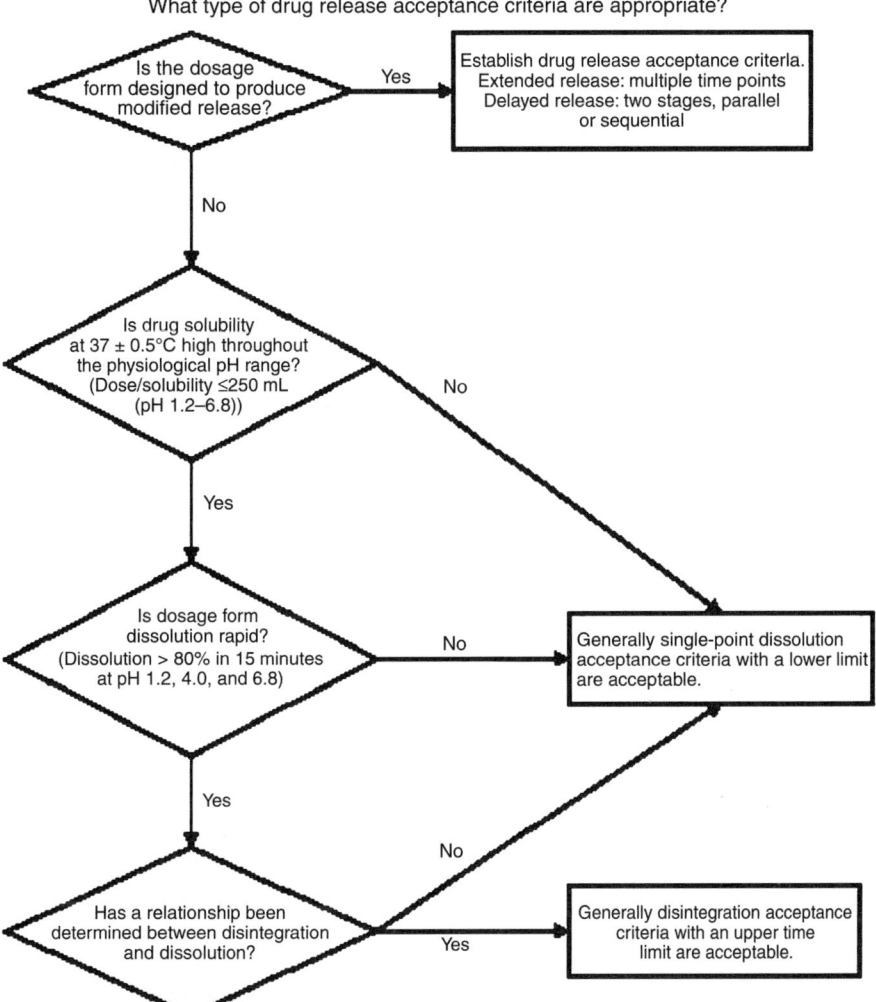

FIGURE 3 Decision tree for acceptance criteria for dosage form dissolution.

For immediate-release dosage forms where changes in dissolution rate have been demonstrated to significantly affect bioavailability, it is desirable to develop test conditions that can distinguish batches with unacceptable bioavailability. Otherwise, test conditions and acceptance criteria should be established that pass clinically acceptable batches as shown in the decision tree in Figure 4. If changes in formulation or process variables significantly affect dissolution, and such changes are not controlled by another aspect of the specification, it may also be appropriate to adopt dissolution test conditions that can distinguish these changes as shown in the decision tree in Figure 4.

For extended-release dosage forms, in vitro–in vivo correlation may be used to establish acceptance criteria when human bioavailability data are available for formulations exhibiting different release rates. Where such data are not available, and drug release cannot be shown to be independent of in vitro test conditions, then acceptance criteria should be established on the basis of available batch data. Normally, the permitted variability in mean release rate at any given time point should not exceed a total

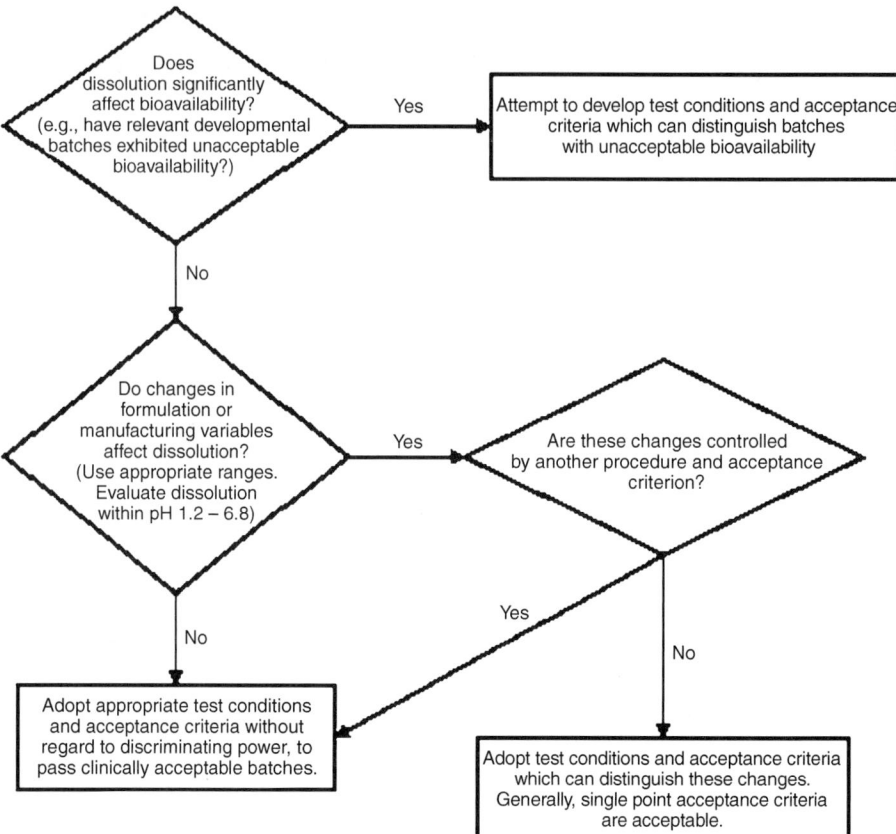

FIGURE 4 Decision tree for acceptance criteria for immediate release dosage form dissolution.

numerical difference of 10% of the labeled content of drug substance (i.e., a total variability of 20%: a requirement of $50 \pm 10\%$ thus means an acceptable range from 40% to 60%), unless a wider range is supported by a bioequivalence study as shown in the decision tree in Figure 5.

Disintegration. For rapidly dissolving (dissolution >80% in 15 minutes at pH 1.2, 4.0, and 6.8) products containing drugs that are highly soluble throughout the physiological range (dose/solubility volume < 250 mL) from pH 1.2 to 6.8, disintegration may be substituted for dissolution. Disintegration testing is considered most appropriate when a relationship to dissolution has been established or when disintegration is shown to be more discriminating than dissolution. In such cases, dissolution testing may not be necessary. It is expected that development information will be provided to support the robustness of the formulation and manufacturing process with respect to the selection of dissolution versus disintegration testing as shown in the decision tree in Figure 3.

Methods for Establishing Shelf Lives

Guidance for evaluation of stability data is provided in ICH Q1E Evaluation of Stability Data. The sections relevant to solid dosage forms are described below.

The purpose of a stability study is to establish, based on testing a minimum of three batches of the product, a shelf life and label storage instructions applicable to all future

Stability Kinetics

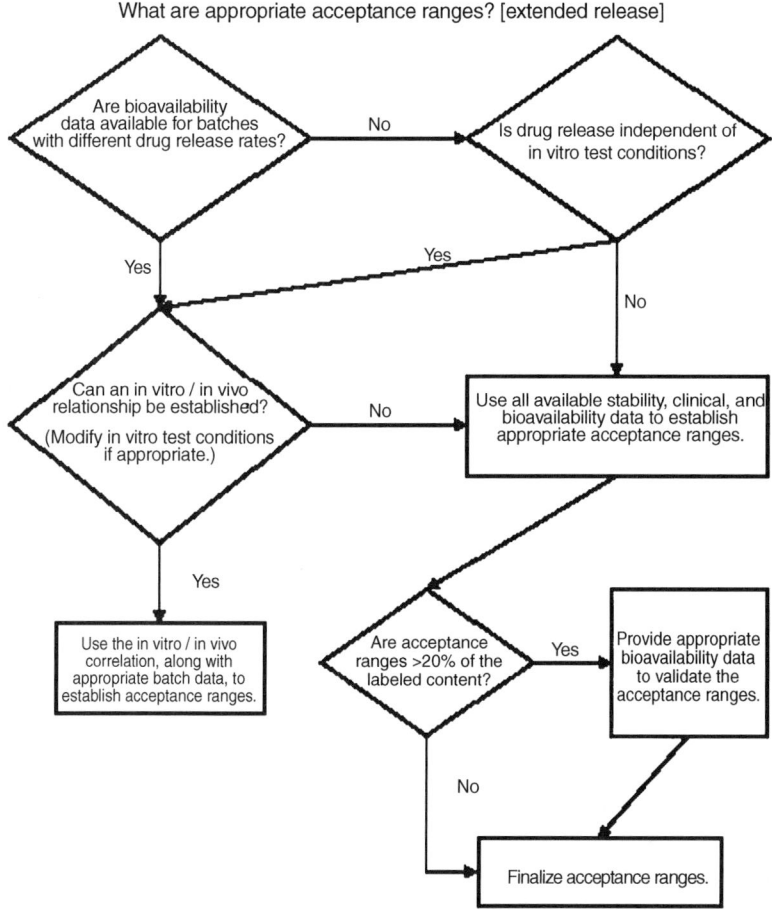

FIGURE 5 Decision tree for acceptance criteria for extended release dosage form dissolution.

batches manufactured and packaged under similar circumstances. The degree of variability of individual batches affects the confidence that a future production batch will remain within acceptance criteria throughout its shelf life.

Although normal manufacturing and analytical variations are to be expected, it is important that the dosage form be formulated with the intent to provide 100% of the labeled amount of the active ingredient at the time of batch release. If the assay values of the batches used to support the registration application are higher than 100% of label claim at the time of batch release, after taking into account manufacturing and analytical variations, the shelf life proposed in the application can be overestimated. On the other hand, if the assay value of a batch is lower than 100% of label claim at the time of batch release, it might fall below the lower acceptance criterion before the end of the proposed shelf life.

A systematic approach should be adopted in the presentation and evaluation of the stability information. The stability information should include, as appropriate, results from the physical and chemical tests, including those related to particular attributes of the dosage form (e.g., dissolution rate). The adequacy of the mass balance should be assessed. Factors that can cause an apparent lack of mass balance should be considered, including, for example, the mechanisms of degradation and the stability-indicating capability and inherent variability of the analytical procedures.

The basic concepts of stability data evaluation are the same for single versus multifactor studies and for full versus reduced-design studies. Data from formal stability studies and, as appropriate, supporting data should be evaluated to determine the critical quality attributes likely to influence the quality and performance of the drug product. Each attribute should be assessed separately, and an overall assessment should be made of the findings for the purpose of proposing a shelf life. The shelf life proposed should not exceed that predicted for any single attribute.

In general, certain quantitative chemical attributes (e.g., assay and degradation products) for a dosage form can be assumed to follow zero-order kinetics during long term storage (71). Data for these attributes are therefore amenable to statistical analysis, including linear regression and poolability testing. Although the kinetics of other quantitative attributes (e.g., dissolution) is generally not known, the same statistical analysis can be applied, if appropriate. Qualitative attributes are not amenable to this kind of statistical analysis.

The recommendations on statistical approaches in the guideline are not intended to imply that use of statistical evaluation is preferred when it can be justified to be unnecessary. However, statistical analysis can be useful in supporting the extrapolation of shelf lives in certain situations and can be called for to verify the proposed shelf lives in other cases.

Extrapolation to extend the shelf life beyond the period covered by long term data can be proposed, particularly if no significant change is observed at the accelerated condition. Whether extrapolation of stability data is appropriate depends on the extent of knowledge about the change pattern, the goodness of fit of any mathematical model, and the existence of relevant supporting data. Any extrapolation should be performed such that the extended shelf life will be valid for a future batch released with test results close to the release acceptance criteria.

An extrapolation of stability data assumes that the same change pattern will continue to apply beyond the period covered by long term data. The correctness of the assumed change pattern is critical when extrapolation is considered. When estimating a regression line or curve to fit the long term data, the data themselves provide a check on the correctness of the assumed change pattern, and statistical methods can be applied to test the goodness of fit of the data to the assumed line or curve. No such internal check is possible beyond the period covered by long term data. Thus, shelf life granted on the basis of extrapolation should always be verified by additional long term stability data.

A systematic evaluation of the data from formal stability studies should be performed. Stability data for each attribute should be assessed sequentially. For products intended for storage at room temperature, the assessment should begin with any significant change at the accelerated condition and, if appropriate, at the intermediate condition, and progress through the trends and variability of the long term data. The circumstances are delineated under which extrapolation of shelf life beyond the period covered by long term data can be appropriate.

No Significant Change at Accelerated Conditions

Where no significant change occurs at the accelerated condition, the shelf life would depend on the nature of the long term and accelerated data.

Where the long term data and accelerated data for an attribute show little or no change over time and little or no variability, it might be apparent that the drug product will remain well within the acceptance criteria for that attribute during the proposed shelf life. In these circumstances, a statistical analysis is normally considered unnecessary but

Stability Kinetics

justification for the omission should be provided. Justification can include a discussion of the change pattern or lack of change, relevance of the accelerated data, mass balance, and/or other supporting data. Extrapolation of the shelf life beyond the period covered by long term data can be proposed. The proposed shelf life can be up to twice, but should not be more than 12 months beyond, the period covered by long term data.

If the long term or accelerated data for an attribute show change over time and/or variability within a factor or among factors, statistical analysis of the long term data can be useful in establishing a shelf life. Where there are differences in stability observed among batches or among other factors (e.g., strength, container size and/or fill) or factor combinations (e.g., strength by container size and/or fill) that preclude the combining of data, the proposed shelf life should not exceed the shortest period supported by any batch, other factor, or factor combination. Alternatively, where the differences are readily attributed to a particular factor (e.g., strength), different shelf lives can be assigned to different levels within the factor (e.g., different strengths).

Where long term data are not amenable to statistical analysis, but relevant supporting data are provided, the proposed shelf life can be up to one-and-a-half times, but should not be more than 6 months beyond, the period covered by long term data. Relevant supporting data include satisfactory long term data from development batches that are (*i*) made with a closely related formulation to, (*ii*) manufactured on a smaller scale than, or (*iii*) packaged in a container closure system similar to, that of the primary stability batches.

If long term data are amenable to statistical analysis but no analysis is performed, the extent of extrapolation should be the same as when data are not amenable to statistical analysis.

However, if a statistical analysis is performed, it can be appropriate to propose a shelf life of up to twice, but not more than 12 months beyond, the period covered by long term data, when the proposal is backed by the result of the analysis and relevant supporting data.

Significant Change at Accelerated Conditions

Where significant change occurs at the accelerated condition, the shelf life would depend on the outcome of stability testing at the intermediate condition, as well as at the long term condition.

Physical changes that can be expected to occur at the accelerated condition but would not be considered significant include failure to meet acceptance criteria for dissolution for 12 units of a gelatin capsule or gelcoated tablet if the failure can be unequivocally attributed to cross-linking.

If there is no significant change at the intermediate condition, extrapolation beyond the period covered by long term data can be proposed; however, the extent of extrapolation would depend on whether long term data for the attribute are amenable to statistical analysis.

When the long term data for an attribute are not amenable to statistical analysis, the proposed shelf life can be up to 3 months beyond the period covered by long term data, if backed by relevant supporting data.

When the long term data for an attribute are amenable to statistical analysis but no analysis is performed, the extent of extrapolation should be the same as when data are not amenable to statistical analysis. However, if a statistical analysis is performed, the proposed shelf life can be up to one-and-half times, but should not be more than 6 months beyond, the period covered by long term data, when backed by statistical analysis and relevant supporting data.

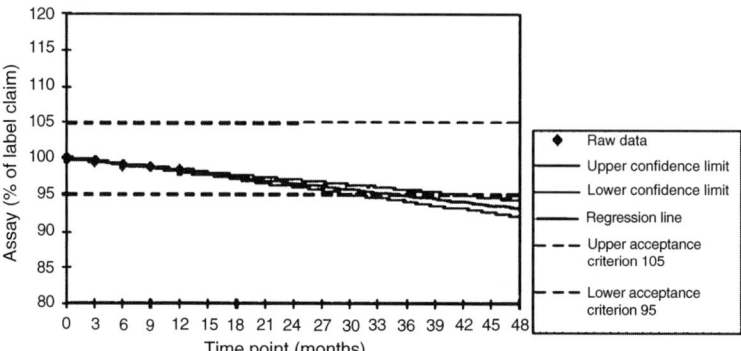

FIGURE 6 Shelf life estimation with upper and lower acceptance criteria based on assay at 25°C/60% RH.

Where significant change occurs at the intermediate condition, the proposed shelf life should not exceed the period covered by long term data. In addition, a shelf life shorter than the period covered by long term data can be appropriate.

STATISTICAL APPROACHES

Where applicable, an appropriate statistical method should be employed to analyze the long term primary stability data. The purpose of this analysis is to establish, with a high degree of confidence, a shelf life during which a quantitative attribute will remain within acceptance criteria for all future batches manufactured, packaged, and stored under similar circumstances.

Regression analysis is considered an appropriate approach to evaluating the stability data for a quantitative attribute and establishing a shelf life. The nature of the relationship between an attribute and time will determine whether data should be transformed for linear regression analysis. The relationship can be represented by a linear or nonlinear function on an arithmetic or logarithmic scale. In some cases, a nonlinear regression can better reflect the true relationship. An appropriate approach to shelf life estimation is to analyze a quantitative attribute (e.g., assay, degradation products) by

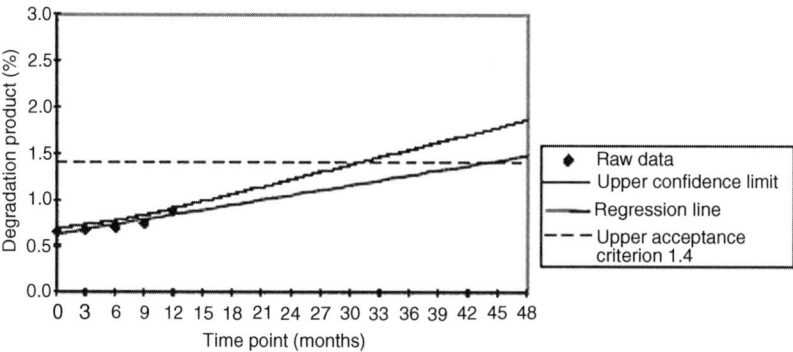

FIGURE 7 Shelf life estimation with upper acceptance criteria based on degradation product at 25°C/60% RH.

determining the earliest time at which the 95% confidence limit for the mean intersects the proposed acceptance criterion.

For an attribute known to decrease with time, the lower one-sided 95% confidence limit should be compared to the acceptance criterion. An example is shown in Figure 6. For an attribute known to increase with time, the upper one-sided 95% confidence limit should be compared to the acceptance criterion. An example is shown in Figure 7. For an attribute that can either increase or decrease, or whose direction of change is not known, two-sided 95% confidence limits should be calculated and compared to the upper and lower acceptance criteria.

The statistical method used for data analysis should take into account the stability study design to provide a valid statistical inference for the estimated shelf life. The approach described above can be used to estimate the shelf life for a single batch or for multiple batches when the data are combined after an appropriate statistical test.

REFERENCES

1. USP General Chapter on Pharmaceutical Stability <1150>, United States Pharmacopeia 30—National Formulary 25, The United States Pharmacopeial Convention, Inc., Rockville, MD, 2007.
2. USP Chapter on Manufacturing Practices for Dietary Supplements <2750>, United States Pharmacopeia 30—National Formulary 25, The United States Pharmacopeial Convention, Inc., Rockville, MD, 2007.
3. Accessed May 2007 at http://www.fda.gov/cder/guidance/index.htm#International%20 Conference%20on%20Harmonisation-Quality.
4. Accessed May 2007 at http://search.emea.europa.eu/search?q=cache:eTpPGROQhgU:http://www.emea.europa.eu/pdfs/human/qwp/18540104en.pdf+185401&restrict=human_medicines &ie=&site=emea_search&output=xml_no_dtd&client=emea_search&access=p&lr=&proxy stylesheet=emea_search&oe=.
5. Garrett ER. The kinetics of solvolysis of acyl esters of salicylic acid. J Am Chem Soc 1957; 79:3401–8.
6. Ip D, Brenner GS. Enalapril Maleate. In: Florey K, ed. Analytical Profiles of Drug Substances, Vol. 16. Orlando: Academic Press, 1987: 207–42.
7. Hamid IA, Parrott EL. Effect of temperature on solubilization and hydrolytic degradation of solubilized benzocaine and homatropine. J Pharm Sci 1971; 60:901–6.
8. Marcus AD, Baron S. A comparison of the kinetics of the acid catalyzed hydrolysis of procainamide, procaine and benzocaine. J Am Pharm Assoc, Sci Ed 1959; 48:85–90.
9. Lund W, Waaler T. The kinetics of atropine and apoatropine in aqueous solutions. Acta Chem Scand 1968; 22:3085–97.
10. Windheuser JJ, Sutter JL, Sarrif A. Analysis of scopolamine and its degradation products by GLC and liquid partition chromatography. J Pharm Sci 1972; 61:1311–3.
11. Siegel S, Lachman L, Malspeis L. A kinetic study of the hydrolysis of methyl DL-alpha-phenyl-2-piperidylacetate. J Am Pharm Assoc Sci Ed 1959; 48:431–9.
12. Patel RM, Chin T, Lach JL. Kinetic study of the acid hydrolysis of meperidine hydrochloride. J Hosp Pharm 1968; 25:256–61.
13. Muhtadi FJ. Cortisone acetate. In: Brittain HG, ed. Analytical Profiles of Drug Substances and Excipients, Vol. 26. San Diego: Academic Press, 1999; 167–245.
14. Florey K. Estradiol Valerate. In: Florey K, ed. Analytical Profiles of Drug Substances, Vol. 4. New York: Academic Press, 1975: 192–208.
15. Mauger JW, Paruta AN, Gerraughty. Consecutive first-order kinetic consideration of hydrocortisone hemisuccinate. J Pharm Sci 1969; 58:574–8.

16. Anderson BD, Taphouse V. Initial rate studies of hydrolysis and acyl migration in methylprednisolone 21-hemisuccinate and 17-hemisuccinate. J Pharm Sci 1981; 70:181–6.
17. Florey K. Estradiol valerate. In: Florey K, ed. Analytical Profiles of Drug Substances, Vol. 4. New York: Academic Press, 1975: 452–65.
18. Bundgaard H, Hansen SH. Hydrolysis and epimerization kinetics of pilocarpine in basic aqueous solution as determined by HPLC. Int J Pharm 1982; 10:281–9.
19. Garrett ER, Lippold BC, Mielck JB. Kinetics and mechanisms of lactonization of coumarinic acids and hydrolysis of coumarins I. J Pharm Sci 1971; 60:396–405.
20. Lippold BC, Garrett ER. Kinetics and mechanisms of lactonization of coumarinic acids and hydrolysis of coumarins II. J Pharm Sci 1971; 60:1019–27.
21. Fassberg J, Stella VJ. A kinetic and mechanistic study of the hydrolysis of camptothecin and some analogues. J Pharm Sci 1992; 81:676–84.
22. Hou JP, Poole JW. Kinetics and mechanism of degradation of ampicillin in solution. J Pharm Sci 1969; 58:447–54.
23. Bundgaard H. Polymerization of penicillins II. Kinetics and mechanism of dimerization and self-catalyzed hydrolysis in aqueous solution. Acta Pharm Suec 1977; 14:47–66.
24. Zia H, Tehrani M, Zargarbasi R. Kinetics of carbenicillin degradation in aqueous solutions. Can J Pharm Sci 1974; 9:112–7.
25. Kreuzig F. Penicillin-G benzathine. In: Florey K, ed. Analytical Profiles of Drug Substances, Vol. 11. New York: Academic Press, 1982: 463–82.
26. Kirschbaum J. Penicillin G, potasium. In: Florey K, ed. Analytical Profiles of Drug Substances, Vol. 15. Orlando: Academic Press, 1986: 427–507.
27. Lorenz LJ. Cefaclor. In: Florey K, ed. Analytical Profiles of Drug Substances, Vol. 9. New York: Academic Press, 1980: 107–23.
28. Tsuji A, Nakashima E, Deguchi Y, et al. Degradation kinetics and mechanism of aminocephalosporins in aqueous solution: Cefadroxil. J Pharm Sci 1981; 70:1120–8.
29. Fabre H, Eddine NH, Berge G. Degradation kinetics in aqueous solution of cefotaxime sodium a third-generation cephalosporin. J Pharm Sci 1984; 73:611–8.
30. Zappala AF, Holl WW, Post A. Cefazolin. In: Florey K, ed. Analytical Profiles of Drug Substances, Vol. 4. New York: Academic Press, 1975: 1–20.
31. Brenner GS. Cefoxitin, sodium. In: Florey K, ed. Analytical Profiles of Drug Substances, Vol. 11. New York: Academic Press, 1982: 169–92.
32. Abounassif MA, Mian NAA, Mian MS. Ceftazidime. In: Florey K, ed. Analytical Profiles of Drug Substances, Vol. 19. San Diego: Academic Press, 1990: 95–121.
33. Wozniak TJ, Hicks JR. Cefuroxime Sodium. In: Florey K, ed. Analytical Profiles of Drug Substances, Vol. 20. San Diego: Academic Press, 1991: 209–36.
34. Marrelli LP. Cephalexin. In: Florey K, ed. Analytical Profiles of Drug Substances, Vol. 4. New York: Academic Press, 1975: 21–46.
35. Badawy SIF, Hussain MA. Microenvironmental pH Modulation in Solid Dosage Forms. J Pharm Sci 2007; 96:948–59.
36. Wasylaschuk WR, Harmon PD, Wagner G, et al. Evaluation of hydroperoxides in common pharmaceutical excipients. J Pharm Sci 2007; 96:106–16.
37. Hovorka SW, Schoneich C. Oxidative Degradation of Pharmaceuticals: Theory, Mechanisms and Inhibition. J Pharm Sci 2001; 90:253–69.
38. Smith GB, DiMichele L, Colwell LF, et al. Autoxidation of simvastatin. Tetrahedron 1993; 49:4447–62.
39. Szulczewski DH, Hong W-H. Epinephrine. In: Florey K, ed. Analytical Profiles of Drug Substances, Vol. 7. Orlando: Academic Press, 1978:193–229.
40. Oyler AR, Naldi RE, Facchine KL, et al. Characterization of autoxidation products of the antifungal compounds econazole nitrate and miconazole nitrate. Tetrahedron 1991; 47:6549–60.
41. Bergh M, Shao LP, Hagelthorn G, et al. Contact allergens from surfactants. atmospheric oxidation of polyoxyethylene alcohols, formation of ethoxylated aldehydes, and their allergenic activity. J Pharm Sci 1998; 87:276–82.

42. Bindra DS, Williams TD, Stella VJ. Degradation of O^6-benzylguanine in aqueous polyethylene glycol 400 (PEG 400) solutions: concerns with formaldehyde in PEG 400. Pharm Res 1994; 11:1060–4.
43. Underberg WJM. Oxidative degradation of pharmaceutically important phenothiazines III: Kinetics and mechanism of promethazine oxidation. J Pharm Sci 1978; 67:1133–8.
44. Timmins P, Jackson IM, Wang YJ. Factors affecting captopril stability in aqueous solution. Int J Pharm 1982; 11:329–36.
45. Hartauer KJ, Arbuthnot GN, Baertschi SW, et al. Influence of peroxide impurities in povidone and crospovidone on the stability of raloxifene hydrochloride in tablets: identification and control of an oxidative degradation product. Pharm Dev Technol 2000; 5:303–10.
46. Waterman KC, Roy MC. Use of oxygen scavengers to stabilize solid pharmaceutical dosage forms: A case study. Pharm Dev Technol 2002; 7:227–34.
47. Kaufman MJ. Applications of oxygen polarography to drug stability testing and formulation development: Solution-phase oxidation of hydroxymethylglutary coenzyme A (HMG-CoA) reductase inhibitors. Pharm Res 1990; 7:289–92.
48. Kasraian K, Kuzniar AA, Wilson GG, et al. Developing an injectable formula containing an oxygen-sensitive drug: a case study of danofloxacin injectable. Pharm Dev Technol 1999; 4:475–480.
49. Won CM, Tang S-Y, Strohbeck CL. Photolytic and oxidative degradation of an antiemetic agent, RG 12915. Int J Pharm 1995; 121:95–105.
50. Miller DM, Buetter GR, Aust SD. Transition metals as catalysts of "autoxidation" reactions. Free Radical Biol Med 1990; 8:95–108.
51. Jackson C, Crabb TA, Gibson M, et al. Studies on the stability of trimelamol, a carbinol-amine-containing antitumor drug. J Pharm Sci 1991; 80:245–51.
52. Won CM. Kinetics of degradation of levothyroxine in aqueous solution and in the solid state. Pharm Res 1992; 9:131–7.
53. Lee YJ, Padula J, Lee H. Kinetics and mechanism of etodolac degradation in aqueous solutions. J Pharm Sci 1988; 77:81–6.
54. Bundgaard H, Mork N. Kinetics of the decarboxylation of foscarnet in acidic solutions and its implication in its oral absorption. Int J Pharm 1990; 63:213–8.
55. Bundgaard H, Hansen SH. Hydrolysis and epimerization kinetics of pilocarpine in basic aqueous solution as determined by HPLC. Int J Pharm 1982; 10:281–9.
56. Butterfield AG, Hughes DW, Wilson WL, et al. Simultaneous high-speed liquid chromatographic determination of tetracycline and rolitetracycline formulations. J Pharm Sci 64:316–20.
57. Ott H, Hoffmann A, Frey AJ. Acid-catalyzed isomerization in the peptide part of ergot alkaloids. J Am Chem Soc 1966; 88:1251–6.
58. Hamilton-Miller JMT. The effect of pH and temperature on the stability and bioactivity of nystatin and amphotericin B. J Pharm Pharmacol 1973; 25:401–7.
59. Cotton ML, Wu DW, Vadas EB. Drug-excipient interaction study of enalapril maleate using thermal analysis and scanning electron microscopy. Int J Pharm 1987; 40:129–42.
60. Gu L, Strickley RG, Chi L-H, et al. Drug-excipient incompatibility studies on the dipeptide angiotensin-converting enzyme inhibitor, moexipril hydrochloride: dry powder vs wet granulation. Pharm Res 1990; 7:379–83.
61. Ahlneck C, Zografi G. The molecular basis of moisture effects on the physical and chemical stability of drugs in the solid state. Int J Pharm 1990; 62:87–95.
62. Landin M, Casalderrey M, Martinez-Pacheco R, et al. Chemical stability of acetylsalicylic acid in tablets prepared with different particle size fractions of a commercial brand of dicalcium phosphate dihydrate. Int J Pharm 1995; 123:143–4.
63. Jakel D, Keck M. Purity of excipients. In: Drugs and Pharmaceutical Sciences, Vol. 103, New York: Marcel Dekker, 1987; 21–58.
64. Dubost DC, Kaufman J, Zimmerman JA, et al. Characterization of a solid state reaction product from a lyophilized formulation of a cyclic hexapeptide. A novel example of an excipient-induced oxidation. Pharm Res 1996; 13:1811–4.

65. Wirth DD, Baertschi SW, Johnson RA, et al. Maillard reaction of lactose and fluoxetine hydrochloride, a secondary amine. J Pharm Sci 1998; 87:31–9.
66. Lessen T, Zhao D-C. Interactions between drug substances and excipients. 1. fluorescence and HPLC studies of triazolophthalazine derivatives from hydralazine hydrochloride and starch. J Pharm Sci 1996; 85:326–9.
67. Jansen PJ, Oren PL, Kemp CA, et al. Characterization of impurities formed by interaction of duloxetine HCl with enteric polymers hydroxypropyl methylcellulose acetate succinate and hydroxypropyl methylcellulose phthalate. J Pharm Sci 1998; 87:81–5.
68. Schildcrout SA, Risley DS, Kleemann RL. Drug-excipient interactions of seproxetine maleate hemi-hydrate: isothermal stress methods. Drug Devel Ind Pharm 1993; 19:1113–30.
69. Descamps M, Willart JF, Dudognon E, et al. Transformation of pharmaceutical compounds upon milling and comilling: the role of Tg. J Pharm Sci 2007; 96:1398–407.
70. Qui Z, Stowell JC, Cao W, et al. Effect of milling and compression on the solid-state Maillard reaction. J Pharm Sci 2005; 94:2568–80.
71. Waterman KC, Adami RC. Accelerated aging: prediction of chemical stability of pharmaceuticals. Int J Pharm 2005; 293:101–25.
72. Mahajan R, Templeton A, Harman A, et al. The effect of inert atmosphere packaging on oxidative degradation in formulated granules. Pharm Res 2005; 22:128–40.
73. Du J, Hoag W. The influence of excipients on the stability of the moisture sensitive drugs aspirin and niacinamide: comparison of tablets containing lactose monohydrate and tablets containing anhydrous lactose. Pharm Dev Technol 2001; 6:159–66.
74. Zografi G, Kontny MJ. The interactions of water and cellulose- and starch-derived pharmaceutical excipients. Pharm Res 1986; 3:187–94.
75. Allinson JG, Dansereau RJ, Sakr A. The effects of packaging on the stability of a moisture sensitive compound. Int J Pharm 2001; 221:49–56.
76. Waterman KC, Adami RC, Alsante KM, et al. Hydrolysis in pharmaceutical formulations. Pharm Dev Technol 2002; 7:113–46.
77. Badawy SIF, Williams RC, Gilbert DL. Chemical stability of an ester prodrug of a glycoprotein IIb/IIIa receptor antagonist in solid dosage forms. J Pharm Sci 1999; 88:428–33.
78. Gordon MS, Rudraraju VS, Rhie JK, et al. The effect of aging on the dissolution of wet granulated tablets containing super disintegrants. Int J Pharm 1993; 97:119–31.
79. Li S, Wei B, Fleres S, et al. Correlation and prediction of moisture-mediated dissolution stability for benazepril hydrochloride tablets. Pharm Res 2004; 21:617–24.
80. Fitzpatrick S, McCabe JF, Petts CR, et al. Effect of moisture on polyvinylpyrrolidone in accelerated stability testing. Int J Pharm 2002; 246:143–51.
81. Rohrs BR, Thamann TJ, Gao P, et al. Tablet dissolution affected by a moisture mediated solid-state interaction between drug and excipient. Pharm Res 1999; 16:1850–6.
82. Meyer MC, Straughn AB, Jarvi EJ, et al. The bioinequivalence of carbamazepine tablets with a history of clinical failures. Pharm Res 1992; 9:1612–6.
83. Wang JT, Shiu GK, Ong-Chen T, et al. Effects of humidity and temperature on in vitro dissolution of carbamazepine tablets. J Pharm Sci 1993; 83:1002–5.
84. Carstensen JT, Rhodes CT. Pellicule formation in gelatin capsules. Drug Dev Ind Pharm 1993; 19:2709–12.
85. Murthy KS, Enders NA, Fawzi MB. Dissolution Stability of Hard-shell Capsule Products, Part I: The Effect of Exaggerated Storage Conditions. Pharm Tech 1989; Mar:72–86.
86. Meyer, MC, Straughn AB, Mhatre RM, et al. The effect of gelatin cross-linking on the bioequivalence of hard and soft gelatin acetaminophen capsules. Pharm Res 2000; 17:962–66.
87. Digenis GA, Gold TB, Shah VP. Cross-linking of gelatin capsules and its relevance to their in vitro–in vivo performance. J Pharm Sci 1994; 83:915–21.
88. Schwier JR, Cooke GG, Hartauer KJ, et al. Rayon: A source of furfural—a reactive aldehyde capable of insolubilizing gelatin capsules. Pharm Tech 1993; 17:78–9.
89. Dey M, Enever R, Kraml M, et al. The dissolution and bioavailability of etodolac from capsules exposed to conditions of high relative humidity and temperatures. Pharm Res 1993; 10:1295–300.

90. Digenis GA, Sandefer EP, Page RC, et al. Bioequivalence study of stressed and nonstressed hard gelatin capsules using amoxicillin as a drug marker and gamma scintigraphy to confirm time and gi location of *in vivo* rupture. Pharm Res 2000; 17:572–582.
91. USP General Chapter on Dissolution <711>, United States Pharmacopeia 30—National Formulary 25, The United States Pharmacopeial Convention, Inc., Rockville, MD, 2007.
92. Murthy KS, Ghebre-Sellassie I. Current perspectives on the dissolution stability of solid oral dosage forms. J Pharm Sci 1993; 82:113–26.
93. Castello RA, Mattocks AM. Discoloration of tablets containing amines and lactose. J Pharm Sci 1962; 51:106.

16
Compaction Simulation

Michael E. Bourland and Matthew P. Mullarney
Pfizer, Inc., Groton, Connecticut, U.S.A.

INTRODUCTION

A quality by design approach to the development of pharmaceutical dosage forms requires the careful characterization and understanding of the properties and limitations of the product and process. In solid dosage form development, tablets are the most common, and often least expensive, vehicle for dosing active pharmaceutical ingredients (API). One of the most significant challenges early in tablet development is the limited quantity and high cost of bulk material (usually API) that is available for laboratory experimentation and manufacturing process scale-up. Therefore, "material sparing" tools for powder characterization and process understanding, such as compaction simulators, are key to the efficient and cost-effective development of tablets.

A compaction simulator is an essential tool for a pharmaceutical scientist when using a material sparing approach to the characterization, scale-up, and troubleshooting of powder compression performance. In the simplest of terms, a compaction simulator is a highly instrumented single station compression machine fitted with an upper punch, lower punch, and die that is capable of mimicking a modeled compaction event. These machines are typically hydraulically, and sometimes mechanically, powered to deliver a range of compression forces (e.g., up to 50 kN) using highly controlled punch displacement profiles. Compaction simulators use sophisticated instrumentation to monitor, at minimum, the displacement and force profiles associated with the compaction event. Therefore, the data generated while using a compaction simulator offers a significant advantage over traditional pharmaceutical unit operations for studying and understanding powder compression behavior.

In the pharmaceutical solid dosage form development process, compaction simulators can be used throughout the life of a compound. Royce and coworkers categorized the lifecycle of a compound into three phases (1).

1. Pre-formulation:
   - characterize the API concerning deformation properties, compactability, sticking tendencies, ejection force, etc...;
   - compare compaction properties of different API salt forms, polymorphs, or hydrates.
2. Formulation:
   - aid in excipient selection (based on deformation properties);
   - compare compaction properties of formulation variants;

- develop robust formulations by simulating production machines or running with dwell times similar to production tablet presses.
3. Scale-up and production:
   - troubleshooting production problems at small-scale;
   - evaluating changes in drug substance (particle size, manufacturing sites, and manufacturing conditions), excipient sources, or processing conditions.

This chapter will provide an overview of compaction simulator theory, construction, experimental design, and applications for the practicing pharmaceutical scientist.

COMPACTION SIMULATOR EVOLUTION AND DESIGN

A compaction simulator must be able to mimic the full compression cycle of the unit operation. Early attempts at compaction simulation utilized mechanical property testing equipment (e.g., Instron and Lloyd type machines) to compact powders into compacts. Although these machines were well suited to apply appropriate compression loads, they were not designed for the high velocities and accelerations necessary to simulate the double-ended compression cycle of a rotary tablet press (2).

The first "true" compaction simulator capable of mimicking the compaction and ejection cycle of a rotary tablet press was reported by Hunter et al. in the 1970s (2). The evolution of such an instrument presented a novel tool for both powder compression research and scale-up of the tableting process. Celek and Marshall report that although compaction simulators are expensive to purchase, they present the following attributes:

- Mimic production conditions
- Mimic cycles of many tablet presses
- Require a small amount of material
- Easily instrumented
- Easy to setup
- Used for stress/strain studies

Compaction simulators are designed to be mechanically robust so that the machines can compress powders into compacts at relatively high punch displacement rates using a significant amount of force. The basic design of simulators has not changed significantly since the 1970s.

Hydraulic compaction simulators are composed of three main components: the hydraulic power unit, the compaction simulator, and a data/information management system. The compaction unit is powered by the hydraulic power pack which delivers pressurized oil to accumulators. The accumulators are necessary to deliver a local high pressure, low volume "burst" of hydraulic oil to the actuators. The oil flow rate and direction are controlled by high-speed servo values, which are electrically integrated into an electronic feedback control system. The servo valves deliver the appropriate oil flow to the upper and lower hydraulic actuators to control their position. Punches mounted on the ends of the actuators compress the powder inside a die, which is fitted within the die table. The die table is positioned in the middle of a rigid load frame between the between the upper and lower hydraulic actuators. Typically machine guarding (e.g., polycarbonate and stainless steel) enclose the compression area to protect critical machine components and ensure the safety of the operator. A block diagram of a hydraulic compaction simulator is shown in Figure 1.

Compaction Simulation

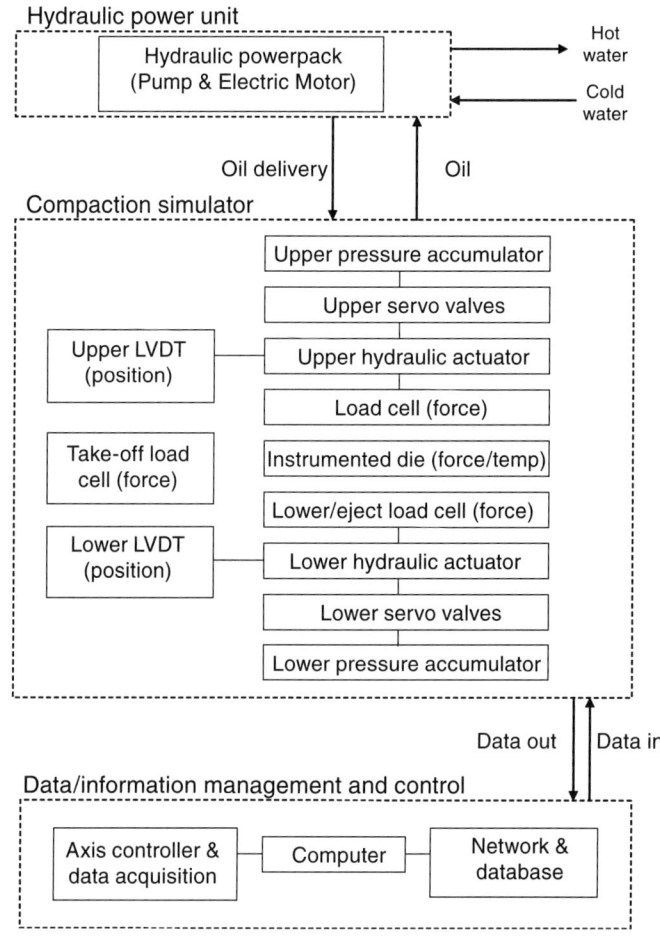

FIGURE 1 Block diagram of a hydraulic compaction simulator.

Mechanically powered compaction simulators are also available to replicate the compression event of tablet presses (3). These machines leverage the design of traditional rotary tablet presses where the punches are forced between a set of roll wheels to enable the compression event. The punch type and roll wheels can be changed to replicate the compression event of different press types. In some models, the fill station, compression station(s), and ejection station are aligned in series on a linear track, where the punches and die travel along this track from station to station to complete the fill–compress–ejection cycle.

It is important to note that compaction simulators are designed to mimic a single compression cycle of a unit operation, not the events prior to compression (e.g., hopper discharge, die filling), effects of production time (e.g., heat buildup, segregation, material adherence), or events after compression (e.g., tablet takeoff and bulk tablet collection). For example, Zinchuk et al. remark that certain features of roller compaction, such as nonhomogeneous compact density, material feeding patterns and bypass, cannot be mimicked using a compaction simulator (4). Therefore, like any unit operation, compaction simulators are robust in what they are designed to do (compression) but are unique in their ancillary features.

TABLE 1 Features of Compaction Simulators Used in the Bateman and Coworker "Round-Robin" Study

Institution	Maximum load (kN)	Maximum compression rate (mm/s)	Displacement LVDT stroke range (mm)		Controlling computer	Manufacturer
			Upper	Lower		
ICI	50	400	±50	±25	Commodore PET	Keelavite
Boots	50	1000	±50	±50	Hewlett Packard Mini	Mand
Wellcome	22.5	400	±12.5	–	Commodore PET	Mand
Smith, Kline & French	50	1000	±5	±5	Apple IIe	Mand
Glaxo	50	3000	±10	±10	Olivetti	ESH
Liverpool School of Pharmacy	50	3000	±10	±10	Apple IIe	ESH

Source: Adapted from Ref. 5.

Bateman and coworkers report a comparative analysis of six different hydraulically powered compaction simulators manufactured by a variety of vendors (Table 1). In their round-robin study, they found that the compaction simulators were comparable when operated within a moderate compression stress range of 50–200 MPa. However, at higher pressures, correction factors needed to be applied because of elastic distortion and differences in loading characteristics of the hydraulic systems (5). These results are not surprising since like rotary tablet presses, compaction simulators are not perfectly rigid. Therefore, compaction simulators should be properly calibrated (including corrections for mechanical flexure and electronic noise) to ensure the collection of quality experimental data.

COMPACTION SIMULATOR ANCILLARY FEATURES

Tooling Types and Design

Most modern compaction simulators are equipped to use different types of tablet tooling. A single "set" of tablet tooling consists of an upper punch, a lower punch, and a die manufactured by expert industrial tooling manufacturers. Tooling can have virtually unlimited tip designs (e.g., shapes, sizes, logos), but are generally categorized by their barrel diameter, head profile, and shaft length. Figures 2 and 3, taken from the *Tableting Specification Manual* (6), show the typical punch and die terminology and some common production rotary press tooling types. Some simulators can also be configured to accommodate single station tablet tooling, such as Manesty "F" type, if the punch head profile is not required to enable the simulation. Compaction simulators that require a cam (a.k.a. roller) to drive the punches (e.g., the Presster™) usually require the use of rotary press tooling with a punch head profile because the punch head tangentially contacts the cam during its travel. However, most hydraulic or uniaxial simulators can be fitted with punch holders to accommodate both single station and rotary press type tooling. In the next section, the importance of how the punch head profile affects the shape of the punch displacement waveform will be discussed.

Powder Feed Mechanism

Compaction simulators are not designed to mimic the powder feeding event of a unit operation. Jackson and coworkers report that die filling on a rotary press involves complex

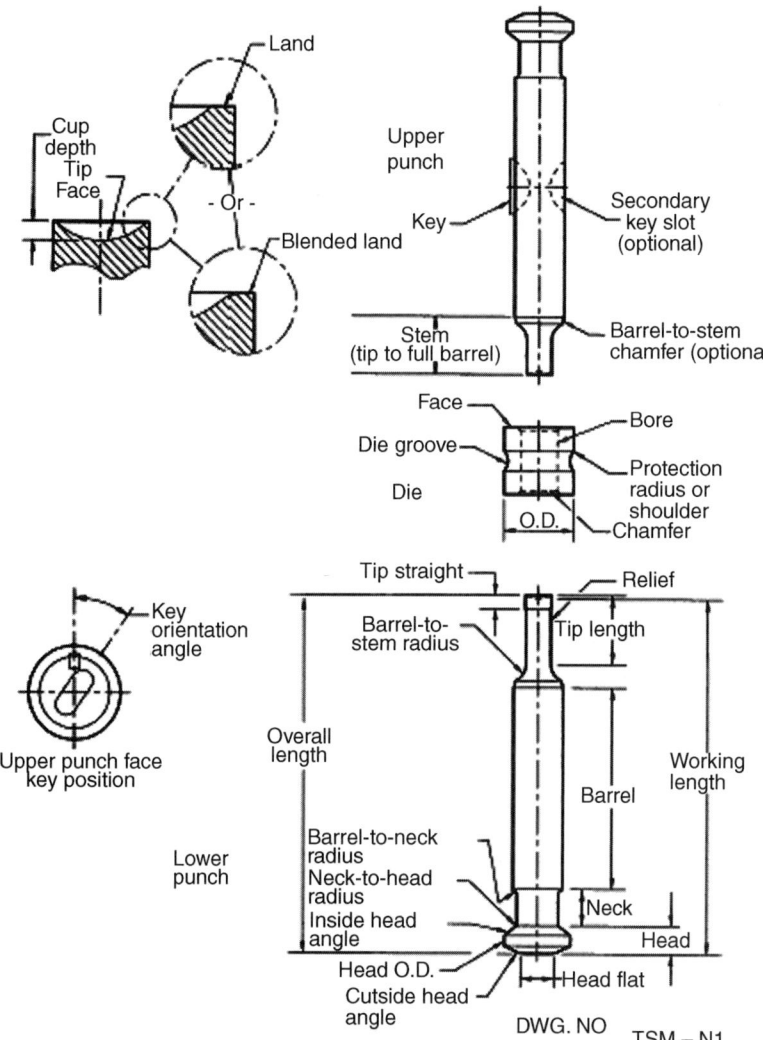

FIGURE 2 Rotary tablet press punch and die terminology. *Source*: Adapted from Ref. 6.

flow phenomena (7). Therefore, for design simplicity, compaction simulators are minimally equipped with a small gravity or agitated hopper that moves over the die as the lower punch is retracted to a predetermined position to enable the correct weight/volume of powder into the die cavity prior to compression. Dies can also be manually filled with a unit dose of powder if material quantity or flow properties are limited.

Lubrication Technique

Lubrication of the die and punches is essential for many solid dosage formulations to prevent material sticking to the equipment surfaces during tablet production. The amount of lubrication, technique to apply the lubrication, and method of addition can have large effects on the die wall friction during the compaction process. Various techniques exist for lubrication of the compaction simulator dies. The most prominent method for manual die lubrication is to brush the die with a magnesium stearate suspension (e.g., in methanol). This technique is easily controlled; however, it can be time intensive and may not be

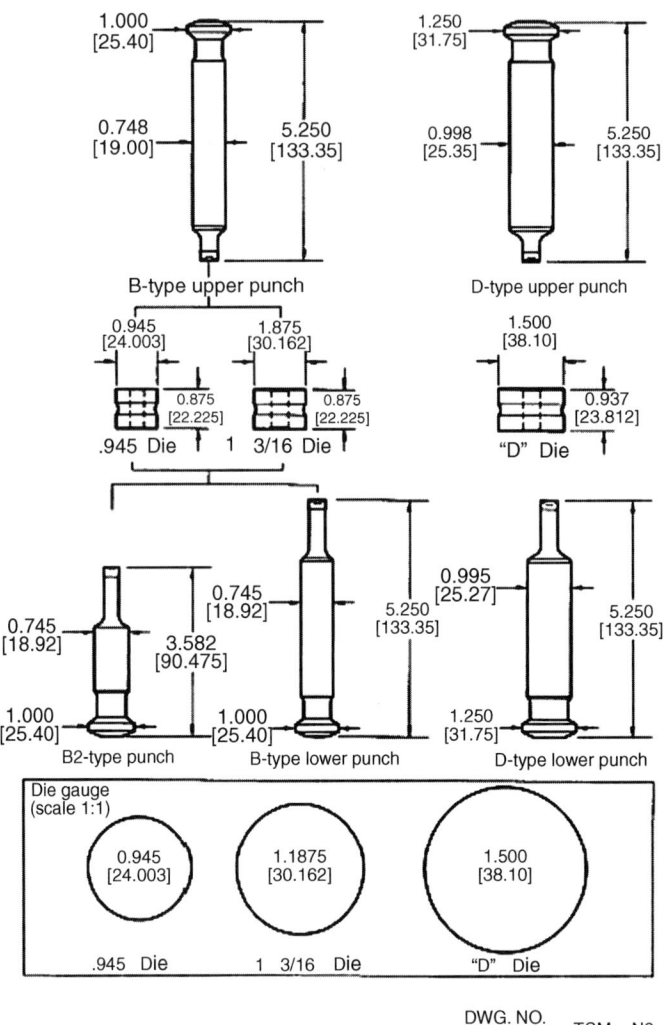

FIGURE 3 Rotary tablet press TSM production tooling types. *Note*: Unless otherwise noted, dimensions shown in figures and tables are given first in inches, followed by the equivalent millimeters in brackets. *Source*: Adapted from Ref. 6.

representative of the production technique. Another common method of lubrication is to blend the magnesium stearate into the formulation (8). This method is more representative of the actual production methodology. However, care must be taken because some blends are sensitive to blend time, blend speed, and proportion of magnesium stearate.

Compaction simulators are a useful tool for the evaluation of the effect of magnesium stearate on the formulation of a drug product (9). Mollan and company investigated various concentrations of magnesium stearate on three types of maltodextrins. The lubricant sensitivity of the materials was determined using the R-values. Nelson developed the "R-value" as a measure of the efficiency of a lubricant (10). The R-value represents the ratio of the maximum lower punch force to the maximum upper punch force. Generally, Mollan et al. were able to demonstrate a decrease in the tablet strength and increase in tablet porosity with an increase in the magnesium stearate concentration. Figure 4 shows the sensitivity of some materials to the addition of magnesium stearate.

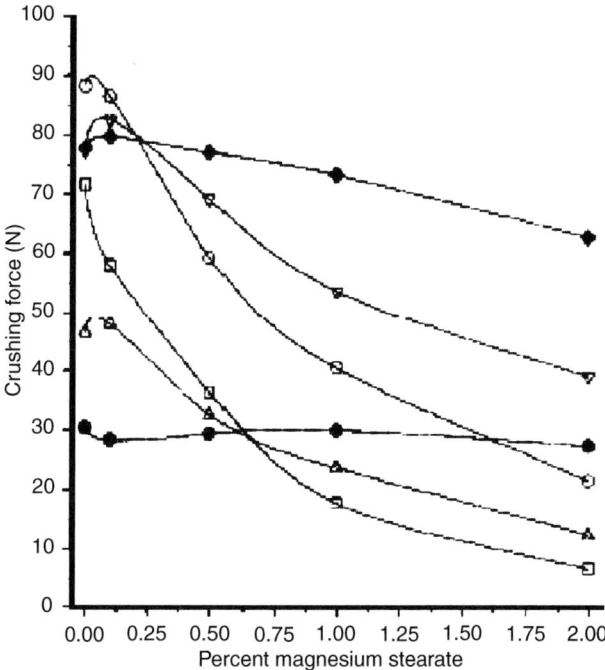

FIGURE 4 The sensitivity of some materials to the addition of magnesium stearate. *Source*: Adapted from Ref. 9.

Safety Concerns

Compaction simulators are relatively safe to operate with proper user training. From a mechanical perspective, the most likely sources of severe physical injury to the operator are the punches and die. However, most modern compaction simulators are equipped with robust (i.e., "bulletproof") machine guarding which prevents the operators from putting their body parts near the moving parts of the instrument and partial/entire components from exiting the compression region (and flying toward the operator) if catastrophic mechanical failure occurs.

In addition to the machine guarding, the control system should be interlocked with an electronically monitored failsafe system. The control software should have an "awareness" of the position and action of all moving parts and measurement devices. Therefore, if an unplanned incident or out-of-protocol action does occur, the system will take action or stop action to minimize the likelihood of additional safety hazards. In some cases, as with system calibration or "super user" access, graded access levels can be custom-built into the design for specialized and infrequent operations.

Because compaction simulators are used to compress powders with API as well as other biologically hazardous materials, powder containment is a significant concern. In terms of laboratory scale pharmaceutical equipment, compaction simulators yield relatively low airborne powder quantities compared to dusty operations such as dry milling. Even so, engineering controls should be designed into the machine to contain the powder compression region, and if possible include a air-extraction system to constantly capture and safely remove any airborne particles. A limited number of surfaces and corners in the product contact regions will also facilitate surface cleaning during and after use.

Tablet Ejection and Takeoff Mechanism

Tablets are ejected from the die by raising the lower punch to the die surface. The lower punch displacement can be controlled to mimic any ejection profile, including a rotary tablet press ejection profile. Typically on a rotary tablet press, an ejection cam or ramp is used to force the lower punch upward during tablet ejection. The tablet production rate and geometry of the ejection cam will dictate the shape of the ejection displacement profile. Several methods have been developed to instrument the compaction simulator to investigate the process of tablet ejection (11–13). Tablets are typically removed from the ejection position using a takeoff actuator which moves across the die tablet to push the tablet to a collection system. Tablets can also be manually removed if tablet sticking or takeoff problems are present with a particular formulation.

INSTRUMENTATION

Most instrumented single station or rotary tablet presses are equipped to measure punch forces, ejection forces, and takeoff forces during tablet manufacturing operations. Compaction simulators are additionally instrumented to measure absolute and relative punch tip positions, which is a significant benefit when studying powder compaction behavior. Compaction simulators can also be easily outfitted with instrumented dies or punches to measure die/punch forces and temperatures. Because each segment of a high-speed tableting operation (e.g., main compaction) typically occurs in 1 to 100 milliseconds, the data acquisition and processing systems for the force and displacement waveforms (i.e., force or displacement vs. time) must be designed to handle data capture rates up to 100 kHz to achieve reasonable control and resolution. This section will discuss the typical instrumentation features on a compaction simulator.

Load Cells

Compaction simulators use load cells to measure the applied and resultant forces from the powder compaction operation. Load cells are available in a variety of configurations (e.g., beam or in-line) and can be used to measure compression, tension, and/or shear. Load cells are typically accurate to 0.1% and designed to operate between –65 and 250°F. Strain gauge load cells are commonly used and measure forces by associating a small deflection in the sensor (e.g., <0.05 mm) to a voltage (e.g., ±10 V DC). The change in voltage as a result of the deflection is proportional to a calibrated force. Load cells can be positioned on a compaction simulator to measure upper punch force, lower punch force, ejection force, die wall force, and takeoff force. In most cases, these load cells are equipped to measure both compression and tension, but primarily measure compressive loads.

On hydraulic compaction simulators the load cells used to measure punch forces are fixed to end of the upper and lower actuator rods, just prior to the punch holders, and therefore are in line with the compression axis. It is desirable for these load cells to be relatively small (e.g., <500 g) to minimize inertial effects and to accommodate typical compression loads (e.g., 0.1–50 kN). Tablet press replicators, which use a roll compression system to apply punch forces, are typically equipped with a shear pin configuration to measure applied upper and lower punch forces. In this case, a set of load cells is required for each compression station (e.g., precompression and main compression).

The lower load cell on a hydraulic compaction simulator is also used to measure ejection force. However, the ejection forces are only a fraction (e.g., <5%) of the compression forces that the lower load cell is equipped to measure. Therefore, the load cell voltage output is usually scaled and filtered through a signal conditioner to improve the precision of the ejection load measurements. On a mechanical tablet press replicator, the ejection load cells are positioned under the ejection cam (ramp) and are a separate unit from the compression load cells.

The takeoff load cells are used to measure the force required to remove the tablet from the lower punch face. Consequently, this is a relative measurement of the tablet to punch adhesive force. An in-line or beam load cell can be attached to a takeoff actuator that moves across long the die table to scrape the tablet off of the lower punch, after which the actuator moves the tablet to a collection area. The magnitude of takeoff force is significantly lower than the ejection force (e.g., < 10 N), and therefore, the takeoff load cell is much more sensitive and fragile than the other load cells on the system. Like a rotary tablet press, a tablet press replicator uses a takeoff load cell that is fixed to a stationary bar. Therefore, this instrument measures both the impact force of the tablet at a high rate of speed and the adhesive force with the punch. Therefore, if the takeoff arm rate could be adjusted to move very slowly, it would be preferred over a high-speed takeoff bar to measure small differences in tablet to punch adhesion.

Displacement Transducers

The absolute position of the each punch on a compaction simulator is typically measured using a linear variable displacement transducer (LVDT). A LVDT operates by moving a magnetic core rod through a sleeve of coils, which results in a detectable change in output voltage. This voltage is proportional to the position of the core rod. The core rod extends beyond the coil housing and if attached to the punch actuator, usually a contacts a stationary reference surface (e.g., the die table) to measure the punch position. Sometimes two LVDTs are used for each punch: one to measure the large actuator strokes (>25 mm) when the punch is outside of the die and the other to measure the small punch position movements (<25 mm) when the punch is inside of the die. This enables high-resolution in-die punch position measurements with the flexibility of long actuator strokes.

Instrumented Punches

In addition to measuring the compression and decompression forces during a compaction cycle, specially designed tablet punches have been developed to measure the degree of tablet adhesion to the punch tip. Schmidt and coworkers developed a functioning instrumented upper punch for the evaluation of a tablet's propensity to stick to the tooling (14,15). Their design operated using an adhesion force sensor instrumented with semiconductor strain gauges and was fitted on a single station eccentric tablet press. Most simply, the punch measures the tension between the punch face and the tablet face during the decompression cycle. Materials that were observed to exhibit more "sticky" behavior during tablet production had increased adhesion force signals (Fig. 5).

Tablet formulations that exhibit punch sticking present a significant robustness challenge as they compromise the appearance and quality of the drug product. If appropriately fitted to a compaction simulator, these punches could be useful for evaluating the effects of formulation composition, compression force, external lubrication, punch tip design and embossing, and run time on the sticking behavior of tablets.

Alternatives to using instrumented punches include punch tip chemical assays to monitor the quantity of material that has adhered to the punch surface (16,17). Additional attempts have been made at using the ejection force and takeoff force instrumentation to monitor tablet adherence to the punch tip. Morris and coworkers reported that tablet

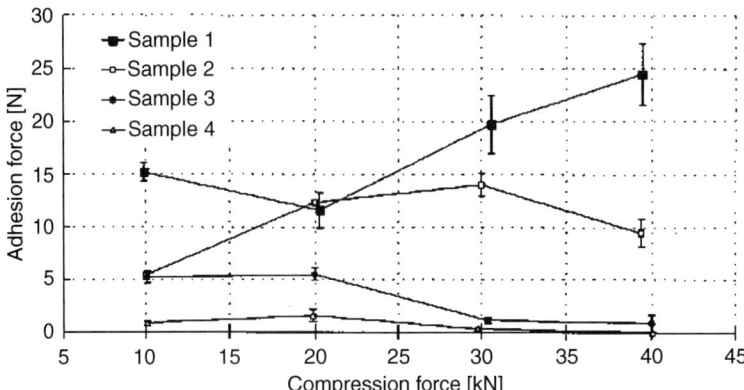

FIGURE 5 Adhesion force versus compression force profile for a formulation at different levels of magnesium stearate. *Source*: Adapted from Ref. 15.

takeoff force and visual inspection of the punch tips was able to correctly rank order the sticking tendency of ketoprofen > ibuprofen > flurbiprofen (18). A compaction simulator may be best suited for takeoff force evaluations of this kind since the rate of impact of the takeoff bar on a compaction simulator is significantly lower than a rotary press (e.g., 1 mm/sec vs. 1000 mm/sec) (Fig. 6). However, it is still unclear whether this method can predictably discriminate the sticking behavior of a new tablet formulation.

Instrumented Dies

Compaction simulators can be fitted with instrumented dies to measure the stress that the powder exerts on the die wall during the compaction and ejection cycle. Different types of instrumented dies have been constructed with single or multiple transducers to measure the die wall stress. The literature reports some examples of different configurations of the pressure transducers within the instrumented die (13), as shown in Figure 7.

The die wall force measurement can be used in combination with the upper punch force, lower punch force, ejection force, and punch position waveform data to calculate useful material parameters, such as maximum/residual die wall pressure, Poisson's ratio, and coefficient of friction. A schematic of the principle force vectors during powder

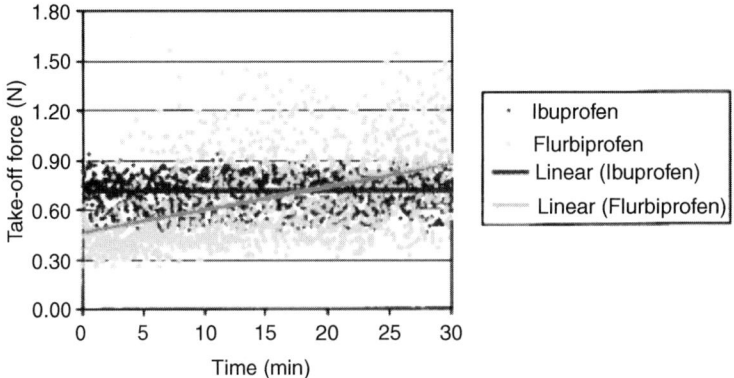

FIGURE 6 Tablet takeoff force versus time for formulated tablets. *Source*: Adapted from Ref. 18.

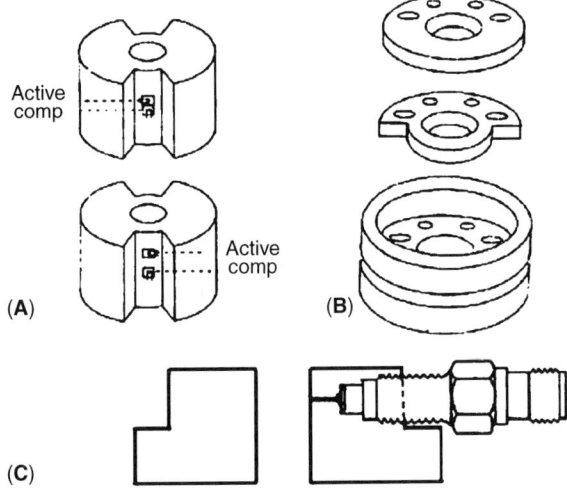

FIGURE 7 Different configurations of the pressure transducers within the instrumented die. *Source*: Adapted from Ref. 13.

compaction are shown in Figure 8 (13) and the measured compaction waveforms are shown in Figure 9. These values can be used to categorize powder compression behavior relative to potential tableting deficiencies (e.g., capping, lamination, die wall friction) where the profile of die wall force reflects the plasticity and friction property of pharmaceutical materials (19).

A common evaluation with an instrumented die involves the study of the axial to radial transmission of forces from the punch surfaces to the die wall. As the punches travel towards one another the powder is compacted axially while it is restricted from radial movement by the die wall. This radial strain constriction causes a radial stress to occur in the die wall. A typical profile for this buildup and release of radial stress during a compaction cycle is shown in Figure 10. The hysteresis is expected of materials which are both compressible and not perfectly elastic, where the decompression part of the waveform shows a higher degree of radial stress than during the compression part of the

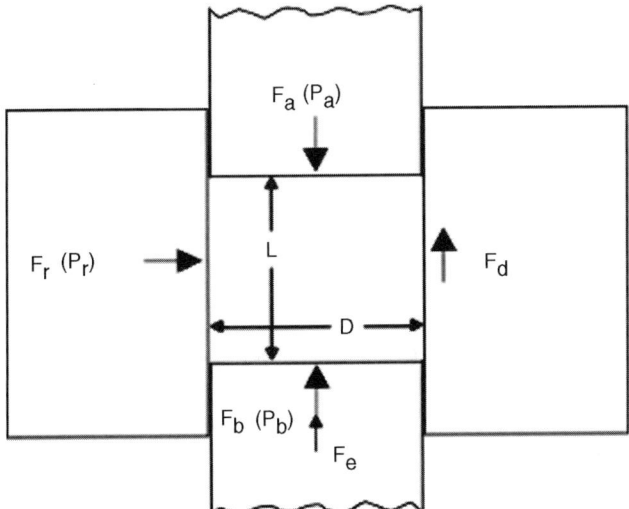

FIGURE 8 Schematic of the principle force vectors during powder compaction. *Source*: Adapted from Ref. 13.

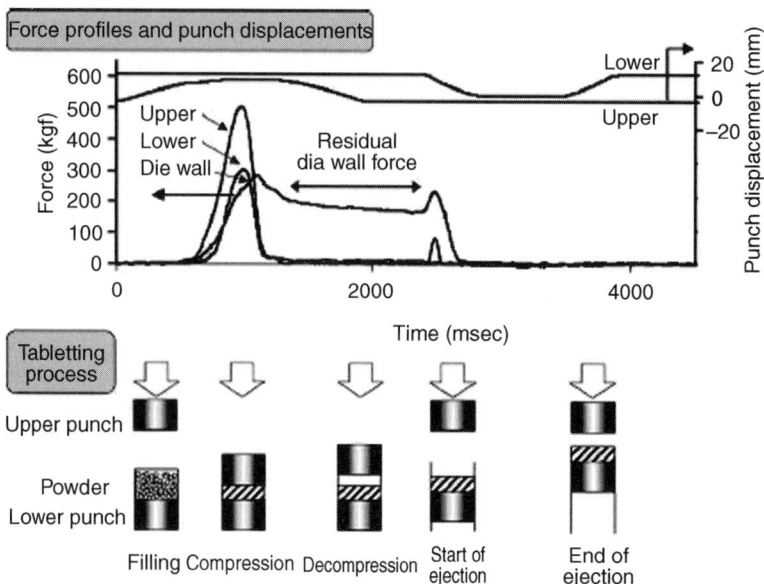

FIGURE 9 Measured compaction waveforms for a compaction simulator equipped with an instrumented die. *Source*: Adapted from Ref. 19.

waveform. As the powder is compressed using higher axial stresses (i.e., punch forces) both the maximum die wall stress and the residual die wall stress typically increase. A significant increase in either can contributed to undesirable die wall friction and/or significant radial expansion of the compact once it is ejected from the die. If the compact is not able to accommodate the rapid release of stress during its ejection from the die (e.g., if it is very brittle) tablet capping or lamination can occur.

These radial and axial stress waveform data are also useful to calculate material property values such as Poisson's ratio. Poisson's ratio is classically defined as the ratio

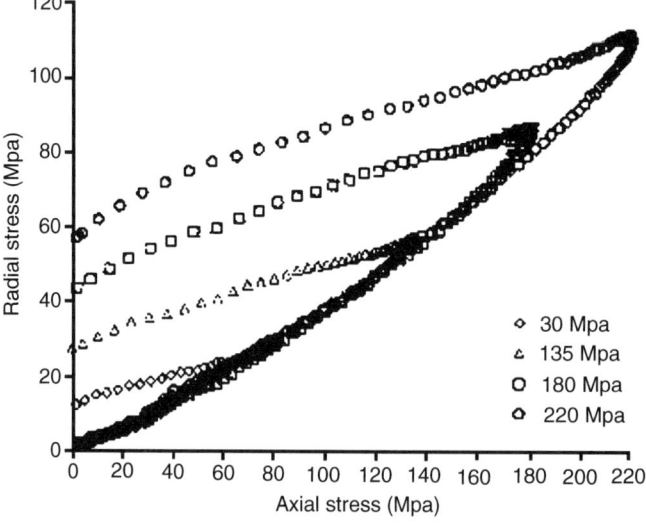

FIGURE 10 Radial versus axial stress plot for sodium chloride tablets prepared on a compaction simulator. *Source*: Adapted from Ref. 12.

of the radial (or transverse) strain to radial strain during compressive or tensile stress application. Long's equation can be used to calculate Poisson's ratio (ν) from the initial slope prior to the elastic limit of the radial stress (σ_r) versus axial stress (σ_a) profile. Values of Possion's ratio typically range from 0.2 to 0.4 for pharmaceutical materials (20) and are useful as input parameters for computational modeling of compression behavior (21).

$$\sigma_a = \sigma_r \left(\frac{\nu}{1-\nu} \right) \tag{1}$$

Data from instrumented die experiments can also be used to calculate the powder's coefficient of friction against the die wall. The coefficient of friction (μ) can be calculated using the data from the following equation described by Unckel where $\eta = \sigma_{radial}/\sigma_{upper}$, L = compact thickness, D = die diameter (22).

$$\frac{\sigma_{upper}}{\sigma_{lower}} = e^{4\mu\eta L/D} \tag{2}$$

In a "round-robin" study of instrumented dies in powder compression, the literature suggests that an accuracy of measurement of friction coefficient of ± 0.01 is preferred, but that an accuracy of ± 0.02 will still give predictions of acceptable levels of accuracy for input to models of the compaction process (23).

The most challenging aspect of using an instrumented die may be its proper calibration. In theory, a perfectly hydrostatic media would apply equal stress to both punch tips and the die wall during compaction. However, interparticulate and particle-tooling frictional influences in powder compaction make powders impractical for use as calibration media. Often perfectly elastic materials (e.g., rubber plugs) are used to calibrate instrumented dies as they generally transmit equal pressure to the die wall and punch tips. Depending on the instrumented die construction, calibration in different positions within the die may be needed to obtain accurate data. Cocolas and Lordi suggest that the use of multiple transducers in the die are preferred for a broader coverage of the response (20).

Calibration (Instrumentation, Elasticity Correction)

Like any laboratory instrument, the force and displacement transducers on a compaction simulator must be routinely calibrated to ensure data quality. Calibration becomes even more important when a compaction simulator is used as a quantitative tool for material property analysis. For example, punch force and displacement data must be accurate and reproducible for studies which require the acquisition of in-die pressure–volume data (e.g., Heckel analysis for yield pressure determinations). Even slight deviations in these measurements can significant magnify the error in certain calculations.

Depending on their function and accessibility, the force transducers are either calibrated in situ or removed for external calibration. Typically, the punch load cells are calibrated in situ by placing a reference load cell between the actuator crossheads and applying incremental static loads over the range of the load cell. The takeoff load cell (typically a button or bar-type) is typically calibrated using an external reference load cell testing apparatus since the load application is not controlled by the takeoff actuator. The instrumented die is calibrated in situ using a "plug" of material (e.g., rubber) that can reasonably induce a hydrostatic stress across the punch tips and die wall without extruding beyond the punch tips. As long as the load cells are not overloaded, their calibration is reasonably robust.

The displacement transducers (LVDTs) which measure the absolute punch positions must also be carefully calibrated. This is particularly important when conducting studies which require accurate in-die tablet thickness measurements. Like the punch load cells, the calibration of the LVDTs are also performed in situ using a reference displacement transducer. Statistical analysis has shown that the displacement versus voltage relationship may not be linear over the full range of some transducers, and could be better described by a third-order polynomial. However, over smaller ranges, the relationship is adequately linear (24). These effects should be taken into account for a particular experiment or application as they could propagate error into in-die tablet thickness measure and subsequent solid fraction calculations. Typically, calibration for both load cells and transducers are conducted once or twice annually.

Perhaps one of the most hotly debated criticisms of in-die tablet thickness measurements is the proper correction for machine and punch deformation. Because the punch system is not perfectly rigid, neglecting to correct for system deformation can also propagate error into punch displacement measurements. To correct for machine deflection, the crossheads or punch tips are brought into contact and the change in the upper and lower LVDT values are monitored as incrementally increasing forces are applied. The machine deflection is dependent on the machine rigidity, punch type, variability in contact area between the punch faces, the variability in the contact area between the punch heads and the punch holders, and the nonlinear elastic deformation of the screw threads along the actuator/punch holder components. Figure 11 shows that the total deformation of a compaction simulator is approximately 0.0075 mm/kN. The deformation is nonlinear and can be described in some systems by a second-order polynomial (24).

COMMON TYPES OF SIMULATION PROFILES

Hydraulic compaction simulators have the unique advantage of mimicking any compaction displacement profile. Common profiles for pharmaceutical studies include sawtooth (or linear), sinusoidal, and rotary tablet press waveforms. In some cases, the profile

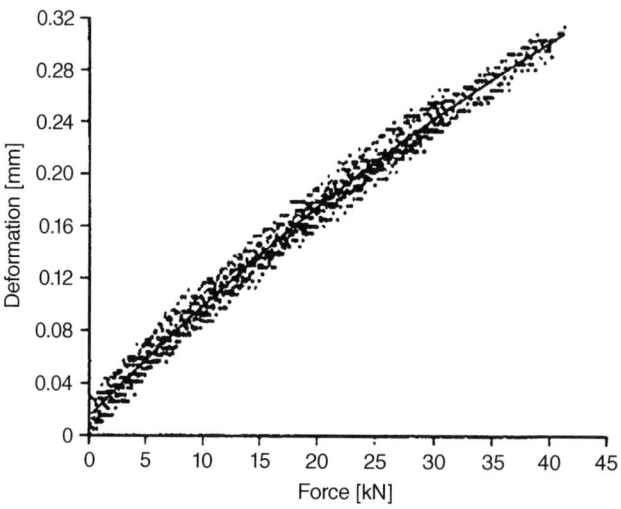

FIGURE 11 Total deformation of punches and machine parts of a compaction simulator under load. *Source*: Adapted from Ref. 24.

Compaction Simulation

requires double-sided compression where both punches are moving. In other cases, the profile requires single-sided compression where the lower punch remains stationary for the compression while the upper punch is moving to compress the powder. Since high-speed machines are operated using "displacement control," these profiles can be generated mathematically and input into the control system software.

Linear Profiles

Linear profiles are the simplest profiles to use for powder compressions. Typically, a sawtooth or v-shaped profile is used where the punch is extended at a constant velocity and retracts at a constant velocity. In theory, during a sawtooth profile, the punch reverses its motion instantaneously between the compression and a decompression strokes. At low speeds (e.g., <1 mm/sec), the hydraulic response system can easily accommodate this discontinuity. However, at high speeds (>100 mm/sec), the control system may show a small lag in the position-time waveform (<10 milliseconds) as it attempts to rapidly reverse the direction of punch. The sawtooth waveform is commonly used for more fundamental compression studies (e.g., Heckel analysis), where the desired powder volume reduction is proportional to time. It is also useful when evaluating instrument performance during factory acceptance testing.

The sawtooth waveform can be augmented to create a trapezoidal profile. Like the sawtooth profile, the trapezoidal profile uses constant compression and decompression rates. However, between the compression and decompression segments an intentional "dwell time" is incorporated. The dwell time is often defined as the time that the moving punches remain stationary at their furthest point of travel. This type of profile is useful when studying either the effects of compression rate or dwell time on powder compression behavior.

Sinusoidal Profiles

Sine curves are relevant to pharmaceutical solid dosage manufacturing unit operations such as modeling the displacement behavior of a roll on a tablet press or roller compactor. Since sine curves have natural (more gradual) acceleration and deceleration regions within their waveforms compared to linear waveforms, it is easier for a compaction simulator to respond accurately to the command profile.

Sinusoidal profiles are used to model the longitudinal (i.e., y) or latitudinal (i.e., x) displacement (D) of a point around the perimeter of a rotating circle. The following equation describes a typical sinusoidal waveform using the circle radius (R), rotation rate (ω), and time (t).

$$D = R \sin(\omega t) \tag{3}$$

This type of simulation has been reported to be effective in mimicking a roller compaction compression cycle as shown in Figure 12 (4). When $t = 0$, the punches begin their travel towards one another and compress the powder at the same strain rate as in the real roller compaction process. The "crest" of the sine wave correlates to the point at which the punches (or roller points) reach their minimum separation and can be used to target the thickness of the simulated ribbons. Once the punches reach their minimum separation, they retract to decompress the ribbon before it is ejected by the lower punch to the die surface. This simulation utilizes a "batch" process to mimic a continuous one. As such, it does not account for roller compaction variables associated with continuous

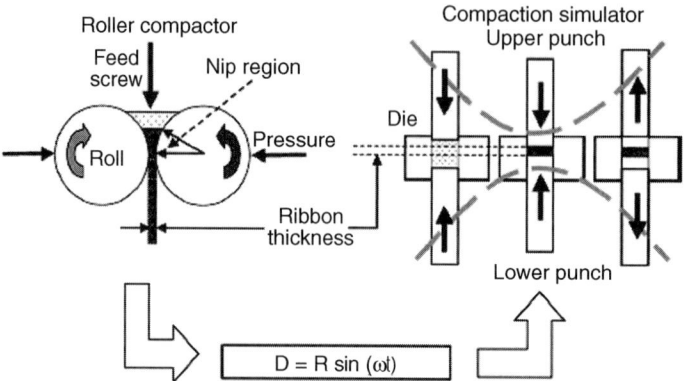

FIGURE 12 Simulating a roller compactor using a compaction simulator. *Source*: Adapted from Ref. 4.

operation such as powder feed mechanisms, the nature of the shear forces experienced by the powder or the transition from the slip to no-slip region of compaction. For the simulation purposes, the contact of the upper punch with the powder during compression can be considered to simulate the onset of the no-slip region. Despite these factors, the simulation is considered as a representative tool for formation of ribbons since it enables control of the critical process variables such as roll separation, speed, pressure and radius. Various tooling shapes and surface designs can be used to produce a representative ribbon sample for further processing (e.g., milling) or physical property testing (e.g., solid fraction and tensile strength).

Eccentric Tablet Press Simulation

Eccentric tablet presses are single station tablet presses that use an eccentric shaft connected to a rotating wheel to control the displacement of the upper punch into the die. The *Encyclopedia of Pharmaceutical Technology* provides a good summary of the construction and function of an eccentric tablet press (25). The details of its operation are not reported here since it is the only simulation of the compression cycle that is of interest to this chapter. In an eccentric press, the displacement profile of the upper punch is sinusoidal and the displacement rate is controlled by adjusting the rotation rate of the eccentric wheel. The lower punch remains stationary during the compression and acts only to enable uniform die filling prior to tablet formation and tablet ejection after tablet formation.

The two most important differences between an eccentric press and a rotary tablet press are (*i*) eccentric presses utilize single-sided compression to make tablets, where rotary presses use double-sided compression, and (*ii*) eccentric press compression cycles do not have a dwell time, where rotary presses typically use a punch head flat which enables a dwell time as the punch passes under the compression roller. Additionally, the degree of machine deflection is different for these different presses. These differences have been reported to have a significant effect on the energy of compaction (26). Figure 13 shows the difference in the pressure displacement waveforms as microcrystalline cellulose is compressed on an eccentric and rotary tablet press. These subtle differences should be taken into consideration when simulating or scaling up powder compression processes using these types of simulations.

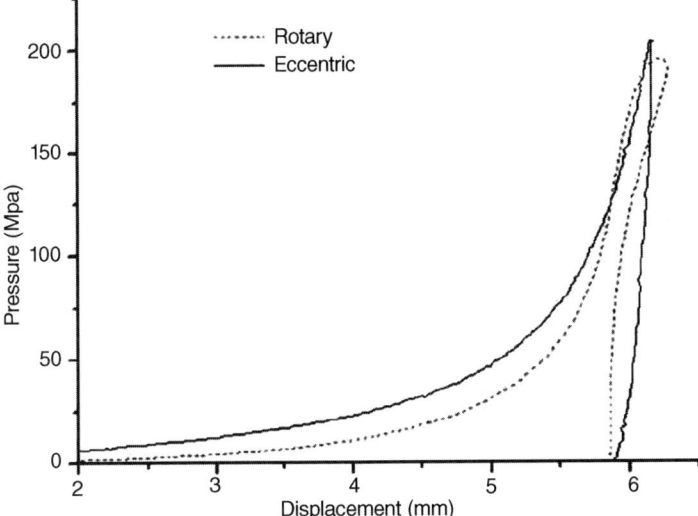

FIGURE 13 The difference in the pressure-displacement waveforms as microcrystalline cellulose is compressed on an eccentric and rotary tablet press. *Source*: Adapted from Ref. 26.

Rotary Tablet Press Simulation

Nearly, all commercial tablets are produced using a rotary tablet press since these machines are designed for high volume and low cost production. However, it is impractical to conduct laboratory scale tableting studies on these relatively large presses since they consume a significant quantity of bulk material and require long setup times. Therefore, compaction simulators are often preferred for studying tableting performance using a rotary press simulation mode.

The basic powder compression operation of a rotary tablet press is rather simple and is essentially the same from machine to machine (Fig. 14). The powders are compressed by passing the upper and lower punch between two rollers (or cams), thus mechanically driving punches towards one another to a specified target tip separation. The distance between the rollers can be adjusted to control the maximum degree of powder consolidation within the die (i.e., minimum tip separation), which has a direct influence on final tablet properties, such as thickness and crushing strength.

In the early 1980s, Rippie and Danielson published their quintessential paper describing the theoretical model for mimicking punch displacement on a rotary tablet press during the compression phase (27). Their model describes the vertical displacement (z) of the punch head as rotates with the turret along path "B" and its radius (r_2) is in contact with the compression roller (A) of radius r_1 (Fig. 15). When the punch head flat is in contact with the roller, there is no vertical displacement of the punch during the "dwell time." During the dwell time the vertical displacement is equal to r_1 plus r_2 and is a function of the punch head flat radius (x_2) and the turret rotation rate (ω). The decompression displacement is a mirror image of the compression displacement.

$$z = \left[(r_1 + r_2)^2 - (r_3 \sin \omega t - x_2)^2\right]^{1/2} \qquad (4)$$

When the compression displacement, dwell time, and decompression displacement profiles are coupled together as command inputs to the control system on a compaction simulator, a compete compression cycle is formed. The command displacement input,

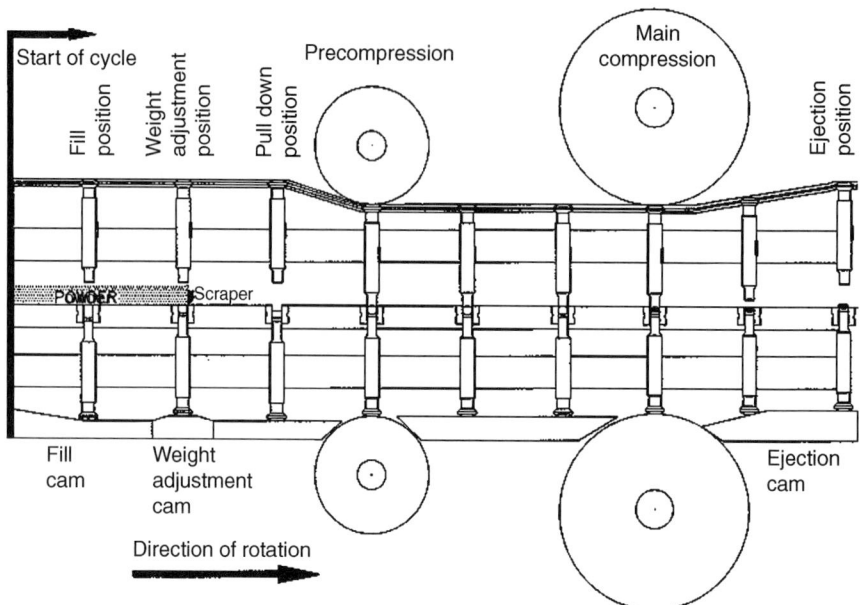

FIGURE 14 Rotary tablet press compression cycle. *Source*: Adapted from Ref. 6.

actual displacement measurement, and force measurement waveforms from a typical compression cycle are shown in Figure 16.

TABLET PRESS DYNAMICS

Compaction simulators are beneficial solid dosage formulation development because of their manufacturing versatility. They can be outfitted with a variety of tooling designs and can simulate a nearly infinite range of realistic compression profiles through the

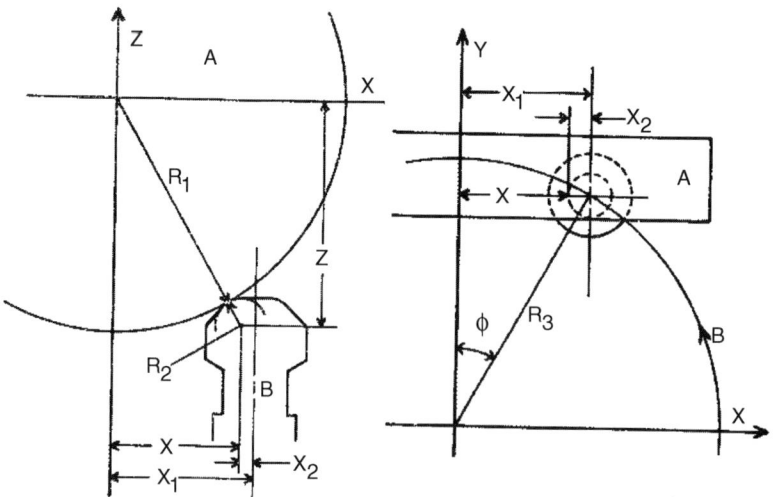

FIGURE 15 Model for vertical displacement of a punch head on a rotary press. *Source*: Adapted from Ref. 27.

Compaction Simulation

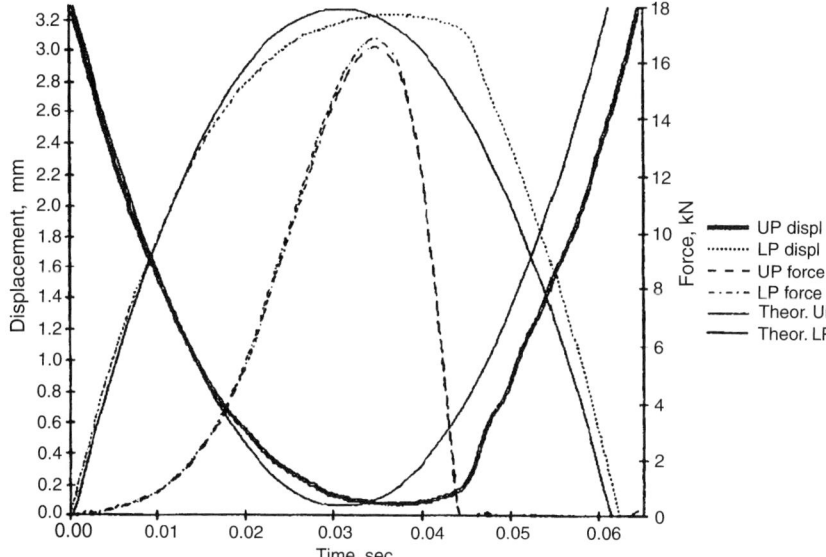

FIGURE 16 Theoretical and simulated punch displacement profiles for a 16-station Manesty Betapress operating at 70 RPM. *Source*: Adapted from Ref. 55.

careful control of punch displacement. The speed, shape, and duration of the punch profile can significantly affect the compression behavior of the powder (e.g., yield pressure) and the resultant tablet properties (e.g., solid fraction and crushing strength). Therefore, during the design of a compaction simulator experiment, the following factors should be considered.

Single- or Double-Ended Compression

Most rotary tablet presses use double-ended compression during the process of tablet manufacturing. This means that during the compaction cycle, both the upper punch and lower punch are moving in unison inside the die—towards each other during compression, holding at a fixed position during any dwell time, and away from each other during decompression. Most single punch tablet presses use single-ended compression during the process of tablet manufacture. In this case, the lower punch remains in a fixed position inside of the die, usually at the fill position, while the upper punch progresses through the compression phase, dwell phase (if any), and decompression phase. Single station tablet presses (or eccentric presses) are designed where a cam and shaft are used to "eccentrically" move the upper punch in and out of the die. This results in a sinusoidal upper punch displacement waveform, which has no dwell time.

The stress and density distribution in uniaxially compacted tablets is non-homogenous (Fig. 17) (28). Particle–particle interaction, particle–punch interactions, intrinsic powder properties, and applied forces all affect the degree of the distributions.

In an ideal case for double-sided compaction, the middle of the powder bed represents the equivalent force plane (29). Therefore, the stress and density distribution above and below this plain should be equivalent. However, in single-sided compaction, the powder in contact with the lower punch may only experience a fraction of the force applied by the upper punch due to punch-die-powder friction. It has been shown that in single-sided compaction the compact surface (i.e., top of the tablet) in contact with the

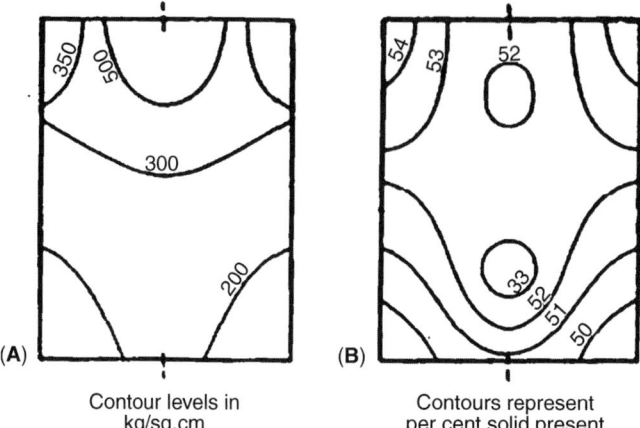

FIGURE 17 Stress and solid fraction distribution of uniaxially compacted powders. *Source*: Adapted from Ref. 28.

moving punch (i.e., upper punch) is harder than the compact surface (i.e., bottom of the tablet) in contact with the stationary punch (i.e., lower punch) (30). These phenomena should be taken into consideration when simulating tablet compression cycles and evaluating tablet manufacturing performance.

Effect of Precompression and Relative Roller Position

Precompression is often used to tamp or apply a small compression force prior to the main compact compression cycle. Rotary tablet presses are often equipped with a separate precompression station, which is positioned between the die-filling feed frame and the main compression station. Typically, precompression is used to improve the quality of tableted products, where it increases the strength of the compact and/or decreases the incidences of capping and lamination. The compact strength is enhanced through the increase in the effective contact time in which the powder particles are in contact under an applied force. During this extended contact time, stronger interparticulate bonds form and stress relaxation occurs.

Akande and coworkers describe a compaction simulator experiment in the literature where they studied the effect of precompression on the quality of a binary tablet formulation (31). They conclude that the application of both a precompression and main compression is preferred over a single main compression for enhancing tablet quality. The improvement in tablet quality was shown to be due to an increase in plastic flow and bond formation with a decrease in elastic energy. Ruegger and Celik concur that precompression can enhance tablet strength (32). Their work showed that the effect on the tensile strength as a function of the ratio and magnitude of the pre and main compression forces is material-dependent. Therefore, each tablet formulation must be evaluated to determine the appropriate force combinations to apply during pre and main compression to optimize tablet strength. Further work by Rugger and Celik showed that the relative position of the pre and main compression stations does not have a significant effect on tablet strength.

Effect of Compression Roller Size

The diameter of the compression roller and punch head geometry can both affect tablet manufacturing performance. The compression roller diameter controls the rate and duration of compression as it forces the punch into the die. Punches traveling around the turret that contact larger diameter compression rollers will have a (*i*) earlier contact time with the roller, (*ii*) lower compression/decompression velocity, (*iii*) longer compression contact time, and (*iv*) later contact break with the roller.

It is reported in the literature that these effects are particularly important for time plasticity dependent materials, such as microcrystalline cellulose, for both low and high degrees of densification. The increased contact time and decreased compression velocity allows for stress relaxation to occur. For brittle materials, such as dibasic calcium phosphate, larger roll wheels enable slower decompression of the compact during elastic recovery and may decrease the tendency for tablet failure at high degrees of densification (33).

Effect of Tablet Press Speed, Dwell Time and Strain Rate

Punch displacement velocity (i.e., strain rate) and dwell time are two factors that can significantly affect the compression behavior of powders. Several authors have published on the fundamentals of these effects in the literature (34–38). As a general rule of thumb, slower compression and decompression speeds and longer dwell times will improve the mechanical properties of a tablet. When particles are subjected to a compression force for a longer period of time, further plastic yielding can occur and the degree of elastic recovery is reduced. Figure 18 shows the range of dwell times that are achievable with a variety of rotary tablet presses (http://www.mcc-online.com/).

Roberts and Rowe studied the effect of compression speed on the yield pressure of a variety of pharmaceutical powders compressed on a compaction simulator (Fig. 19). They found that, in general, powders exhibited an increased resistance to deformation with increasing punch velocity. The influence of punch velocity was dependent on the fragmentation and/or plastic yielding propensity of the material. Materials which consolidate by fragmentation (e.g., calcium phosphate) were less speed sensitive than materials which consolidate by plastic yielding (e.g., microcrystalline cellulose) (39).

If bonding does not occur among particles or the elastic strain recovery is too great, low tablet hardness and capping or lamination are likely to occur. Capping tendency was found to increase significantly with an increase in compaction speed for paracetomol formulations. The increase was attributed to a higher increase in elastic energy relative to

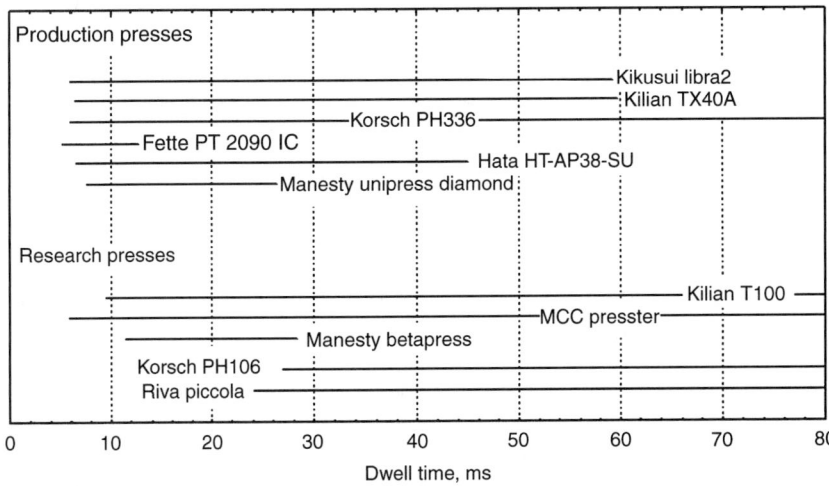

FIGURE 18 Comparison of dwell times for a variety of production and research tablet presses. *Source*: Adapted from Ref. 56.

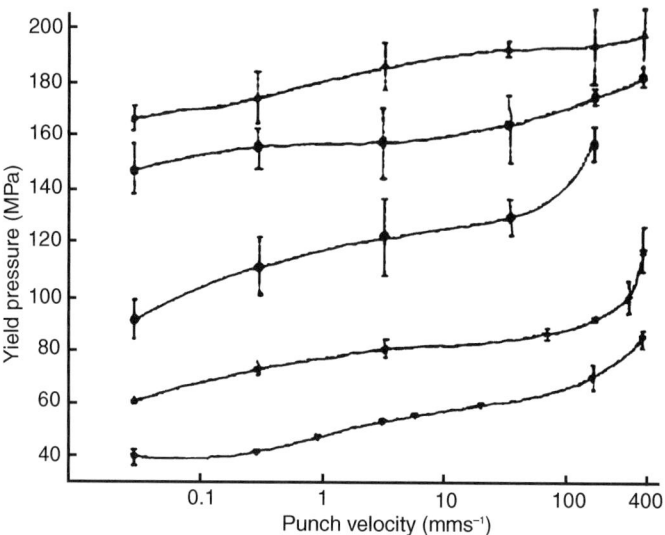

FIGURE 19 Yield pressure versus punch velocity for a variety of pharmaceutical powders. *Source*: Adapted from Ref. 39.

plastic energy. A semi-logarithmic relationship between the applied punch pressure that caused capping to occur and the compression speed has been reported (40).

The simplest method for enabling slower compression/decompression speed and longer dwell times is to reduce the simulated tablet product rate. On a compaction simulator, these parameters can be adjusted independently to study their effects on compact compression performance. If tablet production rate is a concern on a rotary tablet press, increasing the diameter of the punch head flat will result in longer dwell times. Standard or custom punches can be used for this purpose (6).

Compression Modeling

Because compaction simulators are highly instrumented to measure displacement and stresses during the compression of powders, they are well suited to generate material property data necessary to parameterize computational compression models. The detailed discussion of compression modeling is outside of the scope of this chapter, however, it is important to point out that compaction simulators are an integral component to the calibration and validation of the models.

For example, the Drucker–Prager Cap model is commonly used in finite element modeling to model the stress and density distribution of a consolidated powder. Sinka and coworkers have demonstrated that a compaction simulator can be used to parameterize necessary model input parameters such as Young's modulus, Poisson's ratio, cohesion, friction angle, cap eccentricity parameter, and hydrostatic yield stress as a function of relative density and/or volumetric plastic strain (41–43). These material and compression condition specific parameters can be input into finite element modeling software to simulate different compression conditions (e.g., degree of consolidation, tooling shape, and tooling size). A typical output simulation with cutaways of the tablet cross section (used for validation) is shown in Figure 20.

Modeling can also be used to identify the potential failure modes of compacted powders. Wu and coworkers showed that during powder compression of cylindrical tablets an intensive shear band can form from the top corners to the mid-center of the

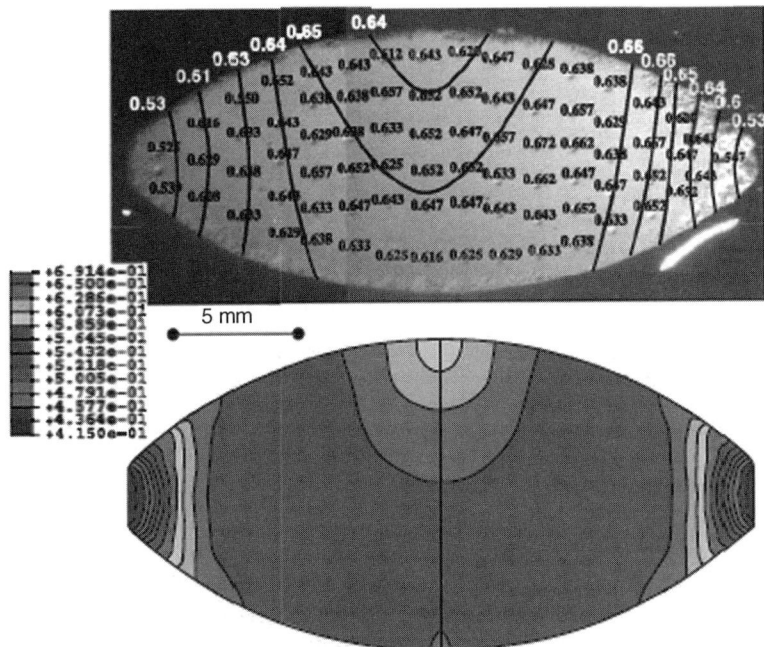

FIGURE 20 Experimental map and numerical simulation of the relative density distribution in a microcrystalline cellulose tablet. *Source*: From Ref. 57.

tablet (44). This stress concentrated region can result in severe capping in the tablet as shown experimentally in tablets made on a compaction simulator (Fig. 21). These and other types of models can be extremely useful for visualizing and understanding phenomenological elements of powder compaction.

EXAMPLES OF COMPACTION SIMULATOR APPLICATIONS

Preformulation

Compaction simulation is a powerful tool early in the solid dosage formulation development process. Compaction simulators are ideal for characterizing powder compression behavior because they can be setup to mimic a range of compression (punch displacement) profiles. Macroscopically, the physics of powder compression seems quite simple

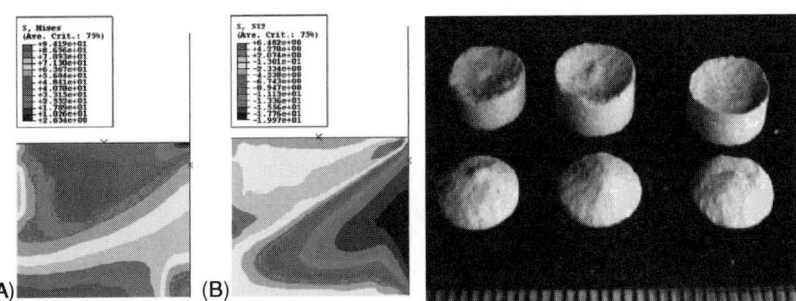

FIGURE 21 Numerical simulations of stress distributions in uni-axially compacted tablets (**A,B**), and the resultant tablet capping phenomenon. *Source*: Adapted from Ref. 44.

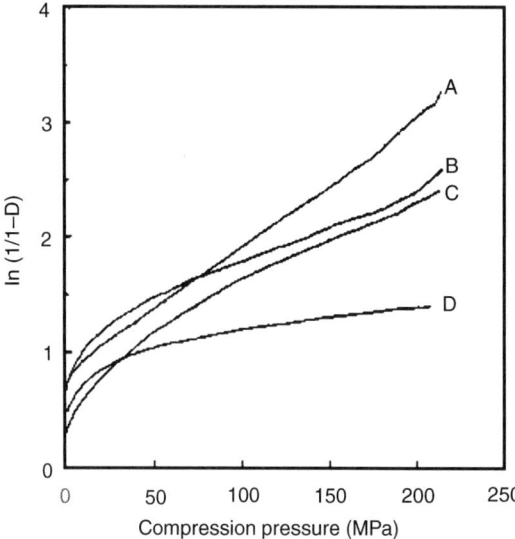

FIGURE 22 Typical Heckel plot for single component materials: A pregelatinized starch, B lactose, C microcrystalline cellulose, and D dicalcium phosphate dihydrate. *Source*: Adapted from Ref. 48.

where a punch and die set are used to apply enough force to the powder to form (and ideally retain) interparticulate bonds in the formed compact. However, powder compression behavior is influenced by a several factors including powder composition, powder moisture content, powder particle size distribution, speed of compaction, applied force, machine elasticity, tooling design, and powder/tooling thermodynamics. Therefore, these experimental parameters must be carefully controlled and monitored to properly characterize powder compression behavior.

One of the most powerful capabilities of a compaction simulator is to measure in real time the applied force and punch displacement profiles. These profile waveforms can be studied to study the stresses and strains applied over the compaction cycle. These waveforms can be used in part or in their entirety to measure or derive semi-intrinsic

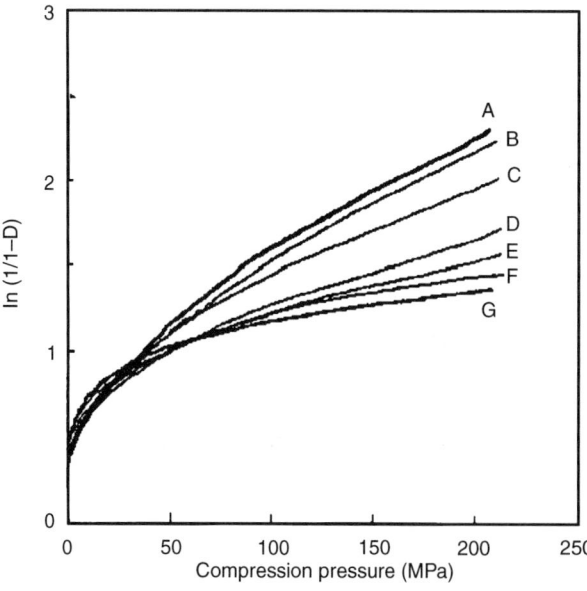

FIGURE 23 Heckel plots for binary mixtures of microcrystalline cellulose. *Source*: Adapted from Ref. 48.

properties of the powder. The term semi-intrinsic is used here because each powder sample, laboratory, machine, and profile are unique. However, when some or all of the testing parameters are standardized, material properties, such as work of compaction, yield pressure, degree of plastic deformation, and elastic recovery can be measured. These types of values are particularly useful for benchmarking material relative performance and as inputs to computer simulations of compression models (i.e., finite element modeling). The details of these measurements and their relevance are discussed in another chapter. Further discussion of the physics of compaction has also been recently reported (45).

It is often difficult to form coherent compacts of single powders that are not designed for direct compression applications (e.g., APIs). Therefore, in-die compression tests can be used to characterize and rank the plastic and/or elastic behavior of powders. These characterization test results can be used to intelligently select complementary formulation components to compensate for any material deficiencies. Heckel analysis is one of the most commonly used in-die compression tests for studying powder densification behavior (46,47). Figure 22 shows that the shape and slope of a "Heckel plot" is material dependent. Materials with smaller slopes along the linear portion of the Heckel plot have a higher yield pressure, indicating that it is more difficult to induce plastic deformation within the powder as it is compressed into a compact.

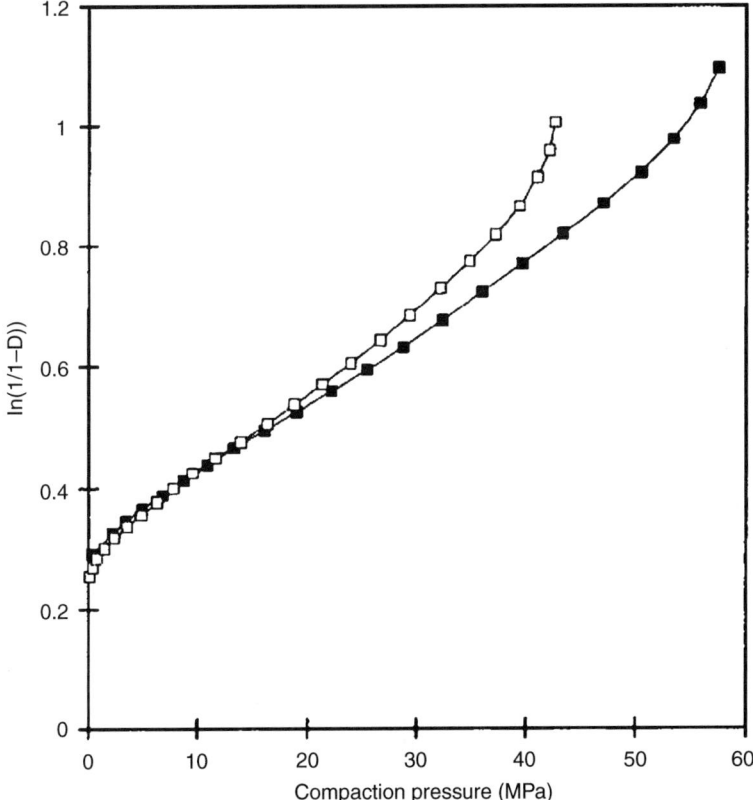

FIGURE 24 Effect of particle size and punch velocity on the compression behavior of polyethylene oxide. *Source*: From Ref. 49.

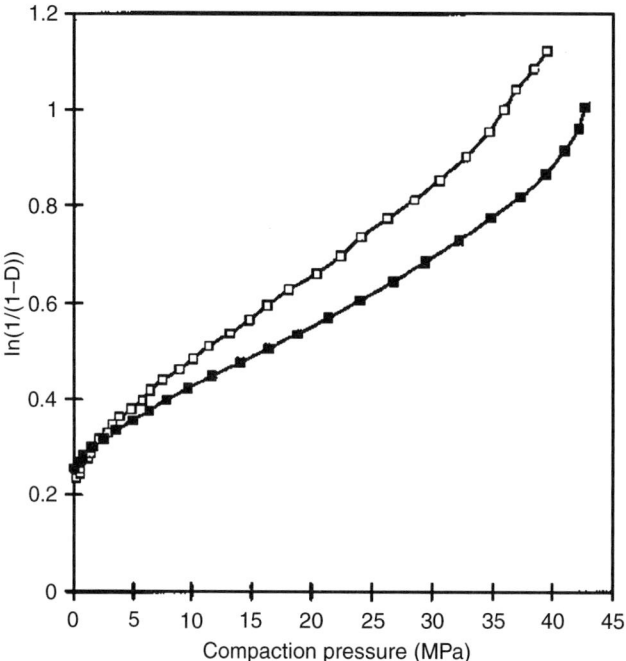

FIGURE 25 Effect of particle size and punch velocity on the compression behavior of polyethylene oxide. *Source*: From Ref. 49.

Ilkka and Paronen used Heckel plots to study the compression properties of binary powder blends mixed in different proportions (48). Their Heckel plot data showed that blended materials act like intermediate materials between the plain mixture components (Fig. 23). However, the binary blend properties could not be modeled using simple arithmetic means of the single components. Typically, one material had a dominant effect on the powder densification behavior.

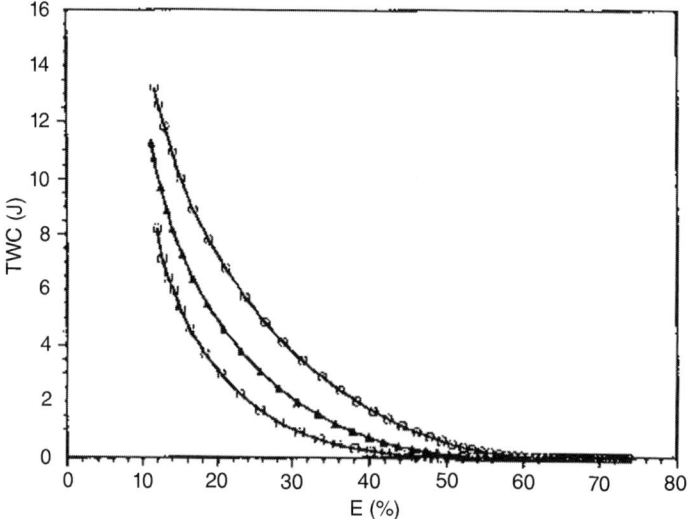

FIGURE 26 Total work of compaction plots for binary mixtures of microcrystalline cellulose and an active pharmaceutical ingredient. *Source*: Adapted from Ref. 50.

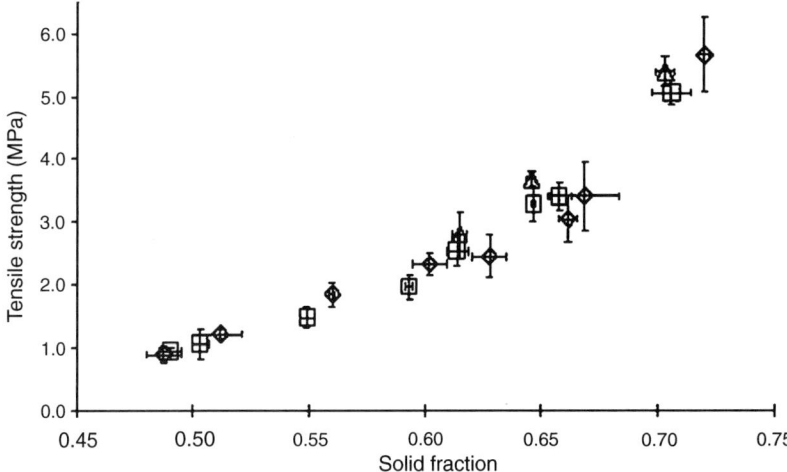

FIGURE 27 Compactability of ribbons produced on a roller compactor and a compaction simulator. *Source*: Adapted from Ref. 4.

Compaction simulators are also useful in the preformulation of a solid oral dosage form to investigate the effect of powder particle size and morphology. Yang et al. report a comparative analysis of eight different grades of polyethylene oxide using Heckel analysis from compaction simulator data (49). Heckel plots revealed that the yield pressure of PEO is relatively low and the yield pressure was significantly dependent on particle size and compression speed (Fig. 24 and 25). The careful characterization of different grades of this excipient enabled a rational approach to the selection of complementary brittle excipients to form tablets with acceptable hardness.

Celik and coworkers demonstrated how additional analysis beyond Heckel analysis can be useful for powder compression characterization with a compaction simulator (50). In addition to the compaction of 100% API compacts, compacts with a range of microcrystalline cellulose additions were tested. It was found that the crystalline API would not form compacts without the addition of the microcrystalline cellulose, regardless of API particle size or crystal structure. Heckel plots, total work of compaction, and net work of compaction plots were used to compare the mixtures of API and microcrystalline cellulose. Celik et al. found that the Heckel plots were not appropriate for discriminating differences in the resulting crushing strength of the tablets formulated with different proportions of MCC. However, the total work of compaction and the net work of compaction plots were discriminating (Fig. 26).

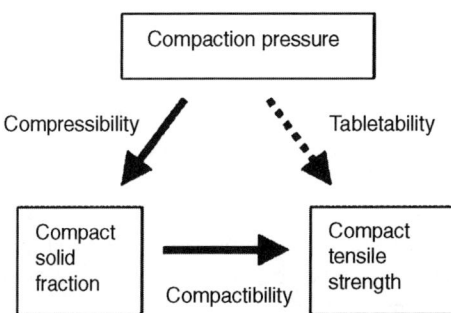

FIGURE 28 Relationships among compaction pressure, solid fraction, and tensile strength for a given powder. *Source*: Adapted from Ref. 52.

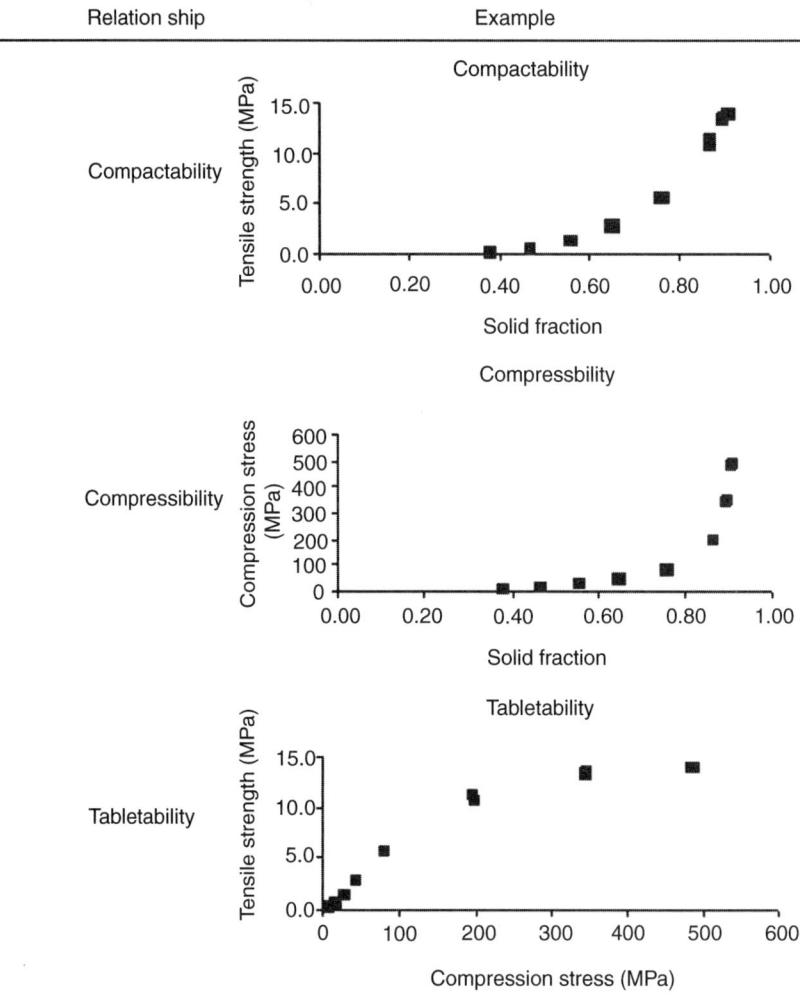

FIGURE 29 Example data for compactability, compressibility, and tabletability relationships.

Formulation

Compaction simulators are also particularly useful for dosage form design experiments, especially when bulk quantities are limited. Compaction simulation allows a small-scale approach to exploring composition and process effects on the manufacturing performance of solid oral dosage forms. Since a compaction simulator can be used to evaluate the manufacturing performance of as little as one tablet's worth of powder using production type conditions, formulations can be screened or evaluated using a fraction of the material required for the laboratory or production scale unit operations.

As reported earlier, compaction simulators can be equipped to replicate the compression process of a roller compactor. Zinchuk et al. describe how a compaction simulator can be used to produce ribbons and determine the formulation specific compactability relationship (tensile strength vs. solid fraction) (Fig. 27) (4). Since compacts produced under equivalent stress–strain conditions exhibit similar mechanical properties, the ribbon solid fraction and/or tensile strength can be used as a scale-up factor for pilot and eventually commercial scale manufacturing.

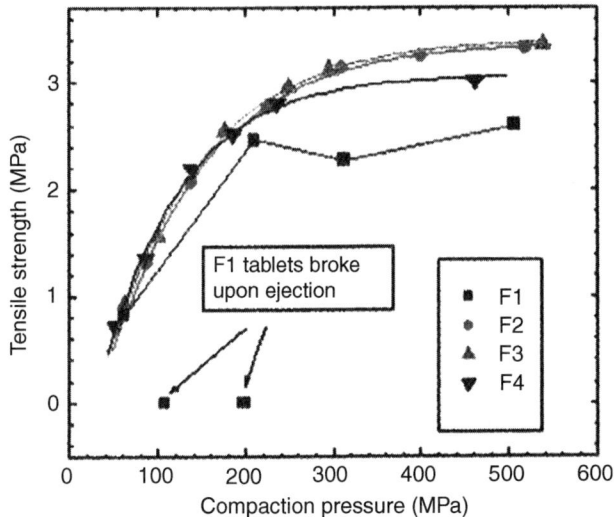

FIGURE 30 Compaction profiles for tablets of different formulations evaluated using a compaction simulator. *Source*: Adapted from Ref. 53.

Mahmoudi et al. used a material sparing approach to develop a formulation and manufacturing process for a drug substance with poor mechanical properties (51). Their work demonstrated how roller compaction parameters and ribbon properties (solid fraction and tensile strength) affected the particle size distribution and tableting performance of four tablet formulations. Although they did not use roller compaction simulation as described by Zinchuk and coworkers, it would have been a material sparing alternative to roller compacting relatively large batches on a roller compactor.

Compaction simulators are most commonly used to replicate the compaction process of a rotary tablet press. Manufacturing parameters, such as production speed, dwell time, compression force, precompression force are often studied using a relatively small quantity of bulk powder. These parameters can significantly affect tablet crushing strength, friability, and disintegration time. The relationship among compaction pressure,

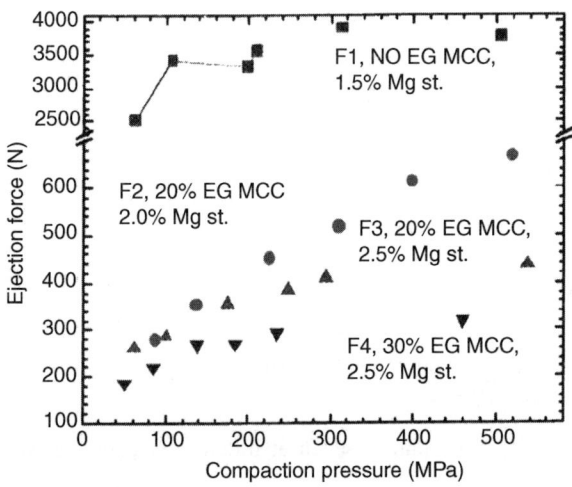

FIGURE 31 Ejection profiles for tablets of different formulations evaluated using a compaction simulator. *Source*: Adapted from Ref. 53.

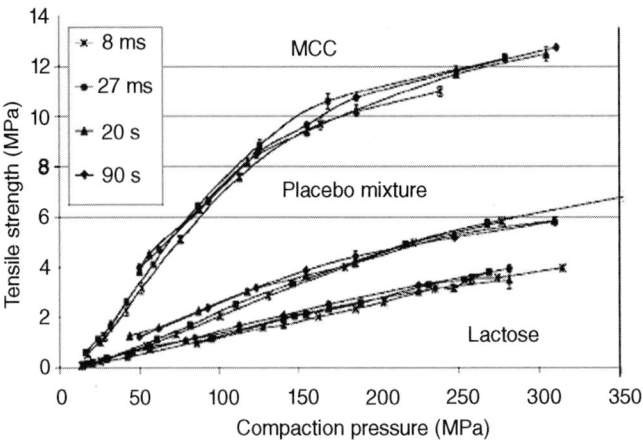

FIGURE 32 Tabletability of various excipients at a range of tableting speeds. *Source*: Adapted from Ref. 52.

compact solid fraction, and compact tensile strength has been described by Tye and coworkers (Fig. 28) (52). The compactability, compressibility and tabletability relationships shown in Figure 29 can be used to evaluate compaction behavior as a function of formulation composition or rotary tablet press operating parameters.

An example of tablet formulation development using a compaction simulator in literature is presented by Fu et al. (53). Fu et al. compare the tableting performance of five formulations. All formulations were wet granulated with 25% active API. By studying relative compaction profiles, tablet ejection forces, and punch force transfer ratios, they were able to probe the robustness of a drug product in early formulation development using very little material and several different compositions (e.g., extragranular microcrystalline cellulose and lubricant level) (Fig. 30 and 31). Upon scale-up to a pilot scale tablet press, the tableting profiles from the compaction simulator and the rotary press were nearly superimposable, demonstrating the predictive power of the

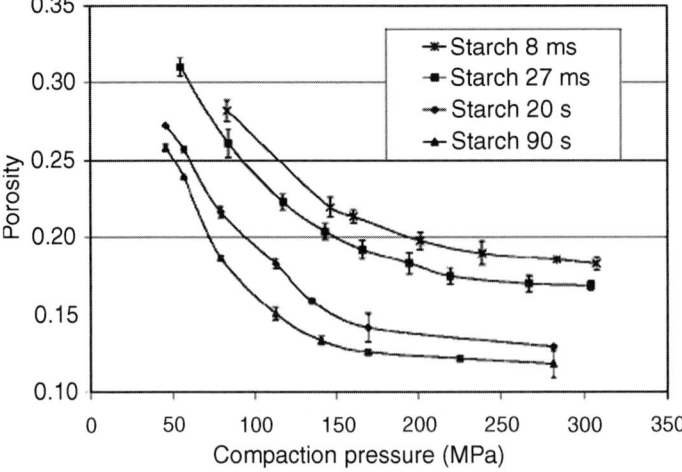

FIGURE 33 Compressibility profiles for pre-gelatinized starch at different tableting speeds. *Source*: Adapted from Ref. 52.

Compaction Simulation

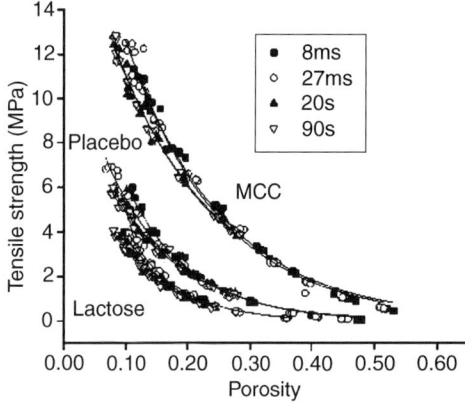

FIGURE 34 Compactability profiles for various excipients at a range of tableting speeds. *Source*: Adapted from Ref. 52.

compaction simulator experiments where the instrument can be used to quantitatively predict tablet manufacturing performance using a fraction of the material normally required for pilot scale runs. The data from these types of small-scale experiments can be used to fingerprint formulation performance and track product changes over the product development lifetime.

Scale-Up and Production

Scale-up of the tableting process is a critical step in tablet manufacturing and often causes time consuming operations. Compaction simulators are designed to mimic high-speed rotary tablet presses with a minimum quantity of material in the early stage of

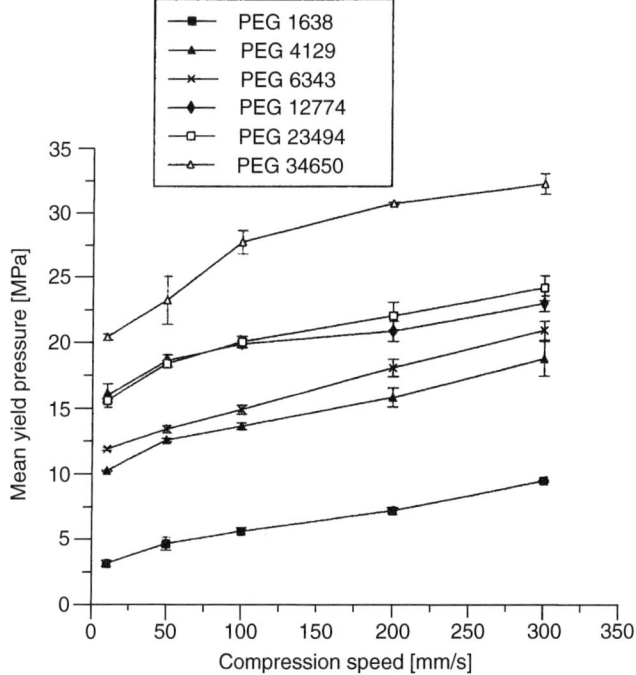

FIGURE 35 Effect of compression speed and molecular weight on mean yield pressure of PEG compacts. *Source*: Adapted from Ref. 37.

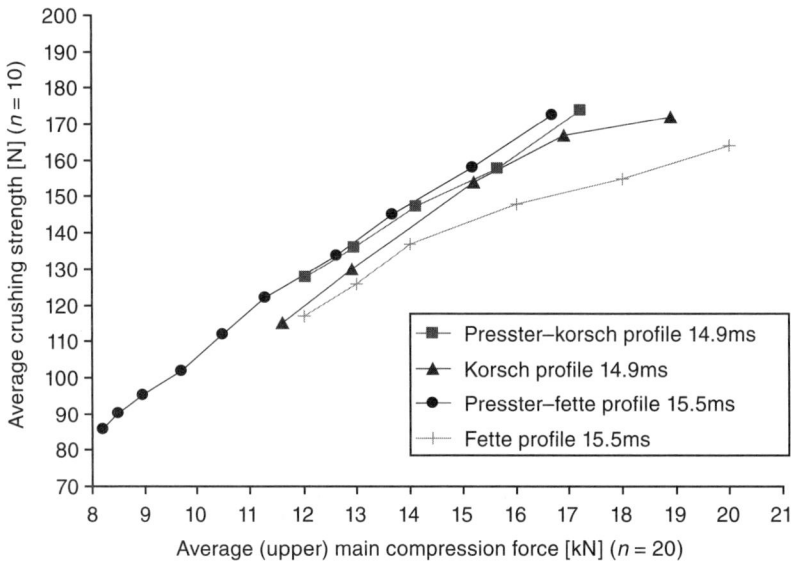

FIGURE 36 Comparison of compression force versus crushing strength for tablets produced on a Presster, Korsch Ph 300e/29 (14.9 milliseconds dwell time) and a Fette PT 2090/29 (15.5 milliseconds dwell time).

development. They are highly versatile for studying the impact of changing tooling designs, production speeds, press types, and formulation composition/process parameters. For example, if a particular tablet demonstrated acceptable manufacturing performance on a pilot scale rotary tablet press, a compaction simulator could be used to evaluate the performance impact of increasing throughput (i.e., compression rate) on the same press or transfer to another type of press.

The effect of production scale tableting speed is a common parameter to explore using the compaction simulator, due to its known influence during scale-up. Tye et al. demonstrate the utility of tabletability, compressibility, and compactability curves for comparison of excipients at a range of compression speeds (52). Several different formulations were tested at a range of dwell times to determine the effect on the resulting tablets. The goal of the study was to show that the compactability of a powder is not affected by the tableting speed. Tye et al. were able to show that over a range of common pharmaceutical powders the compactability profile remains relatively constant over a range of tableting speeds (Figs. 32–34).

The effect of compression speed and compression force was also shown for a series of polyethylene glycols with different molecular weights (37). Larhrib and coworkers showed that the molecular weight of the PEG and the compression speed both interact to affect the mean yield pressure of the material. By using the effect of molecular weight and compression speed, the different molecular weights of PEG were rank ordered by their compressibility (Fig. 35).

An example of the scale-up of a four marketed products from a compaction simulator (Presster) to a production scale press was illustrated by Guntermann. Compression force/crushing strength profiles of routine production batches of four marketed products were replicated on Presster. Figure 36 shows an example of one of these compounds. Compression force/crushing strength profiles are compared between a Presster and a Fette PT 2090/29 at 14.9 milliseconds dwell time and between a Presster and a Korsch

Ph 300e/29 at 15.5 milliseconds dwell time. When the tablets were compressed to the same resulting compression force, the band height (punch to punch distance) set up on Presster partly deviated significantly from the band height set up on a rotary tablet press, leading to differently densified tablets. Compression with the same punch to punch distances on different machines led to comparable thickness and crushing strength of the tablets. Guntermann was able to show that, with proper setup, compaction simulation can be a good model of production scale presses (54).

ACKNOWLEDGEMENTS

The authors thank Bruno C. Hancock for his mentorship and review of this book chapter.

REFERENCES

1. Royce A, et al. Scale-up of the compaction and tableting process. Drugs Pharm Sci 2006; 371–408.
2. Celik M, Marshall K, Use of a compaction simulator system in tabletting research. I. Introduction to and initial experiments with the system. Drug Dev Indust Pharm 1989; 15(5):759–800.
3. Mehrotra A, et al. Influence of shear intensity and total shear on properties of blends and tablets of lactose and cellulose lubricated with magnesium stearate. Int J Pharm 2007; 336(2):284–91.
4. Zinchuk AV, Mullarney MP, and BC, Hancock, Simulation of roller compaction using a laboratory scale compaction simulator. Int J Pharm 2004; 269(2):403–15.
5. Bateman SD, et al. A comparative investigation of compression simulators. Int J Pharm 1989; 49:209–12.
6. Young LL, Tableting Specification Manual, 4th ed. Washington, DC: Americal Pharmaceutical Association, 1995.
7. Jackson S, Sinka IC, Cocks ACF, The effect of suction during die fill on a rotary tablet press. Eur J Pharm Biopharm 2007; 65(2):253–56.
8. Hirai Y, Okada J. Effect of lubricant on die wall friction during the compaction of pharmaceutical powders. Chem Pharm Bull 1982; 30(2):684–94.
9. Mollan MJ, Jr, Celik M. The effects of lubrication on the compaction and post-compaction properties of directly compressible maltodextrins. Int J Pharm 1996; 144(1):1–9.
10. Nelson E.. Physics of tablet compression VIII. Some preliminary measurements of die wall pressure during tablet compression. J Am Pharm Assoc 1955; XLIV(8):494–7.
11. Hoag SW, Nair R, Muller FX. Force–transducer–design optimization for the measurement of die-wall stress in a compaction simulator. Pharm Pharmacol Commun 2000; 6(7):293–8.
12. Yeh C, Altaf SA, Hoag SW. Theory of force transducer design optimization for die wall stress measurement during tablet compaction: optimization and validation of split-web die using finite element analysis. Pharm Res 1997; 14(9):1161–70.
13. Doelker E, Massuelle D. Benefits of die-wall instrumentation for research and development in tabletting. Eur J Pharm Biopharm 2004; 58(2):427–44.
14. Waimer F, et al. The influence of engravings on the sticking of tablets. Investigations with an instrumented upper punch. Pharm Dev Technol 1999; 4(3):369–75.
15. Waimer F, et al. A novel method for the detection of sticking of tablets. Pharm Dev Tech 1999; 4(3):359–67.
16. Roberts M, et al. Effects of surface roughness and chrome plating of punch tips on the sticking tendencies of model ibuprofen formulations. J Pharm Pharmacol 2003; 55(9):1223–8.

17. Roberts M, et al. Effect of punch tip geometry and embossment on the punch tip adherence of a model ibuprofen formulation. J Pharm Pharmacol 2004; 56(7):947–50.
18. Wang JJ, et al. Modeling of adhesion in tablet compression. II. Compaction studies using a compaction simulator and an instrumented tablet press. J Pharm Sci 2004; 93(2):407–17.
19. Takeuchi H, et al. Die wall pressure measurement for evaluation of compaction property of pharmaceutical materials. Int J Pharm 2004; 274(1–2):131–8.
20. Cocolas HG, Lordi NG, Axial to radial pressure transmission of tablet excipients using a novel instrumented die. Drug Dev Indust Pharm 1993; 19(17–18):2473–97.
21. Long W, Special Ceramics. London, New York: Academic Press, 1962: 327–40.
22. Unckel H, Vorgange beim Pressen vol Metallpulvern. Arch Eisenhuttenwesen 1945; 18:161–7.
23. Guyoncourt, DMM, et al. Measurement of friction for powder compaction modelling—comparison between laboratories. Powder Metallurgy 2000; 43(4):364–74.
24. Holman LE, Marshall K. Calibration of a compaction simulator for the measurement of tablet thickness during compression. Pharm Res 1993; 10(6):816–22.
25. Bogda MJ. Tablet Compression: Machine theory, design, and process troubleshooting. In: Swarbrick J, Boylan JC. ed. Encyclopedia of Pharmaceutical Technology. New York: Marcel Dekker, 1999: 249–86.
26. Palmieri GF, et al. Differences between eccentric and rotary tablet machines in the evaluation of powder densification behaviour. Int J Pharm 2005; 298(1):164–75.
27. Rippie EG, Danielson DW. Viscoelastic stress/strain behavior of pharmaceutical tablets: analysis during unloading and postcompression periods. J Pharm Sci 1981; 70(5):476–82.
28. Train D. Transmission of forces through a powder mass during the process of pelleting. Trans Inst Chem Eng 1957; 35:258–66.
29. Munoz–Ruiz A, et al. Frictional Work in Double-Sided Tablet Compression. J Pharm Sci 1997; 86(4):481–6.
30. Aulton ME. Indentation hardness profiles across the faces of some compressed tablets. Pharm Acta Helv 1981; 56(4–5):133–6.
31. Akande OF, Rubinstein MH, Ford JL. Examination of the compaction properties of a 1:1 acetaminophen:microcrystalline cellulose mixture using precompression and main compression. J Pharm Sci 1997; 86(8):900–7.
32. Ruegger CE, Celik M. The influence of varying precompaction and main compaction profile parameters on the mechanical strength of compacts. Pharmaceut Dev Technol 2000; 5(4):495–505.
33. Picker KM. The 3-d model: comparison of parameters obtained from and by simulating different tableting machines. AAPS PharmSciTech 2003; 4(3):E35.
34. Lloyd J, York P, Cook GD. Influence of compression rate on the mechanical properties of compacts. Cong Int Technol Pharm 6th 1992; 4:189–95.
35. Marshall PV, York P, Maclaine JQ. An investigation of the effect of the punch velocity on the compaction properties of ibuprofen. Powder Technol 1993; 74(2):171–7.
36. Nokhodchi A, et al. The effects of compression rate and force on the compaction properties of different viscosity grades of hydroxypropyl methyl cellulose 2208. Int J Pharm 1996; 129(1,2):21–31.
37. Larhrib H, Wells JI, Rubinstein MH. Compressing polyethylene glycols: the effect of compression pressure and speed. Int J Pharm 1997; 147(2):199–205.
38. Kim H, Venkatesh G. Compaction simulator study on pectin introducing dwell time. Yakche Hakhoechi 2005; 35(4):243–7.
39. Roberts RJ, Rowe RC. The effect of punch velocity on the compaction of a variety of materials. J Pharm Pharmacol 1985; 37:377–84.
40. Garr JSM, Rubinstein MH. An investigation into the capping of paracetamol at increasing speeds of compression. Int J Pharm 1991; 72(2):117–22.
41. Cunningham JC, Sinka IC, Zavaliangos A. Analysis of tablet compaction. I. Characterization of mechanical behavior of powder and powder/tooling friction. J Pharm Sci 2004; 93(8):2022–39.

42. Sinka IC, Cunningham JC, Zavaliangos A. Experimental characterization and numerical simulation of die wall friction in pharmaceutical powder compaction. Adv Powder Metallurgy Part Mater 2001: 1/46–1/60.
43. Sinka IC, Cunningham JC, Zavaliangos A. The effect of wall friction in the compaction of pharmaceutical tablets with curved faces: a validation study of the Drucker–Prager Cap model. Powder Technol 2003; 133(1–3):33–43.
44. Wu CY, et al. Modelling the mechanical behaviour of pharmaceutical powders during compaction. Powder Technol 2005; 152(1–3):107–17.
45. Patel S, Kaushal Aditya M, Bansal Arvind K. Compression physics in the formulation development of tablets. Crit Rev Therapeut Drug Carrier Systems 2006; 23(1):1–65.
46. Heckel RW. An analysis of powder compaction phenomena. Trans Metall Soc AIME 1961; 221:1001–8.
47. Heckel RW. Density-pressure relationships in powder compaction. Trans Metall Soc AIME 1961; 221(671–5):1001–8.
48. Ilkka J, Paronen P. Prediction of the compression behavior of powder mixtures by the Heckel equation. Int J Pharm 1993; 94(1–3):181–7.
49. Yang L, Venkatesh G, Fassihi a.R. Characterization of compressibility and compactibility of poly(ethylene oxide) polymers for modified release application by compaction simulator. J Pharm Sci 1996; 85(10):1085–90.
50. Celik M, et al. Compaction simulator studies of a new drug substance: effect of particle size and shape, and its binary mixtures with microcrystalline cellulose. Pharm Dev Technol 1996; 1(2):119–26.
51. Mahmoudi ZN, Alvarez-Nunez FA. Roller Compaction of a Poorly Compressible Drug Substance Chemically Incompatible with Typical Functional Excipients. Am Pharmaceut Rev 2005; 8(5):142–5.
52. Tye CK, Sun C, Amidon GE. Evaluation of the effects of tableting speed on the relationships between compaction pressure, tablet tensile strength, and tablet solid fraction. J Pharm Sci 2005; 94(3):465–72.
53. Fu X-Y, et al. Rational excipient selection for enhanced tablet properties at small formulation scale—case study of compaction simulator application in early phase tablet formulation development. Am Pharm Rev 2005; 8(4):55–6, 58–60.
54. Guntermann A. Untersuchung der Tablettiersimulation mit dem Presster™ in Abhängigkeit von der Formulierung, Chargengrösse und der Tablettenpresse University of Basel, 2007.
55. Ruegger C. An investigation of the effect of compaction profiles on the tableting properties of pharmaceutical materials. New Brunswick, NJ: Rutgers, 1996: 253.
56. MCC—Metropolitan Computing Corporation Website. (Accessed November 7, 2002 at http://www.mcc-online.com/)
57. Sinka IC, Cunningham JC, Zavaliangos A. Analysis of tablet compaction. II. Finite element analysis of density distributions in convex tablets. J Pharm Sci 2004; 93(8):2040–53.

17
Compression and Compaction

Stephen W. Hoag, Vivek S. Dave, and Vikas Moolchandani
School of Pharmacy, University of Maryland,
Baltimore, Maryland, U.S.A.

INTRODUCTION

A tablet is formed by reducing the volume of a set of autonomous particles until they are consolidated into a solid body; a tablet is manufactured by placing a powder in a die and then reducing the volume of the powder with a set of punches. Tablet presses range from small, bench-top single-station presses to large industrial multi-station rotary presses. Most commercially produced tablets are made by rotary tablet presses (Fig. 1). A typical rotary machine runs anywhere from 1 to 200 rpm, and has from 16 to 75 stations or sets of punches and dies. A high speed rotary tablet press can produce over 500,000 tablets per hour, making tablets one of the most cost effective dosage forms. On a rotary tablet press, the die and punches are mounted on a turret. The turret moves the punches and dies simultaneously through the different stages of compaction. Tablet consolidation occurs when the punches and die go between two compression rollers (Fig. 1). The complete tablet manufacturing cycle occurs in four steps: (*i*) the die is filled, (*ii*) the fill weight is adjusted, (*iii*) the tablet is compacted, and (*iv*) the tablet ejected from the die.

A graph of punch stress versus time for Avicel® (FMC Biopolymer, Philadelphia, Pennsylvania, U.S.A.) is displayed in Figure 2. At a slow to medium speed, the total compaction cycle takes between 30 and 50 milliseconds, the dwell phase lasts about 18 milliseconds, and unloading takes about 10 milliseconds. The punch head is shaped liked a torus (doughnut with hole in middle) with the top covered by a flat plate (Fig. 3). It is the location of the compression roll on the punch head which determines the phase of compaction. The loading phase begins when the upper punch first makes contact with the compression roller, and lasts until the compression roller reaches the top of the torus. At this point the dwell phase begins and continues until the compression roller rolls off the top of the torus. During the dwell phase the strain is constant. Unloading begins at roll-off and continues until the punch stress drops to zero; this point is called lift-off. Once the punch stress is zero the relaxation phase begins and continues until the tablet is ejected from the die. The stress created during compaction is a consequence of a reduction in tableting material volume. It is the compression rollers that impart a displacement to the punches, which causes this volume reduction, i.e., the tablet machine produces a strain and the observed stress is the result of this strain. Strain is the independent variable and stress is the dependent variable.

From a material point of view, a compaction process is normally described by a series of sequential phases (Fig. 2). Initially as the volume is reduced, the particles

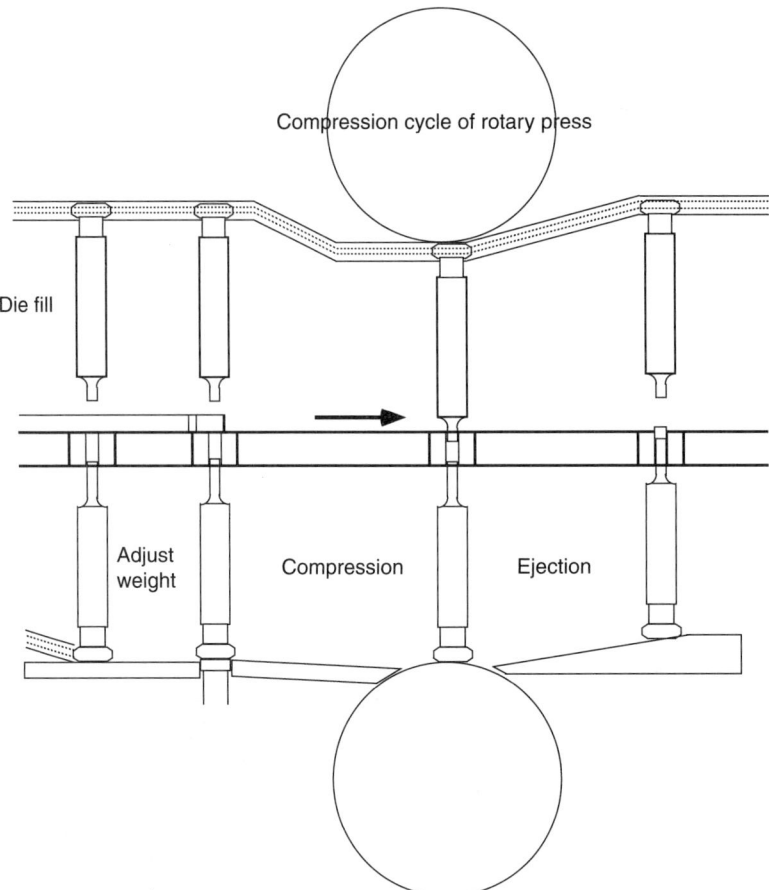

FIGURE 1 Rotary tablet press compression cycle.

rearranged into a closer packing structure. At a certain point, the packing characteristics of the particles and interparticulate friction between particles will prevent any further particle rearrangement. At this point, the further reduction in compact volume results in the elastic, viscoelastic, and plastic deformation of the particles. Elastic deformation is reversible, whereas the plastic deformation is irreversible. In addition, particle fragmentation or breakage results in smaller particles, which further decreases in compact volume. As the volume is further reduced, the smaller particles formed by fragmentation can undergo deformation. As a consequence of these processes, particle surfaces are brought into close proximity to each other which can lead to the formation of interparticulate bonds. These bonds may later break which facilitates further compression. To summarize, the following processes are involved in the compaction of a powder:

1. Particle rearrangement
2. Elastic, viscoelastic, and plastic deformation of particles
3. Fragmentation of particles
4. Formation of interparticulate bonds

Examples of materials that consolidate by predominantly plastic deformation include sodium chloride, starch, and microcrystalline cellulose (MCC) (1–3) and

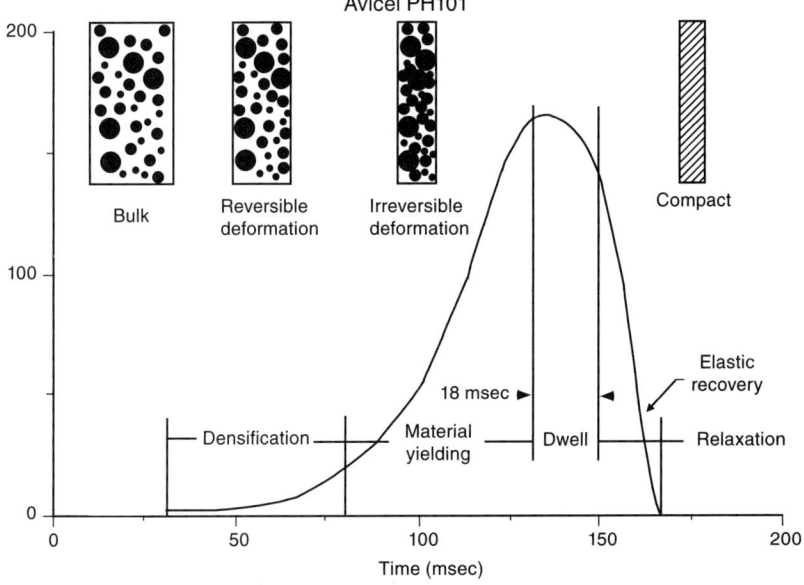

FIGURE 2 Punch and die stress vs. time for Avicel®.

materials that under go fragmenting include crystalline lactose, sucrose, and Encompress (4–8). However, all materials posses some degree of elastic, viscoelastic, plastic, and brittle characteristics. The type of volume reduction mechanism that will predominate for a specific material is dependent on factors such as temperature and compaction rate. Lower temperature and faster loading during compression will generally promote consolidation by fragmentation.

During tablet formation the following types of bond mechanisms are hypothesized to occur:

1. Mechanical interlocking (between irregularly shaped particles)
2. Interparticulate attraction forces (e.g., intermolecular forces, such as Van der Waal forces, electrostatic forces, and hydrogen bonding) (9,10)
3. Solid bridges (due to melting)

In tableting, compact formation occurs due to interparticulate attraction that arises in part from intermolecular bonding forces that act over very short distances. As the

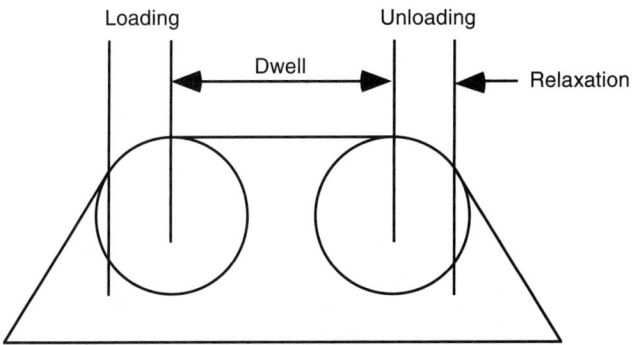

FIGURE 3 Cross section of punch head.

powder bed is consolidated and the particles start to deform around each other this leads to a mechanical interlocking of the particles, and this also increases the number of contact points between the particles. The dominant interaction force between solid surfaces in the Van der Waals force of attraction (10–12) and hydrogen bonding may occur intra and intermolecularly (9). In addition, the applied load gets transmitted from particle to particle through contact points, the pressure at these points can be very high. This may cause heating with a possibility of localized melting, especially of low-melting point solids. Upon unloading, the reduction of local stress at the point of contact could lead to re-solidification, forming a solid bridge between the particles (13). Hence solid bridges that contribute to the overall compact strength can be defined as areas of real contact, i.e., contact at an atomic level between adjacent surfaces in the compact. Different types of solid bridges have been proposed in literature, such as solid bridges due to melting, self-diffusion of atoms between surfaces, and recrystallization of soluble materials in compacts (14–17).

Axial to Radial Stress Transmission

Simultaneous measurement of die-wall pressure and upper punch pressure can be used to examine the behavior of materials during compression. Axial pressure is the force per unit area being applied in the direction in which the punch moves during compression. The radial pressure is the pressure transmitted at right angles to the longitudinal punch axis. For a powder confined in a die, radial pressures during tableting arises due to some of the applied axial stress being transversely transmitted to the die-wall (18). During decompression, the radial pressure exerted on the die-wall decreases; however, upon complete removal of axial pressure some die-wall pressure still remains. This is referred to as the residual die-wall pressure (RDWP) and is inversely proportional to the ejection pressure. Plots of radial versus axial pressure during tableting are referred to as a compaction profile. The relationship between the axial and radial pressures during the compaction in a rigid die was studied by Long in 1960 (19,20). Long investigated compression characteristics of solids under uniaxial compression based upon an analogy to the behavior of a solid isotropic plug. Long defined three types of behavior that could be elucidated using compaction cycles. These are a perfectly elastic body, a body with a constant yield stress in shear, and a Mohr's body. These analyses assume that the die is perfectly rigid, that die-wall friction is negligible and that the die-wall force to be a shearing stress causing deformation of the compact (19–21).

For a perfect elastic body, when axial pressure is applied, the radial pressure is of the same magnitude and related to the axial force via a constant. This constant is known as Poisson's ratio. As illustrated in Figure 4A, the compression and decompression phases of the cycle are straight lines which exhibit no hysteresis and a zero intercept. However, few if any pharmaceutical materials behave as pure elastic bodies. Usually, some amount of force is needed to eject the formed compact from the die. The ejection force (EF) is need to over come the friction between the tablet and die-wall, and for a given coefficient of friction the higher the residual die-wall force the higher the EF that is needed (19–21).

The compaction cycle of a body with constant yield stress in shear is illustrated in Figure 4B. The yield value, A, of the body is independent of the magnitude of the stress. The radial pressure will be determined by the conditions of yield. Until the yield value is reached, the material should transmit force to the die-wall as though it were an elastic body, behaving as previously described. After the yield point, A, is passed, the difference between the axial and radial pressures will have a value of 2S, where S is the yield stress

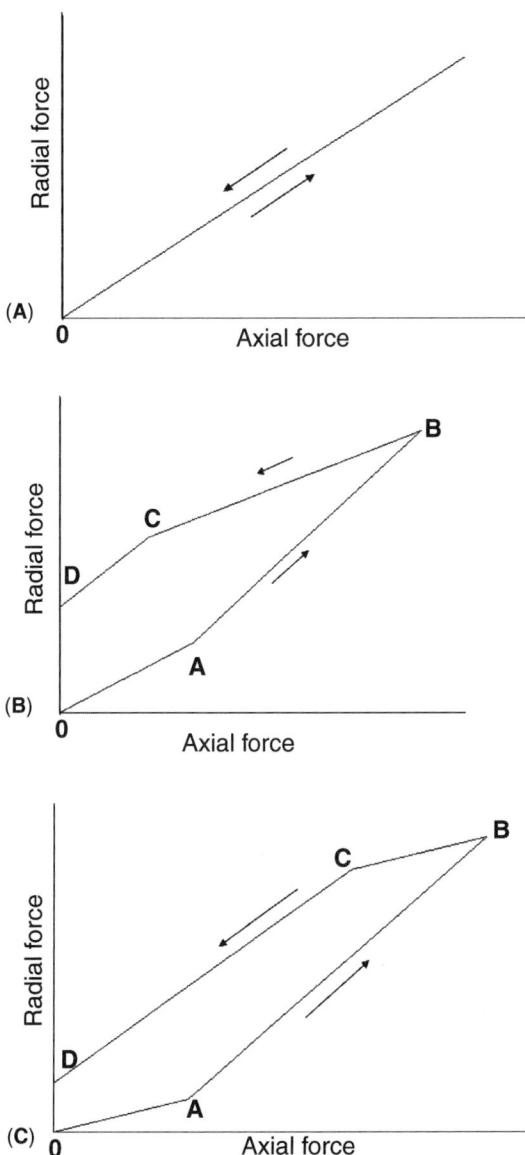

FIGURE 4 Theoretical compression cycles under uniaxial compression within a rigid frictionless die: **(A)** Perfect elastic body; **(B)** body with constant yield stress in shear; and **(C)** Mohr's body. *Source*: Adapted from Ref. 19.

in shear of the material. Thus, the slope of the segment AB should be unity. At point B maximum axial and radial pressure is reached and the decompression phase begins. Since the material is no longer being forced to yield, the radial pressure will fall at a rate equal to the Poisson ratio of the material times the axial load. This results in the slope of segment OA being equal to segment BC. If the maximum applied load was large enough, a point will be reached where the difference between the axial and radial load is equal to the yield value of the material and yielding in shear will begin to occur again. This occurs in Figure 4B at point C. The decompression slope will then again by unity down to the point where the axial load is equal to zero. The radial pressure remaining will be equal to 2S, again where S is the yield strength in shear of the material (19–21).

The third type of material behaves as a Mohr's body where the value of the yield stress in shear is a function of the normal stress on the plane of shear. A theoretical compaction cycle for a Mohr's body is shown in Figure 4C where the slope of section OA and CB is again equal to the Poisson ratio for the material. Slope AB is equal to $(1 - \mu)/(1 + \mu)$ and the slope of segment CD is equal to $(1 + \mu)/(1 - \mu)$ where μ is equal to the coefficient of internal friction as derived by Long (19–21).

FACTORS AFFECTING COMPACT FORMATION

As discussed previously, the bulk volume reduction during compression/compaction is a complex process involving several events: (*i*) transitional repacking/filling the voids between granules, (*ii*) deformation at contact points, (*iii*) fragmentation and/or plastic deformation of granules, (*iv*) filling of voids between primary particles, (*v*) fragmentation and/or plastic deformation of primary particles, and (*vi*) bonding/formation of a compact. Thus, the success and efficiency of compact formation can be influenced by numerous factors. These factors could be product/formulation related, process/equipment related and/or environment related. Some of the most important factors affecting the compressibility/compactibility of pharmaceutical materials are discussed below.

Crystallinity/Polymorphism

Polymorphism, pseudo-polymorphism, and the crystal ordering/disordering of pharmaceutical materials are known to affect their densification behavior and the final compact attributes (22). This influence is brought about by the differences in molecular arrangements, i.e., crystal structure and crystal habit, crystal anisotropy, and particulate properties (22). Typically, crystalline materials undergo brittle fragmentation whereas amorphous materials undergo plastic deformation. Thus, to a certain extent, the degree of crystallinity and the polymorph type of a material determines the mechanism of deformation. Numerous studies have examined the effect of polymorphic forms on the deformation behavior of pharmaceutical actives and excipients (22–28).

Suzuki et al. examined the effect of the degree of crystallinity of MCC on the compactibility of tablets (28). They observed that a decrease in the degree of crystallinity lowered the compression energy (energy required to fracture the crystal region, calculated from a displacement–force curve for the upper punch) of MCC samples (28). Typically, for organic solids the crystalline region with a rigid structure requires considerable energy to be fractured; however, the amorphous region, which tend to deform plastically, with a less ordered and weaker structure requires relatively less energy to fracture (28). A decrease in the degree of crystallinity also lowered the B-value (it reflects the magnitude of fracture caused after densification by movement and reorientation of particles and expressed as the difference between the relative density at the point where measurable force was applied, and the relative density calculated from the intercept of the linear portion Heckel plot) and the yield pressure ($1/k$) during Heckel analysis of MCC. Suzuki et al. also found that the crushing strength of tablets decreased when the crystallinity of MCC granules was reduced.(28). Nichols et al. reported a comparison of compaction properties of two polymorphic forms (monoclinic/form I and orthorhombic/form II) of paracetamol (acetaminophen) (23). They observed that compared to form I, form II (orthorhombic crystals) had lower yield values indicative of plastic deformation, and thus have improved compactibility. This was also confirmed by strain rate sensitivity studies where it was found that form II had greater increase in the yield pressure with increasing punch velocity compared to form I (23).

Suihko et al. examined the densification and deformation behavior of theophylline monohydrate (TMO), a mixture of forms (TMIX), and anhydrous polymorphs I (TA-I) and II (TA-II) using the in-die Heckel method (discussed below) (22). They observed that TMO was the most easily deformable form (lowest K_d, K_{ef}, and K_p values, where K_d is total deformation, including elastic and plastic components) of the material under compression, K_{ef} refers to fast elastic recovery of the material during recovery, and K_p refers to the permanent deformation of the material after viscoelastic recovery); while the other forms showed the following decreasing order of deformability: TMIX > TA-II > TA-I (22). The water present in the crystal lattice of the TMIX and TMO powders was thought to decrease the resistance towards densification and enhance elastic/plastic deformation (22). Moreover, TMO was found to be highly prone to fast elastic recovery on storage compared to other crystalline forms (22). Thus, tableting properties of the various theophylline forms were related to their solid-state structure and crystalline water content; which are the types of changes that can occur with theophylline during storage (22). Thus, a thorough knowledge of the crystal nature and polymorphic forms of pharmaceutical materials and its influence on their physico–mechanical properties is required to understand and predict their deformation/tableting behavior during the pre-formulation as well as the final scale-up stages (22).

For certain materials compression has been shown to change the crystal nature and polymorphic forms (29–32). These effects can significantly alter critical properties of dosage forms like solubility and dissolution profile and might result in a final dosage form with undesirable functionality, e.g., insufficient bioavailability, etc. Brittain published an excellent mini-review on the effects of mechanical processes on phase composition of pharmaceutical materials (29). Although there is a general assumption that the total energy transferred to a formulation during the compression stage is not sufficient to induce a phase transformation, there are several examples where compression causes a change in the crystal nature/polymorphic form of the material. Pirttimaki et al. studied the effects of grinding and compression on crystal structure of anhydrous caffeine using quantitative X-ray diffraction analysis (32). It was found that with progressive increase in compression force (51–357 MPa) there was an increase in conversion of the metastable form I of anhydrous caffeine into stable form II with up to 80% conversion (32). Notably, most of the force transformation occurs on or near the surface of the tablet, suggesting that the transformation decreases with the reduction in applied force. Okumura et al. investigated the polymorphic transitions of Indomethacin under high compression pressures (100 and 400 MPa) (31). They found that with increasing pressure the α- and γ-forms showed amorphization (decrease in the crystalline form) (31). Chan et al. used thermal analysis to conduct a detailed investigation of the polymorphic changes occurring in different regions of compacts under pressure for caffeine, sulfabenzamide, and maprotiline hydrochloride (33). It was found that for all materials, compression caused a conversion from metastable form to the most stable form; this fact was attributed to the assumption that the polymorphic form with the lowest melting point had the weakest attractive forces and possibly the lowest yield values at a given temperature. This assumption is based on previous observations that the main mechanism of polymorphic transitions is nucleation and growth of second phase within the first. Nucleation occurs due to dislocations in a crystal (due to higher free energy). Moreover, compression force induces dislocational strains in a crystal, thus facilitating nucleation. Thus for materials with different crystalline forms, the one having the lowest melting point has the weakest intermolecular attractive forces making them most susceptible to transformation under pressure at a given temperature (33).

In summary, the degree of crystallinity and polymorphic form can be important factors for tableting and care must be taken to ensure that the materials used have consistent crystallinity. Unfortunately, there are no absolute rules to enable the prediction of tableting behavior based on knowledge of a material's crystallinity so data must be considered on a case-by-case basis.

Porosity and Bulk Density

The relative density and hence porosity vary largely among pharmaceutical materials. Moreover, the porosity of these materials may change significantly during processing. Hancock et al. have done an exhaustive study on the absolute and relative densities of a wide range of pharmaceutical materials (34). They also studied the effects of common manufacturing operations, i.e., blending, roller compaction, and tableting, on the relative densities of these materials.

As shown in Figure 5, the powdered active pharmaceutical ingredients (APIs) had the lowest relative densities, suggesting that most APIs must be densified prior to the manufacturing stage so that a sufficient dose can be administered in a reasonably sized dosage form (34). However, most excipients evaluated had densities suitable to processing directly into solid oral dosage forms without the need for densification. A combination of materials (blends) had densities that were intermediate to their component materials. Several of these blends were then subjected to roller compaction and the ribbons were evaluated for their relative densities. As expected, the relative densities of the roller-compacted ribbons were found to be markedly higher than those of the powdered drug, excipients or blends. The ribbons were then granulated and the relative densities of the granulations were studied. The relative densities of granulations fell within a wide range. Although granulating usually increases the apparent densities of many materials, several samples showed either no change or the opposite effect. This was attributed to the processing technique employed as well as changes in the particle packing

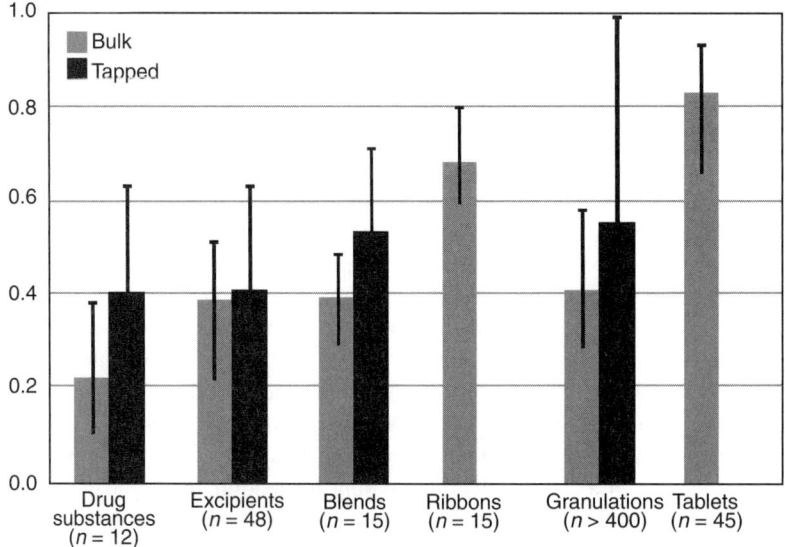

FIGURE 5 Relative density averages and ranges for commonly used pharmaceutical solids. *Source*: From Ref. 34.

efficiency induced by shifts in particle-size distribution (e.g., altered fines content). The tablets were prepared from the dry granulations as well as direct compression blends. The relative densities of the prepared tablets were measured and compared to those of commercially available tablets. The tablet samples were found to have the highest relative densities of all the material types considered, with a mean value of 0.84 g/cm³. This was comparable to the commercially available tablets tested, e.g., Tums® (GlaxoSmithkline London, U.K.), Alka-Seltzer® (Bayer AG Leverkusen, Germany), Motrin® (McNEIL-PPC Morris Plains, New Jersey, U.S.A) etc. (34).

Since the process of compression/compaction is aimed at reducing the porosity of a powder or granule, the initial porosity largely determines the extent to which the porosity can be reduced in a given tablet press. Increases in the original intragranular porosity increased the compressibility at a given applied pressure. Johansson and Alderborn evaluated the compression behavior of two types of granules (irregular and nearly spherical) prepared from MCC (35). The degree of compression (C) was used as a measure of deformation behavior as described by Johansson and Alderborn (36) and given as:

$$C\% = ((H_0 - H_p)/H_0) \times 100 \qquad (1)$$

where H_p is the height of the pellet bed in-die at applied pressure and H_0 is the estimated height before compression (i.e., calculated from the poured bulk density, the powder weight, and the die diameter). An increase in the bulk density was found to cause a decrease in the degree of compression for both granules and pellets of MCC. Thus, the bulk density of the granular material before compression significantly influenced the degree of compression (35). It has also been shown that a decreased bulk density corresponded to an increased tablet tensile strength. When the size and shape of the granules are uniform, the intragranular porosity influences the potential for deformation (35). Both the intragranular porosity (% voidage space in a granule bed within the granules, excluding void spaces between granules) and intergranular porosity (% voidage space in a granule bed between the granules, excluding void spaces within granules) may have a significant effect on the tablet forming ability of granular material. The bulk density of the granules affected both the compressibility and the compactibility of the granules (35). Nicklasson and Alderborn carried out a similar study investigating the effects of porosity on the deformation behavior of MCC and MCC/dibasic calcium phosphate (MCC/DCP) binary mixes (37). As shown in Table 1 it was observed that with increasing agglomerate porosity for all agglomerate types (MCC or MCC/DCP binary mixes) there was a decrease in the yield pressure values as measured with Kawakita ($1/b$) and Adam's (τ_0') compression parameters related to single agglomerate fracture strength equations (37).

Particle Size and Shape

The particle size, size distribution, and shape are among the important determinants of the deformation behavior of pharmaceutical powders and granules. Johansson et al. (35) studied the effect of granule size and shape on the deformation behavior of MCC granules. It was found that increasing the irregularity and roughness of granules changed the compression behavior from plastic deformation towards a more complex process including fragmentation and attrition of the granules (35). For different types of granular material (different particle sizes, shapes, and porosities), the combined effect of the intragranular porosity and the granule shape influences the nature of granule deformation. The dominating mechanism of compression of granules was plastic deformation, however, for highly porous irregular granules some degree of attrition occurred during

TABLE 1 Single Agglomerate and Bed Compression Data

Granule type	Granule porosity ($n = 3$) (%)	Granule fracture strength (τ_{0s}) ($n = 100$) (MPa)	Adams τ'_0 values ($n = 1-3$) (MPa)	Kawakita $1/b$ values ($n = 1-3$) (MPa)	Linear part of Adams equation ($n = 1-3$) (MPa)	Linear part Kawakita + ($n = 1-3$) (MPa)	Heckel σ_y values ($n = 1-3$) (MPa)
MCC	11	25.5	36.4	36.5	21–89	19–200	73.5
14	22.1	25.9	27.6	18–97	5–200	79.5	
27	10.5	9.79	14.7	23–98	13–200	68.5	
40	7.24	3.41	9.01	19–105	10–200	68.5	
46	3.86	1.62	6.66	23–105	8–200	67.1	
DCP/MCC	26	8.73	20.5	23.5	8–78	14–200	167
36	5.42	10.1	17.9	8–109	30–200	161	
42	5.08	8.55	14.9	6–102	18–200	168	
48	7.82	6.08	11.0	10–54	10–200	159	
55	5.42	3.76	7.76	5–56	5–200	156	

Abbreviations: DCP, dibasic calcium phosphate: MCC, microcrystalline cellulose.
Source: Adapted from Ref. 37.

compression (35). Johansson et al. have also shown that relative to uniform spherical particles, irregularly shaped granules had increased compressibility and produced tablets with higher tensile strengths (35).

Kaerger et al. (38) studied the effect of paracetamol particle size and shape on compactibility of binary mixture with MCC. The comparison was made between untreated (irregular, needle-shaped particles with a mean particle size 40 µm), milled (irregular, micronized particles with particle size range of 2–6 µm), and SAXS-treated (solution atomization and crystallization by sonication, spherically shaped with a particle size range of 2–6 µm) samples of paracetamol. They found that compressibility was directly proportional to the particle size of paracetamol. Compressibility was found in the order untreated > milled > SAXS-treated, suggesting that particle processing and shape influenced the apparent mechanical properties such as compressibility and compactibility. The blends containing untreated paracetamol gave tablets with lower tensile strengths than those containing other small particle sized (SAXS-treated or micronized) drugs (38). Garekani et al. studied the compressibility for different particle size fractions from a batch of paracetamol (39). It was observed that a greater degree of densification occurred for the larger particle size fraction (105–210 µm) compared to the smaller size fraction (<90 µm). This was attributed to increased frictional and cohesive forces associated with the smaller size range; which tends to restrict particle flow and thus reduce densification (39).

Compression Force

Compression force is the major driving force in the powder densification process. The rate and extent of the applied force on the powder bed not only affects the way particles physically deform but also determines the integrity of the compact formed (crushing strength/tensile strength).

There are many different descriptions of relationship between crushing strength and compression force, see section "Crushing Strength versus $P_{\max}$"; of these Sonnergaard investigated the relationship between compression pressure and the specific crushing strength (SCS) of pharmaceutical compacts and its applicability to quantify their deformation behavior (40). He proposed a linear relationship between maximum compression pressure and the SCS of the compact (40). The relationship is given by:

$$SCS = C_p \cdot P + b \qquad (2)$$

where P is the maximum (peak) compression pressure and C_p is a dimensionless compactibility parameter known as the compressibility coefficient (calculated from the slope of the linear region obtained between maximum compression pressure and SCS) (40). There was found a positive relationship between compactibility expressed as the C_p and the compressibility expressed as the w coefficient from the Walker equation (40). Rahmouni et al. examined the ability of cross-linked high amylose (CLA) starch to form compacts of a given mechanical strength as a function of compaction pressure (41). As the compaction pressure increased, the diametral crushing force of tablets prepared with granulated CLA increased until a plateau value (about 105 N) was reached. For nongranulated CLA powder the maximum crushing force was reached at 190 N (41). Thus, their exists a positive correlation between compression force and compactibility of the material up to a threshold pressure beyond which either the crushing force of compact remains unchanged, decreases or results in manufacturing problems like capping and lamination.

Lubricants and Glidants

Lubricants are usually added to formulations to reduce die-wall friction, although they may also help improve flow properties (those having a glidant characteristic), as well as function as antiadherents. The amount of lubricant added and the extent or duration of mixing a lubricant have been shown to affect several formulation properties including powder flow, deformation behavior, crushing strength, and dissolution rate. It has been traditionally observed that increasing the concentration of lubricant in a formulation results in tablets with decreased crushing strength. Several studies have been done to characterize the effects of lubricants on the formulation development process. The study by Veen et al. found that compared to unlubricated MCC tablets lubricated MCC tablets demonstrated greater tablet relaxation (porosity–expansion, defined as the difference between the porosity highest applied pressure and the final tablet porosity) during decompression (42). This was ascribed to a reduction of interparticle bonding by the presence of a lubricant film around the MCC particles (42).

Rahmouni et al. (41) studied the effect of Mg stearate (MgSt) and colloidal silicon dioxide (CSD) on the compression and mechanical properties of compacts prepared with granulated CLA starch. The presence of MgSt, even at low concentrations, impaired the compactibility (as measured by tablet tensile strength) of CLA. CSD was found to have a dramatic effect on the compactibility of CLA, but as opposed to MgSt the compactibility was increased with an increase in CSD concentration (41). Mollan and Celik investigated the effects of various concentrations of MgSt as a lubricant on the compaction properties of maltodextrins prepared by different granulation methods (spray drying, fluidized bed agglomeration, and roller compaction) by using R-value (the ratio of the peak lower punch force, F_L, to the peak upper punch force, F_A) to identify lubricant sensitivity (43). The total work of compaction (TWC) and average power consumption (APC) were also used to study the compaction properties of maltodextrins (43). The level of MgSt had a significant effect on the R-value, with R-values increasing with increased lubricant at several pressures and then starting to plateau after MgSt concentrations of 0.5% and above (43). With increases in the MgSt levels, calculated values of TWC and APC decreased at a highest compression pressure of 300 MPa. This effect was attributed to a decrease in the degree of cohesiveness between the particles as well as decreased frictional effects at the punch faces and die-wall. The area under the force–displacement curve decreased because less work was needed to achieve an equivalent mean pressure (43). All the maltodextrins studied (except the roller-compacted sample) showed a decreased tablet crushing force with increased MgSt levels at the pressures studied indicating the lubricant sensitivity of maltodextrins. This is not unexpected considering the fact that MgSt acts at surface and maltodextrins processed via spray drying or fluidized bed granulation deformed plastically; thus, not drastically changing the overall surface area when deforming. Compared to other more plastically deforming maltodextrins, the lower sensitivity of roller compacted samples to MgSt was thought to be due to fact that roller compacted samples mostly deformed by fragmentation during compaction which results in creation of new surfaces thus reducing total surface area covered by MgSt and hence reducing its lubricant effects (43).

In summary, lubricants like MgSt are used in virtually all commercial formulations to reduce die-wall friction. However, the addition of a lubricant can potentially reduced tablet hardness and lower dissolution rates. Adding more MgSt than is necessary has no added benefit and is associated with tableting problems; thus the levels should be kept as low as possible. Typical values for direct compression range from 0.5% to 1.0% (w/w).

Glidants are typically incorporated in solid dosage formulations to improve the flow properties of granules or powders (44,45). There are several mechanisms by with a glidant can increase the flowability of formulations. These include but not limited to (*i*) decreasing surface roughness of the particles by forming a uniform coating around them; thus, reducing the frictional drag between the particles, (*ii*) act as physical barriers between particles which reduces attractive forces between particles, and (*iii*) removing absorbed moisture from the surface of the particles, making them drier and more flowable (44,45).

Apart from their obvious effects on the flow properties glidants may also affect the compaction behavior of a formulation. Chang et al. studied the effect of the glidant CSD on the flowability and tableting behavior of a DMP-504 (a crosslinked polyalkylammonium polymer used as a non-systemic cholesterol lowering agent) (44). They observed that addition of a small amount of CSD (1%) dramatically enhanced the compactibility of DMP-504 (as measured by tablet crushing strength). They speculated that CSD reduced the negative bonding effect of the lubricant (MgSt) by stripping it off the surface of the host particles which facilitated densification of the powder due to its glidants action (44).

Moisture

For pharmaceutical materials, moisture is known to affect a wide range of properties, such as powder flow, compactibility, and stability (physical chemical and microbiological) (8,46–53). The interaction between moisture and a solid is complex and can occur in a variety of ways. For example, water can be stoichiometrically incorporated into a solid's crystal structure in the form of a hydrate (pseudo-hydrate) as discussed previously in this section. In addition, moisture can have non-stroichiometrical, i.e., non-specific interactions with a solid by adsorbing on the surface or being absorbed into the material and acting as a plasticizer. These non-specific interactions are more common in amorphous or semi crystalline materials, and are the subject of this section.

Moisture interactions can have a significant effect on the physico–mechanical properties of pharmaceutical formulations including flow, compression, hardness of granules and tablets, particle surface energy, die-wall friction, and Young's elastic modulus (49). Sebhatu et al. studied the effect of moisture content on the compression and bond formation properties of amorphous lactose particles (50). They observed that absorbed moisture increased the deformability of the material by facilitating a temporary transition of the amorphous material from a glassy to a rubbery state (particularly for long chain polymeric materials), occurring during the compression phase thus affecting the bond-formation process (50). This results in the formation of solid bridges (due to evaporation of moisture during processing)with a subsequent increased interparticulate bonding area, which increases the deformability of the particles (50). Nokhodchi published a comprehensive review on the effects of moisture on compression and compaction (49); it was pointed out that increased moisture content usually results in a reduction in tablet porosity and an increased tablet fracture resistance. This is thought to occur due to a decrease in the density variation within the tablet, and by recrystallization of granules within the tablet (49). The reduced tablet density variation can be ascribed to the uniform die-filling and lubrication of the die-wall by the expressed moisture during compaction resulting in uniform force transmission through the compact onto the lower punch (49). Bravo et al. examined the effect of moisture on the mechanical properties of methyl methacrylate-starch copolymers (46). They observed a general decrease in the mean yield pressure of total deformation (K_d) of methyl methacrylate-starch copolymers with a progressive increase in relative humidity (46). At intermediate moisture contents (25–50% RH) the plasticizing effect of water promoted an improvement in the plastic consolidation mechanism combined with an elastic deformation component (46). At higher moisture contents (>75% RH), the effect of multilayer adsorbed water at the surface hindered the bond formations and resulted in weak tablets (46). Elkhider et al. studied the effect of moisture on the compaction behavior of tablets using a controlled humidity cell (47). Formation of condensed water in the tablet and an increase in tablet density were observed with tablets [ibuprofen+HPMC (hydroxypopyl methylcellulose)] that were exposed to a higher relative humidity (>60%) (47). This was attributed to the formation of a multilayer of water around ibuprofen particles, an increase in the intermolecular attraction forces and this resulted in the facilitation of bond formation between closely placed particles (47). HPMC is a hydrophilic polymer with many polar sites and is known to have high affinity for water. Thus, the absorbed/adsorbed moisture is thought to act as a lubricant and a plasticizer between particles at points of contact and reduce resistance and increases the cohesiveness of the powder (47).

The importance of moisture in pharmaceutical solid dosage forms can also be appreciated from the fact that an excessive loss of moisture can have deleterious effects on the functionality of a formulation. Nieuwmeyer et al. studied the effect of drying phase of wet-granulation on the granule breakage phenomena and generation of fines (54); they found that as the moisture content decreased the granules tended to break and generate a significant amount of fines (particularly at moisture levels below 2%) (54). They also observed that the mean granule size decreased with decreasing moisture levels, due to granule breakage and fines generation (54). Song et al. compared the effect of freeze-drying and conventional hot air oven-drying on the physical characteristics of extrusion–spheronization granules, i.e., appearance, compaction behavior, tablet voidage, and crushing strength (51). They observed that the mode of drying had a noticeable impact upon the compaction characteristics of extrusion-spheronized granules, with the freeze-dried granules being more deformable in compaction, and producing tablets of lower voidage for a given compaction pressure. The yield points for the freeze-dried granules and the conventional oven dried samples were found to be 1.5 and 2.7 MPa, respectively (51). It was also found that freeze-dried granules had crushing strength ≈70% higher than the oven dried samples. As a general rule, there is an optimal moisture level in a formulation with very low moisture levels having poor compaction properties and high friability and conversely very high moisture levels having problems with compaction, flow, and processing; also, there is a concern with moisture induce stability problems. Thus, knowledge of the type and level of moisture in pharmaceutical materials is critical for understanding its impact not only on deformation behavior but also on the attributes of the final compact.

Granule Type

Typically, tablets are prepared by one of the three techniques: wet granulation, dry granulation, or direct compression. Other novel techniques like hot melt granulation, extrusion-spheronization, and compression of beads are less commonly used. The choice of the technique is determined by the ease, efficiency, stability, and cost. The type of granulation does have an impact on the granule deformation behavior. This impact could be due to moisture levels as in wet granulation, changes in particle size and size distribution, work hardening or reworking as in dry granulation or tableting and possible changes in crystalline nature induced by wet granulation, to name a few possible effects of granulation type. Much work has been done to investigate the effects of granulation technique on the deformation behavior of formulations and this research is described below.

Rahmouni et al. studied the effect of granulation method on compactibility of CLA starch (41). Wet-granulation was found to substantially decrease the compactibility of CLA as indicated by a reduction in tablet strength at an equivalent compaction pressure. This was attributed to a decrease in the bonding surface area which can develop intermolecular forces between particles (41). It was also thought to be related to the increase in crystallinity (to crystalline B form) during wet granulation. This crystalline form of CLA is known to have increased stiffness and less plastic deformability(41). However, compression force–displacement studies found that the non-granulated powder offered much more resistance to consolidation and required more input energy to form compacts than granulated CLA (41).

Zuurman et al. evaluated the effects of a binder on the relationship between the bulk density and compactibility of lactose granules by comparing binderless granules with granules containing hydroxypropylcellulose (55). The presence of a binder resulted in an increased tablet crushing strength, as compared with tablets without binder. The crushing strength was found to be dependent on the granule bulk density and independent of the type of lactose (α- or β-lactose) used (55). Mattson et al. studied the influence of various binders on the tensile strength and porosity of tablets made from binary mixtures with sodium bicarbonate (56). The addition of a binder resulted in increased tensile strength and a decrease in the porosity of the sodium bicarbonate tablets. For tablets made of pure sodium bicarbonate and a granulated mixture of sodium bicarbonate with MCC, sodium microcrystalline cellulose, PEG-3000 (polyethylene glycol), polyvinyl pyrrolidone, or pre-gelatinized starch (PGS) the fracture, during strength testing was thought to occur around the particles rather than through them (since the sodium bicarbonate particles are difficult to break), which explains the increase in tablet tensile strength after binder addition (56). Horisawa et al. studied lactose and MCC granules prepared by various granulating methods and compared with nonpareil sugar spheres for their effects on the compression and strength of tablets (48). Within the compression pressure range of 2–10 MPa, MCC granules showed a distinct difference between the granulation methods, whereas lactose (lactose) and NP (non-Pareil) granules did not show any such distinction (48). Since MCC granules were considered to deform via plastic deformation, a positive correlation was found between the crushing force and yield pressure among all the granulation methods used (48). While in lactose and NP granules, which are thought to deform by brittle fracture there was no obvious correlation found, suggesting that the lactose granules fractured into nearly primary particles under pressure (48).

For brittle lactose granules the tablet strength was found to be low and not influenced much by the granulating method and the tablet strengths of lactose granules were not much different from those prepared by direct compression of lactose powder (48). In contrast, the tablet strength prepared from MCC granules using various granulating methods were lower than those of tablets prepared by direct compression of MCC powder. It was observed from the stereomicroscopic studies that the surface of the tablets prepared from direct compression of MCC powder was smooth, while that of the tablets prepared from granules was rough. These studies also revealed that during tensile test the tablet's fracture at the granule boundaries suggesting lower degree of plastic deformation compared to powdered MCC (48). The contact area between the granule particles within the tablet was also found to be smaller with granulated MCC (48).

The effect of roll compaction on the tableting behavior of some materials has also been studied. Freitag et al. (57) found that for all the materials they tested, the relative tap density of the granules increased with increasing roll pressure. The flowability of granules improved, which was attributed to the increase in mean particle size, and the tensile strength of the tablets decreased with increasing roll pressure. The degree of densification (ratio of the relative tablet density to the relative tap density) decreased with increasing roll pressure. Roller compaction affected the ability of the material to be compacted to the same degree of densification during tableting (57). Roller compaction also modified the compactibility of the materials, as increasing the roll pressure resulted in higher apparent mean yield pressures (as obtained from Heckel plots) of all analyzed samples (57). One possible explanation for these observations is discussed in the section "Constitutive Equations: Material Properties".

Tableting Speed

The deformation behavior of many pharmaceutical materials is time-dependent and the nature of this time dependency is often related to the mechanism of compaction for a given material. It is thought that time dependency or speed sensitivity arises from the viscoelastic or viscoplastic characteristics of a material. In contrast, studies have shown that brittle materials are much less speed dependent that ductile materials because yielding and fragmentation are not as dependent on the rate of compression. It is also believed that the particle size and size distribution of the powder or granules have an important role in the speed sensitivity due to the fact that this property affects the predominant mechanism of deformation (6,58–60).

The speed sensitivity of pharmaceutical materials can have serious implications on the final tablet attributes. The effect of punch velocity can be pronounced when a material is transferred from a single station laboratory press to a rotary press or scaled up to a very high speed industrial press. Several studies have found that materials that have a high degree of elastic recovery or deform via plastic deformation tend to show a decrease in tablet strength with increase in tableting speed, and problems like capping and lamination are more likely to occur when such materials are scaled up to a high-speed press.

The effect of tableting speed on compressibility and compactibility is well known. Akande et al. studied the effect of compression speeds on the compaction properties of a 1:1 paracetamol–MCC mixture prepared by two methods (6). The tablets were compressed at pressures of 80, 160, 240, or 320 MPa for single compression and combinations of 80:160, 160:80, 240:320, or 320:240 MPa, were used for pre-compression: main compression. The plastic and elastic energies of compression were determined as described by Ragnarsson and Sjögren (61,62) from the plots of the compression force-displacement data captured during compression and the ratios of the elastic energy to plastic energy were determined at each compression speed (6). An increase in tableting speed caused the tensile strength of tablets to decrease at a constant compression pressure. A combination of pre- and main-compression also resulted in a decrease in tablet tensile strength with an increase in tableting speed (6). This was ascribed to the time-dependent consolidation of the paracetamol and MCC powder mixture; at higher compression speeds there was a lack of sufficient time required for stress relaxation and plastic deformation to take place. The amount of energy dissipated via plastic deformation during compression generally increased and the ratios of the elastic energy to plastic energy also increased (6).

The effects of tableting speed on the compressibility, tabletability, and compactibility of MCC, lactose, PGS and DCP were studied over a wide range of dwell-times from 8 millisecond to 90 second by Tye et al. (60). However, they found rather contradictory results that showed that the compaction behavior of MCC was independent of the compression speeds. The compaction behavior of lactose was also found to be independent of compression speeds and this was attributed mainly to its brittle properties. Compactibility of PGS was substantially affected by compression speed since it is considered to exhibit viscoelastic behavior. The tabletability or ability to form strong tablets of DCP increases as the compaction speed increases. However, this again is contradictory to the traditional belief that DCP as a brittle material is expected to have the least strain rate sensitivity. The explanation given for such behavior is that at higher tableting speeds there is more extensive fragmentation of DCP; thus, resulting in the formation of a large number of clean sites available for bonding. This was supported by the fact that the porosity of tablets decreased with increasing compression speeds (60).

David and Augsburger (63) studied the effects of the compression cycle duration and of the duration of the maximum compressive force on tablet strength using an instrumented rotary tablet press. Various direct compression fillers were evaluated. Increasing the overall compression cycle duration to 10 seconds resulted in significantly greater tablet tensile strength with MCC and compressible starch but not with lactose or compressible sugar. Increasing the duration of the maximum compressive force to 20 seconds significantly increased the tensile strength in all cases, but MCC and compressible starch tablets were affected more than lactose or compressible sugar.

Ruegger and Celik (59) investigated the effects of compression and decompression speed on the compaction behavior of several pharmaceutical powders. In general, it was found that if the compression and decompression speeds are equal, then the tablet crushing strength was inversely proportional to the punch velocity. It was also found that the percent viscoelastic recovery increased with increasing speed, resulting in increased percent ejected porosity ($\varepsilon\%$) and decreased crushing strength values. Heckel analysis showed that as the speed of compaction increases, there is a reduction in plastic deformation and plastic flow or an increase in brittle behavior. For plastically deforming materials like MCC and pregelatinized starch, at a given compression speed, the increase in decompression speed reduced the crushing strength of tablets. However, brittle materials like directly compressible acetaminophen showed no effect of decompression speed (59).

In summary, the rate of compaction has been known to have an effect on the compactability of materials (59,64). The consolidation mechanism of compacted powder highly depends on the time of compaction. Materials undergoing plastic and/or viscoelastic deformation generally produce stronger tablets at reduced speeds, whereas brittle fragmenting materials are relatively unaffected by compaction speed because fragmentation occurs rapidly. In reality, it is tough to categorize any one type of deformation behavior to one material; therefore, combinations of deformation mechanisms are applicable in most of the cases. Materials that deform elastically or exhibit time-dependence are more susceptible to capping and lamination as the punch velocity increased. The effect of punch velocity mostly shows up when transferring a material from a single station press to a rotary tablet press or when scaling up to a larger tablet press. Often, problems such as capping and lamination, which were not present during development, begin to surface during the scale-up process as the speed of production increases. It should be noted that the literature on this subject is sometimes contradictory, which the authors believe result from a lack of standardization of test methods and test protocols.

Tablet Press Type

The compaction behavior of pharmaceutical materials could be significantly altered by the type of tablet press used. Palmieri et al. (65). investigated the differences in the powder densification at different compression speeds between single station (eccentric) and rotary tablet presses by compressing several commonly used pharmaceutical excipients at different compression pressures and obtaining the corresponding stress strain data from both machines. In general, it was found that the deformation behavior of plastically deforming materials like MCC was more sensitive to the effect of longer dwell times of the rotary machine, whereas, compaction of brittle materials like DCP was more sensitive to the compression mechanism of the rotary machine (compared to the eccentric machine) based on the Heckel plot (65).

Miscellaneous

Roueche et al. investigated the influence of temperature on the compaction behavior of an organic powder (66). It was shown that a change in compaction temperature modifies the microstructure and the mechanical behavior of the tablets, and this influence of temperature mainly occurs during the isobaric stage (constant pressure) of the compression cycle and not during the stages of pressure changes. Within the range of temperatures studied (20–140°C) it was found that the tensile strength of tablets increased with an increase in temperature, reaching a maxima at 60°C and then decreased despite further increases in temperature (66). Newton et al. studied the influence of punch face curvature on the compactibility of MCC (67). They found that at a given compaction pressure, compacts with different thicknesses and face curvatures showed differences in diametrical crushing strength (tensile strength). This was attributed to differences in the internal structure of the compacts due to different stress distributions during the formation process. It was also observed that the tensile strength of compacts was maximum when the compact diameter to face curvature ratio was 0.67, corresponding to "normal" concave tablets (67).

ANALYSIS OF POWDER COMPACTION DATA

The consolidation of a powder bed into a tablet is a process of porosity reduction and the formation of an intact compact. During compression, the structure of the powder bed changes and consolidation is brought about mainly by particle rearrangement, plastic deformation, and fragmentation. The compression of powdered or granular material into a cohesive mass is a complex and irreversible dynamic process.

The study of compression/compaction mechanisms of powders or granules have become an important part in the design and development of solid dosage forms. These types of studies are greatly facilitated by the availability of instrumented tablet presses, universal testing machines and integrated compaction research systems, commonly known as compaction simulators. Various parameters are monitored during the compression process to assess powder behavior. These parameters are obtained from the measurement of punch force and displacement for the upper and lower punches, axial to radial load transmission, i.e., die-wall stress, die-wall friction, EF, and temperature changes. Several relationships between stress–strain, pressure–volume, pressure–porosity or pressure–density have been proposed to define the compaction behavior of powders, since natural strain is proportional to the changes in the powder-bed height or volume under applied pressure. Thus, a compaction equation relates a property of the state of consolidation of a powder bed, such as porosity, volume, density or void ratio, as a function of the compaction pressure. Compaction data analysis is usually carried out with two major purposes; initially it is used to linearize the plots to make comparisons easier between different sets of data, secondly it is used for predicting the pressure used to obtain a required density. Usually compaction studies are performed over a wide range of compression pressures and the pressures plotted logarithmically so as to spread out the data in reasonable and meaningful form (68).

When interpreting compaction data it is important to know what compaction mechanisms operate over different levels of pressure; thus, a good compaction plot should be able to describe material behavior and determine when material behavior changes. One of the earliest studies done to investigate the compaction behavior of powders was by Walker in 1923; he plotted the relative volume (V_r) of the powder compact against the logarithm of the applied axial pressure (P) using the relationship (69):

$$V_r = a_1 - K_1 \ln P \tag{3}$$

Following Walker's analysis, several other compaction relationships have been proposed by different workers and currently more than a dozen different mathematical descriptions of the compaction process can be found in the literature, each having its own set of benefits and drawbacks. Among the most widely used for pharmaceutical systems include those of Heckel (68–70), Kawakita (70), and Adams (4,71). These different methods will be reviewed in this section.

Athy–Heckel Equation

The Heckel equation is among the most popular methods used in pharmaceutical research to determine the volume reduction mechanism during compression (4,36,37,40,43,69–82).

Compression and Compaction

It is based on the assumption that powder compression follows first-order kinetics with the interparticulate voids as the reactants and the densification of the powder as the product. According to the relationship, the degree of compact densification with increasing compression pressure is directly proportional to the porosity:

$$\frac{d\rho_r}{dP} = k\varepsilon \tag{4}$$

where ρ_r is the relative density at pressure, P and ε is the porosity.

The relative density is defined as the ratio of density of the compact at pressure P, to the density of the compact at zero porosity; which is the true density of the material. The porosity (ε) is given by:

$$\varepsilon = \frac{(V_p - V_0)}{V_p} = 1 - \rho_r \tag{5}$$

where V_p and V_0 are the volume at any applied pressure and the volume at theoretical zero porosity (i.e., true volume of material), respectively. Thus, Equation (4) can also be expressed as:

$$\frac{d\rho_r}{dP} = k(1 - \rho_r) \tag{6}$$

and by solving this differential; Equation (6) is transformed to:

$$\ln\left[\frac{1}{(1-\rho_r)}\right] = kP + A \tag{7}$$

Plotting the value of $\ln[1/(1-\rho_r)]$ against applied pressure, P, yields a graph with a linear portion having slope, k and intercept, A (Fig. 6).

The reciprocal of k gives a material dependent constant known as the yield pressure P_y, which is inversely related to the ability of the material to deform plastically under pressure (83). Typically, lower values of P_y indicate the onset of plastic deformation at lower applied pressures (42,69,82). This relationship has been extensively used to differentiate between forms of pharmaceutical solids like powders, granules, and other multi-component systems (5,8,35,69,71,72,74–77,84–87). The intercept of the extrapolated linear region, A, is a function of the original compact volume. The Heckel plot can be divided into three stages of densification. In the first stage densification occurs via particle rearrangement and possibly some particle fragmentation, in the second stage plastic deformation or brittle fracture are the primary modes of densification and in the third stage work hardening can affect the densification behavior (Fig. 6). From the value of A, the relative density, ρ_A, which represents the total degree of densification at zero pressure, can be calculated using the equation:

$$A = \ln\frac{1}{(1-\rho_A)} \tag{8}$$

Thus,

$$\rho_A = 1 - e^{-A} \tag{9}$$

The relative density of a powder bed at a point when the applied pressure equals zero, ρ_0, is used to describe the initial rearrangement phase of compaction as a result of die filling. ρ_0 is determined experimentally and is equal to the ratio of the bulk density at zero pressure to the true density of the powder. The relative density, ρ_b, indicates the

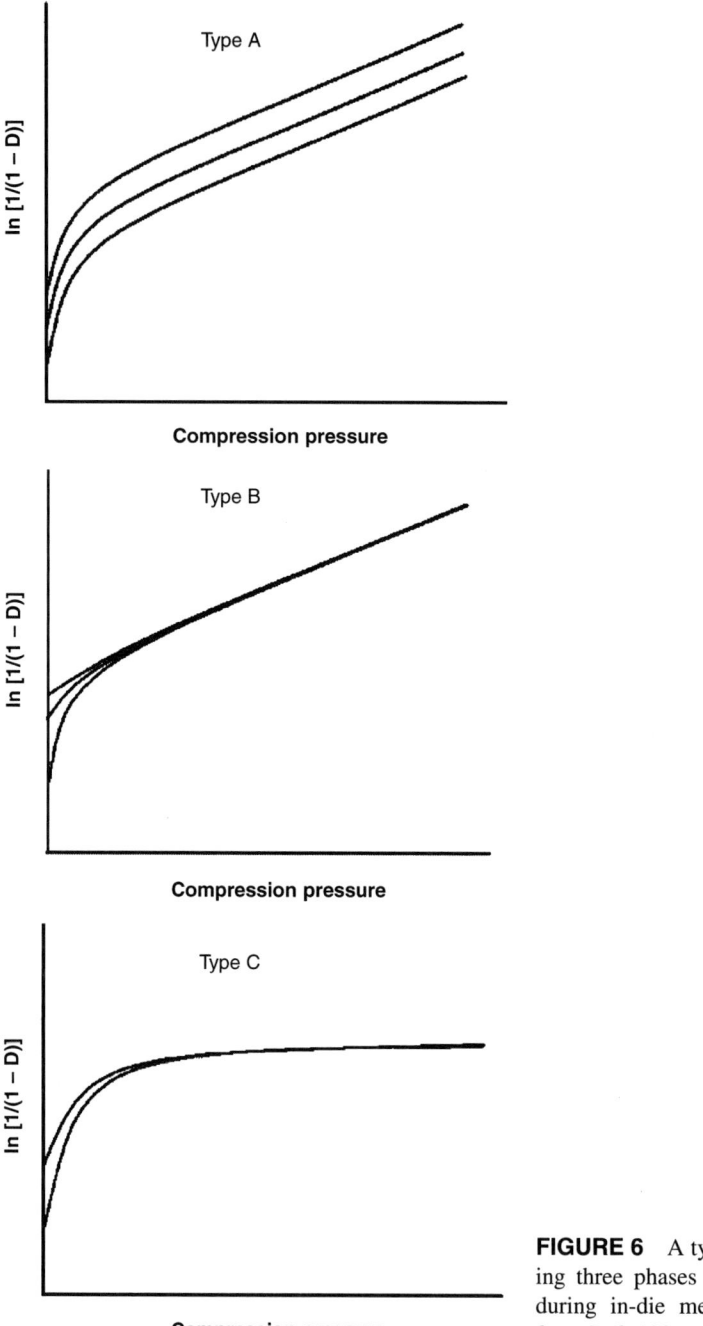

FIGURE 6 A typical Heckel plot showing three phases of particle deformation during in-die method. *Source*: Adapted from Ref. 180.

phase of rearrangement of particles in the early stages of compression and tends to indicate the extent of particle or granule fragmentation, although fragmentation can occur concurrently with plastic and elastic deformation of the constituent particles. ρ_b can be obtained from the equation:

$$\rho_b = \rho_A - \rho_0 \tag{10}$$

Compression and Compaction

The main utility of Heckel plots arises from their ability to identify the predominant deformation behavior of the material. The relationship is mostly used to distinguish between substances that consolidate by fragmentation and those that consolidate by plastic deformation.

Empirical evidence shows that materials with low mean yield pressures undergo plastic deformation, whereas, tableting materials with high mean yield pressure have a tendency to be brittle and consolidate via fragmentation. Based on Heckel plots and the compaction behavior of materials can be classified into three types, A, B, and C (Fig. 6) (88,89).

Type A materials show a linear relationship with the plots remaining parallel (for example, if three different particle size fractions were used they would have different initial packing densities) as the applied pressure is increased; which indicates deformation occurring due to plastic deformation. Examples of materials that exhibit type A behavior include MCC, corn starch, maize starch. Type A materials are usually comparatively soft and readily undergo plastic deformation with different degrees of porosity depending on the initial packing of the powder in the die. This in turn is dependent on the particle size, size distribution, shape, etc. of the original material.

Compression of type B materials show an initial curved region followed by a straight line in which all curves superimpose onto the same line. As with type A materials if three different particle size fractions were used, particle fragmentation would reduce the porosity of all three fractions to the same level causing the curves to superimpose. Type B plots are typical of harder materials with higher yield pressures which usually undergo compression by fragmentation to increase packing density. These two regions (initial curved region followed by a straight line) of a Heckel plot in type B are thought to represent the initial rearrangement stage and subsequent deformation process, the point of intersection corresponding to the lowest force at which a coherent tablet is formed. Common examples of type B materials include lactose and DCP.

For type C materials, there is an initial steep linear region after which the curves superimpose and flatten out as the applied pressure is increased. This behavior is ascribed to the absence of a rearrangement stage and densification is due to plastic deformation and asperity melting (88,89). Usually type A plots exhibit a higher final slope than type B plots indicating that the former materials have a lower yield pressure. This can be attributed to the fact that fragmentation with subsequent percolation of the broken particles is a less efficient process than filling in of voids by plastic deformation. The crushing strength of tablets can be correlated with the values of k from the Heckel plot; larger k values usually indicate harder tablets. This information can be useful for selecting a binder during the formulation development of tablets.

The most common variables affecting Heckel analysis are the rate and duration of compression, the degree of lubrication, and even the size and shape of the dies and punches (86); hence these variables should be taken into consideration during analysis. Although the use of the Heckel relationship to study the compression behavior of pharmaceutical powders/granules has been criticized (81), it still remains one of the most commonly used methods in the field of formulation research and development of pharmaceutical solids.

Kawakita Equation

The Kawakita equation was developed to study powder densification using the degree of reduction in volume, C, and expressed as (70):

$$C = \frac{(V_0 - V_p)}{V_0} = \frac{abP}{(1+bP)} \tag{11}$$

Equation (11) can be rearranged to give:

$$\frac{P}{C} = \frac{P}{a} + \frac{1}{ab} \tag{12}$$

where V_0 is the initial volume of the powder bed and V_p is the powder volume after application of pressure P. a and b are constants which are obtained from the slope and intercept of the $\frac{P}{C}$ versus P plots, respectively as shown in Figure 7. The constant a is equal to the minimum porosity of the powder system prior to compression while b, also known as the coefficient of compression, is related to the plasticity of the material.

Values of $(1-a)$ give the initial relative density of the material, ρ_0 which has been shown to provide a measure of the initial packed density of tablets with the application of small pressure (also referred to as tapping) (90). The reciprocal of b gives a pressure term, P_k, which is the pressure required to reduce the powder bed by 50% (80). For plastic materials, the value of P_k, is inversely proportional to the degree of plastic deformation during the densification process. Lower the value of P_k, the higher the degree of plastic deformation occurring during compression (37,69–71,80). Some of the limitations of the Kawakita relationship as reported by Celik (72) are that the Kawakita equation is applicable to materials in powder form only. The equation can be modified by substituting the initial compaction volume with an initial bulk volume in order to have a better correlation to the Kawakita equation for granulated materials. Also, he reported that with using this equation, the compaction process can be described only up to a certain pressure, above which the linearity of the equation is lost. Thus, it is now commonly accepted that the Kawakita equation is best applicable to low pressures and high porosities (69). It has been reported that the Kawakita equation can be used to determine the tensile strength of granules provided that the influence of die-wall friction has been

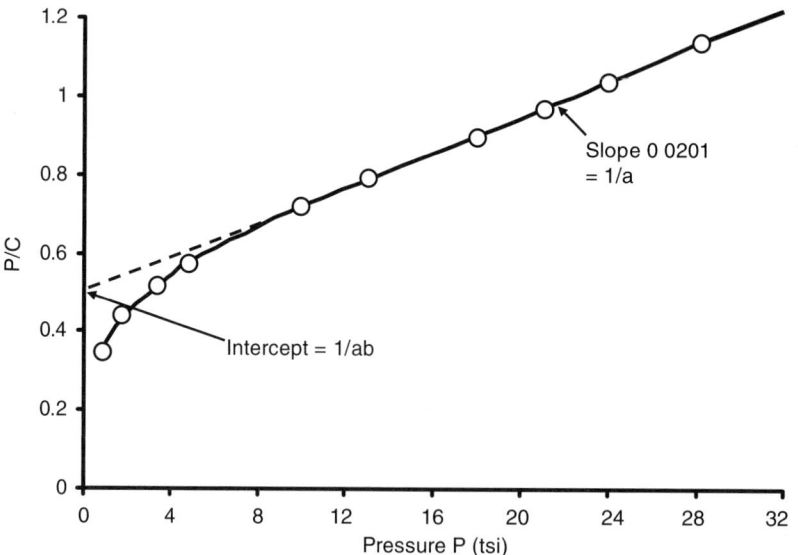

FIGURE 7 Graphical representation of Kawakita equation. A plot of P/C vs. P. *Source*: From Ref. 70.

Compression and Compaction

taken into account since it is well established that die-wall friction significantly increases resistance to deformation (70,71).

Despite their limitations, the Heckel and Kawakita plots have been extensively used to evaluate and explain the compression behavior of single- and multi-component systems at high and low pressures, respectively (72). Thus, to obtain more accurate information on the compression characteristics of a given system, both relationships can be used together and analyzed.

Adams Equation

The Adams equation was derived to estimate the fracture strength of single granules from in-die compression data. It assumes the bed of granules in the die as a series of parallel load-bearing columns (4,71). The equation derived was expressed as:

$$\ln P = \ln \frac{T_0'}{\alpha'} + \alpha' \varepsilon + \ln\left(1 - e^{(-\alpha' \varepsilon)}\right) \tag{13}$$

Where P is the applied pressure and is the natural strain which is given by:

$$\varepsilon = \ln\left[\frac{H_0}{H_p}\right] \tag{14}$$

and H_0 and H_p are the initial and current height of the powder bed, respectively. The quantity T_0' is the apparent single agglomerate strength which is related to the actual strength, T_0, as:

$$T_0' = k_1 T_0 \tag{15}$$

where k_1 is a constant. The quantity α' is related to the pressure coefficient, α of the agglomerate strength by the following expression:

$$\alpha' = k_2 \alpha \tag{16}$$

where k_2 is a constant.

At higher values of natural strain, the last term of the Equation (13), becomes negligible and can be omitted, leaving a linear function. The intercept and slope of this linear part of the profile were used to calculate the compression parameter, T_0'. Nicklasson and Alderborn (37) have used the Adams and Kawakita equations to analyze the compaction behavior of pharmaceutical granules (Fig. 8). They found that both $1/b$ and P_k from Kawakita and T_0' from Adams were related to the intergranular porosity and tensile strength of the tablets formed from the agglomerates (Table 1). They concluded that $1/b$ and T_0' may be interpreted as a measure of agglomerate shear strength during uniaxial confined compression and as such may be used as indications of tableting performance of the agglomerates.

Cooper–Eaton Equation

The Cooper–Eaton equation is based on the assumption that compression of powders follows a two-step process. Firstly rearrangement occurs whereby particles fill up the interparticulate voids that are larger than or of the same size as that of the particles. Secondly, deformation (elastic, plastic or fragmentation) occurs whereby particles fill up the voids smaller than that of the particles due to applied pressure. The relationship is given by (79,91),

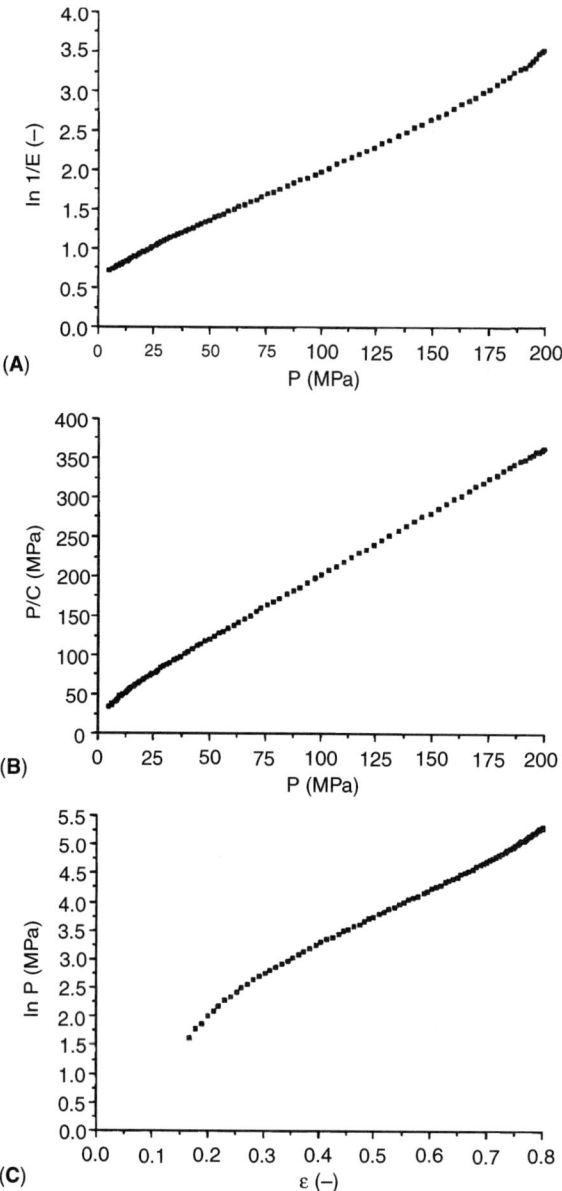

FIGURE 8 Examples of linearized compression equations: (**A**) Heckel equation; (**B**) Kawakita equation; and (**C**) Adams equation. All examples are for MCC granules having same porosity. *Abbreviation*: MCC, microcrystalline cellulose. *Source*: From Ref. 37.

$$\frac{1/\rho_0 - 1/\rho_r}{1/\rho_0 - 1} = a_1 \exp\left(-\frac{k_1}{P}\right) + a_2 \exp\left(-\frac{k_2}{P}\right) \tag{17}$$

where ρ_0 is the relative density at zero pressure, ρ_r the relative density at pressure P, a_1, a_2 are constants indicating the fraction of the total densification achieved by filling voids of the same size (a_1) and of a smaller size (a_2) than the actual particles and k_1 and k_2 are the pressures at which this two-stage densification is thought to occur. The relationship is plotted as pressure versus fractional volume compression (Fig. 9).

A wide variety of pharmaceutical excipients have been studied for their deformation behavior using the Cooper–Eaton relationship (92). The estimation of constants, a_1 and a_2, are used as measures of deformability of the materials. If the sum of $(a_1 + a_2)$

Compression and Compaction

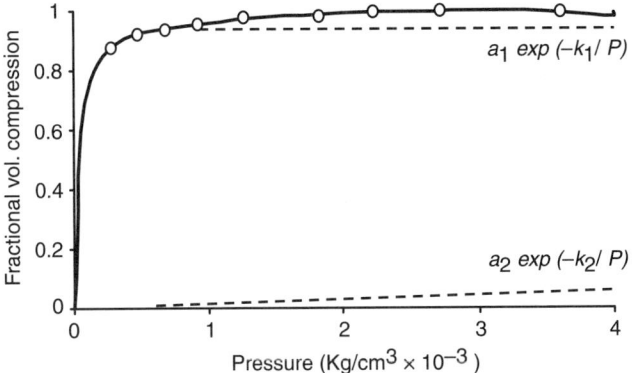

FIGURE 9 A Cooper–Eaton plot of a tromethamine salt of (±)-5-Benzoyl-1,2-dihydro-3H-pyrrolo(1,2a)pyrrole-1-carboxylic acid. *Source*: From Ref. 73.

is greater than unity a nonporous compact is expected to be obtained at lower pressures (92). Pharmaceutical powders with different particle size and shape were also studied to estimate the usefulness of this relationship in studying their compression behavior (73). It was found that the different density values and the yield pressure values from Heckel analysis were in excellent agreement with the coefficients of the Cooper–Eaton equation, thus proving the usefulness of the relationship (73). The same group further investigated the compression properties of granulations using the Cooper–Eaton relationship (93). The fractional volume compression versus applied pressure plots were used to calculate the coefficients of Cooper–Eaton equation (93). Again, the sum of coefficients ($a_1 + a_2$) ranged from 0.97 to 1.01, indicating that compression is achieved by the two probabilistic processes of filling large and small voids successively by rearrangement, fragmentation and plastic flow (93).

The Gurnham Equation

Considering the several limitations of the Heckel equation (lack of correlation between the mean yield pressure and the plasticity of a material, clear identification of the linear region of a Heckel plot etc.), recently, a new relationship using the Gurnham equation was proposed to characterize the deformation behavior of pharmaceutical material by Zhao et al. (94). This relationship was introduced in chemical engineering by Gurnham and Masson (95). They proposed that the rate of applied pressure is directly proportional to the apparent density of a given mass of material (94). Thus,

$$dP/P = Ad\rho \tag{18}$$

where P is pressure, ρ apparent density based on solid weight and total volume, and A is a constant. By integration, Equation (18) gives,

$$\rho = a \ln(P) + b \tag{19}$$

where a and b are constants. Porosity is a more commonly used parameter in the study of compressibility/compactibility of pharmaceutical material:

$$\varepsilon = 1 - \left(\frac{\rho}{\rho_{\text{true}}}\right) \tag{20}$$

where ε is porosity, ρ_{true} is true density. Thus, replacing density with porosity in Equation (19) yields:

$$\varepsilon = -c\ln(P) + d \qquad (21)$$

where c and d are constants. Equation (21) describes a linear relationship between ln (P) and porosity (ε) for powder compression. Writing Equation (21) in its differential form gives:

$$d\varepsilon = \frac{-cdP}{P} \qquad (22)$$

The constant c represents the effect of change in applied pressure on the compact porosity. The authors examined several pharmaceutical powders (Acetaminophen, Emcompress® or DCP, lactose, MCC, and corn starch) to estimate the value of c and determine if it is a true representation of the compressibility of a given material (Fig. 10) (94). It was found that the parameter, c, provides a good representation of material compressibility for single- and multi-component systems. Thus, the relationship promises to be a useful quantitative descriptor of deformation behavior of pharmaceutical powders (94).

Apart from the above mentioned relationships (pressure–porosity, pressure–volume, pressure–density) several less common methods to quantify compactibility of pharmaceutical powders have been explored and can be found in the literature. These relationships are briefly summarized by Sonnergaard (40) as shown in Table 2.

MECHANICAL ANALYSIS OF TABLET COMPACTION

Analysis of tablet compaction involves force and displacement, which can be normalized to stress and strain and the material relationships between stress and strain. The study of these factors comes under the study of solid or continuum mechanics. Many key concepts used in this chapter have their origin in continuum mechanic so in this section we will give a very brief overview of the main points needed to understand the basics of tablet

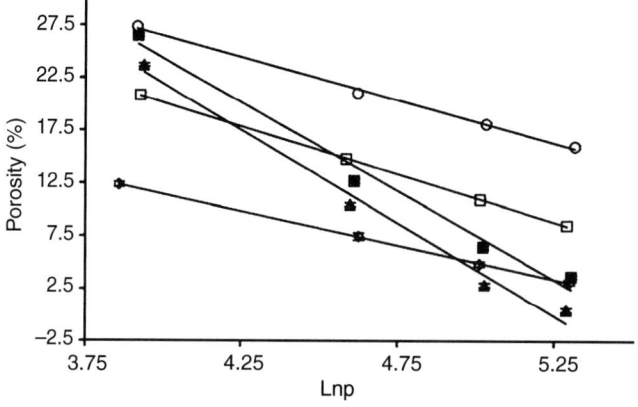

FIGURE 10 A typical Gurnham plot [Porosity vs. ln P for (■) MCC, (▲) corn starch, (o) emcompress, (□) lactose, and (♦) acetaminophen]. *Abbreviation*: MCC, microcrystalline cellulose. *Source*: From Ref. 94.

TABLE 2 Relationship Between Pressure and Porosity

Relationship	Group
One-point methods	
Pressure at CF = 8 Kp	Fraser
CS at pressure = 150 MPa	Duberg and Nystrom
CS at porosity = 15%	Van Veen et al.
Pressure profile	
$CS = a*P + b$	Newton et al.
$CS = a*\log(P) + b$	Higuchi et al.
$\log(CS) = a*\log(P) + b$	Newton and Grant
$CS = k*P^{T/2}$	Kuentz and Leuenberger
$\ln[-\ln(1 - CS/CS_{max})] = a*\ln P + b$	Castillo and Villafuerte
$F1 = \log(\sqrt{2})*(CF_i + 2CF_{i+1} + CF_{i+2})/2$	Amidon et al.
$H = H_{max}[1 - \exp(-\gamma\rho P)]$	Leuenberger and Jetzer
Porosity profile	
$CS = CS_0 * \exp(-k*\varepsilon)$	Ryshkewitch
$CS = k(\rho - \rho_c)^{2.7} + CS_0$	Ramirez et al.

Abbreviations: CF, crushing force; CS, crushing strength, including tensile strength; H, indentation hardness (Brinell); P, maximum compaction pressure; ε, porosity of the compact; ρ, density of the compact. All other symbols are constants.
Source: Adapted from Ref. 40.

compaction. Continuum mechanics is a well developed field with numerous excellent treatises on the subject; thus, this section will follow the presentation outline used by Fung (96), Fluggie (97), Shames and Cozzarelli (98), and some parts of this section were taken from the authors' previous work (99). This section will start out with basic definitions of stress and strain in one- and three-dimensions and then discuss elastic, viscoelastic, and plastic constitutive relations between stress and strain, and use this theory to do a three-dimensional viscoelastic stress analysis of tablet compaction.

Stress and Strain in One and Three–Dimensions

As mentioned previously single station and rotary presses impart a displacement onto the powder bed and the response to the displacement is the force the tablets resist compression with. Thus, the basic variables of any mechanical analysis are the stress and strain. Numerous definitions of stress (σ) and strain (ε) that have been developed for a discussion of these different types of analyses (96,98); in this section we will only cover the basic definitions needed for our analysis of tablet compaction.

The most commonly used stress, and the stress that will be used in this chapter, is the engineering stress:

$$\sigma = \frac{F}{A} \quad (23)$$

where the force (F) on an object is divided by the initial area (A) (Fig. 11A). This definition differs from the true stress which is the force divided by the current area. For small deformations, the difference between the different areas is not significant, but as the extent of deformation increases these differences can become significant. By convention compression forces are defined as forces that push into the body and by definition are negative and tension forces are forces that pull on an object and by definition are positive. The engineering strain is the normalized change in length:

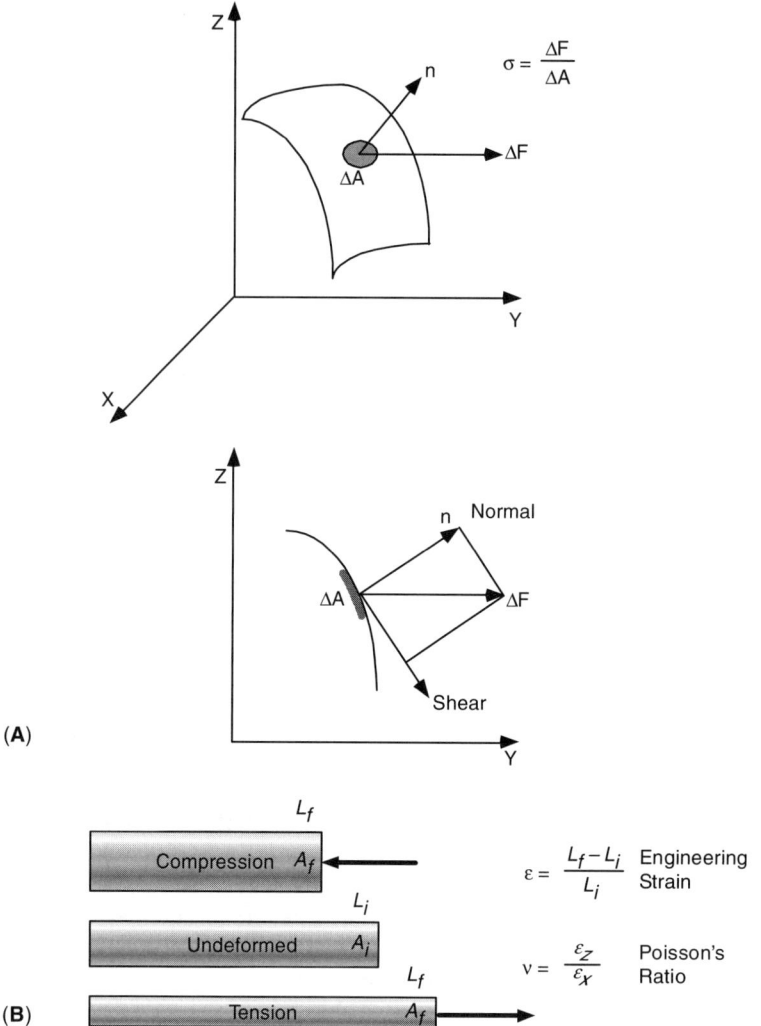

FIGURE 11 The calculation of strain for the deformation of a bar of original length of L_i showing compression, tension, and the change in diameter used to calculation of Poisson's ratio.

$$\varepsilon = \frac{L_f - L_i}{L_i} \qquad (24)$$

where L_i is the initial length of the specimen and L_f is the final length of the specimen (Fig. 11B). Like the stress, there are many other definitions of strain (98). If the specimen is longer after the test, i.e., $L_f > L_i$ the strain is positive and object is said to be in tension; conversely if the $L_f < L_i$ the strain is negative and the object is said to be in compression. A Cartesian coordinate system is utilized with z as the axial direction within the tablet, and x and y as radial directions. Compressional stresses and strains are negative, and tensional stress and strain is positive. The work computed is the work done by the environment on the tablet. A negative sign indicates that energy is going from the tablet to the environment whereas a positive sign indicates the tablet is absorbing energy.

Compression and Compaction

When a specimen is loaded in tension, the sample becomes longer in the axial direction and narrower in the radial direction transverse to the axial loading, and when the sample is compressed it becomes shorter and wider in the transverse direction (Fig. 11B). The ratio of axial to radial (transverse) dimension change is constant for a given material, and can be expressed by Poisson's ratio:

$$v = -\frac{\varepsilon_{radial}}{\varepsilon_{axial}} = -\frac{\varepsilon_{xx}}{\varepsilon_{zz}} \tag{25}$$

The negative sign is by convention so that v is positive (some specialty materials have negative Poisson's ratios). Poisson's ratio typically varies from 0 to 0.5 for incompressible materials. For many materials Poisson's ratio is about $v \sim 0.3$.

As written, Equations (23) and (24) are for the one-dimensional case; these basic concepts can be extended to three dimension. If one considers the three-dimensional vector in Figure 11A, this vector for the sake of illustration can be projected onto a two-dimensional plane. The force acting on the surface can be resolved into its normal and shear components. Normal stresses and strains are perpendicular to a surface and shear is parallel to a surface (Figs. 11A and 12). Thus, any force acting a body can be resolved into its normal shear components. The details of how this is done are beyond the scope of this chapter; the interested reader can refer to (96,98) for example. For a three-dimensional body, the distribution of stress and strain can be represented mathematically by a symmetric matrix also called a second order tensor:

$$\begin{bmatrix} \sigma_{xx} & \sigma_{xy} & \sigma_{xz} \\ \sigma_{yx} & \sigma_{yy} & \sigma_{yz} \\ \sigma_{zx} & \sigma_{zy} & \sigma_{zz} \end{bmatrix} = \sigma_{ij} \tag{26}$$

$$\begin{bmatrix} \varepsilon_{xx} & \varepsilon_{xy} & \varepsilon_{xz} \\ \varepsilon_{yx} & \varepsilon_{yy} & \varepsilon_{yz} \\ \varepsilon_{zx} & \varepsilon_{zy} & \varepsilon_{zz} \end{bmatrix} = \varepsilon_{ij} \tag{27}$$

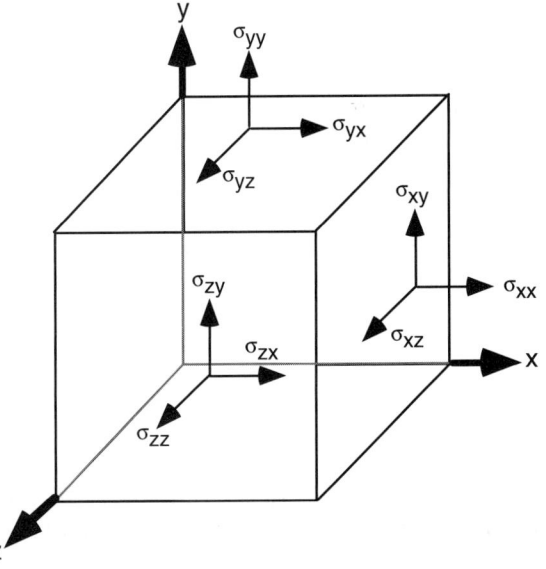

FIGURE 12 Three-dimensional state of stresses.

The normal components have repeated indices and appear on the diagonal of the tensor. The shear components indices are not repeated and appear over the remainder of the tensor.

For a powder to become a tablet it must undergo a volume reduced and a change in shape which introduces shear stresses into the tablet (Fig. 13). These two types of deformations are referred to as dilation a change in volume and distortion a change in shape. Just like any surface force can be resolved into normal and shear forces. The compression of a powder can be resolved into volume and shape changes. Dilation is a change in volume without change in shape. Mathematically, dilation is computed from the average of normal stresses or strains:

$$s_{ij} = \frac{1}{3}\sigma_{\alpha\alpha}\delta_{ij} = \frac{1}{3}\left(\sigma_{xx} + \sigma_{yy} + \sigma_{zz}\right) \tag{28}$$

$$e_{ij} = \frac{1}{3}\varepsilon_{\alpha\alpha}\delta_{ij} = \frac{1}{3}\left(\varepsilon_{xx} + \varepsilon_{yy} + \varepsilon_{zz}\right) \tag{29}$$

In tensor notation the repeated index is summed. The s_{ij} and e_{ij} are dilational tensors in stress and strain, respectively, and δ_{ij} is Kronecker's delta which equals 1 when $i = j$ and 0 when $i \neq j$. Distortion is a change in shape without a change in volume. Distortion is

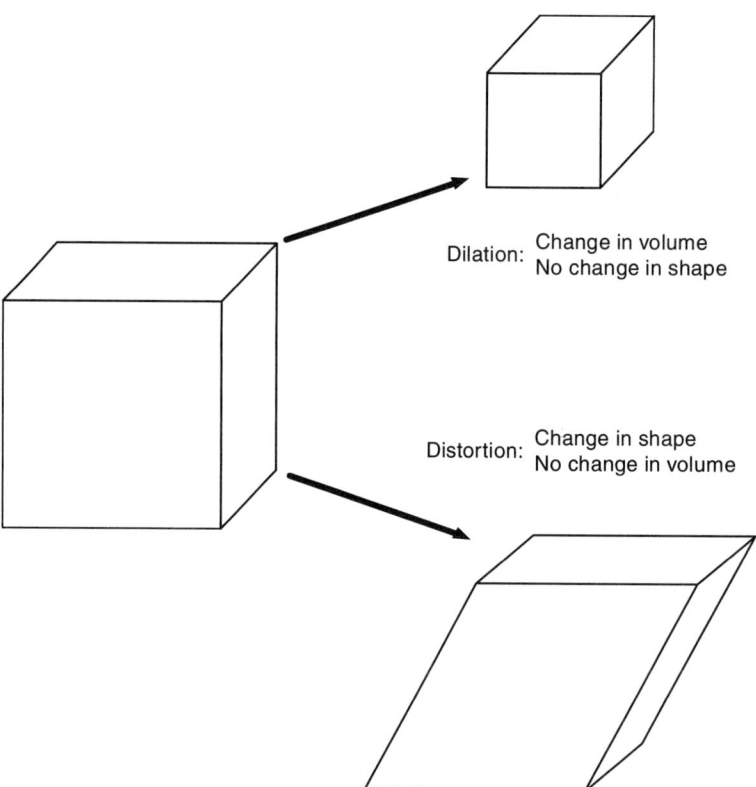

FIGURE 13 The deformation of a cube under hydrostatic stress causes a change in volume without a change in shape and the pure shearing of a cube causes a change in shape without a change in volume as shown in the top and bottom cubes, respectively.

Compression and Compaction

computed from the difference between original stress or strain and the corresponding dilation component:

$$S_{ij} = \sigma_{ij} - \frac{1}{3}\sigma_{\alpha\alpha}\delta_{ij} \tag{30}$$

$$E_{ij} = \varepsilon_{ij} - \frac{1}{3}\varepsilon_{\alpha\alpha}\delta_{ij} \tag{31}$$

where S_{ij} and E_{ij} are the stress and strain distortional tensors, respectively. The two material constants needed to describe distortion and dilation are independent of each other. For example, hydraulic fluids can be elastic in dilation and viscous in shear. Fluids used in hydraulic systems can withstand large hydrostatic stress but cannot support their own weight when a shear is applied.

The distribution of stress and strain, as described above, is independent of material and based only on geometric arguments, but the relationship between stress and strain is related by a class of material dependent equations called constitutive equations. For small deformations, an isotropic elastic body requires two material constants to completely describe the relationship between stress and strain (100). The most common elastic constants in use are the shear modulus, bulk modulus, Poisson's ratio, elastic modulus, and Lame's modulus. The bulk and shear modulus can be used to analyze tablet compaction. The bulk modulus relates dilational stress to dilational strain, and the shear modulus relates distortional stress to distortional strain.

Constitutive Equations: Material Properties

The discussion of material properties is a vast subject that no section of a chapter can do justice; the interested reader can review (96,98). As mentioned previously, a constitutive equation is a class of equations that relate stress to strain. The concept of a constitutive equation can be introduced by considering what would happen if a specimen were pulled apart in uniaxial tension and the stress and strain were continuously measured. For example, if one took a piece of plastic (like the plastic that holds a six pack together) between their fingers and pulled it till it broke. The results of such an experiment are shown in Figures 14 and 15. These idealized results show how the stress strain curve goes through three phases: (*i*) elastic, (*ii*) viscoelastic, and (*iii*) plastic.

The initial elastic phase is characterized by reversible deformation. For elastic materials, any deformation of the specimen is completely reversible and when the specimen is unloaded it will return to its original configuration or shape. In addition, elastic deformations are time independent that is the nature of the deformation doesn't depend upon the speed of compaction, and any energy put into the material during loading will be completely returned with no energy dissipation (i.e., no heat production) during unloading. As shown in Figure 14, elastic deformations take place in the initial portion of the curve and are only applicable for small strains after which the material begins to exhibit viscoelastic behavior.

The next phase is when the material starts to exhibit viscoelastic behavior. Viscoelastic deformations can be divided into viscoelastic solids and viscoelastic fluids. When a viscoelastic fluid like the Maxwell model is load and the load is removed the material does not return to its original configuration (Fig. 16); this is true for even the smallest deformations; typically viscoelastic fluids are not used to model solid behavior, although there are exceptions to this generalization. In contrast viscoelastic solids do return to there original configuration when unloaded. The key features of viscoelastic

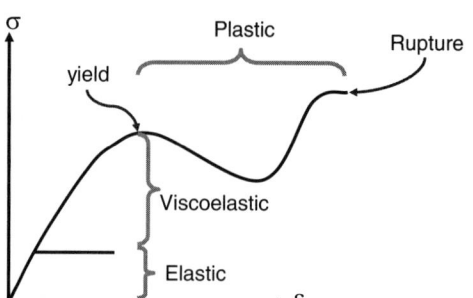

FIGURE 14 Idealized stress–strain curve for uniaxial tension experiment.

solid deformations are that they are time dependent and a portion of the energy put into the system is irreversibly dissipated. That is viscoelastic materials are history dependent and the past loading can affect current loadings. This type of behavior is very common with materials used in tableting.

In the final phase once the yield stress has been exceeded plastic deformation begins to occur (Fig. 14). The yield stress is the point where the deformation becomes permanent. For example, when you bend a coat hanger or stiff wire if you bend it a little it bounces right back to its original configuration; however, as you continue bending the wire, a point is reached where the coat hanger has a permanent bend in the wire; this point is called the yield point. Once a material has reached its yield point there are different ways the material can behave post yield. For example, a brittle material like chalk, once it exceeds it yield stress it immediately breaks. This type of behavior is called brittle material fracture and is illustrated in Figure 15A. The key feature is that little deformation occurs post yield. In contrast, ductile materials have a great deal of flow post yield (Fig. 15B). Brittle and ductile behaviors are the two extremes of material behavior post yield. Plastic deformations are characterized by an irreversible permanent set in the material. In other words when the specimen is unloading the deformation is permanent. Also, plasticity deformations can be either time independent or time dependent depending on the nature of the material.

Viscoelastic constitutive equations are used to model material properties. Viscoelastic theory combines the elements of elasticity and Newtonian fluids. The theory of viscoelasticity was developed to describe the behavior of materials which show intermediate behavior between solids and fluids.

The constitutive equation of elasticity is represented by the Hookian spring (Fig. 16). Hook's law states that the stress is proportional to the strain

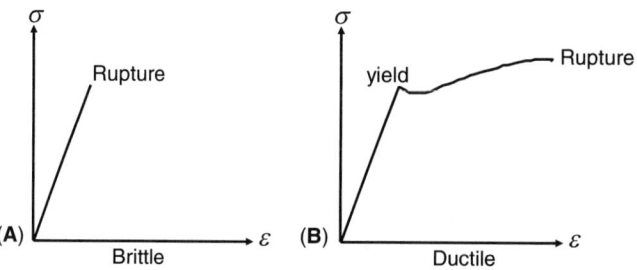

FIGURE 15 The difference between a brittle and ductile stress strain profile.

Compression and Compaction

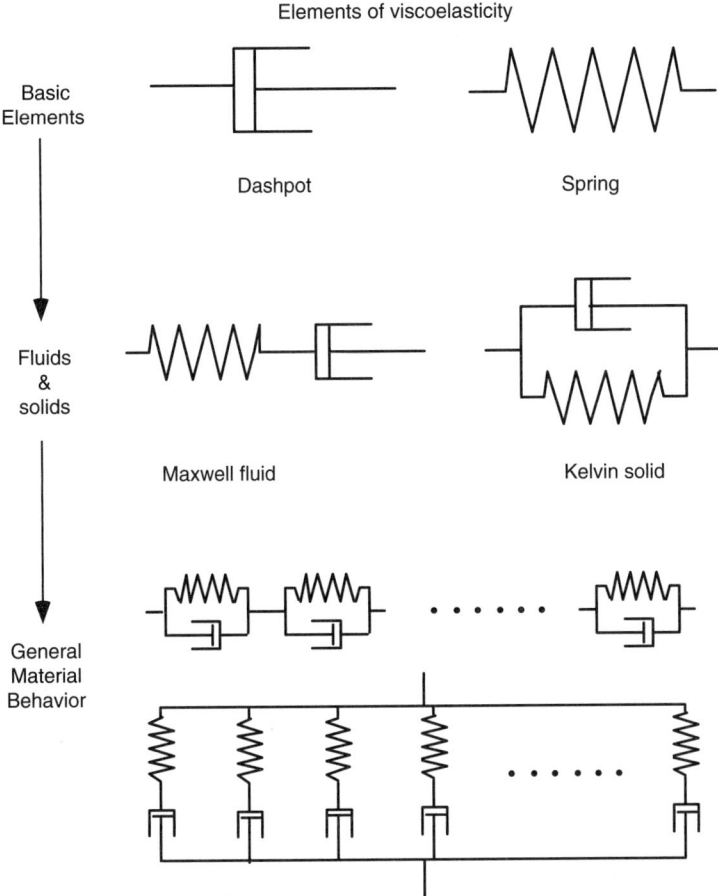

FIGURE 16 Viscoelasticity outline.

$$\sigma = \kappa \cdot \varepsilon \tag{32}$$

The proportionally constant κ is called Young's elastic modulus. The constitutive equation for a Newtonian fluid is represented by the dashpot Figure 16. For a Newtonian fluid, the stress is proportional to the strain rate:

$$\sigma = \eta \dot{\varepsilon} \tag{33}$$

where the dot above the strain ε stands for derivative with respect to time:

$$\dot{\varepsilon} = \frac{d\varepsilon}{dt} \tag{34}$$

and the proportionally constant η is called the viscosity. For dashpots, the faster you go the greater the resistance, which is typical of fluids like water. Anyone that has done a belly-flop in the pool is immediately aware of this property of Newtonian fluids.

The spring and dashpot provide a method for representing mathematical ideas or concepts. By combining springs and dashpots, a differential equation can be derived which describes the relationship between stress and strain (i.e., providing a description of material behavior). The most basic viscoelastic bodies are the Kelvin or Voigt solid and the Maxwell fluid (Fig. 16). The Maxwell body is a combination of a spring and dashpot in series. When elements are in series the strain of each element is added (Fig. 16):

$$\varepsilon = \varepsilon_s + \varepsilon_d \tag{35}$$

The subscript s and d refer to the elastic spring and viscous dashpot, respectively. The differential equation for a Maxwell body is obtained by first differentiating the sum of the strains Equation (35). This allows the viscous Equation (33) to be directly inserted in the differentiated form of Equation (35). Then by differentiating elastic Equation (32) it can also be inserted into the differentiated form of Equation (35) giving the final result:

$$\dot{\varepsilon} = \frac{\dot{\sigma}}{\kappa} + \frac{\sigma}{\eta} \tag{36}$$

The Kelvin body is a combination of the spring and dashpot in parallel. When elements are in parallel the stress of each element is added.

$$\sigma = \sigma_s + \sigma_d \tag{37}$$

The differential equation of a Kelvin element is obtained by directly inserting the elastic Equation (32) and the viscous Equation (33) into (37):

$$\sigma = \kappa\varepsilon + \eta\dot{\varepsilon} \tag{38}$$

For a more complete discussion of Maxwell and Kelvin models and viscoelasticity (96–98,101).

When examining material properties over long periods of time or at high loading rates as in tablet compaction it is often apparent that a Maxwell or Kelvin models are inadequate. To overcome this limitation, more complicated combinations of springs and dashpots have been used. It can be shown that the differential equation resulting from any combination of springs and dashpots will have the general form (97,101):

$$\sigma + p_1\dot{\sigma} + p_2\ddot{\sigma} + \ldots = q_0\varepsilon + q_1\dot{\varepsilon} + q_2\ddot{\varepsilon} + \ldots \tag{39}$$

where the ps and qs are combinations of the spring and dashpot constants. In this p and q notation it is customary to set the coefficient of the stress equal to one, thus p_0 is often not included. For example, if Equation (38) of a Kelvin element is written in p and q notation like Equation (39), then $q_0 = k$, $q_1 = \eta$ and $p_0 = 1$. The Maxwell elements in series or Kelvin elements in parallel (Fig. 16) are the most common way to represent general viscoelastic behavior (97,101). The more complicated models allow a greater range of frequencies and longer stress histories to be modeled. Equation (39) can be written in operator form:

$$\mathbf{P}\sigma = \mathbf{Q}\varepsilon \tag{40}$$

where $\mathbf{P}$ and $\mathbf{Q}$ are given by

$$\mathbf{P} = \sum_{i=1}^{n} p_i \frac{d^i}{dt^i} \tag{41}$$

$$\mathbf{Q} = \sum_{i=1}^{n} q_i \frac{d^i}{dt^i} \tag{42}$$

Compression and Compaction

A key characteristic of plastic deformations is that they are irreversible. The difference between a viscoelastic fluid and a plastic material is the presence of a yield stress. The yield stress is the stress at which the deformation becomes irreversible and once the yield stress has been exceeded then the deformation is irreversible (Figs. 14 and 15). For example, brittle materials often behave elastically until the yield point has been reached; once this point has been exceeded, the material will irreversibly deform or fracture like a piece of chalk (Fig. 15A). The key feature of a brittle material is that there is little deformation after the yield point. In contrast to a brittle material are a ductile materials (Fig. 15B); ductile materials undergo a lot of deformation after the yield point.

For plastic materials, the strain for a plastic material can be expressed as:

$$\varepsilon = \varepsilon_e + \varepsilon_p \tag{43}$$

where ε is the total strain, ε_e the elastic strain, and ε_p is the plastic strain. The plastic strain can be expressed as:

$$\varepsilon_p = \begin{cases} 0 & \text{if } \sigma < \sigma_y \\ f(\sigma) & \text{if } \sigma \geq \sigma_y \end{cases} \tag{44}$$

where $f(\sigma)$ is the flow function, which describes the material behavior post yield, i.e., after the yield stress has been exceeded. The nature of $f(\sigma)$ is matter of much research and there are almost as many flow rules as materials. For example, there are rate independent, rate dependent materials that show hardening, power law hardening and, the Bauschinger effect; a more detailed account of these different flow rules is given in (98,102).

One idealized material is the elastic perfectly plastic material a typically stress strain curve is shown in Figure 17A. For this curve we can substitute Equation (32) into Equation (43) to yield:

$$\dot{\varepsilon} = \dot{\varepsilon}_e + \dot{\varepsilon}_p = \frac{\dot{\sigma}}{\kappa} + \dot{\varepsilon}_p \tag{45}$$

where plastic strain rate can be expressed as

$$\dot{\varepsilon}_p = \begin{cases} 0 & \text{if } \sigma < \sigma_y \\ \text{Const.} & \text{if } \sigma = \sigma_y \\ 0 & \text{if } \sigma < \sigma_y \end{cases} \tag{46}$$

For perfectly plastic materials, post-yielding the strain rate is a constant function of the stress and the stress is constant and never exceeds σ_y (Fig. 18A). The extent of plastic deformation ε_p depends upon the proportionality between plastic strain rate and the stress and the how long the stress is applied as shown in Figure 17A. The elastic perfectly plastic material is highly idealized and not many materials exhibit this type of behavior.

Many materials show some type of strain hardening post yield, sometimes called work hardening; in other words, post-yield the material becomes harder to deform as the modulus increases. The power law strain hardening is the simplest model for strain hardening. The equations for power law strain hardening can be expressed as:

$$\varepsilon = \frac{\sigma}{\kappa} \quad \text{if } \sigma < \sigma_y \tag{47}$$

for pre-yielding and for post-yielding, i.e., $\sigma \geq \sigma_y$, is used

$$\varepsilon = \frac{\sigma}{\kappa} + \left(\frac{\sigma - \sigma_y}{\mu_p}\right)^n \quad \text{where } n \geq 1 \tag{48}$$

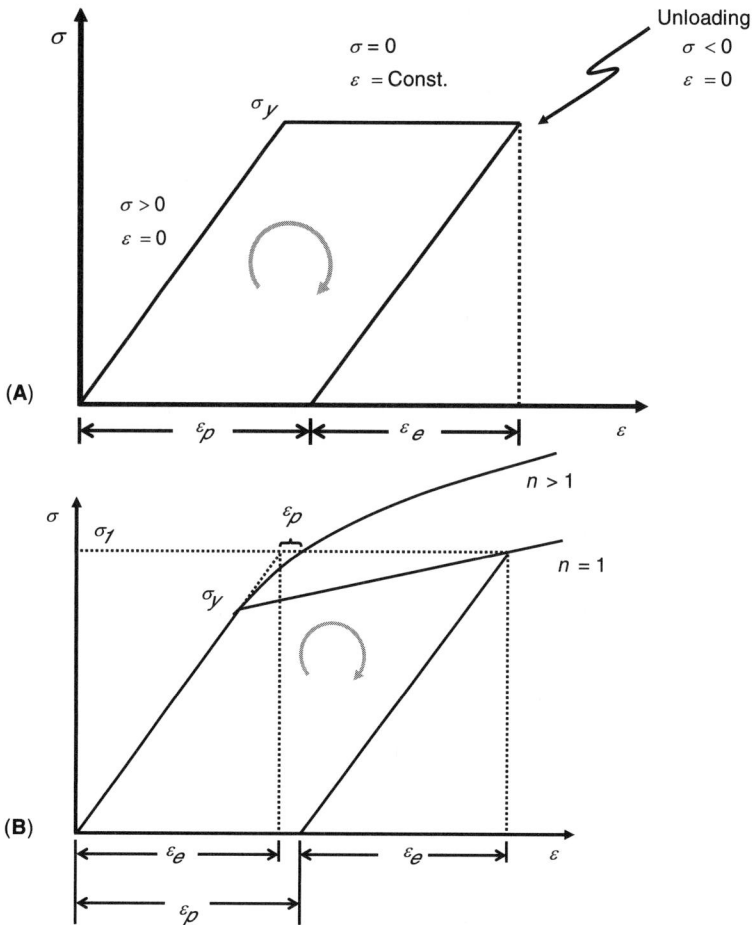

FIGURE 17 (**A**) Stress–strain diagram of elastic perfectly plastic material and (**B**) stress–strain diagram of elastic material power law with strain hardening. *Source*: Adapted from Ref. 98.

where n and μ_p are material constants for plastic materials. The stress strain diagram for a power law strain hardening material is shown in Figure 17B. The shape of the stress strain curves can be determined by taking the derivative of Equations (47) and (48) for pre- and post-yielding. For pre-yielding the stress strain profile is obviously a straight line with a slope of κ. For post-yielding the derivative of Equation (48) is

$$\frac{d\varepsilon}{d\sigma} = \frac{1}{\kappa} + n\left(\frac{\sigma - \sigma_y}{\mu_p}\right)^{n-1}\frac{1}{\mu_p} \qquad (49)$$

As can be seen by this equation when $n = 1$ the post yield curve is a straight line with a slope that is a function of the elastic and plastic material properties. For $n > 1$ the slope is a function of σ i.e., not a straight line.

For elastic perfectly plastic models there is no elastic deformation in the post-yielding phase; however, with the power law strain hardening there is continued elastic and plastic deformation combined. The extent of elastic and plastic deformation post-yielding can be determined by looking at some arbitrary stress σ_1 as shown on Figure 17B. For this stress the elastic and plastic deformations are

Compression and Compaction

$$\varepsilon_e = \frac{\sigma_1}{\kappa} \text{ and } \varepsilon_p = \left(\frac{\sigma_1 - \sigma_y}{\mu_p}\right)^n, \tag{50}$$

respectively. Thus, if the load were removed at $\sigma = \sigma_1$ then ε_e would be the amount of deformation recovered and ε_p would be the amount of permanent set in the material.

This type of material behavior is very important in tableting especially when materials like MCC are reworked. For example, it is hypothesized that when roller compacting MCC if the material is over compressed when going through the rollers that it will work harden and not deform as readily when compacted into tablets. The reduced compactibility results in less contact between the particles, and thus, weaker tablets, and in fact this type of behavior is often observed.

Three-Dimensional Viscoelastic Analysis

The main difference between three-dimensional viscoelastic stress analysis and three-dimensional elastic stress analysis is the time dependency of the modulus. A general way to solve these time dependent problems is to use the correspondence principle. The correspondence principle transforms the time dependent problem into a domain that removes time from the equations; in this domain the elastic time independent solution is calculated. This elastic solution is then transformed back into a time dependent domain yielding a time dependent solution. An analogous strategy is the use of logarithms to solve multiplication problems. By using logarithms the multiplication problem is converted into an addition problem which is easier to solve. Once the addition solution has been obtained, the multiplication answer can be found by taking the inverse logarithm. This method was very useful in the days before calculators and computers. The correspondence principle uses a Laplace or Fourier transform to remove the time dependency from the viscoelastic problem, then in the Laplace or frequency domain the problem is solved as an elasticity problem. The viscoelastic solution is obtained by inverting the elastic solution, which is dependent on s or $i\omega$ back into the time domain which is dependent on time (t) (96,98,101).

To avoid these mathematical details and focus on the key concepts of tablet stress analysis this discussion will examine the simplest of viscoelastic models using the method outlined by Fluggie (97). To begin the analysis, the boundary conditions which apply to tablet compaction, will be used to set up the stress and strain tensors Equations (26) and (27). Then the dilation and distortion Equations (28–31) will be used to obtain dilation and distortion tensors. After obtaining the dilational and distortional stress and strain tensors, a Kelvin viscoelastic model will be used to relate the distortional stress to distortional strain and the dilational stress to dilational strain.

When setting up tensor Equations (26) and (27), the tablet is considered a viscoelastic right circular cylinder in a rigid die under initial stress at the beginning of roll-off. For these conditions, Equations (26) and (27) take the following form if the shear stresses and shear strains are neglected:

$$\begin{bmatrix} \sigma_{xx} & 0 & 0 \\ 0 & \sigma_{yy} & 0 \\ 0 & 0 & \sigma_{zz} \end{bmatrix} = \begin{bmatrix} s & 0 & 0 \\ 0 & s & 0 \\ 0 & 0 & s \end{bmatrix} + \begin{bmatrix} S_{xx} & 0 & 0 \\ 0 & S_{yy} & 0 \\ 0 & 0 & S_{zz} \end{bmatrix} \tag{51}$$

$$\begin{bmatrix} \varepsilon_{xx} & 0 & 0 \\ 0 & \varepsilon_{yy} & 0 \\ 0 & 0 & \varepsilon_{zz} \end{bmatrix} = \begin{bmatrix} e & 0 & 0 \\ 0 & e & 0 \\ 0 & 0 & e \end{bmatrix} + \begin{bmatrix} E_{xx} & 0 & 0 \\ 0 & E_{yy} & 0 \\ 0 & 0 & E_{zz} \end{bmatrix} \tag{52}$$

For this analysis, the shear stresses and shear strains can be neglected because the die-wall is assumed to be lubricated with sufficient lubrication to render the die-wall friction negligible. The assumption of negligible die-wall friction is consistent with experimental results found in the literature. It has been shown that if the die-wall stress is small compared to the punch pressure the die-wall friction can be neglected. In addition, die-wall friction is created by the interaction of the tablet and the die-wall, and these interactions are minimized in a rotary tablet press. The compression cycle on a rotary machine is symmetric, so that the middle of the tablet experiences no significant frictional forces. The ends only are subjected to frictional forces resulting from material sliding along the die-wall.

To simplify the notation, the subscript yy will be written as xx since the radial directions are equivalent. Using tensor Equations (28) and (29) the dilation becomes,

$$s = \frac{1}{3}(2\sigma_{XX} + \sigma_{ZZ}) \tag{53}$$

$$e = \frac{1}{3}(2\varepsilon_{XX} + \varepsilon_{ZZ}) \tag{54}$$

Using tensor Equations (30) and (31) the distortion becomes:

$$S_{ZZ} = \frac{2}{3}(-\sigma_{XX} + \sigma_{ZZ}) \tag{55}$$

$$S_{XX} = \frac{1}{3}(\sigma_{XX} - \sigma_{ZZ}) \tag{56}$$

$$E_{ZZ} = \frac{2}{3}(-\varepsilon_{XX} + \varepsilon_{ZZ}) \tag{57}$$

$$E_{XX} = \frac{1}{3}(\varepsilon_{XX} - \varepsilon_{ZZ}) \tag{58}$$

The formation of a tablet during the loading phase causes the system to be under initial stress at the beginning of the deformation analysis. The initial stress has many important implications to the analysis of tablets during unloading and relaxation (99,103,104). For three-dimensional multi-axial loading conditions, Hook's law can be written as:

$$s = 3\,K\,e \tag{59}$$

$$S_{ij} = 2\,G\,E_{ij} \tag{60}$$

K is the bulk and G is the shear modulus. The equivalences between Equation (40) and Equations (59) and (60) indicate that K and G are given by Equations (61) and (62). Where the dilational parameters are abbreviated by a double prime in the superscript and distortional parameters by a single prime, respectively:

$$3K = \frac{\mathbf{P}''}{\mathbf{Q}''} \tag{61}$$

$$2G = \frac{\mathbf{P}'}{\mathbf{Q}'} \tag{62}$$

Compression and Compaction

Using the bulk and shear modulus to relate dilational stress to dilational strain and distortional stress to distortional strain yields:

$$\mathbf{P}''s = \mathbf{Q}''e \tag{63}$$

$$\mathbf{P}'S_{ij} = \mathbf{Q}'E_{ij} \tag{64}$$

Inserting the dilational Equations (53), and (54) into the dilation operators Equation (63) yields:

$$2\mathbf{P}''\sigma_{XX} + \mathbf{P}''\sigma_{ZZ} = 2\mathbf{Q}''\varepsilon_{XX} + \mathbf{Q}''\varepsilon_{ZZ} \tag{65}$$

There is only one distortional Equation because of the linear dependence between the x and z directions. Substituting distortional Equations (56) and (58) into the distortional operators Equation (64) produces:

$$\mathbf{P}'\sigma_{XX} - \mathbf{P}'\sigma_{ZZ} = \mathbf{Q}'\varepsilon_{XX} - \mathbf{Q}'\varepsilon_{ZZ} \tag{66}$$

Solving Equations (65) and (66) for σ_{xx} and σ_{xx} yields:

$$3\mathbf{P}''\mathbf{P}'\sigma_{XX} = 2\mathbf{P}'\mathbf{Q}'' + \mathbf{P}''\mathbf{Q}'\varepsilon_{XX} + \mathbf{P}'\mathbf{Q}'' - \mathbf{P}''\mathbf{Q}'\varepsilon_{ZZ} \tag{67}$$

$$3\mathbf{P}''\mathbf{P}'\sigma_{ZZ} = 2\mathbf{P}'\mathbf{Q}'' - \mathbf{P}''\mathbf{Q}'\varepsilon_{XX} + \mathbf{P}'\mathbf{Q}'' + \mathbf{P}''\mathbf{Q}'\varepsilon_{ZZ} \tag{68}$$

The viscoelastic operators for Kelvin dilation $\mathbf{P}''$ and $\mathbf{Q}''$ are

$$\mathbf{P}'' = 1$$

$$\mathbf{Q}'' = q_0'' + q_1'' \frac{\mathrm{d}}{\mathrm{d}t} \tag{69}$$

The viscoelastic operators for Kelvin distortion $\mathbf{P}'$ and $\mathbf{Q}'$ are

$$\mathbf{P}' = 1$$

$$\mathbf{Q}' = q_0' + q_1' \frac{\mathrm{d}}{\mathrm{d}t} \tag{70}$$

where q_0'' abbreviates elastic dilation, q_1'' viscous dilation, q_0' elastic distortion, and q_1' viscous distortion. The q's are the viscoelastic parameters to be determined from the experimental stress/strain data. Inserting the operators Equations (69) and (70) into Equations (67) and (68) yields:

$$\sigma_{ZZ} = \frac{1}{3}(q_0'' + 2q_0')\varepsilon_{ZZ} + \frac{1}{3}(q_1'' + 2q_1')\dot{\varepsilon}_{ZZ} + \frac{2}{3}(q_0'' - q_0')\varepsilon_{XX} + \frac{2}{3}(q_1'' - q_1')\dot{\varepsilon}_{XX} \tag{71}$$

$$\sigma_{XX} = \frac{1}{3}(q_0'' - q_0')\varepsilon_{ZZ} + \frac{1}{3}(q_1'' - q_1')\dot{\varepsilon}_{ZZ} + \frac{1}{3}(2q_0'' + q_0')\varepsilon_{XX} + \frac{1}{3}(2q_1'' + q_1')\dot{\varepsilon}_{XX} \tag{72}$$

Stress Relaxation in the Die

The relaxation equations are calculated in a similar manner to the unloading equations, except that during the relaxation phase the punch stress is zero. When the punch stresses are zero, stress and strain tensors become:

$$\begin{bmatrix} \sigma_{xx} & 0 & 0 \\ 0 & \sigma_{yy} & 0 \\ 0 & 0 & 0 \end{bmatrix} = \sigma_{ij} \qquad (73)$$

$$\begin{bmatrix} \varepsilon_{xx} & 0 & 0 \\ 0 & \varepsilon_{yy} & 0 \\ 0 & 0 & \varepsilon_{zz} \end{bmatrix} = \varepsilon_{ij} \qquad (74)$$

Recalling the dilational Equations (28) and (29) and the distortional Equations (30) and (31). These equations can be adjusted for stress relaxation boundary conditions shown in Equations (73) and (74). Thus, using the tensor Equations (73) and (74) and Equations (28) and (29) to compute the dilational and distortional stresses and strains. Once the dilational and distortional stresses and strains are computed, the shear and bulk modulus Equations (63) and (64) can be used to relate stress to strain yielding:

$$2\mathbf{Q}'\mathbf{P}''\sigma_{XX} = 2\mathbf{Q}'\mathbf{Q}''\varepsilon_{XX} + \mathbf{Q}'\mathbf{Q}''\varepsilon_{ZZ} \qquad (75)$$

$$\mathbf{Q}'\mathbf{P}''\sigma_{XX} = \mathbf{Q}''\mathbf{Q}'\varepsilon_{XX} - \mathbf{Q}''\mathbf{Q}'\varepsilon_{ZZ} \qquad (76)$$

Using Equations (75) and (76) to eliminate ε_{zz} produces an equation which relates σ_{xx} to ε_{xx}.

$$3\mathbf{Q}''\mathbf{Q}'\varepsilon_{XX} = \mathbf{P}'\mathbf{Q}'' + 2\mathbf{P}''\mathbf{Q}'\sigma_{xx} \qquad (77)$$

Then using the Kelvin operators as in Equations (69) and (70), and assuming $\varepsilon_{xx} = \dot{\varepsilon}_{xx} = 0$ produces the following differential equations to describe relaxation:

$$(q_0'' + 2q_0')\sigma_{XX} + (q_1'' + 2q_1')\dot{\sigma}_{XX} = 3q_0''q_0'\varepsilon_{XX} \qquad (78)$$

The boundary condition for this differential equation is

$$\sigma_{XX}(0) = \sigma_0 \qquad (79)$$

where $\sigma_{xx}(0)$ is the die stress when the punch stress goes to zero (i.e., lift-off) and is a constant. Solving Equation (78) yields:

$$\sigma_{XX}(t) = C_1 + \sigma_0 - C_1 e^{-C_2 t} \qquad (80)$$

where

$$C_2 = \frac{q_0'' + 2q_0'}{q_1'' + 2q_1'} \qquad (81)$$

$$C_1 = \frac{3q_0''q_0'\varepsilon_{XX}}{q_0'' + 2q_0'} \qquad (82)$$

Because there are only two equations and four unknowns, values for the individual q's cannot be solved for. Only C_1 and C_2 can be obtained by nonlinear parameter estimation techniques. C_1 and C_2 are important parameters, C_2 is the retardation time (101) and C_1 is the equilibrium die stress.

Compression and Compaction

Work Equations

During the loading phase, the tablet machine is doing force displacement work on the tablet (7). Some of this energy is stored and some is dissipated as heat (103). While the punches are on the flat, there is no force displacement work being exchanged with the environment, but the tablet is dissipating energy through irreversible processes. During unloading the tablet is releasing stored elastic energy to the tablet machine and internally dissipating stored energy through irreversible processes. Finally, during the relaxation phase no force displacement energy is being exchanged with the environment, but the tablet is relaxing and dissipating energy. The tablet is always irreversibly dissipating stored energy. The internal energy only increases during the loading phase and other phases then dissipate this stored energy either irreversibly or through force displacement work.

It can be shown (97) that the rate of work per unit volume is given by

$$\dot{W} = \sigma_{ij}\dot{\varepsilon}_{ij} \tag{83}$$

For a tablet machine, all of the energy exchange with the environment (neglecting heat flux) occurs thorough the punches reducing Equation (83) to

$$\dot{W} = \sigma_{zz}\dot{\varepsilon}_{zz} \tag{84}$$

The work input can be divided into dilation and distortion, Equation (84) can be written as:

$$\dot{W} = \sigma_{zz}\dot{\varepsilon}_{zz} = 3s\dot{e} + 2S_{XX}\dot{E}_{XX} + S_{ZZ}\dot{E}_{ZZ} \tag{85}$$

Inserting the axial stress Equation (71) and the radial stress Equation (72) into Equation (85), and assuming $\dot{\varepsilon}_{xx} = 0$, yields:

$$\dot{W} = \frac{1}{3}q_0''\varepsilon_{zz}\dot{\varepsilon}_{zz} + \frac{2}{3}q_0''\varepsilon_{xx}\dot{\varepsilon}_{zz} + \frac{2}{3}q_0'\varepsilon_{zz}\dot{\varepsilon}_{zz} - \frac{2}{3}q_0'\varepsilon_{xx}\dot{\varepsilon}_{zz} + \frac{1}{3}q_1''\dot{\varepsilon}_{zz}^2 + \frac{2}{3}q_1'\dot{\varepsilon}_{zz}^2 \tag{86}$$

Alternatively, Equation (86) can be obtained by inserting the axial stress Equation (71) into the left side of Equation (83). Equation (86) is divided into four parts. Separating the four individual q terms in Equation (86) and integrating with respect to time over an interval starting with α and ending with β yields on can break up the work into four parts:

$$W_0'' = \frac{1}{3}\int_\alpha^\beta q_0''\varepsilon_{zz}\dot{\varepsilon}_{zz} + 2q_0''\varepsilon_{xx}\dot{\varepsilon}_{zz}\,d\tau \tag{87}$$

$$W_0' = \frac{2}{3}\int_\alpha^\beta q_0'\varepsilon_{zz}\dot{\varepsilon}_{zz} - q_0'\varepsilon_{xx}\dot{\varepsilon}_{zz}\,d\tau \tag{88}$$

$$W_1'' = \frac{1}{3}\int_\alpha^\beta q_1''\varepsilon_{zz}\dot{\varepsilon}_{zz}\,d\tau \tag{89}$$

$$W_1' = \frac{2}{3}\int_\alpha^\beta q_1'\varepsilon_{zz}\dot{\varepsilon}_{zz}\,d\tau \tag{90}$$

where the following abbreviations are used: W_0'' elastic dilation, W_1'' viscous dilation, W_0' elastic distortion, and W_1' viscous distortion. Viscoelastic materials store and dissipate energy simultaneously during deformation. During the loading phase, the tablet is absorbing energy from the environment. At approximately the time the punches reach the start of the dwell phase, the internal energy is at a maximum and then starts to decrease. The internal free energy decreases during the dwell phase, because while there is no force displacement work being exchanged with the environment there is internal viscous flow. This loss in internal free energy occurs with heat generation which is small during the 18 milliseconds dwell phase. The stress relaxation that occurs during the dwell phase will reduce the amount of elastic free energy available for subsequent expansion (103).

The amount of work done on a tablet during loading is relatively constant for a given P_{max}. However, the amount of elastic free energy stored during this process is quite variable. Different formulations and manufacturing conditions affect the way energy is stored and released during loading. Also, additives such as binders, disintegrating agents, and lubricants may affect the amount of elastic free energy.

HIESTAND TABLETING INDICES

Pharmaceutical compacts are complex structures that present difficult challenges when measuring their mechanical properties. Hiestand was a pioneer who quantified the compaction properties of pharmaceutical powders and (105–109) the result of his work are indices known as the Hiestand Tableting Indices. These indices are dimensionless numbers used to describe the mechanical properties and consolidation behavior of materials under compression and decompression. The three main Hiestand Tableting Indices are the bonding index, brittle fracture index (*BFI*), and strain index.

The Hiestand bonding index (*BI*) is related to the ability of bonds formed during compression to survive the decompression process. It is a measure of the material's ability to form bonds and produce a suitable tablet. The Hiestand bonding index can be calculated by taking a ratio of the tensile strength (σ_T) to the dynamic or static indentation hardness (*H*):

$$BI = \frac{\sigma_T}{H} \tag{91}$$

Tensile strength represents the strength of a compact after ejection from the die, which directly relates to the bonds remaining after the elastic recovery process. Tensile strength can be measured by diametrical compression test described by Fell and Newton (110), and is described in the section "Mechanical Strength of Tablets". Indentation hardness is indicative of the resistance of the material to deformation under a compressive load. Using the dynamic pendulum method of Hiestand et al. (107) the dynamic indentation hardness (H_0), is obtained from a pendulum impact device and is calculated using the following equation:

$$H = \frac{4mgrh_r}{\pi a^4}\left(\frac{h_i}{h_r} - \frac{3}{8}\right) \tag{92}$$

where m is the mass of the indenter, g the gravitational constant, r the radius of the sphere, a the chordal radius of the indent, h_i the initial height of indenter, and h_r is the rebound height of the indenter. In addition, the static indentation hardness can be measured; for these measurements, the indenter is applied to the tablet surface for longer periods using a material testing machine like an Instron®. In terms of notation when the indenter is pressed into the surface for 30 minutes the measured hardness is the H_{30} value. Although tableting manufacturing doesn't involve long dwell times, comparison of the hardness for these different times gives information about the time dependent properties of a material. A ratio of H_0 and H_{30} can be used to assess the viscoelastic behavior of a material. For example, the ratio of H_0/H_{30} for APAP (acetaminophen) is only 1.2. This is relatively small value and indicates non-viscoelastic nature of APAP and therefore it has poor tableting characteristics.

The *BFI*, is a measure of the brittleness of a material, and indicates the ability or inability of a compact to relieve stress by plastic deformation or plastic flow, which reflects a materials propensity towards capping and lamination. The *BFI* is given by:

$$BFI = \frac{1}{2}\left(\frac{\sigma_T}{\sigma_{T0}} - 1\right) \quad (93)$$

where σ_T is the tensile strength of compact without a hole in the center, σ_{T0} is the tensile strength of a compact with a small axially oriented hole in the center of the compact, which are typically square. When a hole or macroscopic (relative to the particle size) flaw is in a compact, this hole concentrates the stress on the sides parallel to the applied stress. For round holes, the stress concentration is 3.2 times more than the stress if no hole was present. Thus, for very brittle materials $\sigma_T > \sigma_{T0}$ by a factor of approximately 3; however, if a material can deform plastically this plastic flow relives the stress at the edges of the hole which reduces the stress concentration. Typically, *BFI* values less than 0.20 are indicative of a low capping propensity.

The third Hiestand Index is the stain index. It is a measure of the strain, associated with the release of elastic stresses after plastic deformation. It can be calculated by taking a ratio of H_0/E' where H_0 is the dynamic indentation hardness of the compact including particles and pores,

$$\frac{1}{E'} = \frac{(1-v_1^2)}{E_1} + \frac{(1-v_2^2)}{E_2} \quad (94)$$

where is the Poisson's ratio, E is the Young's modulus of elasticity for materials 1 and 2, respectively. The SI index does not as correlated to material properties as well as the *BI* and *BFI*; thus, its use is less.

By determining these indices for drugs and excipients a portfolio of material properties can be assembled, and by using these indices, excipients can be rationally chosen to overcome an undesirable characteristic of the API. In other words the indices of the individual components and the final formulation can be used to assess the mechanical properties; thus, providing an important tool to predicting the quality of the final formulation.

Williams and McGinity (111) examined how the amount of MgSt affected the three indices for calcium sulfate powders. They found that as the level of MgSt in the compacts was progressively increased up to 5%, the magnitude of the tensile strength, dynamic indentation hardness, and bonding index decreased. They concluded that the compacts composed of calcium sulfate and MgSt were unable to maintain the extensive areas of true contact that were established under maximum compressive stress during decompression. Similar trends were observed on *BFI*. The presence of increasing levels of MgSt reduced the *BFI* to a value where the propensity for brittle fracture was minimal. The accumulation of MgSt at the surfaces of the host particles reduced the shear strength of the compact. Wurster et al. (112) also studied the effect of MgSt on the Hiestand indices and consolidation mechanisms of single component maltodextrins. Their findings were in agreement with William and McGinity, MgSt was shown to lower the tensile strengths of maltodextrin compacts. Also, MgSt lowered both the bonding index and *BFI*. They concluded that the lower values of the Hiestand *BFI* indicate that MgSt promotes greater plastic behavior in maltodextrin compacts.

Wurster et al. (113) predicted Hiestand bonding indices of binary powder mixtures from single-component bonding indices. By combining the properties of individual components they developed an equation that was able to satisfactorily predict the bonding indices of mixtures with varying compositions using only the single-component bonding indices.

DIE-WALL FRICTION AND AXIAL TO RADIAL STRESS TRANSMISSION

Die-wall stress measurements are useful for elucidating frictional phenomenon occurring during compaction and is important in assessing compaction related problems like capping, lamination, chipping, and tooling wear. For a single station press in which the lower punch is stationary, the applied upper punch force is transmitted though the powder bed where some of the force is transmitted radially to the die-wall, which in direct proportion to the force increases friction between the tablet and the die-wall (Fig. 18). The term, F_d is the force lost due to friction between the tablet and the die-wall and is calculated by the difference between the upper and lower punch forces:

$$F_d = F_a - F_b \tag{95}$$

where F_a and F_b are the applied upper punch force and the force transmitted to the lower punch (in a single-punch press), respectively. F_d is called the frictional loss whereas F_e is the EF experienced by the lower punch. The radial force, F_r arises as a result of the horizontal transmission of force in response to the axial compression force (114).

The radial stress generated by axial compression of a body in a die has been described by numerous equations. For compaction in a single station press, the lower punch is fixed and the upper punch moves through the compression cycle, which has been described above. When there is die-wall friction not all of the force transmitted from the upper punch reaches the lower punch due to frictional losses (Fig. 18). The difference in

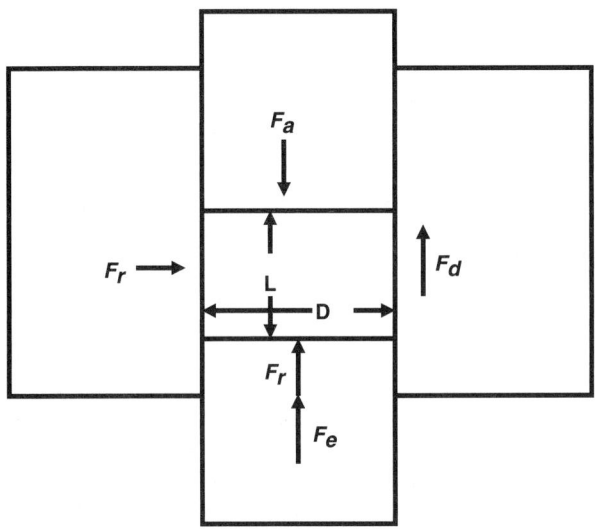

FIGURE 18 Forces and pressures operating on a powder under compression in a punch and die assembly. Key: F_a, force applied by the upper punch; F_b, force transmitted to the lower punch; F_d, force lost to the die (axial frictional force); F_r, force radially transmitted to the die-wall; F_e, EF; D, die diameter; L, height of the compact. *Abbreviation*: EF, ejection force. *Source*: Adapted from Ref. 114.

Compression and Compaction

force or pressure between the upper punch stress P_a and lower punch stress P_b is given by:

$$\frac{P_a}{P_b} = e^{4\mu\eta L/D} \quad (96)$$

where μ is the coefficient of die-wall friction; η the stress ratio, defined as the ratio between the radial pressure, P_r, and the applied pressure, P_a; L the compact length, and D is the diameter of the die. A well known derivation of this equation is given by Unckel (114,115).

The coefficient of friction μ between a powder mass and the die-wall is given by:

$$F_d = \mu F_r \quad (97)$$

Equation (96) describes an exponential decay of the applied pressure down the compact length and assumes a constant μ and η values. However, it has been suggested that μ and η may vary along the length of the compact depending upon the extent of relative interfacial movement, even though the product $\mu \cdot \eta$ may remain constant. This could help to explain the experimentally observed uneven stress (and density) distribution in compacts. In fact, both axial and radial stress gradients are present although short compacts (like pharmaceutical tablets) are supposed to be reasonably homogenous along the axial axis, especially when the die is lubricated (114).

Effect of Compression Force on EF

The EF is the force required to overcome the friction between the die-wall and the tablet; the EF is directly related to the RDWP resulting from compression [Equation (97)] (98,99). By making tablets at different applied pressures, one can obtain different residual die-wall forces and different EFs. It has been observed that the EF is directly proportional to the residual die-wall force (Fig. 19).

Nelson et al. (116) performed a study using sulfathiazole and lactose granules. They studied the effect of upper punch force and a difference between the upper and lower punch forces (R values) on the EF. Upon adding lubricant to a formulation, the upper punch force was lowered from 1390 to 1010 kg and the difference between the upper and lower punch forces was reduced significantly from 630 to 30 kg, and they

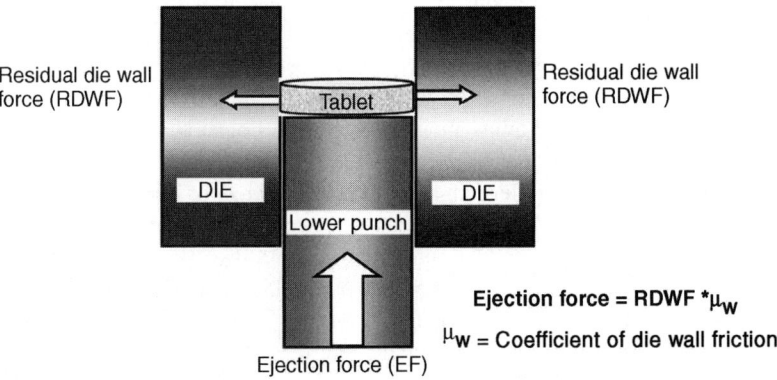

FIGURE 19 Schematic showing relationship between EF, residual die-wall force and coefficient of die-wall friction (μw). *Abbreviation*: EF, ejection force.

found a similar reduction in EFs from 210 to 20 kg for the unlubricated and lubricated granulations, respectively. Therefore, for these formulations, there is a direct relationship between the force difference between the upper and lower punch forces and EFs.

Khan and Rhodes (117) studied the effect of variation in compression force, e.g., increasing the P_{max}, on properties of six direct compression tablet formulations in which the material properties ranged from very plastic to very brittle. The first formulation contained spray-dried lactose, and it had a very high EF, which increased linearly with an increase in compression force in spite of having 1% MgSt in it. The second formulation was a commercially available direct compression matrix that underwent plastic deformation at high compression forces; for this formulation the EF was independent of the compression force. The third and fourth formulations contained two different types DCP dihydrate salts (milled and unmilled), and both formulations exhibited an excellent pressure-crushing strength profile and their EF profiles increased linearly with an increase in compression force. The fifth formulation had a higher amount of MCC and the EF was independent of compression force. The sixth formulation used a calcium phosphate–carbonate complex and they found a sharp increase in EF with an increase in compression force. Based on the above observations it appears that brittle materials like spray dried lactose, DCP and calcium phosphate–carbonate showed a linear relationship between EF and compression force. However, for materials showing plastic deformation like MCC and certain polymers the EF was independent of compression force. Hence, it is important to consider the nature of the drug and the excipient before undertaking formulation development.

CALCULATION OF NET WORK OF COMPACTION FROM THE FORCE–DISPLACEMENT PROFILE

The calculation of work requires accurate measurements of force and displacement. Higuchi et al. were the first in pharmacy to develop a system for measuring punch force and displacement during compression (118–121). Using instrumented tablet presses like Higuchi's and De Blaey and Polderman (122) and others the work of compaction can be calculated. The work of compaction is represented by the total area ABC (E_1) (Fig. 20) i.e., the total work done on the tablet during the compression phase is give by the area ABC. The areas E_1, E_2, and E_3 (note: $E_1 = E_2 + E_3$) will be used in the discussion to follow (123). The origin represents the point where the upper punch first contacts the powder in the die. The energy recovered during decompression as expansion work (W_{exp}) done on the punches by the tablet is represented by the area DBC (E_3), in Figure 20. The area ABD (E_2) represents the apparent net work (W_{net}) used in the formation of the compact and the work needed to overcome die-wall friction; this area is given by $E_1 - E_3$. As mentioned in the introduction the areas shown in Figure 20 have been related to the deformation and binding properties of a material (123).

As defined by De Baley and Polderman et al. (122), the work of compaction is the amount of work done by upper and lower punches to compress a powder mass into a consolidated tablet. This work can be divided into W_f, W_{exp}, and W_{net} (Fig. 21); where W_f is the amount to work required to overcome interparticulate and die-wall friction. According to De Baley and Polderman et al. (122) energy is consumed during compaction by: particle rearrangement, interparticulate friction, die-wall friction, plastic deformation and elastic deformation. When calculating W_{net} they felt the magnitude of particle rearrangement and interparticulate friction were negligible but subtracted the work used to overcome die-wall friction and the work recovered during decompression

Compression and Compaction

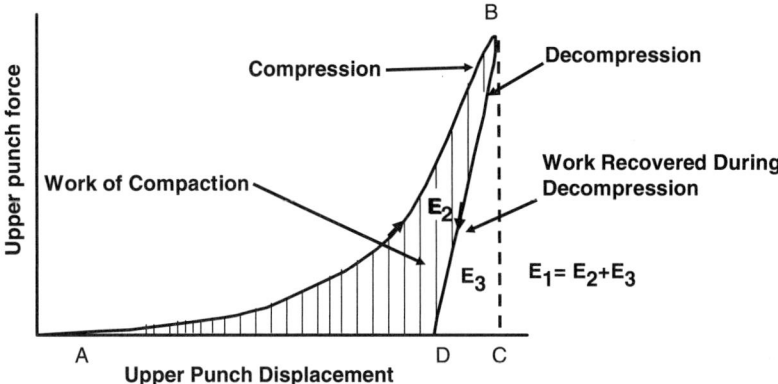

FIGURE 20 Plot of upper punch force vs. upper punch displacement during compression and decompression. *Source*: Adapted from Ref. 65.

due to elastic recovery from the total work input, see W_{net} in Figure 21. This calculation method assumes that the calculated W_{net} represented the energy used for plastic deformation, brittle fracture and bond formation. Thus W_{net} calculation could be used to characterize a material's mechanical properties.

For the formation of compact, the energy used can be calculated from the punch force and displacements. As mentioned above, there are some key factors that affect W_{net} value out of which friction against die-wall is very useful in the derivation of total work input. There are few equations proposed to derive the relationship between work of friction and total work input among which De Blaey–Polderman and Jarvinen–Juslin equations are common and widely used, the later one being more applicable.

Using the scenario shown in Figure 22 De Blaey and Polderman (122) have calculated the work of die-wall friction using:

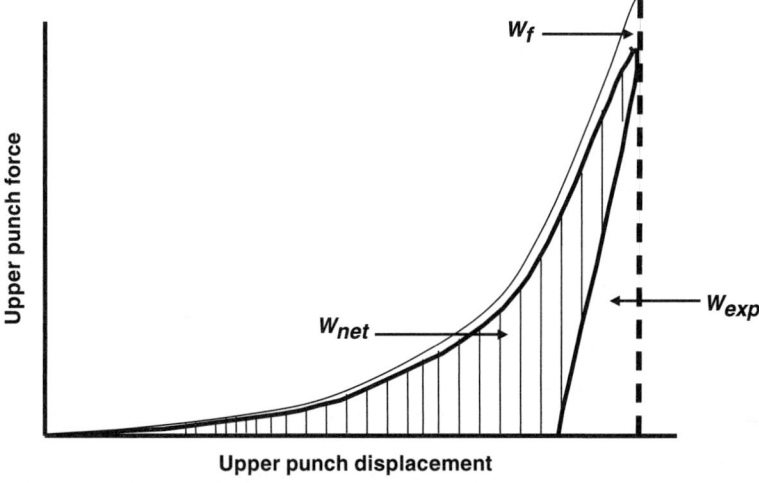

FIGURE 21 Force–displacement plot illustrating the net work (W_{net}), work of friction (W_f) and work recovered during expansion (W_{exp}, expansion work).

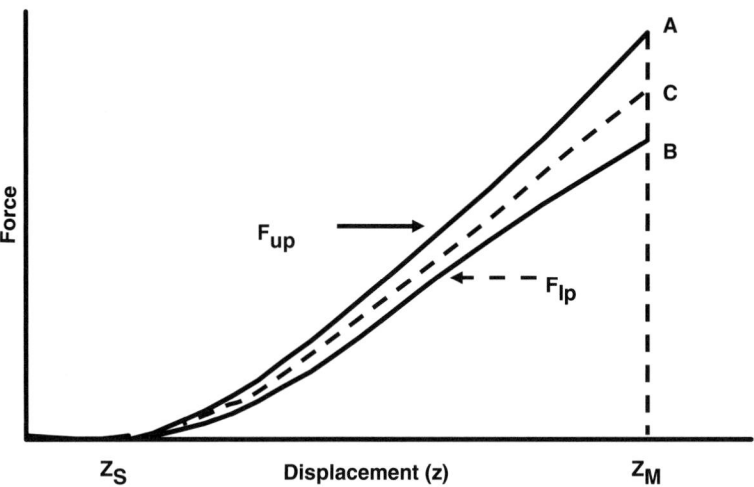

FIGURE 22 Calculation of work needed to overcome die-wall friction. Z, the displacement of the upper punch, measured relative to the lower punch; Z_S the point at which the force rises from zero; Z_M, the maximum displacement of the upper punch; F_{up}, the upper punch force; F_{lp}, the lower punch force. *Source*: Adapted from Ref. 123.

$$W_f = \int_{Z_s}^{Z_M} (F_{up} - F_{lp}) dz \tag{98}$$

where z is the displacement of the upper punch, measured relative to the lower punch, Z_S the displacement at the point where the force rises from zero, Z_M the maximum displacement of the upper punch, F_{up} the upper punch force, F_{lp} is the lower punch force. This method has been criticized by Jarvinen and Juslin (124), who also calculated a work of friction based on the movement of the particles in contact with the die-wall and the force acting on the particles rather than the force and displacement of the upper punch:

$$W_f = \int_{Z_s}^{Z_M} \left[F_{up} - (F_{up} - F_{lp})/\ln(F_{up}/F_{lp}) \right] dz \tag{99}$$

By using Equation (99), they found that frictional work obtained was 46% less than that obtained by the calculation method used by DeBlaey and Polderman (122). Jarvinen and Juslin (124) concluded that friction only occurs at the true areas of interparticulate contact between the compact and the die-wall. Thus, only the movement of these particles and not the movement of the upper punch should be used in the calculation of the work of friction. Therefore, the assumption that the frictional force does not completely coincide with the movement of the upper punch appears plausible. In addition, only the particles in the upper layer of the compact adjacent to the punch are capable of moving the same distance as the upper punch. The particles in the middle of the tablet in double side compression or adjacent to the lower punch in single sided compaction remain stationary.

The net work of compaction is a function of material properties. For example, the energy needed to deform an ideal elastic material will be completely recovered during the decompression phase and there will be zero net work compact. On the other hand, for plastic deformation, with or without fragmentation, the energy input will be dissipated and there will be a sizable net work of compaction. Thus, study of the net work of compaction gives info about the extent of elastic recovery, viscoelastic deformation, plastic deformation, and bond formation.

Energy Balance During Compaction

The liquid-surface film theory attributes bonding to the presence at the particular interfaces of thin liquid films, which may be the consequence of fusion or adsorbed moisture. For materials that may be compressed directly, the liquid-surface film theory proposes that the liquid film is a result of fusion or solution at the surface of the particle induced by the energy of compression. Gross melting does not occur during the compression of most tablets because the energy expended causes only a small temperature rise, which is sufficient to melt the material being tableted (125).

The relation of pressure and melting point is expressed by the Clausius–Clapeyron Equation (126),

$$\frac{dT}{dP} = T\frac{(V_1 - V_s)}{\Delta H} \tag{100}$$

in which dT/dP is the change in melting point with pressure, T the absolute temperature, ΔH the molar latent heat of fusion, and V_1 and V_s are the molar volumes of the liquid melt and the solid, respectively. As the latent heat of fusion is positive, the Clapeyron equation states that for a solid, which expands on melting ($V_1 > V_s$), the melting point is raised by increasing the pressure. Most solids expand on melting. Thus, the Clapeyron equation predicts that during compression it would be unlikely that fusion would occur. The Clapeyron equation is derived from a thermodynamically reversible process in which the solid is uniformly exposed to a pressure. In fact, the compression of pharmaceutical tablet is nonreversible, and the pressure is not uniformly exerted on each granule.

Skotnicky (127) derived an equation relating the heat of fusion, volumes of the liquid and solid phases, temperature, and the pressures applied to the liquid and solid phases. For an ideal process in which the material is exposed to a uniform pressure, the relation reduces to the Clapeyron equation. If the pressure at the points of contact is exerted only on the solid, and the liquid phase is subjected to a constant atmospheric pressure, the relationship simplifies to

$$\frac{dT}{dP_s} = \frac{-V_s T}{\Delta H} \tag{101}$$

where ΔH is the heat of fusion, V_s the volume of the solid, and T is the temperature. As dT/dP_s is always positive regardless of the expansion or contraction of the solid, the pressure acting locally at the points of contact lowers the melting point.

For surface fusion at the points of contact, a localized temperature at least equal to the melting point of the material must be attained. With some mixtures the melting point may be depressed by other ingredients and fusion will occur at a temperature lower than the melting point of the pure material. For most pharmaceutical solids, the specific heat is low and the thermal conductivity is relatively slow. The heat transfer to the surface can be estimated by dividing the compressional energy by the total time of compression. Using the derivation of Carslaw and Jaeger (128) for heat transfer, Rankell and Higuchi (129) estimated for the compression of 0.4 g of sulfathiazole that if the area of contact were

0.01–0.1% of the total area, the surface temperature would reach the melting point of most medicinal compounds and pharmaceutical excipients, and fusion would occur. Then upon release of the pressure, solidification of the fused material would form solid bridges between the particles.

All energy used to compress a material will be released as heat if no change in the energy content of the material takes place. The work of compaction, Wc, will then be equal to the heat released during compaction, Qc, i.e.,

$$Ec = Wc - Qc \tag{102}$$

where Ec is the energy change during compression, Wc the work done on the powder (work of compression) and Qc is the heat released by the system.

Fuhrer and Parmentier (130) estimated that about 90% of the work of compression was released as heat. Coffin–Beach and Hollenbeck (130,131) found that the energy released as heat was larger than the energy of compression phase and not during decompression but efforts were made to compensate for energy changes associated with the deformation of machine parts. The extent to which the heat released exceeded the work of compression was termed as the energy of formation as it was assumed that this energy was equal to the reduction in surface energy due to bonding. For example, MCC, Avicel, gave a high energy of formation while DCP, di-Tab, known to fragment to a large extent during compression, gave considerably lower values. It was further suggested that fracture and bonding balanced each other at forces below approximately 10 kN for DCP, while particle recombine and bond at higher pressures resulting in increased energy of formation. The energy of formation correlated with the tensile strength for each material but it appears not to be a simple general correlation.

At very high compressional forces, there are chances of error to occur due to elastic deformation of the punches and other parts of press. Altaf and Hoag studied the influence on deformation of tablet press during tablet compaction on DCP dihydrate and MCC (7). It was found that the press deformation absorbs energy during the loading phase and then releases this energy later in the compaction cycle. The rate at which the press stores energy depends in part upon the viscoelastic properties of the tablet. They concluded that the coupling between press elasticity and a tablet's viscoelastic properties should be accounted for when analyzing tablet compaction or trying to simulate the punch displacement profile of a tablet press that deforms during compaction (7).

Effect of Lubricant on W_{net} of Compaction

Ragnarsson and Sjogren (61) reported the effect of lubricants on the crushing strength and net work done (W_{net}). They found that MgSt reduced the crushing strength and W_{net} of all the formulations studied and the effect was very pronounced in NaCl and Sta-Rx-1500. They also found that a 30-minutes mixing time eliminated the bonding properties of Sta-Rx and reduced W_{net} by 30%, which they attributed to a decrease in particle interaction i.e., friction and bonding. However, a brittle material like Emcompress did not showed a significant reduction in W_{net} even after mixing it with MgSt for 30 minutes and there was a linear relationship between W_{net} and applied load at all three settings (Fig. 23) (62,130).

From these studies and other similar studies there is a general consensus in the literature that the main effect of the MgSt over mixing is to form a film or thin layer on the particles and this layer reduces intermolecular, bonding which decreases compact strength. If intermolecular forces were the only bond type present and no fragmentation

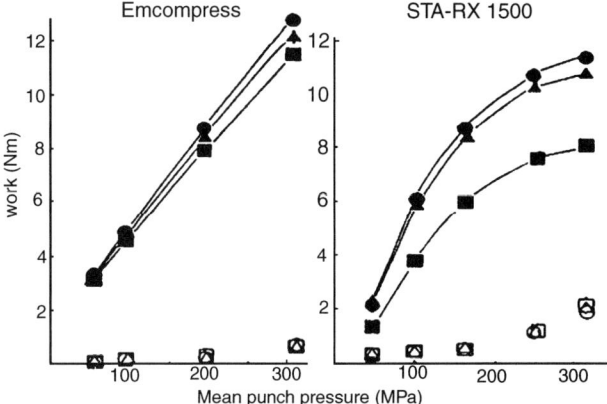

FIGURE 23 The effect of MgSt admixture on net work (filled symbols) and expansion work (open symbols) in the tabletting of Emcompress and Sta-Rx 1500. (●) pure substance; (▲) 0.5% MgSt blended for 1 minute; (■) 0.5% MgSt admixed for 30 minutes. *Source*: Adapted from Ref. 62.

of the particles or rupture of the lubricant film occurred, a compact strength close to zero would be expected (132). In contrast, when there is particle fragmentation this creates clean surfaces that are free of MgSt and can readily bond with other clean surfaces; thus, as a general rule brittle materials are not as sensitive to lubricants as materials that undergo a lot of plastic deformation and hence less surface area creation.

Effect of Moisture on W_{net} of Compaction

For many materials, the moisture content is a critical factor in their performance, and powders with low moisture content often produce tablets with very poor mechanical strength. For example, moisture affects the compaction properties of MCC, moisture acts as a plasticizer that facilitates plastic flow within the individual particles. Sjogren et al. (61) found that increased moisture levels gave a lower yield pressure, tablet height, and reduced W_{net}. Their sample with low moisture content (1.1%) gave considerably lower crushing strength than tablets with normal moisture content (4.9%) throughout the pressure range test. The bonding property of the moist sample (8.2% water) was good at low pressure but less affected by moisture at higher pressures. Thus, controlling moisture content is a critical quality parameter that must be controlled when making tablets.

PEAK COMPRESSION FORCE: QUANTITATIVE ANALYSIS

Crushing Strength vs. P_{max}

The tensile strength is an indirect measure of bond strength. Tablets must have sufficient tensile strength so that they can maintain their integrity during postcompaction processes, such as coating, packing, and shipping. Therefore, adequate particle bonding is required for a tablet to meet these requirements. Heistand and Peot (108) reported that the tensile strength is an important measurement for characterizing the interaction between solid particles. The particles inside the die are of irregular shapes and sizes and have very little true contact between the particles. In this context, the term true contact refers to the surfaces being close enough such that molecular interactions can occur between the atoms (Fig. 24), it is at these points of true contact where strong bonds form, because molecular forces such as Van der Waals forces act over very short distances that are on the order of atomic dimensions. During compression the particles deform or fracture which increases the area of true contact between the surfaces and hence the attractive force between the particles is greatly. The amount of the true contact area between particles after elastic recovery is dependent on the magnitude of maximum stress applied and the amount of plastic deformation and brittle fracture that has occurred during compression (108).

The most common method for measuring the tensile strength is the diametrical compression test (called the Brazilian test in the engineering literature); with this test, force is applied to the tablet as shown in Figure 25 and the load is steadily increased until the tablet fractures this peak load is recorded as the crushing strength, which is also called the crushing force or breaking strength. In the older literature the crushing strength was know as tablet hardness, but current terminology reserves the term hardness for indentation tests like the H_0 and H_{30} tests described previously in the Hiestand tableting indices section. It turns out that when a circular tablet is compressed as shown in Figure 25 that along the load diameter, i.e., the center line between the applied forces, that a tensile force actually develops, and when a tablet fails along this line you are actually measuring the tensile strength of the material. To obtain reproducible results the tablet must break in such a manner that the tensile stress is the major stress. If the tablet does not fail primarily along the load diameter then other fracture mechanisms are probably responsible for the tablet failure, and care must be taken when comparing results, because direct comparisons between different failure mechanisms is problematic. This is particularly true when capping and lamination begin to occur.

Fell and Newton (110) made use of the diametrical-compression test to assess the tensile strength of lactose tablets. The determination of tensile strength from this procedure depends upon the correct state of stress developing within a specimen of known shape and dimensions. For the case of ideal line loading across the tablet, the tensile σ_1, compressive σ_2, and shear τ stresses can be calculated using elasticity theory [Fig. 25A]. The maximum tensile stress σ_0 is constant over the whole of the load diameter and has a magnitude. In Figure 25B, y axis represents the distance along the load diameter from

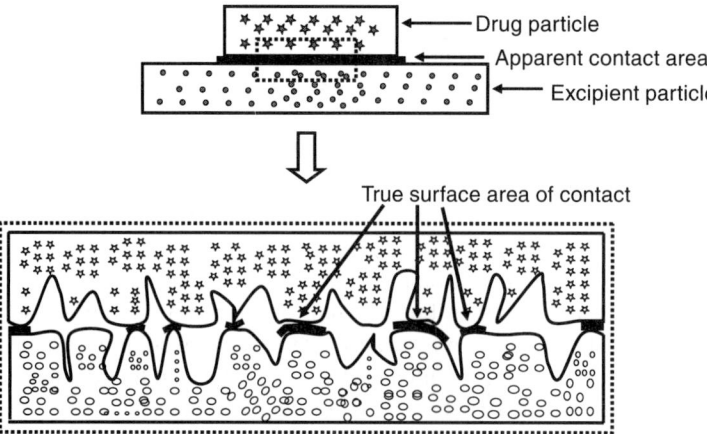

FIGURE 24 Apparent and true surface contact area.

Compression and Compaction

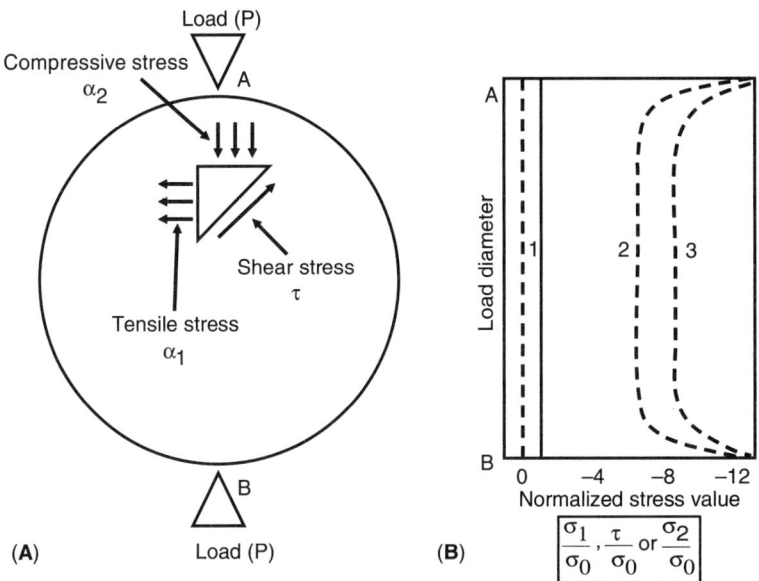

FIGURE 25 Stress distribution across loaded diameter for a cylindrical tablet: (**A**) Line Loads are applied at points A and B; and (**B**) relative magnitude of tensile σ_1, shear τ stresses and compressive σ_2; using the maximum tensile stress σ_0 for normalization. Curve 1 = σ_1/σ_0; Curve 2 = τ/σ_0; Curve 3 = σ_2/σ_0. *Source*: Adapted From Ref. 110.

Figure 25A and the *x* axis gives the normalized tensile, shear, and compressive stress values (110). The equation that gives the tensile stress based upon the applied load and tablet dimensions is given by:

$$\sigma_0 = \frac{2P}{\pi Dt} \tag{103}$$

where σ_0 is the tensile strength, P the applied load, D the tablet diameter, t is the tablet thickness. The values for the compressive and shear stresses are a minimum at the center of the tablet along the loading diameter and in theory for line loading the other stresses are infinitely high immediately under the line loading points; obviously in practice this does not occur.

An idealized the crushing strength versus peak applied compression pressure P_{max} used to make the tablet has a profile like that shown in Figure 26. P^*_{max} is the maximum practical pressure applicable to the tablet; at this point the maximum crushing strength is achieved and at higher compression pressures ($P_{max} > P^*_{max}$), the crushing strength decreases often due to capping and lamination. As shown in Figure 26, when setting specification for tablets it is best to choose pressures in the range from A to B, when working in region between points B and C there is the possibility that the tablets could begin to cap and laminate, i.e., this region may not be as robust as the region from A to B and have a higher risk or product failure.

The effect of compression force on the tensile strength is dependent on the material properties of excipients. The five most commonly used fillers in formulation development are: MCC, lactose monohydrate, DCP dihydrate, pregelatinized starch, and coprocessed sucrose. MCC shows a rapid increase in tensile strength with the increase in compression force (Fig. 27) whereas pregelatinized starch shows minimum sensitivity under compaction and its tensile strength is independent of compression force.

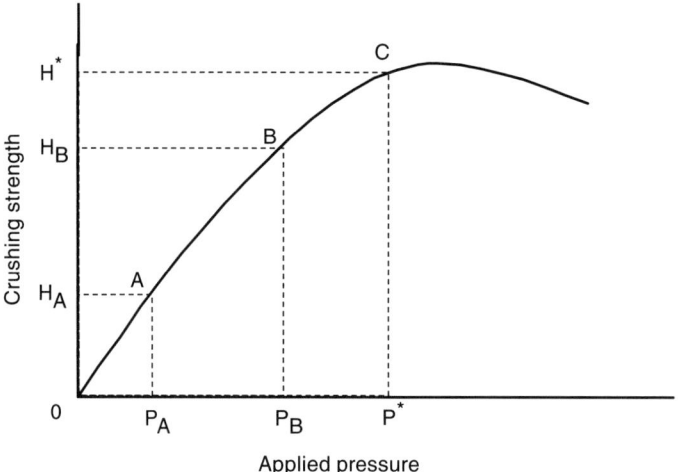

FIGURE 26 Idealized crushing strength vs. applied compression pressure plots. *Source*: Adapted from Ref. 159.

Higuchi et al. (119) found that tablet crushing strength varies directly with the logarithm of compressional force but leveled off at higher forces. While working on aspirin, lactose, and lactose–aspirin mixtures, they found the properties of the mixtures were in between those of the neat materials (Fig. 28).

Rawas-Qalaji et al. (133) studied the effect of compression force with increasing concentration of epinephrine bitartrate tablets (0%, 6%, 12%, and 24% of drug load in microcrystalline tablets). They found an exponential increase in crushing strength with the increase in compression force. They correlated the exponential increase in tablet crushing strength to reduction in tablet porosity (134). Interestingly, higher compression force was required to achieve the same crushing strength in high drug-load tablets (Fig. 29). They attributed this behavior to the poor compressibility of epinephrine bitartrate. In summary, there are many different type of P_{max} versus crushing strength profiles and the type of profile depends upon the nature of the materials used in formulation.

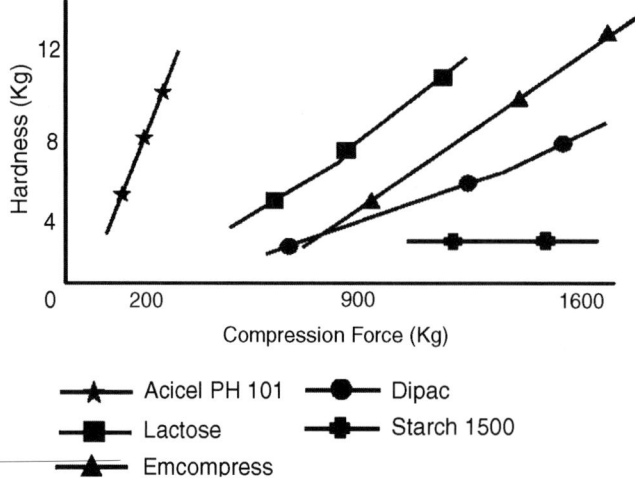

FIGURE 27 Compaction profiles of some direct compression fillers (0.75% MgSt).

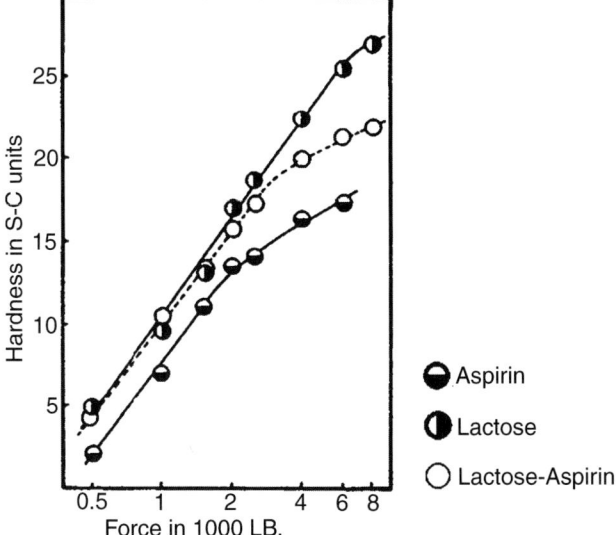

FIGURE 28 Effect of compressional force on the hardness (crushing strength) of various tablets. *Source*: From Ref. 119.

The fracture strength of compressed tablets varies inherently as a property of the material. The Weibull distribution (125) can be used to describe this variability in tablet strength and to characterize the formulation. The probability P_f that a tablet from a large batch of tablets will exhibit a tensile strength of σ_t is expressed by:

$$P_f = 1 - \exp\left[-\left(\frac{\sigma_t - \bar{\sigma}_t}{\beta}\right)^k\right] \tag{104}$$

where k (the Weibull modulus) is the reciprocal of variability in material strength (also called as shape parameter), $\bar{\sigma}_t$ the mean tensile strength of the batch and β is the scale parameter. Sonnergaard (135) while studying the distribution of crushing strength of

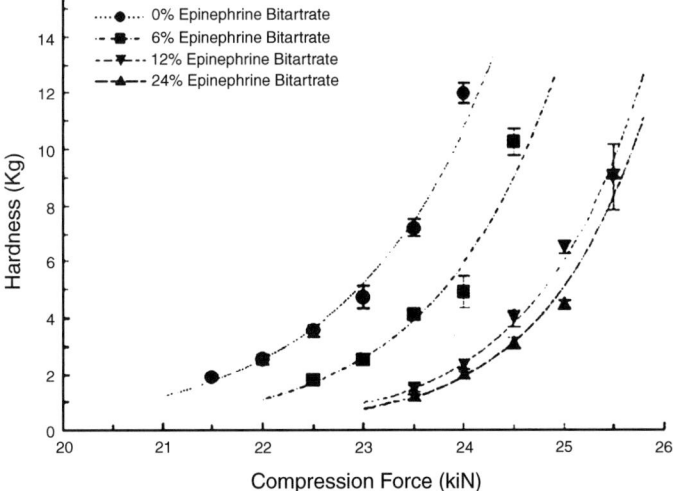

FIGURE 29 Effect of increasing compression force on tablet hardness (crushing strength) of 0%, 6%, 12%, and 24% epinephrine bitartrate tablet formulations. *Source*: From Ref. 133.

tablets found a strong and significant relationship between the Weibull modulus and the coefficient of variation of Weibull distributed data was found by theoretically based calculations.

Specific Surface Area vs. P_{max}

Specific surface area is the total surface area per unit of mass or volume of material. It is the surface area that promotes interparticulate bonding between powder particles under compression. Higuchi et al. (119) observed the influence of compression force on the specific surface area of the sulfathiazole granules. Initially, an increase in the maximum compressional force resulted in a larger specific surface area. This relation continued until a certain force was reached after which increasing the force apparently reduced the specific surface area (Fig. 30). When lactose granules are compressed into a tablet, the specific surface increased to a maximal value (four times that of the initial granules), indicating the formation of new surfaces due to granule fragmentation. However, a further increase in compressional force produce a progressive decrease in specific surface as the particles undergo interparticulate bond formation.

Amorphous lactose produced tablets of higher tensile strength than crystalline lactose and there was a tendency for reduced particle size to increase tablet strength. Hence tablet strength was correlated with the effective area of contact for each material.

Sebhatu et al. (136) studied the relationships between effective interparticulate contact area and the tensile strength of amorphous and crystalline lactose tablets with varying particle size and compression forces. They measured the area of interparticulate contact within the tablet using a model proposed by Eriksson and Alderborn (137), which is based upon measuring the deformation properties of the particles during compression. This relationship is given by:

$$\sigma_t = \sigma_b \frac{P_a - P_o}{D} \tag{105}$$

where σ_t is the tensile strength of tablet (N/m^2), σ_b the tensile strength of interparticulate bond (N/m^2), P_a the applied pressure during compaction (N/m^2), P_o the minimum

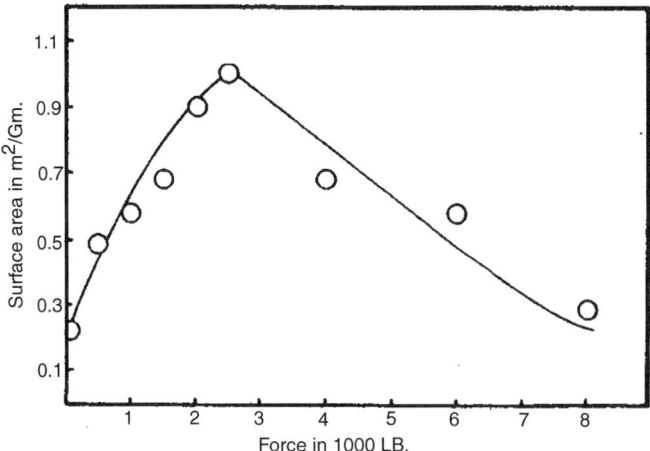

FIGURE 30 Effect of compression force on specific surface area of sulphadiazine tablet. *Source*: From Ref. 119.

applied pressure required to form a coherent compact (N/m^2), D is the particle deformability (N/m^2). The ratio of (P_a/D) gives the total contact area between particles in a cross section of the tablet while the ratio (P_o/D) represents the contact area in a cross section of the tablet needed to form a coherent tablet. This contact area will be formed at an applied pressure of P_o, i.e., the critical formation pressure. D as an indication of the plastic deformability of the particles and can be replaced by P_y (yield pressure derived from Heckel profiles (N/m^2) (136). Using this approach, it was concluded that the tensile strength of lactose tablets is mainly controlled by the degree of deformation of the particles, rather than the degree of fragmentation which occurs during compaction, and that the different compactabilities of amorphous and crystalline lactose are to some degree due to differences in particle deformability but also to differences in inter-particulate bonding capacity.

Disintegration vs. P_{max}

Tablet disintegration is often a prerequisite for dissolution and drug absorption. During tablet manufacturing the compression force results in both fragmentation and consolidation of the particles. Particle fragmentation tends to be more common at low compression forces whereas particle consolidation tends to occur at higher compression forces. Therefore, as a general rule tablets prepared at high forces have a smaller specific surface area, lower porosity, higher tablet density, higher crushing strength, and increased disintegration time than tablets prepared at low compression forces (119,121).

Khan et al. studied the effect of compressional force on the disintegration time of tablets prepared from DCP dihydrate containing various disintegrants. They found that disintegration time initially shows dramatic decrease; however, after a certain force further increases in compressional force have no effect on disintegration time. They hypothesized that this behavior was due to a decrease in porosity at higher compression forces, which reduces the fluid penetration into the tablet (138).

The relationship between compression force and disintegration time can be of linear or exponential nature, depending on the type of formulation. Rawas-Qalaji et al. (133) studied the effect of increase in drug load (epinephrine bitartrate) on disintegration and wetting of four different batches. These four tablet formulations, A, B, C, and D, were containing 0%, 6%, 12%, and 24% of epinephrine bitartrate in a MCC and low-substituted hydroxypropyl cellulose (HPC) (9:1) matrix. They found that linear increase in compression force resulted in linear increase in disintegration and wetting times of formulation A, and an exponential increase in disintegration and wetting times of B, C, and D formulations (Fig. 31). Typically, as compression force increases disintegration time also increases, however this is not always the case. Massimo et al. (139) reported an inverse relationship between P_{max} and disintegration time, and the tablets made at higher P_{max} values exhibited shorter disintegration times, and similar results have been found in other studies (140).

Dissolution Rate vs. P_{max}

The effect of compression force on dissolution rate is dependent on the pressure range used and on the properties of the drug, filler, and binder. Generally increasing the compression force increases the density, disintegration time, and crushing strength and decreases porosity; consequently water penetration into the tablet is reduced, which reduces wettability. Conversely higher compression forces have been shown to cause deformation, crushing or fracture of drug particles into smaller ones or convert spherical

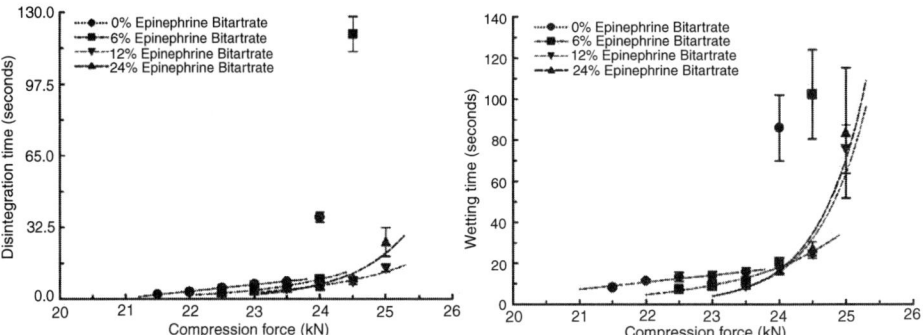

FIGURE 31 Effect of increasing compression force on (**A**) tablet disintegration time and (**B**) tablet wetting time of 0%, 6%, 12%, and 24% epinephrine bitartrate tablet formulations. *Source*: From Ref. 133.

granule into a disc-shaped particle with a larger surface area, which can result in an increase in the dissolution rate of the tablet (141). Both bonding of particles and cleavage or crushing of particles occurs upon increasing force of compression and which property predominates varies among drugs and excipients (142). When particle bonding is the predominating phenomenon during the compression event, dissolution rate generally diminishes and when particle cleavage predominates, the dissolution rate generally increases (141).

The four general dissolution-compression force relations are: (*i*) the dissolution is more rapid as the compressional force is increased; (*ii*) the dissolution is slowed as the compressional force is increased; (*iii*) the dissolution is faster, to a maximum, as the compressional force is increased, and then further increases in compressional force slow dissolution; (*iv*) the dissolution is slowed to a minimum as the compressional force is increased, and then further increases in compressional force increases dissolution as shown in Figure 32 (142).

Iranloye and Parrott (143) studied the effects of compression force on the dissolution rate of compressed disks of salicylic acid, aspirin, and an equimolar mixture of aspirin and salicylic acid. They found that increase in compression force from 450 to 9100 kg had no effect on dissolution rates. Also, upon incorporating 5% starch

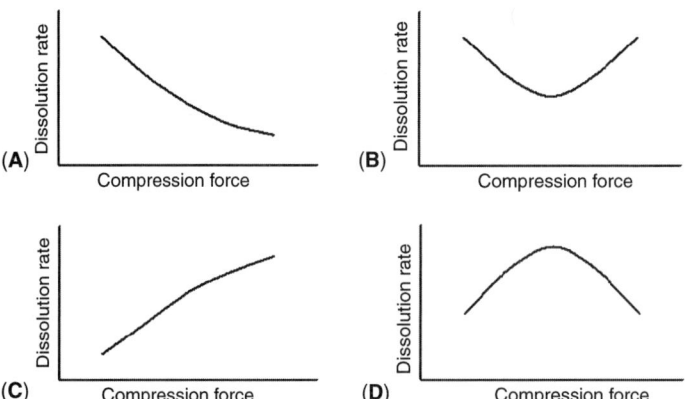

FIGURE 32 Various types of relations observed between applied compressional force during tableting and dissolution rate of tablets.

(disintegrant) into an equimolar mixture of aspirin and salicylic acid, the dissolution rates were independent of compression force from 910 to 9100 kg no effect on dissolution of compressed disks (tablets) of salicylic acid, aspirin, and an equimolar mixture of aspirin and salicylic acid at varied range of compression force (450–9100 kg). They reported progressive decrease in dissolution rate upon addition of lubricants (MgSt, stearic acid, glyceryl monostearate) (143).

Yu et al. (144) found that disk intrinsic dissolution rate of model drugs metoprolol [a Bio-pharmaceutics Classification System (BCS) high solubility drug] and furosemide (a BCS low solubility drug) did not vary significantly with the increase in compression force (Table 3).

The presence of excipients (binder) play an important role in dissolution rate of drug. SY Lin (145) studied the effect of compression force on dissolution behavior of theophylline-tableted microcapsule with and without excipients (lactose and HPC). The dissolution characteristics of theophylline from tableted microcapsules without excipients were independent of the applied compression force as was the tablet crushing strength. Upon adding lactose and hydroxypropyl cellulose they found rapid and zero order release of theophylline from tablets containing lactose and HPC, respectively with the increase in compression force (145). A linear correlation between dissolution efficiency and the logarithm of force was found to exist over the compression range studied (146).

Koparkar et al. (147) found that the filler having a higher intrinsic dissolution rate permitted faster drug release than the filler having a lower intrinsic dissolution rate. For example, the dissolution rate of Hydrochlorothiazide from the direct compression formulations containing DCP dihydrate (Di-Tab) was faster than that from the formulation containing tricalcium phosphate (Tri-tab). In this study all the formulations were compressed to control the crushing strength to the same value of 6 kg. Similar results were found by Du and Hoag (148).

Shimizu et al. reported that higher compression force can cause cleavage and crushing of the enteric layer of Lansoprazole fast-disintegrating tablet leading to faster dissolution. This unwanted property was later counteracted by increasing the quantity of methacrylic polymer and adding plasticizer (149).

TABLE 3 The Effect of Disk Compression Force on Disk Dissolution Rate

Drug	Compression force (psi)	Intrinsic dissolution (mg/min/cm^2)		
		Mean	S.D.	CV(%)
Metoprolol	600–700	19.9	1.345	6.76
	900–1000	20.3	0.939	4.57
	2000	22.4	0.252	1.12
	3000	22.7	0.608	2.68
	4000	21.6	0.379	1.75
	5000	21.7	0.503	2.32
Furosemide	600–700	0.019	0.0006	2.99
	900–1000	0.020	0.0010	5.00
	2000	0.018	0.0015	8.33
	3000	0.021	0.0006	2.79
	4000	0.019	0.0010	5.26
	5000	0.022	0.0012	5.33

Source: Adapted from Ref. 147.

The effect of compression force on in vivo dissolution rate of drug has been also studied. John S Kent (150) studied the dissolution of 95% delmadinone acetate pellets at three different compression forces in rats. He found that the dissolution rate for the lot with the lowest density made at the lowest compression was statistically higher from the lot compressed a higher compression force which had higher density. The possible explanation for this phenomenon was that increased rate in dissolution from these pellets could be attributed to possible channel formation between particles inside pellets. But after certain compression force and density, the dissolution was equivalent between the lots (150).

Application of Ryshkewitch–Duckworth Equation
Prediction of Tensile Strength

Pharmaceutical tablets are made from a number of components, and each component contributes to the tablet's final properties. Therefore, it is important to study the physical properties of the individual components and their mixture rules in order to predict the mechanical properties of the final tablet. Tensile strength is one of the crucial properties that assess mechanical strength; the most common method for measuring tensile strength is the diametrical compression test discussed above (110). In this section the application of the Ryshkewitch–Duckworth equation to the analysis of tensile strength of mixtures will be discussed (151,152).

Ryshkewitch (152) investigated the tensile strength of porous sintered alumina and zirconia and showed that the logarithm of the tensile strength is inversely proportional to the porosity. Based upon this, Duckworth (151) developed an equation that correlates tensile strength and porosity, which is called the Ryshkewitch–Duckworth equation:

$$\ln\left(\frac{\sigma_t}{\bar{\sigma}}\right) = -k\varepsilon \tag{106}$$

or

$$\sigma_t = \bar{\sigma}e^{-k\varepsilon} \tag{107}$$

where ε is the porosity of compact ($\varepsilon = 1 - D$), $\bar{\sigma}$ the tensile strength of the material at zero porosity, and k is a constant representing the bonding capacity and indicates the effect of a change in porosity on the tensile strength. Note in this section the symbol D is used for relative density, where earlier in this chapter the symbol ρ_m is used, while confusing the symbol most commonly used in a particular body of literature will be used. A higher value of k corresponds to stronger bonding. From these equations, the tensile strength of each component can be described.

For binary mixtures, assuming that the volumes of constituent powders do not change during compression, the tensile strength at zero porosity can be calculated using a linear mixing rule:

$$\bar{\sigma}_m = \bar{\sigma}_1 \delta_1 + \bar{\sigma}_2 \delta_2 \tag{108}$$

A similarly mixture rule can be used for the bonding capacity:

$$k_m = k_1 \delta_1 + k_2 \delta_2 \tag{109}$$

where $\bar{\sigma}$ and k_m are the tensile strength at zero porosity and the bonding capacity of binary mixture, respectively. The terms $\bar{\sigma}_1$ and $\bar{\sigma}_2$ are the tensile strengths of the constituents in a binary mixture at zero porosity, respectively, and k_1 and k_2 are the bonding capacity of

Compression and Compaction

the constituent powders of single component, respectively. $\bar{\sigma}_1$, $\bar{\sigma}_2$, k_1 and k_2 can be determined by fitting the experimental data for the single-component powders using Equation (106). In Equations (108) and (109), δ_1 and δ_2 are the volume fractions of the constituent powders, which can be expressed in terms of weight fractions:

$$\delta_1 = \frac{V_1}{V_m} = \frac{n_1 G_m/\rho_1}{G_m/\rho_m} = \frac{n_1 \rho_m}{\rho_1} \tag{110}$$

$$\delta_2 = \frac{V_2}{V_m} = \frac{n_2 G_m/\rho_2}{G_m/\rho_m} = \frac{n_2 \rho_m}{\rho_2} = \frac{(1-n_1)\rho_m}{\rho_2} \tag{111}$$

where V_1, V_2, and V_m are the volume of single-component powder (1 and 2) and their mixture, respectively. ρ_1, ρ_2, and ρ_m are the corresponding true densities. n_1 and n_2 are the weight fractions of the constituents powders, respectively. G_m is the weight of the binary mixture. By applying mixing rule, the true density of binary mixtures ρ_m can be expressed as a function of the true densities of the constituent single-component powders, ρ_1 and ρ_2, as follows:

$$\frac{1}{\rho_m} = \frac{n_1}{\rho_1} + \frac{n_2}{\rho_2} \tag{112}$$

Wu et al. found a close resemblance in the measured true density (using pycnometer) and predicted true density for the binary mixtures, as given in Table 4.

Therefore, Equation (112) can be used to predict the true density of binary mixtures. After calculating predicted true densities [Equation (112)] and substituting Equations (110) and (111) into Equations (108) and (109), we can obtain $\bar{\sigma}_m$ and k_m for the binary mixture based upon the corresponding values of n, $\bar{\sigma}$, and k of the constituent powders and the true densities. Upon obtaining the values of $\bar{\sigma}_m$ and k_m, the tensile strength of binary tablets (σ_{tm}) can be derived for a given relative density of the mixture (D_m) using Equation (106), i.e.,

TABLE 4 Measured True Densities for Powder Systems Considered

Notation	Powder	Measured true density (g/cm³)	Predicted true density (g/cm³)
MCC	MCC (Avicel PH-102)	1.5897±0.0028	–
HPMC	HPMC	1.3160±0.0003	–
Starch	Starch 1500	1.4934±0.0014	–
MixA	50% MCC + 50% HPMC (w/w)	1.4420±0.0003	1.4400
MixB	10% MCC + 90% HPMC (w/w)	1.3440±0.0008	1.3390
MixC	90% MCC + 10% HPMC (w/w)	1.5540±0.0004	1.5573
MixAs	50% MCC + 50% starch (w/w)	1.5425±0.0014	1.5400
MixBs	20% MCC + 80% starch (w/w)	1.5215±0.0014	1.5117
MixCs	80% MCC + 20% starch (w/w)	1.5643±0.0013	1.5695

Abbreviation: MCC, microcrystalline cellulose.
Source: Adapted from Ref. 155.

$$\ln\left(\frac{\sigma_{tm}}{\bar{\sigma}_m}\right) = -k_m(1 - D_m) \tag{113}$$

or

$$\sigma_{tm} = \bar{\sigma}_m e^{-k_m(1 - D_m)} \tag{114}$$

Wu et al. (153,154) used Ryshkewitch–Duckworth equation to successfully predict the tensile strength of tablets made from multi-component mixtures. Michrafy et al. (155) had success with the application linear and power law mixing rules for calculating the parameters of the Ryshkewitch–Duckworth equation and the prediction of tensile strength. Thus, the Ryshkewitch–Duckworth equation shows promise as a tool for understanding the tensile strength of tablets.

MECHANICAL STRENGTH OF TABLETS

Common problems with the mechanical integrity of tablets include capping, lamination, chipping, stress cracking, and picking. Capping is the phenomenon where the upper part, cap, of the tablet breaks off, typically, during ejection (Fig. 33A,B). Lamination occurs when the tablet splits apart into horizontal layers typically upon ejection. The common causes of capping and lamination are extensive elastic recovery with insufficient interparticulate bonding. Chipping is when small pieces break away from the edges of tablet [Fig. 33B]. Chipping can result from incorrect machine setting or poor material bonding. In addition, tablet shape can affect edge chipping sharp edges are more prone to chipping that rounded edges. Stress cracking is when small fine cracks form on the upper and lower surface of tablets. It occurs mainly because of formulation problems or the use of poor tooling. Picking occurs when a small amount of the material sticks to a punch faces (13).

Theories of Capping

Several theories have been proposed to describe the causes of capping and lamination. One theory suggests that the elastic properties of a material are responsible for the failure of a tablet. When the punches lift-off during unloading the compressed tablet expands axially in the rigid die, and as a result of this confined expansion shear stresses develop as the material elastically rebounds. Some theories are based upon material properties as the reason for capping and lamination (46,50,117,136,152). The mechanisms involved in capping were examined by Nystrom et al. (156). They measured both the axial and the radial tensile strengths of different compacts and found that these two values were not equal. The axial strength often decreases at higher compaction pressures. They proposed

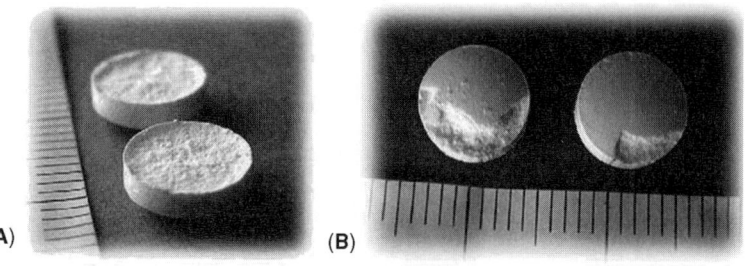

FIGURE 33 (A) Capping and (B) Chipping. *Source*: From Ref. 181.

Compression and Compaction

that the ratio of axial to radial tensile strength should be close to unity to minimum capping.

Train (157) proposed that lamination was the result of radial elastic recovery during ejection. The top of the compact expands while the bottom is still confined in the die, creating a shear plane which causes the top layer to cap or laminate. This widely accepted theory for lamination (19,158) attributes capping to the RDWP, which causes internal shear stress in the tablet during ejection. The stresses cause initiation and propagation of cracks, which result in lamination and capping. However, the propagation of cracks can be prevented by plastic relaxation of shear stresses which means that materials having sufficient plasticity are not as susceptible to lamination.

During decompression, the elastic recovery component is responsible for breaking the bonds that are formed during the compression process; an excess of elasticity can result in capping and lamination phenomenon. At punch speed of 100 mm/sec, residual die-wall forces for all the formulations were higher than those at a punch speed of 1 mm/sec (18).

It is commonly known that the stresses leading to capping and lamination problems are most likely to develop during the unloading phase of compaction, during which the expansion of elastically deformed particles disrupts interparticulate bonds (117,133,149). It has also been observed that the capping tendency increases with increasing rates of decompression. A slower removal of force during decompression was suggested to produce a less detrimental effect on binding forces between the particles. Therefore, it might also be useful to alter the decompression rate in order to improve the mechanical properties of tablets. Materials that deform elastically or exhibit time-dependence are more susceptible to capping, lamination, and strength reduction as the punch velocity is increased (59). Hiestand et al. (109) showed that the problem of capping is to a large degree associated with uniaxial relaxation in the tablet die at the point where upper punch force drops to zero. Rue et al. demonstrated that some capping problem may occur at ejection (159). Mann et al. (160) suggested that the capping pressure is related to the amount of air present in the granule bed prior to compression; although this theory is not universally accepted.

Stress Relaxation

The degree of stress relaxation can be used to predict the capping tendency of a formulation. It occurs when the upper punch begins to move upwards in the die after reaching P_{max}. Upon removal of upper punch the tablet when outside the die will expand in the axial and radial directions to relieve stress resulting from elastic recovery after compaction which could eventually lead to problems like capping and lamination (163).

David and Augsburger (63) studied the decay of compressional forces for a variety of excipients, compressed with flat-faced punches on a Stokes rotary press. They found that initial compressive force could be subject to a fairly rapid decay and that this rate was dependent on the deformation behavior of the excipient for the materials studied, they found that maximum loss in compression force was for compressible starch and MCC, which was followed by compressible sugar and DCP. This was attributed to differences in the extent of plastic flow. The decay curves were analyzed using the Maxwell model of viscoelastic behavior. Maxwell model implies first order decay of compression force.

Peleg and Moreyra (164) looked at the effect of moisture on stress relaxation. They found that the presence of moisture increased the rate of post-compressional relaxation.

Rippie and Danielson (104) and later Danielson et al. (165) re-examined the stress relaxation aspect both from the mathematical and the practical aspects. The measurements were carried out on an instrumented rotary press with strain gages on the punches and the die-wall. They compressed the range of compounds and excipients, in order to see which three-dimensional viscoelastic model provided the best statistical agreement with the physical measurements. They suggested that the dynamics of tablet compression could be divided into dilation and distortion. Of the models investigated, the simplest was the model that characterized as "elastic in dilation, Kelvin in distortion". The authors felt that the viscoelastic properties of the compact were functions of the compression conditions, and that informed adjustments of those conditions could help to avoid such problems as capping and lamination (60,157).

Ruegger and Celik (59,64) found that during tablet compression it is possible to improve tablet strength and reduce capping and lamination by reducing the rate of compaction. They found that by determining the effect of reducing either the loading or unloading speeds on the individual materials, it was possible to increase crushing strength and reduce capping and lamination to greater extent than was possible by simply reducing the overall compaction speed. Some other interesting work on compaction and relaxation can be found in references 161 and 162.

Acoustic Emission in the Detection of Capping

When any material is deformed, sonic energy is produced which is called an acoustic emission (AE). AEs occur when a surface displacement produces sound waves that can be detected by transducers. In practice, much of the emitted energy lies in the ultrasonic region which extends from 10 Hz to much higher frequencies.

Sometimes it is possible to detect an unambiguous sharp peak that appears just as the punch stress falls to zero. Joe Au et al. (166) came up with a method that could discriminate between capped (faulty) and non-capped (good) tablets based on comparing the measured level of acoustic energy against a threshold value. They use AE energy obtained from compressing lactose powder to monitor the condition and formation of good intact tablets. The method was based on the setting of an AE energy decision threshold such that problems of tablet capping and lamination were successfully identified. To assess the performance of their system, they used receiver operating characteristic curve (ROC) obtained by plotting the correct detection probability against the false alarm probability based on AE energy distributions for capped and non-capped tablets. The value of area under ROC curve, referred to as the area under the curve (AUC) model classifies as faulty or acceptable. A value of 1 indicates a high probability of detecting capped tablets. Their approach of AE energy monitoring for tablet capping gave an AUC value of 0.96, thereby suggesting the possibility of high accurate classifier [Fig. 34A] (166).

The ROC of a classifier is an important indicator of the classifier's performance in terms of differentiating between false alarm and detection rates. Considering three different scenarios regarding the relative positions of the two distributions:

1. Two identical overlapping distributions represented by curve 1 in Figure 34A. A diagonal passing in the center is merely an exercise of random guessing.
2. Two distinct distributions with some degree of overlap represented by curve 2 [Fig. 34A] above the diagonal there will be false alarm and missed detection.
3. Two distinct non-overlapping distributions represented by curve 3 in [Fig. 34A] comprising the left-vertical and top-horizontal axes-there will be correct classification every time (166).

Figure 34B shows the probability distributions of AE energy derived from the experimental results for non-capped and capped tablets.

Compression and Compaction

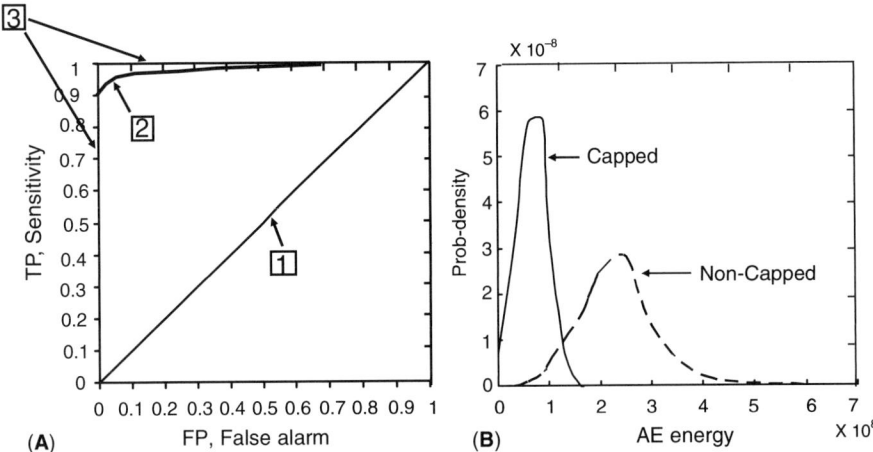

FIGURE 34 (A) ROC plot on AE for lactose; AUC of classifier at 0.96 and (B) AE energy distributions for capped and non-capped tablets. *Abbreviations*: AE, acoustic emission: ROC, receiver operating characteristic curve. *Source*: From Ref. 166.

Compaction Conditions and Capping

Cartensen et al. (159) carried out the unique experiment by applying Hiestand's triaxial compression method to a product which is prone to capping in a manner that will eventually give a noncapping product. In this study, tablets of Probucol (159) were first prepared in a single punch machine, under light pressure that would not induce capping; they were then transferred carefully to a compression coating machine and were re-compressed in a powder bed of incompressible polymeric material (any substance with an elastic limit higher than the second compression stress could be used). The outer bed, being incompressible, did not bonded with the tablet under pressure, but merely fell away loosely from the central tablet on ejection (Fig. 35). This shows that a non-compressible outer coat in a double compression procedure constitutes a means in imparting three-dimensional relaxation and allows compression of a product which otherwise could not be produced at acceptable crushing strength and/or without excessive capping. The data obtained from this experiment was in agreement with Hiestand principle, that capping can be prevented if relaxation can be made three-dimensional (159).

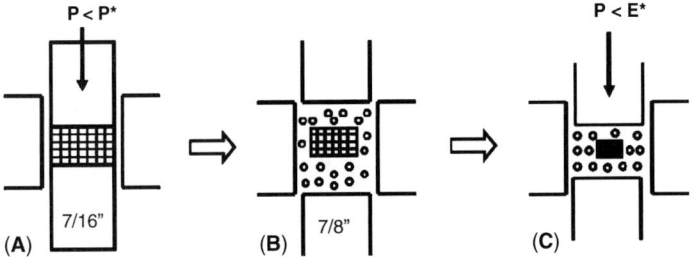

FIGURE 35 (A) Compression of inner tablet and (B) Positioning of inner tablet in polymer bed; and (C) Double compression. *Source*: From Ref. 159.

Parmentier (167,168) commented that capping was caused by inhomogenous density distribution, coupled with low binding forces in the capping zone. To rectify this problem he came up with two suggestions: First, the particle size of the original material, before granulation should be kept as small as possible. Second, the moisture content of the material should be kept carefully to such a level that binding is optimized (168). To solve the capping problem Krycer et al. (169) suggested a "Capping Index" C, defined as the slope of the percentage elastic recovery versus RDWP, could be used to predict capping tendencies.

Granulation Binders and Capping Prevention

Besides controlling compaction conditions the addition of binder to the formulation may mitigate tablet capping. Binders are added to materials having poor adhesive property to strengthen intergranular binding; thus, reducing the tendency to cap. For elastic materials the elastic energy released, when the punch pressure is relieved, overcomes the bonds present between particles in that region and capping occurs. Binders tend to be plastic materials and under compression these materials undergo plastic deformation. The total energy of compression is dissipated throughout the entire material being compressed. A greater part of the total energy of compression is absorbed by the binder at greater concentrations and less energy is stored elastically by the elastic deformation of the other materials in the formulation, Upon removal of the compressional force, there is less elastic recovery and reduced tendency toward capping (170).

PERCOLATION THEORY

Percolation theory was developed by Broadbent and Hammersley to mathematically describe disordered media in which the disorder was defined by a random variation in the degree of connectivity (172). Percolation theory deals with the random occupation of a (one-, two-, three-dimensional, or n-dimensional) lattice by different items (e.g., drug or excipient particles). If the lattice is having d dimensions together with each edge of lattice to be opened with probability p and closed otherwise, the resulting process is called as bond model since the random blockages in the site lattice are associated with the edges (Fig. 36). Another type of percolation process is the site percolation model, in which the vertices rather than the edges are randomly declared to be open or closed; the closed vertices acting as junctions that block the passage or flow between sites (Fig. 36). Hence

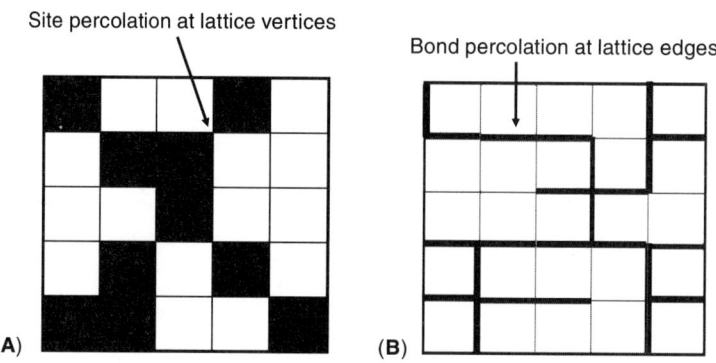

FIGURE 36 (A) Site percolation phenomenon and (B) Bond percolation phenomenon.

a bond percolation considers the lattice edges as the relevant entities whereas site percolation considers the lattice vertices as the relevant entities. For the case of a site percolation in the pharmaceutical arena, the sites are occupied at random by drug particles for example. Thus, the unoccupied sites may be empty i.e., porous, or may be occupied by another material, e.g., an excipient. Such a system is a binary system (173). This random occupation of either drug or excipient particles at one site can lead to the formation of a group of contiguous particles, which are called clusters. On the other hand if all the sites are occupied by identical isometric (equal in dimensions) particles a "bond percolation" phenomenon occurs. This bond percolation may occur because of the existence of interparticulate forces leading to the formation of infinite lattice, which is all the clusters are connected (Fig. 36).

A key aspect of percolation theory is the existence of a percolation threshold (p_c), defined in the following way. Suppose p is a probability parameter that defines the average degree of occupancy of a sites or bonds in a lattice, as p increases it reaches some point where all the clusters become connected which leads to the formation of an infinite lattice with long range connectivity between all the clusters in the lattice; the critical point where this transition occurs is the percolation threshold p_c. For example, when $p = 0$, all sites are totally empty and when $p = 1$, all the sites are full and all the sub-units are connected to some maximum number of neighboring sub-units. As p increases from zero the probability that two random sites are connected to form a cluster increases; and as the occupancy increases further the probability of two clusters connecting increases, and as the system become more and more interconnected. At some p value between 0 and 1 there is a critical point (threshold point) above which all clusters are connected to each other and since there are paths that go completely across the system, it will link one sub-unit to the next throughout the entire system.

In percolation theory, a tablet formed by compression is imagined to have a combination of site and bond percolation phenomenon. The concept of percolation theory can be illustrated using an example of drug dissolution from a tablet. Consider a rectangular tablet, where each site is randomly occupied with water of probability p or empty with probability $1-p$. Occupied and empty sites may have very different physical properties. For example, assume that occupied sites are hydrophilic excipients (e.g., lactose) whereas empty sites represents hydrophobic drug (e.g., Hydrochlorothiazide). Here the water can flow between nearest neighbor hydrophilic lactose sites. At a low concentration p, the hydrophilic lactose sites are either isolated or form small clusters of nearest neighbor sites. Two hydrophilic lactose sites belong to the same cluster if they are connected by a path of nearest neighbor hydrophilic sites, and water can flow between them. At low p values, the mixture is hydrophobic, since hydrophilic paths connecting opposite edges of the lattice are very unlikely to exist and hence no infinite cluster is formed. At large p values, on the other hand, many hydrophilic paths between opposite edges exist, where water can flow, and the mixture is hydrophilic due to formation of an infinite cluster. At some concentration in between these extremes is the threshold concentration p_c where for the first time water can percolate from one edge to the other. Thus, below p_c, is a hydrophobic mixture whereas above p_c it gives hydrophilic mixture. The threshold concentration is called the percolation threshold as it separates two different properties of mixture in tablet, the critical concentration of drug and excipients particles.

Generally percolation theory deals with the number and properties of clusters. A system at the percolation threshold is considered as a single cluster which occupies bordering sites in the particulate system. In the case of bond percolation, a group of particles is considered to belong to the same cluster only when bonds are formed between neighboring particles (Fig. 37). The bond probability p_b can assume values between 0 and 1. When $p_b = 1$, all possible bonds are formed and tablet strength is at its maximum, i.e., a tablet should show maximal strength at zero porosity when all bonds are formed. In order to form a stable compact it is necessary that the bonds percolate to form an infinite cluster within the ensemble of powder particles filled in a die and put under compressional stress.

According to percolation theory, a system property X follows a power law at the percolation threshold p_c:

$$X = S|p - p_c|^q \tag{115}$$

S is the scaling factor and q is the critical exponent. This equation is strictly valid only close to the percolation threshold. In some cases, the validity is limited to a range of ± 0.1 of the p_c.

APPLICATION OF PERCOLATION THEORY IN PHARMACEUTICAL INDUSTRY

Leuenberger and Leu (174) used percolation theory to examine tablet compaction, and they found that the Heckel equation (74,75) was in good agreement with the results of power law of percolation theory. Kuentz and Leuenberger (175) investigated the tensile strength of tablets made from binary mixtures comprising good and poorly compactable substances and developed a model using percolation theory. It was assumed that a tablet can only be produced with a relative density higher than a critical relative density (D_c) which is threshold required to build a percolating cluster in the tablets (153). Blattner et al. (176) found that compactibility of tablets obtained from binary powder systems of PEG powder and lactose monohydrate is highly dependent on geometrical arrangement of the particles (particle size and particle size distribution). The later was in fact a function of percolation threshold for tensile strength and compressibility which they found highly dependent on the ratio of PEG and lactose powder. Hence the expected two percolation thresholds can be distinguished as a function of ratios of different particle size distributions. The results of the compaction behavior of binary powder systems was satisfactorily explained with the help of percolation theory (176).

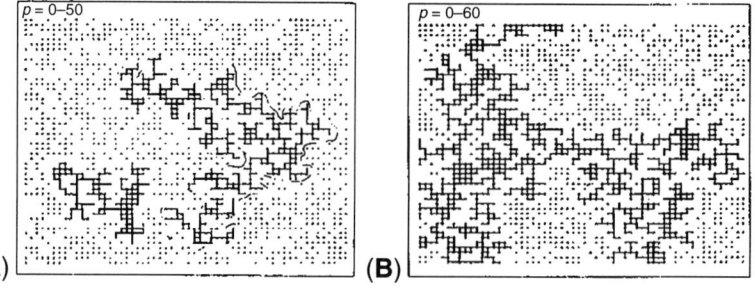

FIGURE 37 Site percolation with an occupation probability p below the critical concentration, i.e., percolation threshold p_c. No infinite cluster is formed. Two finite clusters are shown. (**B**) Site percolation with an occupation probability p above the critical concentration, i.e., percolation threshold p_c. An infinite cluster percolates the system. *Source*: From Ref. 176.

In addition, some studies have been done to study the quantitative effect of packing parameters (like particle size and particle size distribution) on percolation threshold. Caraballo et al. (177) found a linear relationship between drug particle size and the drug percolation threshold. Later Millan et al. (178) also studied the effect of the excipients particle size on the drug percolation threshold. They found that it is not the absolute particle size but the drug/excipients particle size ratio that is the main factor influencing the drug percolation threshold (178). Recently, Kimura et al. (179) reported the application of percolation theory on ternary mixture. They showed the utility of percolation threshold p_c (volumetric ratio of the starch based disintegrant) to the mixture of caffeine and mefenamic acid formulations being equal to $p_c = 0.2$ (v/v) in which both drugs have similar average particle size. Hence with the help of percolation threshold they were able to mathematically model disintegration time (179).

REFERENCES

1. Duberg M, Nystrom C. Porosity-pressure curves for the characterization of volume reduction mechanisms in powder compression. Powder Technol 1986; 46:67.
2. Hardman JS, Lilley BA. Deformation of particles during briquetting. Nature 1970; 228(5269):353–5.
3. Sixsmith D, The compression characteristics of microcrystalline cellulose powders. J Pharm Pharmacol 1982; 34(5):345–6.
4. Adams MJ, Mullier MA, Seville JPK. Agglomerate strength measurement using a uniaxial confined compression test. Powder Technol 1994; 78(1):5–13.
5. Akande OF, Ford JL, Rowe PH, et al. The effects of lag-time and dwell-time on the compaction properties of 1:1 paracetamol/microcrystalline cellulose tablets prepared by pre-compression and main compression. J Pharm Pharmacol 1998; 50(1):19–28.
6. Akande OF, Rubinstein MH, Rowe PH, et al. Effect of compression speeds on the compaction properties of a 1:1 paracetamol microcrystalline cellulose mixture prepared by single compression and by combinations of pre-compression and main-compression. Int J Pharm 1997; 157(2):127–36.
7. Altaf SA, Hoag SW, Deformation of the stokes b2 rotary tablet press: Quantitation and influence on tablet compaction. J Pharm Sci 1995; 84(3):337–43.
8. Amidon GE, Houghton ME. The effect of moisture on the mechanical and powder flow properties of microcrystalline cellulose. Pharm Res 1995; 12(6):923–9.
9. Israelachvili JN. Intermolecular and surface forces. In: Intermolecular and Surface Forces. London: Academic Press, 1985: 98.
10. Israelachvili JN, Tabor D. The shear properties of molecular films. Prog Surf Membr Sci 1973; 7:1.
11. Derjaguin BV. The force between molecules. Sci Am 1960; 203:47–53.
12. Derjaguin BV, Abrikosova II, Lifshitz EM, Direct measurement of molecular attraction between solids separated by a narrow gap. Quart Rev Chem Soc 1956; 10:295–329.
13. Marshall K. Compression/compaction. 1999 [cited 1999; Available from: http://www.fmcbiopolymer.com/Portals/bio/content/Docs/Pharmaceuticals/Problem%20Solver/PS-Section%203.pdf].
14. Ahlneck C, Alderborn G. Moisture adsorption and tableting. ii. The effect on tensile strength and air permeability of the relative humidity during storage of tablets of 3 crystalline materials. Int J Pharm 1989; 56:143–50.
15. Down GRB, McMullen JN. The effect of interparticulate friction and moisture on the crushing strength of sodium chloride compacts. Powder Technol 1985; 42:169–74.
16. Mitchell AG, Down GRB. Recrystallization after powder compaction. Int J Pharm 1984; 22:337.
17. Rumpf H. The strength of granules and agglomerates. In: Knepper WA, ed. Agglomeration. New York: Interscience, 1962.

18. Tatavarti AS, Muller FX, Hoag SW. Evaluation of the deformation behavior of binary systems of methacrylic acid copolymers and hydroxypropyl methylcellulose using a compaction simulator. Int J Pharm 2007.
19. Long WM. Radial pressures in powder compaction. Powder Metall 1960; 6:73.
20. Long WM Alderton JR. The displacement of gas from powders during compaction. Powder Metall 1960; 6:52–72.
21. Fletcher MG. Determination of compaction cycles on a rotary tablet press development of digitally interfaced instrumentation for continuous, at speed monitoring of die wall and punch pressures and the clarification of lag time as a confounding variable. Department of Pharmaceutics, University of Maryland Baltimore, 1983:1–216.
22. Suihko E, Lehto VP, Ketolainen J, et al. Dynamic solid-state and tableting properties of four theophylline forms. Int J Pharm 2001; 217(1–2):225–36.
23. Gary Nichols CSF: Physicochemical characterization of the orthorhombic polymorph of paracetamol crystallized from solution. J Pharm Sci 1998; 87(6):684–93.
24. Leung SS, Padden BE, Munson EJ, et al. Solid-state characterization of two polymorphs of aspartame hemihydrate. J Pharm Sci 1998; 87(4):501–7.
25. Liebenberg W, de Villiers MM, Wurster DE, et al. The effect of polymorphism on powder compaction and dissolution properties of chemically equivalent oxytetracycline hydrochloride powders. Drug Dev Ind Pharm 1999; 25(9):1027–33.
26. Otsuka M, Nakanishi M, Matsuda Y. Effects of crystalline form on the tableting compression mechanism of phenobarbital polymorphs. Drug Dev Ind Pharm 1999; 25(2):205–15.
27. Sun CQ, Grant DJW. Influence of crystal structure on the tableting properties of sulfamerazine polymorphs. Pharm Res 2001; 18(3):274–80.
28. Suzuki T, Nakagami H. Effect of crystallinity of microcrystalline cellulose on the compactibility and dissolution of tablets. Eur J Pharm Biopharm 1999; 47:225–30.
29. Brittain HG. Effects of mechanical processing on phase composition. J Pharm Sci 2002; 91(7):1573–80.
30. Chakravarty P, Alexander KS, Riga AT, et al. Crystal forms of tolbutamide from acetonitrile and 1-octanol: Effect of solvent, humidity and compression pressure. Int J Pharm 2005; 288(2):335–48.
31. Okumura T, Ishida M, Takayama K, et al. Polymorphic transformation of indomethacin under high pressures. J Pharm Sci 2006; 95(3):689–700.
32. Pirttimaki J, Laine E, Ketolainen J, et al. Effects of grinding and compression on crystal-structure of anhydrous caffeine. Int J Pharm 1993; 95(1–3):93–9.
33. Chan HK, Doelker E. Polymorphic transformation of some drugs under compression. Drug Dev Ind Pharm 1985; 11(2&3):315–32.
34. Hancock BC, Colvin JT, Mullarney MP, et al. The relative densities of pharmaceutical powders, blends, dry granulations, and immediate-release tablets. Pharm Technol 2003; 27(4):64–80.
35. Johansson B, Alderborn G. The effect of shape and porosity on the compression behavior and tablet forming ability of granular materials formed from microcrystalline cellulose. Eur J Pharm Biopharm 2001; 52:347–57.
36. Johansson B, Wikberg M, Ek R, et al. Compression behavior and compactability of microcrystalline cellulose pellets in relationship to their pore structure and mechanical-properties. Int J Pharm 1995; 117(1):57–73.
37. Nicklasson F, Alderborn G. Analysis of the compression mechanics of pharmaceutical agglomerates of different porosity and composition using the Adams and Kawakita equations. Pharm Res 2000; 17(8):949–54.
38. Kaerger JS, Edge S, Price R. Influence of particle size and shape on flowability and compactibility of binary mixtures of paracetamol and microcrystalline cellulose. Eur J Pharm 2004; 22:173–9.
39. Garekani HA, Ford JL, Rubinstein MH, et al. Effect of compression force, compression speed, and particle size on the compression properties of paracetamol. Drug Dev Ind Pharm 2001; 27(9):935–42.

40. Sonnergaard JM. Quantification of the compactibility of pharmaceutical powders. Eur J Pharm Biopharm 2006; 63(3):270–7.
41. Rahmouni M, Ienaerts V, Massuelle D, et al. Influence of physical parameters and lubricants on the compaction properties of granulated and non-granulated cross-linked high amylose starch. Chem Pharm Bull 2002; 50(9):1155–62.
42. Veen BV, Bolhuis GK, Wu YS, et al. Compaction mechanism and tablet strength of unlubricated and lubricated (silicified) microcrystalline cellulose. Eur J Pharm Biopharm 2005; 59:133–8.
43. Mollan MJ, Celik M. The effects of lubrication on the compaction and post-compaction properties of directly compressible maltodextrins. Int J Pharm 1996; 144:1–9.
44. Chang RK, Leonzio M, Hussain MA, Effect of colloidal silicon dioxide on flowing and tableting properties of an experimental, crosslinked polyalkylammonium polymer. Pharm Dev Technol 1999; 4(2):285–9.
45. Ohta KM, Fuji M, Takei T, et al. Effect of geometric structure and surface wettability of glidant on tablet hardness. Int J Pharm 2003; 262(1–2):75–82.
46. Bravo-Osuna I, Ferrero C, Jimenez-Castellanos MR, Influence of moisture content on the mechanical properties of methyl methacrylate-starch copolymers. Eur J Pharm Biopharm 2007; 66:63–72.
47. Elkhider N, Chan KLA, Kazarian SG. Effect of moisture and pressure on tablet compaction studied with FTIR spectroscopic imaging. J Pharm Sci 2007; 96(2):351–60.
48. Horisawa E, Danjo F, Sunada H. Influence of granulating method on physical and mechanical properties, compression behavior, and compactibility of lactose and microcrystalline cellulose granules. Drug Dev Ind Pharm 2000; 26(6):583–93.
49. Nokhodchi A. An overview of the effect of moisture on compaction and compression. Pharm Technol 2005: 46–66.
50. Sebhatu T. The effect of moisture content on the compression and bond-formation properties of amorphous lactose particles. Int J Pharm 1997; 146:101–14.
51. Song B, Rough SL, Wilson DI. Effects of drying technique on extrusion-spheronisation granules and tablet properties. Int J Pharm 2007; 332(1–2):38–44.
52. Tsukamoto T, Chen CY, Okamoto H, et al. The effects of adsorbed water on tensile strength and Young's modulus of moldings determined by means of a three-point bending method. Chem Pharm Bull 2000; 48(6):769–73.
53. Wu C, McGinity JW. Influence of relative humidity on the mechanical and drug release properties of theophylline pellets coated with an acrylic polymer containing methylparaben as a non-traditional plasticizer. Eur J Pharm Biopharm 2000; 50:277–84.
54. Nieuwmeyer FJS, Maarschalk KV, Vromans H. Granule breakage during drying processes. Int J Pharm 2007; 329(1–2):81–7.
55. Zuurman K, Bolhuis GK, Vromans H. Effect of binder on the relationship between bulk density and compactibility of lactose granulations. Int J Pharm 1995; 119:65–9.
56. Mattsson S, Nystrom C. Evaluation of critical binder properties affecting the compactibility of binary mixtures. Drug Dev Ind Pharm 2001; 27(3):181–94.
57. Freitag F, Kleinebudde P. How do roll compaction/dry granulation affect the tableting behavior of inorganic materials? Comparison of four magnesium carbonates. Eur J Pharm 2003; 19:281–9.
58. Roberts RJ, Rowe RC. The effect of punch velocity on the compaction of a vareity of materials. J Pharm Pharmacol 1985; 37:377–84.
59. Ruegger CE, Celik M. The effect of compression and decompression speed on the mechanical strength of compacts. Pharm Dev Technol 2000; 5(4):485–94.
60. Tye CK, Sun CC, Amidon GE. Evaluation of the effects of tableting speed on the relationships between compaction pressure, tablet tensile strength, and tablet solid fraction. J Pharm Sci 2005; 94(3):465–72.
61. Ragnarsson G, Sjögren J. Work of friction and net work during compaction. J Pharm Pharmacol 1983; 35:201–4.

62. Ragnarsson G, Sjögren J. Force–displacement measurements in tableting. J Pharm Pharmacol 1985; 37:145–50.
63. David ST, Augsburger LL. Plastic flow during compression of directly compressible fillers and its effect on tablet strength. J Pharm Sci 1977; 66(2):155–9.
64. Ruegger CE, Celik M. The influence of varying precompaction and main compaction profile parameters on the mechanical strength of compacts. Pharm Dev Technol 2000; 5(4):495–505.
65. Palmieri GF, Joiris E, Bonacucina G, et al. Differences between eccentric and rotary tablet machines in the evaluation of powder densification behavior. Int J Pharm 2005; 298(1):164–75.
66. Roueche E, Serris E, Thomas G, et al. Influence of temperature on the compaction of an organic powder and the mechanical strength of tablets. Powder Technol 2006; 162(2):138–44.
67. Newton JM, Haririan I, Podczeck F. The influence of punch curvature on the mechanical properties of compacted powders. Powder Technol 2000; 107(1–2):79–83.
68. Odeku OA. The compaction of pharmaceutical powders [review] 2007 [cited 2007 March 29th]; Available from: http://www.pharmainfo.net/exclusive/reviews/the_compaction_of_pharmaceutical_powders/.
69. Denny PJ. Compaction equations: A comparison of the Heckel and Kawakita equations. Powder Technol 2002; 127(2):162–72.
70. Kawakita K. Some considerations on powder compression equations. Powder Technol 1971; 4(2):61.
71. Adams MJ, McKeown R. Micromechanical analyses of the pressure–volume relationships for powders under confined uniaxial compression. Powder Technol 1996; 88(2):155–63.
72. Celik M. Overview of compaction data-analysis techniques. Drug Dev Ind Pharm 1992; 18(6–7):767–810.
73. Chowhan ZT, Chow YP. Compression behavior of pharmaceutical powders. Int J Pharm 1980; 5:139–48.
74. Heckel RW. Density–pressure relationships in powder compaction. Trans Metall Soc AIME 1961; 221(4):671–5.
75. Heckel RW. An analysis of powder compaction phenomena. Trans Metall Soc AIME 1961; 221(5):1001–8.
76. Heda PK, Muller FX, Augsburger LL. Capsule filling machine simulation. I. Low-force powder compression physics relevant to plug formation. Pharm Dev Technol 1999; 4(2):209–19.
77. Ilkka J, Paronen P. Prediction of the compression behavior of powder mixtures by the Heckel equation. Int J Pharm 1993; 94:181–7.
78. Muller FX, Augsburger LL. The role of the displacement–time wave-form in the determination of Heckel behavior under dynamic conditions in a compaction simulator and a fully-instrumented rotary tablet machine. J Pharm Pharmacol 1994; 46(6):468–75.
79. Paronen P, Ilkka J. Porosity–pressure functions. In: Alderborn G, Nystrom C, eds. Pharmaceutical Powder Compaction Technology. New York: Marcel Dekker, Inc., 1996: 55–75.
80. Shivanand P, Sprockel OL. Compaction behavior of cellulose polymers. Powder Technol 1992; 69(2):177–84.
81. Sonnergaard JM. A critical evaluation of the Heckel equation. Int J Pharm 1999; 193(1):63–71.
82. Wikberg M, Alderborn G. Compression characteristics of granulated materials. 4. The effect of granule porosity on the fragmentation propensity and the compactibility of some granulations. Int J Pharm 1991; 69(3):239–53.
83. Tavakoli AH, Simchi A, Reihani SMS. Study of the compaction behavior of composite powders under monotonic and cyclic loading. Compos Sci Technol 2005; 65(14):2094–104.
84. Antikainen O, Yliruusi J. Determining the compression behavior of pharmaceutical powders from the force–distance compression profile. Int J Pharm 2003; 252(1–2):253–61.

85. Briscoe BJ, Rough SL. The effects of wall friction on the ejection of pressed ceramic parts. Powder Technol 1998; 99(3):228–33.
86. Kiekens F, Debunne A, Vervaet C, et al. Influence of the punch diameter and curvature on the yield pressure of MCC-compacts during Heckel analysis. Eur J Pharm 2004; 22(2–3):117–26.
87. Lin MC, Duncanhewitt WC. Deformation kinetics of acetaminophen crystals. Int J Pharm 1994; 106(3):187–200.
88. Hersey JA, Rees JE. Particles-deformation of particles during briquetting. Nature 1971; 230:96.
89. York P, Pilpel N. The effect of temperature on the mechanical properties of some pharmaceutical powders in relation to tableting. J Pharm Pharmacol 1972; 24:47P–56P.
90. Podczeck F, Sharma M. The influence of particle size and shape of components of binary powder mixtures on the maximum volume reduction due to packing. Int J Pharm 1996; 137(1):41–7.
91. Cooper AR Jr, Eaton LE. Compaction behavior of several ceramic powders. J Am Ceram Soc 1962; 45(3):97–101.
92. Zhang Y, Law Y, Chakrabarti S. Physical properties and compact analysis of commonly used direct compression binders. AAPS Pharm Sci 2003; 4(4-Article 62):1–11.
93. Chowhan ZT, Chow YP. Compression properties of granulations made with binders containing different moisture contents. J Pharm Sci 1981; 70(10):1134–9.
94. Zhao J, Burt HM, Miller RA. The Gurnham equation in characterizing the compressibility of pharmaceutical materials. Int J Pharm 2006; 317(2):109.
95. Gurnham CF, Masson HJ. Expression of liquids from fibrous materials. Ind Eng Chem 1946; 38(12):1309–15.
96. Fung YC. In: Fung YC, ed. Foundations of Solid Mechanics. Prentice-Hall International Series in Dynamics. Englewood Cliffs NJ: Prentice-Hall, Inc. 1965: 525.
97. Fluggie W. Viscoelasticity. Waltham, MA: Blaisdell, 1967.
98. Shames IH, Cozzarelli FA. Elastic and Inelastic Stress Analysis. Philadelphia, PA: Taylor & Francis Ltd., 1997.
99. Hoag SW. Physics of tablet compaction: Viscoelastic and thermodynamic analysis of internal tablet structure. In: Department of Pharmaceutics, University of Minnesota, Twin Cities Minneapolis, 1990.
100. Lekhnitskii SG. Theory of Elasticity of an Anisotropic Body. 2nd ed. Moscow: Mir Publishers, 1981:430.
101. Findley WN, Lai JS, Onaran K. Creep and Relaxation of Nonlinear Viscoelastic Naterials: With an Introduction to Linear Viscoelasticity. Amsterdam: North-Holland, 1976:371.
102. Hill R. The Mathematical Theory of Plasticity. London: Oxford University Press 1998:366.
103. Hoag SW, Rippie EG. Thermodynamic analysis of energy dissipation by pharmaceutical tablets during stress unloading. J Pharm Sci 1994; 83(6):903–8.
104. Rippie EG, Danielson DW. Viscoelastic stress/strain behavior of pharmaceutical tablets: Analysis during unloading and postcompression periods. J Pharm Sci 1981; 70(5):476–82.
105. Hiestand EN. Principles, tenets and notions of tablet bonding and measurements of strength. Eur J Pharm Biopharm 1997; 44(3):229–42.
106. Hiestand EN, Smith DP. Indices of tableting performance. Powder Technol 1984; 38:145–59.
107. Hiestand EN, Bane JM Jr, Strzelinski EP. Impact test for hardness of compressed powder compacts. J Pharm Sci 1971; 60(5):758–63.
108. Hiestand EN, Peot CB. Tensile strength of compressed powders and an example of incompatibility as end point on shear yield locus. Pharm Technol 1974; 63(4):605–12.
109. Hiestand EN, Wells JE, Peot CB, et al. Physical processes of tableting. J Pharm Sci 1977; 66(4):510–9.
110. Fell JT, Newton JM. Determination of tablet strength by the diametral-compression test. J Pharm Sci 1970; 59(5):688–91.

111. Williams RO, McGinity JW. The use of tableting indices to study the compaction properties of powders. Drug Dev Ind Pharm 1988; 14(13):1823–44.
112. Wurster DE, Likitlersuang S, Chen Y. The influence of magnesium stearate on the Hiestand tableting indices and other related mechanical properties of maltodextrins. Pharm Dev Technol 2005; 10(4):461–6.
113. Wurster DE, Majuru S, Oh E, Prediction of the Hiestand bonding indices of binary powder mixtures from single-component bonding indices. Pharm Dev Technol 1999; 4(1):65–70.
114. Doelker E, Massuelle D. Benefits of die-wall instrumentation for research and development in tableting. Eur J Pharm Biopharm 2004; 58(2):427–44.
115. Train D, Hersey JA, Some fundamental studies in the cold compaction of plastically deforming solids. Powder Metall 1960; 6:20.
116. Nelson E, Naqvi SM, Busse LW, et al. The physics of tablet compression. IV. Relationship of ejection, and upper and lower punch forces during compressional process: Application of measurements to comparison of tablet lubricants. J Am Pharm Assoc 1954; 43(10):596–602.
117. Khan KA, Rhodes CT. Effect of variation in compaction force on properties of six direct compression tablet formulations. J Pharm Sci 1976; 65(12):1835–7.
118. Higuchi T, Arnold RD, Tucker SJ, et al. The physics of tablet compression. I. A preliminary report. J Am Pharm Assoc 1952; 41(2:1):93–6.
119. Higuchi T, Elowe LN, Busse LW. The physics of tablet compression. V. Studies on aspirin, lactose, lactose-aspirin, and sulfadiazine tablets. J Am Pharm Assoc 1954; 43(11):685–9.
120. Higuchi T, Nelson E, Busse LW. The physics of tablet compression. III. Design and construction of an instrumented tableting machine. J Am Pharm Assoc 1954; 43(6:1):344–8.
121. Higuchi T, Rao AN, Busse LW, et al. The physics of tablet compression. II. The influence of degree of compression on properties of tablets. J Am Pharm Assoc 1953; 42(4):194–200.
122. de Blaey CJ, Polderman J. Compression of pharmaceuticals. I. The quantitative interpretation of force–displacement curves. Pharm Weekblad 1970; 105(9):241–50.
123. Ragnarsson G. Force–displacement and network measurements. In: Alderborn G, Nystrom C, eds. Pharmaceutical Powder Compaction Technology. New York: Marcel Dekker, 1996: 77–97.
124. Jarvinen MJ, Juslin MJ. Comments on "Evaluation of force–displacement measurements during one-sided powder compaction in a die; the influence of friction with die wall and of the diameter of punches and die on upper and lower punch pressure". Powder Technol 1981; 28:115.
125. Parrott EL. Compression. In: Lieberman HA, Lachman L, eds. Pharmaceutical Dosage Forms: Tablets New York: Marcel Dekker, 1981.
126. Wikipedia (2007) Clausius-clapeyron relation.
127. Skotnicky J. The dependence of melting point on pressure. Czech J Phys 1953; 3:225–30.
128. Carslaw HS, Jaeger JC. In: Carslaw HS, Jaeger JC, eds. Conduction of Heat in Solids, 2nd ed. London: Oxford University Press. 1959:75.
129. Rankell AS, Higuchi T. Physics of tablet compression XV. Thermodynamic and kinetic aspects of adhesion under pressure. J Pharm Sci 1968; 57(4):574–7.
130. Fuhrer C. Interparticulate attraction mechanisms. In: Alderborn G, Nystrom C, eds. Pharmaceutical Powder Compaction Technology, New Tork: Marcel Dekker, 1996:1–15.
131. Coffin-Beach DP, Hollenbeck RG. Determination of the energy of tablet formation during compression of selected pharmaceutical powders. Int J Pharm 1983; 17:313.
132. Karehill PG, Nystrom C. Studies on direct compression of tablets XXI. Investigation of bonding mechanisms of some directly compressed materials by strength characterization in media with different dielectric constants (relative permittivity). Int J Pharm 1990; 61(3):251–60.
133. Rawas-Qalaji MM, Simons FE, Simons KJ. Fast-disintegrating sublingual tablets: Effect of epinephrine load on tablet characteristics. AAPS Pharm Sci 2006; 7(2):E41.
134. Marshall K. In: Lachman L, Lieberman HA, Kanig JL, eds. Compression and consolidation of powdered solids. In: The Theory and Practice of Industrial Pharmacy, Philadelphia: Lea & Febiger, 1986:66–99.

135. Sonnergaard JM. Distribution of crushing strength of tablets. Eur J Pharm Biopharm 2002; 53(3):353–9.
136. Sebhatu T, Alderborn G. Relationships between the effective interparticulate contact area and the tensile strength of tablets of amorphous and crystalline lactose of varying particle size. Eur J Pharm 1999; 8(4):235–42.
137. Eriksson M, Alderborn G. The effect of particle fragmentation and deformation on the interparticulate bond formation process during powder compaction. Pharm Res 1995; 12(7):1031–9.
138. Khan KA, Rhodes CT. Disintegration properties of calcium phosphate dibasic dihydrate tablets. J Pharm Sci 1975; 64(1):166–8.
139. Massimo G, Santi P, Colombo G, et al. The suitability of disintegrating force kinetics for studying the effect of manufacturing parameters on spironolactone tablet properties. AAPS Pharm Sci 2003; 4(2):E17.
140. Tatavarti AS, Fahmy R, Wu HQ, et al. Assessment of NIR spectroscopy for nondestructive analysis of physical and chemical attributes of sulfamethazine bolus dosage forms. AAPS Pharm Sci 2005; 6(1):9.
141. Khan KA, Rhodes CT. Effect of compaction pressure on dissolution times of some direct compression systems. J Pharm Pharmacol 1971; 23:262S.
142. Banakar UV. Factors that influence dissolution testing. In: Pharmaceutical Dissolution Testing. New York: Marcel Dekker, 1992:133–87.
143. Iranloye TA, Parrott EL. Effects of compression force, particle size, and lubricants on dissolution rate. J Pharm Sci 1978; 67(4):535–9.
144. Yu LX, Carlin AS, Amidon GL, et al. Feasibility studies of utilizing disk intrinsic dissolution rate to classify drugs. Int J Pharm 2004; 270(1–2):221–7.
145. Lin SY. Effect of excipients on tablet properties and dissolution behavior of theophylline-tableted microcapsules under different compression forces. J Pharm Sci 1988; 77(3):229–32.
146. Ibrahim HG. Observations on the dissolution behavior of a tablet formulation: Effect of compression forces. J Pharm Sci 1985; 74(5):575–7.
147. Koparkar AD, Augsburger LL, Shangraw RF. Intrinsic dissolution rates of tablet filler–binders and their influence on the dissolution of drugs from tablet formulations. Pharm Res 1990; 7(1):80–6.
148. Du JP, Hoag SW. Characterization of excipient and tableting factors that influence folic acid dissolution, friability, and breaking strength of oil- and water-soluble multivitamin with minerals tablets. Drug Dev Ind Pharm 2003; 29(10):1137–47.
149. Shimizu T, Nakano Y, Morimoto S, et al. Formulation study for lansoprazole fast-disintegrating tablet. I. Effect of compression on dissolution behavior. Chem Pharm Bull 2003; 51(8):942–7.
150. John SK. Implant pellets I: Effects of compression pressure on in vivo dissolution of delmadinone acetate pellets. J Pharm Sci 1976; 65(1):89–92.
151. Duckworth W. Discussion of Ryshkewitch paper. J Am Ceram Soc 1953; 36:68.
152. Ryshkewitch E. Compression strength of porous sintered alumina and zirconia. J Am Ceram Soc 1953; 36:65–8.
153. Wu CY, Best SM, Bentham AC, et al. A simple predictive model for the tensile strength of binary tablets. Eur J Pharm 2005; 25(2–3):331–6.
154. Wu CY, Best SM, Bentham AC, et al. Predicting the tensile strength of compacted multi-component mixtures of pharmaceutical powders. Pharm Res 2006; 23(8):1898–905.
155. Michrafy A, Michrafy M, Kadiri MS, et al. Predictions of tensile strength of binary tablets using linear and power law mixing rules. Int J Pharm 2007; 333(1–2):118–26.
156. Nystrom C, Malmqvist K, Mazur J, et al. Measurement of axial and radial tensile strength of tablets and their relation to capping. Acta Pharm Suec 1978; 15(3):226–32.
157. Train D. An investigation into the compaction of powders. J Pharm Pharmacol 1956; 8:745–61.
158. Ritter A, Sucker HB. Methods of measuring tablet capping. Pharm Technol 1980; 4(3):56–65.

159. Carstensen JT, Alcorn GJ, Hussain SA, et al. Triaxial compression of "cappable" formulations. J Pharm Sci 1985; 74(11):1239–41.
160. Mann SC, Roberts RJ, Rowe RC, et al. The effect of high speed compression at subatmospheric pressure on the capping tendency of pharmaceutical tablets. J Pharm Pharmacol 1983; 35(12):44.
161. Leuenberger H, Rohera BD. Fundamentals of powder compression. II. The compression of binary powder mixtures. Pharm Res 1986; 3(2):65–74.
162. Tousey M. Basic technologies for tablet making. Pharm Technol 2002: 8–12.
163. Maarschalk KVVD, Zuurman K, Vromans H, et al. Stress relaxation of compacts produced from viscoelastic materials. Int J Pharm 1997; 151:27–34.
164. Peleg M, Moreyra MR. Effect of moisture on the stress relaxation pattern of compacted powders. Powder Technol 1979; 23(2):277–9.
165. Danielson DW, Morehead WT, Rippie EG. Unloading and postcompression viscoelastic stress versus strain behavior of pharmaceutical solids. J Pharm Sci 1983; 72(4):342–5.
166. Joe Au YH, Eissa S, Jones BE. Receiver operating characteristic analysis for the selection of threshold values for detection of capping in powder compression. Ultrasonics 2004; 42(1–9):149–53.
167. Parmentier W. Warcum deckeln tabletten. Pharm Ind 1980; 42(7).
168. Watt PR, ed. Tablet Machine Instrumentation in Pharmaceutics: Principle and Practice. New York: John Wiley & Sons, 1988:357–96.
169. Krycer I, Pope DG, Hersey JA. An evaluation of the techniques employed to investigate powder compaction behaviour. Int J Pharm Tech Prod Manuf 1982; 3:93.
170. Jarosz PJ, Parrott EL. Factors influencing axial and radial tensile strengths of tablets. J Pharm Sci 1982; 71(6):607–14.
171. Naito SI, Masui K, Shiraki T. Prediction of tableting problems such as capping and sticking: Theoretical calculations. J Pharm Sci 1977; 66(2):254–9.
172. Broadbent SR, Hammersley JM. Percolation processes, I and II. Math Proc Cambridge Philos Soc 1957; 53:629–45.
173. Holman LE, Leuenberger H. The effect of varying the composition of binary powder mixtures and compacts on their properties: A percolation phenomenon. Powder Technol 1990; 60:249–58.
174. Leuenberger H, Leu R. Formation of a tablet: A site and bond percolation phenomenon. J Pharm Sci 1992; 81(10):976–82.
175. Kuentz M, Leuenberger H. A new theoretical approach to tablet strength of a binary mixture consisting of a well and a poorly compactable substance. Eur J Pharm Biopharm 2000; 49(2):151–9.
176. Blattner D, Kolb M, Leuenberger H. Percolation theory and compactibility of binary powder systems. Pharm Res 1990; 7(2):113–7.
177. Caraballo I, Millan M, Rabasco AM. Relationship between drug percolation threshold and particle size in matrix tablets. Pharm Res 1996; 13(3):387–90.
178. Millan M, Caraballo I, Rabasco AM. The role of the drug/excipient particle size ratio in the percolation model for tablets. Pharm Res 1998; 15(2):216–20.
179. Kimura G, Puchkov M, Betz G, et al. Percolation theory and the role of maize starch as a disintegrant for a low water-soluble drug. Pharm Dev Technol 2007; 12(1):11–9.
180. Gabaude CMD, Guillot M, Gautier JC, et al. Effects of true density, compacted mass, compression speed, and punch deformation on the mean yield pressure. J Pharm Sci 1999; 88(7):725–30.
181. Wu Z, Lagorio C, Braunstein LA, et al. Numerical evaluation of the upper critical dimension of percolation in scale-free networks. Phys Rev E Stat Nonlin Soft Matter Phys, 2007; 75(6 Pt 2):066110.

Index

Absolute humidity, definition, 199
Acrylic polymers, 285
Adams equation, 577
Aerodynamic properties, 247
Alveolus sacks, 247
Athy–Heckel equation, 572–575
Atomization, 230–236, 277, 394
   automizer selection, 232–236
   effect on protein stability, 251
   rotary atomizer, 234–236
   twin-fluid atomizer, 232–234
Atomized binder, 277

Bifurcated press feed chute, 81f
Binder functionality, 265–268
Binder selection, 283–291
   ethylcellulose, 287–288
   hydroxypropyl methylcellulose, 288–289
   hydroxypropylcellulose, 290–291
   methylcellulose, 289–290
   polyethylene glycol, 286–287
   polymethacrylates, 285–286
   polyvinylpyrrolidone, 284–285
   starch, 283–284
   sugars, 283
Blenders
   continuous blenders, 169–170
   convection blenders, 164, 167
   extruders, 169
   high shear mixers, 167
   pneumatic blenders, 168
   tumble blenders, 161–164
Blending, 111, 112
   definition, 112
   demixing, 117

[Blending]
   importance, 111
   kinetics, 116
   mechanism, 112
      convection, 113
      diffusion, 113
      shear, 114
   principles, 114, 115
Blending equipment, 156
   advantages and disadvantages, 158t
   classification, 160
   equipment requirements, 156–160
      logistical considerations, 159
      materials considerations, 156, 157
Blending processes, affecting factors, 121–124
   blender rotation speed, 124
   cohesivity, 121–123
   density, 121
   electrostatic charge, 124–125
   humidity, 123
   shape, 121
   size, 121
   temperature, 123
   time, 116
Blending techniques, 112
   Low dose blends, 125
   spatulation, 112
   trituration, 112
   tumbling, 112
Blend uniformity, assessment, 141–147
   good blending practice, 146
   sample locations, 146–147
   sampling error, 143–145
   sampling thieves, 141–142
      plug thief, 142
   size of sample, 145–146
Bottom spray processing, 376–380

---

f = location of figures.
t = location of tables.

[Bottom spray processing]
   basic design considerations, 376–378
   HS Wurster technology, 379–380
Bound moisture, 202
Bovine Spongiform Encephalopathy, 266
Buckingham-Pi theorem, 331
Bulk container, 79f
Bulk flow, 101–109
   factors affecting, 98
      chemical composition, 101
      moisture content, 98–99
      particle shape and size distribution, 99
      storage time, 100
      temperature, 100
      vibration and overpressures, 100–101
   funnel flow design, 102–103
   mass flow designs, 103–108
   two-phase flow effects, 108–109
Bulk solids handling, 75, 77–81
   discharge from a blender, 78
   equipments, 77
   final blending, 78
   flow from IBC to press, 80
   flow to die cavity, 80–81
   intermediate bulk containers, 79–80
   processing steps, 77

Cellulose-based polymers, 287–291
   ethylcellulose, 287–288
   hydroxypropyl methylcellulose, 288–289
   hydroxypropylcellulose, 290–291
   methylcellulose, 289–290
CFD. *See* computational fluid dynamic.
Chemical stability, 487–494
   chemical reactions, types, 489
      dehydration, 491
      elimination, 490
      hydrolysis, 489
      isomerization, 491
      oxidation, 490
   impact of processing, 492
   interaction with excipients, 491–492
   photostability, 494
   role of microenviromental pH, 494
   role of moisture, 492–494
   solution kinetics, 487–489
      complex reactions, 488–489
      reaction order, 487–488
      role of pH, 489
      role of temperature, 489
Chemometrics, 329–333
   application of roller compaction, 330
      critical raw material properties, 330
      density monitoring, 330
   definition, 329
   scale-up, 330–333

Comil™, 323
Compact formation, 560–572
   bulk density, 562–563
   compression force, 564–565
   crystallinity/polymorphism, 560–562
   granule type, 568–569
   lubricants and glidants, 565–566
   moisture, 566–568
   particle size and shape, 563–564
   porosity, 562–563
   tablet press type, 571
   tableting speed, 569–571
Compaction, 555
   axial to radial stress transmission, 558–560
   bond mechanisms, 557
   factors affecting compact formation, 560–572
   mechanisms of powders, 572–580
   processes, 556
Compaction simulator, 519–526
   ancillary features, 522–526
   applications
      formulations, 546–549
      preformulations, 542–546
   block diagram, 521f
   design, 521
   evolution, 520
   instrumentation for, 526–532
      calibration, 531–532
      displacement transducers, 527
      instrumented dies, 528–531
      instrumented punches, 527–528
      load cells, 526–527
Compaction simulator ancillary features, 522–526
   lubrication technique, 523–524
   powder feed mechanism, 522–523
   safety concerns, 525
   tablet ejection, 526
   tooling types and design, 522
Compendial requirements, 486
   stability kinetics, 486
Computational fluid dynamic (CFD), 239
Countercurrent drying, 209–210
Conduction, definition, 197
Conical concept trigonometry, 180f
Conical mill, 179–180
Constant rate period, 203–204
Contamination of samples, 14
   abrasion, 14
   alteration, 14
   cleanliness, 14
   intentional tampering, 14
   unintentional mistakes, 14
Continuous blenders, 169–170
Convection, definition, 197
Convection blenders, 164
Cohesive strength, 87–92
Cooper–Eaton equation, 577–579

Index

Correct sampling principles, 1–2
Coulter counter, 24
Critical equipment variables, 312–320
   dwell time, 317
   feed system, 314–316
   mill, 317–320
   roll design, 312–314
   roll gap, 317
   roll pressure, 316–317
   roll speed, 316–317
Critical formulation variables, 320–323
   binder properties and, 323
   impact of micromeritic, 321–322
   lactose grade, 322
Critical milling factors, 182–185
   feed conditions, 185
   impeller/screen gap, 182–185
   tip velocity, 185
Critical moisture content, 204–205
Critical rathole diameter (D_t), 91
Cryogenic and dry ice milling, 190–192
   carbon dioxide, 191–192
   cryogens, 191
   dry ice, 192
   heat sensitive products, 191
   liquid nitrogen, 191
   soft products, 190–191

Dallavalle's shape factor, 47
DEA. *See* dielectric analysis
Deformation, pharmaceutical powders, 303–309
   bonding, 306–308
   fragmentation, 306
   micromeritics, 308–309
   stress–strain relationships, 304–305
   yield behavior, 305–306
Delimitation error (DE), 11–12
Design space, 324
Density 6–10, 13, 18–23, 37, 46, 216, 231, 242, 348
   Bulk, 66, 85, 90, 94, 96, 98, 253
   Tapped, 94, 100
   true, 20, 32, 46
Dew point, 199
Diameter 17, 20
   Mean, 32
   See particle size statistics
Dielectric analysis (DEA), 473
Dielectric drying, 216–218
Die-wall stress, 598–600
Differential thermal analysis (DTA), 441
Dissolution rate, 242, 466
   Effect of particle size, 18
Droplet size, 230–236, 393–395
   factors governing, 393
   measurement, 231
Drug release from pellets, 355–356

Drug release rate, 18
Dry powder inhalers (DPI), 247–248
Dry-bulb temperature (T_{db}), 199, 201
Dry granulation, methods, 309–312
Drying, 195, 196, 345
   classification, 196
   definition, 195
   formulation issues, 221–223
   mechanisms, 202–204
   methods, 205–218
      countercurrent drying, 209–210
      fluid bed drying, 210–213
      microwave drying, 216–218
      tray drying, 206–209
      vacuum drying, 213–215
Drying process, 202, 204
Drying profiles, 202–203
DTA. *See* differential thermal analysis.
Dye, 207, 429–432

El-Shanawany and Lefebvre equation, 234
Electrostatic changing, 124
Endpoint determination, 218–219, 291–292
   drying, 218–219
Ethylcellulose, 287–288, 416–419
Eudragit® RL 100, 286
Eudragit®RS 100, 286
Eudragit® RL 30, 285
Eudragit®RS 30, 285
Excipients, 256, 262
Extrusion, 339
Extraction error (EE), 12
   sampling, 12–13

Falling rate Ferel's diameter, 23
FBRM. *See* focused beam reflectance measurement.
Film coating, 399–401
   for immediate release applications, 401–407
   latex coating, 399–400
   origins of, 399
   problems of, 430–432
   period, 205
Fast dissolving/disintegrating tablets (FDDT), 252
Feedstock preparation, 229–230
   pseudolatexes coating, 400
   substrates, 401
      coating defects, 431–432
      physical aging, 430
Film coating additives, 424–430
   anti-taking agents, 427–428
   coloring agents, 428–429
   flavoring agents, 429–430
   opacifiers, 428–429
   plasticizers, 424–426

[Film coating additives]
  pore forming agents, 426–427
Film coating for immediate release, 401–407
  coating materials, 403
    Eudragit® E 100, 406–407
    Kollicoat IR, 407
    polyethylene glycol, 400
    povidone, 407
    water-soluble cellulose ethers, 403–406
  cosmetic applications, 402
  ease of injection/swallowing, 403
  insulating barrier, 402–403
  subcoats and topcoats, 403
  taste masking, 401–402
Film coating for modified release, 407–422
  for enteric release, 407–414
    cellulose derivatives, 409–412
    methacrylic acid copolymers, 412–414
    polyvinyl acetate phthalate, 414
  for sustained release, 414–424
    ethylcellulose, 416–419
    multiparticulate coating, 422–424
    polymethacrylates, 419–421
    polyvinyl acetate, 421–422
Film coating, general processing, 389–396
  droplet size, 393, 394f, 395
  evaporation rate, 387–393
  solids application rate, 395–396
Film formation, 412–420
Fine milling, 188–190
  Fine Grind F10, 188–189
Fitzmill models, 179t
Flowability, 76
  bulk solid, 76
  definition, 76
Flow patterns, 84–85
  mass flows, 85
  funnel flows, 84–85
Flow problems, 81–84
  arching, 82–83, 83f
  flooding, 84
  flow rate limitation, 84
  no-flow, 82
  steady flow, 84
Flow properties, 98–101
  influencing factors, 98–101
Flow properties, measurement of, 86–98
  bulk density, 94–95
  cohesive strength tests, 87–92
  permeability, 95–96
  wall friction test, 92–94
Fluid bed drying, 210–213
Fluid bed granulators, 276–282
Focused beam reflectance measurement (FBRM), 261
Formulas for Var (FE), 7–10
  example calculation, 9

[Formulas for Var (FE)]
  general formula, 7–9
  particle size distribution, 10
Frasier equation, 235
Free moisture content, 202
Frewitt oscillator, 179f
Froude number, 129

Gelatin, 267
Gibbs free energy, 469
Granulation, 77, 255, 261
  definition, 261
Granulation binders, 262t, 620
Granulation formulation, 265, 283
Granulation, dry, 303
Granulation processes, 272–283
Grouping and segregation (GE) error, 10–11
Gurnham equation, 579–580
Gy's sampling errors, 5–6

Hammer mills, 177–178
Hatch–Choate equations, 24, 42
Heat transfer, 196–197
  conduction, 197
  convection, 197
  radiation, 197
Heckel plots, 544, 545, 575
Heywood's factors, 47
Hiestand tableting indices, 596–598
  bonding index (BI), 596
  brittle fracture index (BFI), 596, 597
  stain index, 597
High-shear mixers, 167, 273, 281, 282
  advantages of, 273
  challenges to, 274
  process variables, 274
Hooke's law, 304
Hookian spring, 586
Horizontal feed screw (HFS), 314
Humidity, 123, 199
  absolute humidity, 201
  definition, 199
  dew point, 199
  relative humidity, 199
  saturation humidity, 199
Hydroxyethyl cellulose (HEC), 404
Hydroxypropyl cellulose (HPC), 404
Hydroxypropyl methylcellulose (HPMC), 288–289, 404, 458

Inert milling, 187
Intermediate bulk containers, 79–80

Index

Jenike direct shear test, 87–89
Joule–Thomson throttling effect, 236
Jones riffler splitter, 13

Kauzmann temperature (TK), 472
Kinetics of blending, 115–121
   blending model, 115–117
   demixing, 117–121
      blending times, 119–121
Kubelka–Munk function, 326, 327
Kawakita equation, 575–577

Lactose monohydrate, 265, 321, 342, 493, 607, 622
Laser diffraction instrument, 24, 70, 71f, 231, 232
Lens aberrations, 54
   chromatic aberrations, 54
   spherical aberrations, 54
Linear variable differential transformer (LVDT), 527
Low-shear granulation, 275
Low dose blends, manufacture of, 125–126
   geometric dilution, 125
   spraying solvent drug, 126
   wet granulation processes, 126

Mad cow disease, 266
Martin's diameter, 23
Mass flow, 103
Maxwell and Kelvin models, 588
Mean dissolution time (MDT), 354
Meaningful analysis of the data, 147–149
Melt granulation, 282–283
   advantages of, 283
Methylcellulose, 289–290
Micro- and nanoparticles, 252–253
Microcrystalline cellulose (MCC), 264, 303, 342, 539, 556
   role in wet granulation, 264
Micromeritics, 17, 308–309
   definition of, 17
Micronization, 188
Microwave drying, 216–218
MIE. *See* minimum ignition energy.
Mill, 317–320
   collection of materials, 319–320
   fluid energy, 189
   hammer design, 319
   location, 317–318
   screen, 319
   speed, 319
   type, 318f, 318–319
Mill selection criteria, 185–187
Milling, 175

[Milling]
   applications of, 175
   particle size, 176
   size reduction, 175
Milling technologies, 177–179
   comparative analysis, 187
   conical screen mill, 179
   hammermills, 177–178
   oscillating granulators, 178–179
Minimum ignition energy (MIE), 187
Mixing, ordered, 126–128
   adhesional, 127–128
   coated, 128
   mechanical, 127
   (*see also* Blending)
Modes of internal mass transfer, 197, 198
   capillary flow, 198
   external conditions, 198
   liquid diffusion, 198
   vapor diffusion, 198
Mohr's circle, 88

Natural polymers, 283–284
   starch, 283–284
Noyes–Whitney dissolution model, 18f
Nucleation, 270, 271

One plane critical stability (OPCS), 45, 49–50, 348
Ordered mixing, 126–128

Partial least squares projection (PLS), 329
Particles, 17
   definition, 19
   properties, 17
Particle collection, 244
   baghouse filtration, 245
   cyclone separation, 244
Particle formation, 236–238
   definition, 236
   stages, 236–238
Particle interactions, 268–270
   immobile liquids, 268
   intermolecular forces, 268
   mechanical interlocking, 268
   mobile liquids, 268
   solid bridges, 268
Particle properties, 17
   shape, 17, 43, 99
   size, 17
   size distribution, 17
Particle size, 17, 18, 20–23
   definition, 20–23

[Particle size
  definition]
    by equivalent diameters, 21–23
    by physical properties, 22
    by statistical diameters, 23
Particle size distribution, 262
Particle size, characterization, 19
  definition, 20
    equivalent diameters, 20
    statistical diameters, 20
  overview, 19
Particle size, measurement of 51
  laser diffraction, 70–71
  microscopy, 51
    eye pieces, 58
    illumination, 58
    light microscope, 53
    resolutions, 58
    sample preparation, 59
  sieving, 59–70
    automatic, 65
    manual, 64
    motion, 68
    properties, 67
    purposes, 59
    sonic sifter, 66
    standards of USP and Tyler, 61, 62t, 63t
    time, 68
Particle size, statistics of 24–42
  distribution, characterization of, 29
  linearization of the cumulative distribution curve, 38–42
  arithmetic mean, 30
  geometric mean, 31
  harmonic mean, 31
  probability distributions, types of, 24
    cumulative distribution, 26
    Gaussian (normal) distribution, 25
    log normal distribution, 35–38
    Hatch–Choate equations, 24, 42, 47
  weighted diameter averages, 32–35
Particle shapes, 43
  effect on powder flow, 44t
Particle surface, 17
Particulate solids, 1
Peak compression force, 605–616
  crushing strength, 605–610
  disintegration, 611
  dissolution rate, 611–614
  specific surface area, 610–611
Peclet number, 228
Pellets, mechanical properties of, 350–352
  shape, 347–348
  elastic modulus, 351, 425
  fracture by diametral compression, 351
  friability, 350
  shear strength, 351

[Pellets, mechanical properties of]
  viscoelasticity, 351–352
    elements of viscoelasticity, 587f
  yield value, 352
Pellets, preparation of, 338–345
  extrusion, 339–342
  mixing, 339
  spheronization, 342–345
  stages, 338
Pellets, properties of, 345–347
  density/porosity, 348–349
  shape, 347
  size, 345–347
  size distribution, 345–347
Percolation theory, 620–623
  application in pharmaceutical industry, 622–623
Perforated pan processing, 384–389
  mixing, 387
  spraying, 387–389
Permeability test-set up, 97–98
Pharmaceutical granulation drying methods, 205–218
  countercurrent drying, 209–210
  dielectric or microwave drying, 216–218
  fluidized bed drying, 210–213
  tray drying, 206–210
  vacuum drying, 213–215
Pharmaceutical powders deformation, 303–309
  bonding, 306–308
  fragmentation, 306
  micromeritics, 308–309
  stress–strain relationships, 304–305
  yield behavior, 305–306
Phase doppler velocimetry, 231
Physical instability, 495–497
Pigment 402, 405, 407, 429
Plackett–Burmann experimental design, 274
Planetary blender, 166f
Plastic, 303–306
  Plasticity, 206
  plastic flow 538, 570
Pneumatic blenders, 168–169
Podczeck factor, 50
Poisson ratio, 331, 583
Polymethacrylates, 285
Polyvinylpyrrolidone (PVP), 265, 284, 311, 458, 496
Polyethylene glycol, 286–287
Powder beds, 17
Powder flowability, 75
Powder bed cohesion, 19
Powder compaction data, analysis of, 572–580
  Adams equation, 577
  Athy–Heckel equation, 572–575
  Cooper–Eaton equation, 577–579
  Gurnham equation, 579–580
  Kawakita equation, 575–577
Preformulation
  objectives, 465

Index

[Preformulation]
   physico-chemical parameters, influence on tablet formulation, 466
   processing-induced phase transformation studies, 477
  solid-state properties, 468
   polymorphs, 449
   solvate, 468
   salt, 242, 405, 408
Preparation error (PE), 13
Principal component analysis (PCA), 329, 359
Process analytical technology (PAT), 154–156, 196, 219–220, 261
Processing-induced phase transformation, 477–481
Property, 348, 350
Protein stabilization, 249–251
  Air–liquid interface, 251
  effect of atomization, 251
  effect of temperature, 250
Psychrometric chart, 200, 200f, 201–202
Psychrometry, 198–202
  definition, 198

Quadro comil, 180f
Quadro comil U10, 182f
Quadro comil U5, 182f

Random, sampling, 5
  stratified, 5
  systematic, 5
Regulatory guidelines, 486–487
Regulatory requirements, 485–486
Relative humidity (RH), 237, 275
  definition of, 199
  Mean Annual Relative Humidity, 487
Ribbons characterization, 323–324
Ring-die extruder, 339
Roller compactors, 312–323
  designing of, 312–323
   critical equipment variables, 312–320
   critical formulation variables, 320–323
Rotary atomizer, 234, 235f, 236
Rotor (centrifugal) processing, 381–382, 382f, 383–384
Ro-Tap® machine, 65–66
Ryshkewitch–Duckworth equation, 614–616

Sample integrity, 2, 13
Sampling, 1
  dimension, 1–3
  Frequency, 4
  instruments (tools), 1, 3, 4

[Sampling]
  mode, 1, 4
  Mode, 4
  problems, 1
  random, 1
  techniques of, 1
  types, 1
Sampling dimension, 1, 2–4, 11, 12
  one-dimensional sampling, 3, 11, 12, 13
  three-dimensional sampling, 2, 3, 11
  two-dimensional sampling, 3, 11
  zero-dimensional sampling, 2
Sampling error, 5–16, 136, 143, 145
Sampling instruments, 4
  cutter, 4, 13, 318
  riffle splitter, 11, 12
  thief probe, 4f, 12, 13, 141, 142
Sampling technique, 11
  coning and quartering, 13
  fractional shoveling, 10
  grab (convenience), 11, 12
  Jones riffler, 13
  scooping, 13
  spinning riffler, 13
  table sampler, 13
Sauter mean diameter droplet size, 234
Scaling, 292–294
  factors, 292
Scaling of blenders, 128–130
  numerical modeling, 128, 129
  parameter, 129
Schneiderhöhn's aspect ratio, 48
Semi-synthetic polymers, 284–287
Sieving, 59
Sieve Standards, 62
Segregation, 130
  definition, 130
Segregation mechanisms, 130–133
  dusting, 133
  fluidization, 132–133
  material properties, 131
  processing conditions, 131
  sifting, 131–132, 132f
Segregation problems, 135
  equipment changes, 137–139
  material changes, 136
  process changes, 137–139
Segregation testing, 133
  fluidization method, 134–135
  sifting method, 133–134
Seven sampling, Errors of Gy, 5
  delimitation error (DE), 6
  extraction error (EE), 6
  fundamental error (FE), 6, 7, 8
  grouping and segregation error (GE), 6
  long-range, 6
   nonperiodic heterogeneity fluctuation error, 6

[Seven sampling, Errors of Gy long-range]
   periodic heterogeneity fluctuation error, 6
  preparation error (PE), 6
Shape of particles, 43–51
  definition, 43
  importance, 43
  kinds, 44t
  quantitative factors, 45–51
    correction, 46
    Dallavalle's, 47
    fractal dimension, 48
    Heywood's, 47
    one plane critical stability, 49
    Podczeck's factor, 50
    Schneiderhöhn's ratio, 48
    Wadell's, 45
Shelf life determination, 504–512
  methods for establishing shelf lives, 508–512
  specifications, 504–508
    assay, 505
    description, 505
    disintegration, 508
    dissolution, 506–508
    impurities, 505–506
Simple random sampling (SRS), 1
Simulation profiles, 532–536
  eccentric tablet presses, 534
  linear profiles, 533
  rotary tablet press, 535–536
  sinusoidal profiles, 533–534
Single pot processor (SPP), 196, 214f, 275–276
  commercially, 276t
Size distribution, 230
Sonic sifter, 66–67
Solid dispersions, 253, 255
Solid dosage manufacturing process layout, 176f
Solid state control, 253
Solid–liquid interface, 270–272
Solid-state properties, 468–477
  amorphous pharmaceuticals, 470–477
    hydrates, 474–476
    interaction with water, 476–477
  crystalline pharmaceuticals, 468–470
Spatulation, 112
Spherical particle, 17, 18
  Volume, 8
  surface area, 17
Spheronization, 342–344
  formulation aspects, 356
  mechanism, 344
  operating conditions, 342–344
Spheronization binders, 357–360
SPP. *See* single pot processor.
Spray drying, 227
  applications in the pharmaceutical industry, 227
  definition, 227

Spray drying applications, 247–256
  coating and encapsulation, 251–252
  excipients, 256
  fast dissolving/disintegrating tablets, 252
  granulation, 255
  micro- and nanoparticles, 252–253
  protein stabilization, 249–251
  solid dispersions, 253, 255
  solid state control, 253
  spray dried powders for inhalation, 247–249
Spray drying process, 228
  definition, 228
  droplet drying, 228
  feedstock atomization, 228
  feedstock preparation, 229, 230
  particle formation, 229, 236–238
  particle separation, 229
  schematic of, 229f
SRS. *See* simple random sampling.
Stability
  Regulatory guidelines, 486
  Regulatory requirements, 485
  Compendial requirements, 486
Stability study design, 498–504
  batch selection, 498–499
  bracketing, 499–501
  matrixing, 499, 501–504
  storage conditions, 498–499
Stairmand design, 244
Starch-dextrin mixtures, 360
Starch, 283–284
  binder selection, 283–284
Statistical approaches to stability analysis, 512–513
Statistical diameters, 20, 23
  Feret's diameter, 23
  Martin's diameter, 23
Stratified sampling, 149–150, 150f, 151–153
  comparison of blend, 151–152
  troubleshooting, 152–153
Strain
  Normal, 304
  shear, 114
Stress
  Normal, 559
  shear, 87,
Suragam SA®, 354
Surface area, 18
Sugars, 283
  binder selection, 283
Synthetic polymers, 284–287
  polyethylene glycol, 286–287
  polymethacrylates, 285–286
  polyvinylpyrrolidone, 284–285

Tablets, mechanical strength of, 616–620
  acoustic emission, 618

Index

[Tablets, mechanical strength of]
  compaction conditions, 619–620
  granulation binders, 620
  stress relaxation, 617–618
  theories of capping, 616–617
Tablet formulation process, 466–467
  influence of physicochemical properties, 466–467
    particle size and shape, 466–467
Tablet manufacturing cycle, 555
Tablet compaction, mechanical analysis of, 580–596
  material properties, 585
    elastic phase, 585
    plastic phase, 589
    viscoelastic phase, 587
  stress and strain, 581–585
  three-dimensional viscoelastic analysis, 591–596
Tablet press dynamics, 536–540
  double-ended compression, 537–538
  precompression, 538
  roller position, 538–539
  roller size, 538–539
  single-ended compression, 537–538
  tablet press speed, 539–540
Tensile strength, 323
The Parenteral Drug Association, 140
Thermal analysis, 439–441
  definition, 439
  uses of, 439–441
Thermal analysis of formulation, 449–458
  drug excipient compatibility, 457–458
  glassy systems, 453–457
  pharmaceutical hydrates, 452–453
  polymorphism, 449–452
Thermal analysis of polymeric systems, 458–461
  characterization of polymer films, 459–460
  polymeric dosage forms, 460–461
  use of polymers in design, 458–459
Thermoanalytical methods, 441–448
  differential scanning calorimetry (DSC), 441–444
  emerging thermal techniques, 447–448

[Thermoanalytical methods]
  hot stage microscopy, 445–446
  microcalorimetry, 446–447
  thermogravimetric analysis (TGA), 444–445
Third stage of particle formation, 237
TK. See Kauzmann temperature.
Tools, sampling. See instruments sampling.
Top spray process, 374–376
Tray drying, 206–209
Triethyl citrate (TEC), 285
Trituration, 112
Tumble blenders, 161–164
Tumbling, 112
Twin-fluid atomizer, 232–234
Twin-screw extruder, 339
Two fundamental processes, 196

Van der Waals forces, 268, 306
Vertical feed screw (VFS), 314
Vaccum drying, 213–215
Variance, See formulas for variance

Wadell's factor, 45
Wadell's true sphericity, 45
Weibull distribution, 609
Weibull modulus, 609
Wall friction test, 92–94
Wet granulation processes, 126
Wet granulation, 195, 263
Wet-bulb temperature (T_{wb}), 199
Wolin decision, 139
Work, 310
Wurster system. See Bottom spray processing

Young's modulus, 304, 323